HEALTH PROMOTION

HEALTH PROMOTION

PLANNING AND STRATEGIES

JACKIE GREEN and KEITH TONES

SECOND EDITION

SAGE

Los Angeles | London | New Delhi
Singapore | Washington DC

First edition published 2004
Reprinted 2004, 2005 (twice) 2006 and 2009
This edition first published 2010
Reprinted 2011

SAGE Publications Ltd
1 Oliver's Yard
55 City Road
London EC1Y 1SP

SAGE Publications Inc.
2455 Teller Road
Thousand Oaks, California 91320

SAGE Publications India Pvt Ltd
B 1/I 1 Mohan Cooperative Industrial Area
Mathura Road
New Delhi 110 044

SAGE Publications Asia-Pacific Pte Ltd
33 Pekin Street #02-01
Far East Square
Singapore 048763

Library of Congress Control Number 2009943932

British Library Cataloguing in Publication data

A catalogue record for this book is available from the British Library

ISBN 978-1-84787-489-4
ISBN 978-1-84787-490-0 (pbk)

Typeset by C&M Digitals (P) Ltd, Chennai, India
Printed in Great Britain by TJ International Ltd, Padstow, Cornwall
Printed on paper from sustainable resources

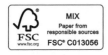

CONTENTS

LIST OF FIGURES AND TABLES

Figures

Tables

ACKNOWLEDGEMENTS

The publisher is grateful to the following for their kind permission to reproduce material:

Figure for box in Appleton, J. (1992) 'Notes from a food and nutrition PRA in a Guinean fishing village', *RRA Notes (No. 16): Special Issue on Applications for Health*: 77–85, from the *Participatory Learning and Action Series*.

Figure 2.3 from *Health Promotion Models and Values* edited by Downie R.S, Tannahill C. and Tannahill A. (1996) by permission of Oxford University Press.

Figure 2.4 and Table 2.4 from Alan Beattie, Marjorie Gott, Linda Jones and Moyra Sidell, *Health and Wellbeing*, published 1992 by Macmillan in association with the Open University. Reproduced with permission of Palgrave Macmillan.

Figure 2.5 derived from Raeburn J.M. and Rootman I (1989) 'Towards an expanded health field concept: conceptual and research issues in an era of health promotion', *Health Promotion*, 3 (4): 383–92 by permission of Oxford University Press.

Figure 2.6 © Institute of Future Studies, Stockholm, 1991.

Figure 2.7 by Green et al 1997 from *Oxford Textbook of Public Health Vol 1* (3rd edn). By permission of Oxford University Press.

Figure 4.2 by Dignan, M.B. and Carr, P.A. (1992) *Program Planning for Health* (2nd edn), Malvern, PA: Lee & Febiger. By permission of Lippincott Williams and Wilkins.

Figure 4.3 from Green and Kreuter, *Health Promotion Planning: An Educational and Environmental Approach* (3rd edn) © 1999, The McGraw-Hill Companies.

Figure 4.8 from Laverack G. and Labonte R., 'A planning framework for community empowerment goals within health promotion' Health Policy Plan, Sep 2000; 15: 255–62 by permission of Oxford University Press.

Figure 4.13 from Haglund B.J.A., Jansson B., Pettersson B. and Tillgren P. (1998) 'A quality assurance instrument for practitioners', in J.K. Davies, and G. Macdonald (eds), *Quality, Evidence and Effectiveness in Health Promotion*. London: Routledge.

Figure 5.3 from Len Doyal and Ian Gough, *A Theory of Human Need*, published 1991, The Guilford Press. Reproduced with permission of Palgrave Macmillan.

Figure 5.6 from Arnstein S., *Journal of the American Planning Association*, Jan 7, 1969, Taylor & Francis.

Figure 5.7 from *Community Organising*, by Brager and Specht © 1973 Columbia University Press. Reprinted with permission of the publisher.

Figure 5.8 from Annett, H. and Rifkin, S. 'Improving Urban Health: Guidelines for rapid appraisal to assess community health needs. A focus on health improvements for low-income urban areas' © WHO, 1990.

Figure 5.9 and Figure 6.1 from Beattie A. (1991) 'Knowledge and control in health promotion: a test case for social policy and social theory', in J. Gabe, M. Calnan, and M. Bury (eds) The *Sociology of the Health Service*. London: Routledge.

Figure 6.2 from Tones K. and Tilford S. (1994) *Health Education: Effectiveness, Efficiency and Equity*. London: Chapman & Hall.

Figure 7.3 reprinted from *Advances in Experimental Social Psychology*, Volume 3, Michael Argyle and Adam Kendon, The Experimental Analysis of Social Performance © 1967 with permission from Elsevier.

Figure 7.5 from Kolb, David A.; Oxland, Joyce S.; Rubin, Irwin M., *Organizational Behavior: An Experiential Approach* (6th edn) © 1995, p.49. Reprinted by permission of Pearson Education, Inc., Upper Saddle River, NJ.

Figure 7.6 and 10.4 from Anderson, J. (undated) *The HEA Health Skills Dissemination Project: A Whole School Approach to Life Skills and Health Education*. Leeds: Counselling and Career Development Unit.

Figure 7.10 © Turner, C.M. (1978) *Interpersonal Skills in Further Education*. Blagdon: Further Education Staff College, Coombe Lodge. Every effort has been made to contact the copyright holder.

Figure 7.11 © Macdonald, J.U. and Warren, W.G. (1991) 'Primary health care as an educational process: a model and a Freirean perspective', *International Quarterly of Community Health Education*, 12 (1): 35–50. By permission of Baywood Publishing Company, Inc.

Figure 7.12 © Hopson, B. and Scally, M. (1981) *Lifeskills Teaching*.

Figure 9.2 © Popay J (forthcoming) 'Community Engagement for Health Improvement: questions of definition, outcomes and evaluation', in Morgan A, Barker, R. Davies, M. Ziglio, E (eds). *International Health and Development: Investing in Assets of Individuals, Communities and Organisations*. New York: Springer.

Figure 10.1 © Parsons, C., Stears, D., Thomas, C., Thomas, L. and Holland, J.

Figure 10.2 © Christine Beels, Jen Anderson and Derek Powell.

Figure 10.3 from D. Lawton, *School Curriculum Planning*, Hodder & Stoughton © 1986. Reproduced by permission of Hodder & Stoughton Ltd.

Table in Box: 'Which Health Differences are Inequitable?' from Dahlgren G, Whitehead M. *Policies and Strategies to Promote Equity in Health*. Copenhagen, WHO Regional Office for Europe, 1992:4.

Table 2.3 from Doll, R., Peto, R., Wheatley, K., Gray, R. and Sutherland, I. 'Mortality in relation to consumption of alcohol: 13 years' observations on male British doctors', *British Medical Journal*, Oct 8, 1994, BMJ Publishing Group Ltd.

Table 6.1 from Chapman, S. (1994) 'The A–Z of public health advocacy', in S. Chapman and D. Lupton, (eds), *The Fight for Public Health: Principles and Practice of Media Advocacy*. London: BMJ Publishing Group.

Table 6.2 from Douglas, M.J., Conway, L., Gorman, D., Gavin, S. and Hanlon, P. (2001) 'Developing principles for health impact assessment', *Journal of Public Health Medicine*, 23 (2): 148–54 by permission of Oxford University Press.

Table 7.1 from McLeroy, K. (1992) 'Editorial: Health education research: theory and practice – future directions', *Health Education Research*, 7 (1–8) by permission of Oxford University Press.

Table 7.4 from Ryder, J. and Campbell, L. (1988) *Balancing Acts in Personal, Social and Health Education: A Practical Guide for Teachers*. London: Routledge.

Table 7.5 © John Fien 1994.

Table 9.3 from Batten, T.R. (1967) *The Non-Directive Approach in Group and Community Work* by permission of Oxford University Press.

Table 10.1 © Scottish Health Education Group 1989.

Data on Gambia from United Nations Development Programme, Human Development Report 2007/08, published 2007, reproduced with permission of Palgrave Macmillan.

INTRODUCTION

The poor health of the poor, the social gradient in health within countries, and the marked health inequities between countries are caused by the unequal distribution of power, income, goods, and services, globally and nationally, the consequent unfairness in the immediate, visible circumstances of people's lives — their access to health care, schools, and education, their conditions of work and leisure, their homes, communities, towns, or cities — and their chances of leading a flourishing life. This unequal distribution of health damaging experiences is not in any sense a 'natural' phenomenon but is the result of a toxic combination of poor social policies and programmes, unfair economic arrangements, and bad politics.

Commission on Social Determinants of Health, 2008: 1

Contemporary public health problems are all too frequently attributed to individual behaviour such as poor diet, lack of exercise, unsafe sex and smoking, drinking alcohol and using other addictive substances. Interpretations of this sort tend to be associated with a biomedical discourse and a deficit model of health which equates it with the absence of disease, rather than more holistic interpretations of health which encompass positive well being. Such attributions are clearly overly simplistic. Nonetheless they are still potentially damaging with regard to public health practice as responsibility for unhealthy behaviour, and therefore by implication health, becomes delegated to the individual. Health promotion has challenged such a narrow focus on behaviour and has supported a more comprehensive analysis of the factors which influence health and wellbeing. In particular, it recognizes the fundamental importance of environmental influences on health and the complex interplay between these factors and health-related behaviour. Environmental factors are taken to include not only the physical environment, but also psycho-social aspects and, importantly, the socio-economic environment. Acknowledging the importance of these wider determinants moves the primary focus of health promotion towards creating the conditions supportive of health and health behaviour. It also effectively involves the state in responsibility for tackling the so-called upstream determinants of health and draws attention to the essentially political nature of health promotion. Rather than being a matter of individual responsibility, health therefore becomes an issue of social justice.

The 'big issues' which are a threat to health at the global level include poverty and deprivation, climate change, environmental degradation, discrimination and exploitation, and violence in all forms including terrorism. Inequalities in health persist between high and low income countries. A child born in Japan or Sweden can today expect to live to over 80 years of age whereas in some African countries life expectancy would be less than 50. It is also anticipated that the effects of global recession and climate change will be experienced disproportionately by poorer countries – despite the fact that the most affluent nations carry the major share of blame for the problem. Tackling global health inequalities demands international commitment and coordinated action.

At the national level, there are also major inequalities. Life expectancy for men in one area of Glasgow in Scotland is only 54 compared to 82 in another nearby area (Commission on Social Determinants of Health, 2008). However, it is not only the poorest in society who experience worse health. There are gradations in health at all levels of the socioeconomic scale. This appears to be the case in all countries – the only difference being the steepness of the gradient (Commission on Social Determinants of Health, 2008). Furthermore, Wilkinson and Pickett (2009) argue that those countries with less income inequality experience fewer health and social problems than those where the differential is greater. They suggest that more equal societies have less stress and higher levels of trust. Friedli graphically encapsulates the problem in her report on mental health: 'It is abundantly clear that the chronic stress of struggling with material disadvantage is intensified to a very considerable degree by doing so in more unequal societies' (2009: iii).

Attempts to improve public health may fail to be effective for a number of reasons – notably by focusing on individual behaviour rather than the social and environmental determinants of health and ill health. Clearly, inadequate understanding of the key determinants will risk interventions addressing inappropriate variables. In some instances, they are a knee-jerk reaction to addressing an emerging issue. They may, therefore, be poorly planned with insufficient attention to relevant theory and existing research and evaluation evidence. Interventions may also be under-resourced with unreasonable expectations of what might be achieved within the time frame.

Responses to tackling contemporary health problems are often driven by the political imperative to be seen to be doing something – regardless of whether or not it is the most appropriate means of achieving significant and sustainable improvements in health. They are often concerned with demonstrating early high profile wins to fit in with political time frames dictated by electoral cycles rather than achieving long-term sustainable change. Furthermore, there is a marked reluctance to adopt unpopular measures which might risk alienating the electorate, for example by requiring the majority to make cutbacks or major changes to their behaviour – hence the muted (some would argue wholly inadequate) response to tackling world poverty or climate change. We are advised to switch off the standby light on our televisions rather than take any serious action to reduce energy expenditure. Efforts to reduce health inequality tend to focus downstream on mitigating the effects of poverty and unequal life chances rather than upstream on tackling disadvantage itself through redistributive policy.

One of the success stories of recent years has been the prohibition of smoking in enclosed public places in a number of countries following years of campaigning to overcome political opposition. The effect of high pricing on reducing tobacco consumption is also recognized. However, at the time of writing, there appears to be considerable resistance to adopting a similar policy response to curb the alcohol problem. The Chief Medical Officer of England, Sir Liam Donaldson recently proposed the introduction of a minimum price per unit of alcohol sold (Donaldson, 2009) with the intention of reducing the availability of cheap alcohol, excessive consumption and associated harm. However, politicians across the political spectrum argued that the majority of the population who use alcohol sensibly and responsibly should not be made to suffer because of the excesses of the minority – despite the fact that economic projections showed that moderate drinkers, unlike their heavy drinking counterparts, would be only minimally affected by the pricing change.

Health promotion has been characterized by a concern to create supportive environments for health through healthy public policy. Effectively, this shifted the emphasis away from health education. For many, health education had become associated with attempts to persuade individuals to change their behaviour and was criticized for failing to take account of the wider influences and, therefore, being victim-blaming in orientation. However, health promotion has been encapsulated as the synergistic interaction between health education and healthy public policy summed up as:

health promotion = health education × healthy public policy

The marginalization of health education effectively stifled debate about its continuing relevance to health promotion (Green, 2008). Yet a broader conceptualization of health education recognizes its potential for contributing to the major goals of health promotion – equity and empowerment. This broader conceptualization is concerned with enabling individuals and communities to gain control over their health and is, therefore, more radical and political in intent. We use the term 'new health education' to distinguish it from more traditional forms.

A basic premise of this text is that the new health education can be a major driver within health promotion with the capacity to:

- develop the knowledge, values and skills required for individual decision-making and voluntary action and, importantly, contribute to individual empowerment
- raise awareness of the need for environmental and policy change to support health and health choices
- develop critical awareness among communities about factors influencing their health and the skills and motivation required to take collective action – thereby contributing to critical consciousness raising and community empowerment
- be part of professional education and training to enable professionals across a range of sectors to contribute to the health and wellbeing of their client groups and engage in advocacy on their behalf.

Our rationale for producing the first edition of this book was that in order to be effective health promotion must be systematically planned. This second edition updates our argument by drawing on contemporary examples and revisiting the various debates. It remains our contention that planning should be more than a mere technical exercise. It should provide a framework which allows initiatives to be grounded in the core values and principles of health promotion. Accordingly, we begin by identifying these values and principles to establish a foundation for detailed discussion of planning and its application to practice. Throughout, we emphasize the importance of theory and demonstrate its application through the use of examples and case studies from a range of different countries.

We make no apology for including reference to older 'classic sources' and seminal work; we see this as a major strength of the book. Health promotion is in danger of losing sight of its roots and there is an emerging tendency to 'reinvent the wheel' – not always as well as the first time round! It is therefore our aim to maintain the visibility of some of the early innovative and radical thinking, which continues to be of relevance to contemporary health promotion.

Since the first edition of the book was published, some specific issues such as social marketing and health literacy have achieved more prominence and these are now given greater attention.

At a more fundamental level, Wills and Douglas (2008) note that health promotion is struggling to remain true to the ideals set out in the Ottawa Charter (WHO, 1986) and maintain its focus on tackling the social determinants of health. This is attributed to current neo-liberal political climates which favour individualistic lifestyle approaches rather than efforts to address social determinants of health. There is increasing concern in some parts of the world that the discourse of health promotion is being obscured and replaced – for example in England by 'health improvement' (Wills and Douglas, 2008) and in Canada by 'population health' (Raphael, 2008). What is all the more surprising is that this is happening in countries which have, historically, been at the forefront of the development of health promotion. Tackling complex public health problems requires a multidisciplinary response. We see health promotion as having an essential and pivotal role in orchestrating that response. However, if it is to make a significant contribution to tackling contemporary health issues, it needs to re-engage with its radical agenda and core values and maintain its distinctive identity and purpose. This edition looks at the relationship between health promotion and modern multidisciplinary public health and sets out its unique contribution. The International Union of Health Promotion and Education and Canadian Consortium for Health Promotion Research (2007) identifies building a competent health promotion workforce among its priorities for the future. We therefore include discussion of the position of health promotion as a profession.

A number of key themes run throughout the whole text. These are:

- the need to adopt a systematic approach to planning
- the importance of theory and other forms of evidence
- support for an empowerment model of health promotion
- health education as a major driving force within health promotion
- acknowledgement of the upstream social determinants of health – the 'causes of the causes'
- the complex interplay between agency and structure – between individuals and their environment
- the need to tackle health inequalities.

Health is a nebulous and contested concept meaning different things to different people. Clearly those working to promote health should have a clear view of what they are aspiring to. We therefore begin by considering alternative conceptualizations of health and develop a simple working model. This includes physical, mental and social dimensions. It also recognizes the existence of health – or its absence – at individual and societal levels. It acknowledges the split between negative approaches to conceptualizing health which focus on the absence of disease and positive approaches which incorporate wellbeing. However, we contend that empowerment should be central to definitions of health and, further, that an emphasis on empowerment supports the achievement of both disease prevention and positive health goals.

The term health promotion has variously been used to refer to a social movement, an ideology, a discipline, a profession and a strategy or field of practice delineated by commitment to key values. Chapter 1 discusses the ideology of health promotion and seeks to identify its core values. It also reviews the major WHO documents which have contributed to shaping its development – and, in particular, the Ottawa Charter (WHO, 1986). It identifies different models of health promotion and argues on ethical, ideological and even pragmatic grounds that health promotion should subscribe to an empowerment model. Empowerment approaches recognize the reciprocal relationship between individuals and their environment and the complex interplay between agency and structure – one of the themes of this text.

Following on from discussion of health and health promotion, Chapter 1 then locates health promotion within the context of modern multidisciplinary public health and identifies its distinctive contribution to the public health endeavour. It also considers the importance of maintaining a separate identity for health promotion. This chapter concludes by examining the relationship between health education and health promotion. We argue that the 'new critical health education' is the driving force within health promotion – another of the major themes which run through the book.

Chapter 2 focuses on identifying the determinants of health and various ways of assessing them. Importantly, it looks at the value of incorporating lay perspectives and distinguishes salutogenic from pathogenic explanations of health and ill health. It concludes by considering inequality and social exclusion and social capital.

Chapter 3 begins by looking at the uptake of new ideas and practices at the community level. It then goes on to consider, at the micro-level, how various factors interact to influence decisions and behaviour. In order to do so, it draws on a number of psycho-social theories and particularly the Health Action Model (HAM). In line with our support for an empowerment model of health promotion, it pays particular attention to the dynamics of empowerment. It considers issues associated with power and control and the reciprocal determinism between individuals and their environment.

Chapter 4 sets out the argument supporting systematic planning and introduces a number of planning models. It emphasizes the central importance of developing clear objectives. It also recognizes that partnerships across different sectors are needed to tackle the multiple and complex determinants of health and looks at what is involved in developing successful partnerships.

Chapter 5 focuses on the first stage of the planning cycle – identifying health needs. It looks at different conceptualizations of need. Consistent with the values of health promotion, it supports participatory approaches to identifying and prioritizing health needs.

We emphasize throughout the book the importance of environmental determinants of health. Chapter 6 explores in detail the role of healthy public policy in establishing supportive environments for health. It considers the process of policy development and identifies the important contribution of health education and advocacy. Clearly, policies across a whole range of areas – including, for example, education, agriculture, planning and transport – will potentially influence health. The chapter concludes by discussing the use of Health Impact Assessment to assess the potential effects on health of policies at all levels, from the macro-level down to local policies.

One of the major themes of the book is the central importance to health promotion of what we have termed the 'new' health education. Chapter 7 focuses specifically on the role of health education. It begins by examining the communication process and the design of messages before looking at different models of health education and types of learning. It then looks at methods of facilitating learning and specifically at the use of peer education and creative arts. It briefly discusses the use of health education for persuasion and attitude change – recognizing the potential conflict with empowerment. The chapter concludes by looking at health education as a strategy for social and political change, including reference to Freirean approaches.

Health education has, in the past, been associated with mass media campaigns. Chapter 8 analyses the potential and limitations of mass media interventions. It discusses relevant theory and also the technical issues involved in mass media campaigns. It also considers the more general influence of mass media on behaviour. A separate section looks at the contribution of social marketing, which is currently receiving considerable attention. The chapter concludes by considering the use of mass media for advocacy purposes to shape public opinion and influence policy makers.

Chapter 9 focuses on working with communities and in particular on community development and empowerment approaches. It identifies key aspects of good practice in working with communities and considers some of the challenges of putting the rhetoric of community development into practice. In particular, it draws attention to the need to ensure that disadvantaged and socially excluded groups are able to participate.

Chapter 10 looks at the settings approach and its potential for improving health. By focusing on the conditions which are supportive of health, the approach shifts the emphasis away from individual behaviour and towards organizations and structural factors. Having examined the principles of the approach, it goes on to consider in detail the health promoting school as an example, as well as making observations about a range of different settings.

Evaluation is an essential element of health promotion practice and the development of an evaluation strategy is clearly integral to systematic programme planning. Chapter 11 distinguishes between formative evaluation which contributes to the development and quality of programmes and summative evaluation to assess their overall effectiveness. It emphasizes that, in addition to measuring outcomes and the extent to which the goals of a programme have been achieved, evaluation should also comment on the process and identify those factors which may have contributed to the success and sustainability of programmes – or equally have resulted in failure. Chapter 11 considers the methodological debates about evaluation in order to make recommendations about appropriate methodology – that is a methodology which is capable of identifying the range of potential health promotion outcomes and unpicking the complex pathways which lead towards them. Importantly, it must also be consistent with the values of health promotion and conform with ethical principles.

Following on from the discussion of evaluation, Chapter 11 considers the contribution of evaluation and empirical research findings to the evidence-base for health promotion and the use of systematic reviews to synthesize the evidence. It notes the tendency for systematic reviews to favour quantitative evidence and evidence relating to simple interventions rather than the complex interventions more typical of health promotion and calls for greater attention to qualitative evidence. It also argues that the development of the evidence-base should include practitioner expertise and insights and, importantly, should also incorporate theory. Indeed, theory should constantly be updated and refined in the light of emergent empirical evidence as part of a continuing cycle of development. Finally, the chapter considers how evidence can be put into practice. By looking at how evidence can be used in systematic planning, we effectively come full circle.

Health promotion has been referred to as an idea whose time has come. It has the potential to make a major contribution to tackling contemporary health problems and improving the health of individuals and communities. The purpose of this book is to demonstrate how that potential can be maximized through systematic planning, with due regard to evidence, theory and values at each stage of the planning cycle.

1

HEALTH AND HEALTH PROMOTION

It is no measure of health to be well adjusted to a profoundly sick society.

Jiddu Krishnamurti

OVERVIEW

This chapter focuses on three broad areas – the concept of health, setting out the distinctive features and values of health promotion and establishing the position of health promotion vis-à-vis modern multidisciplinary public health and health education. It will:

- explore alternative conceptualizations of health
- develop a working model of health
- consider the ideology and core values of health promotion
- identify different models of health promotion
- set out the rationale for an empowerment model of health promotion
- locate health promotion within modern multidisciplinary public health
- propose a new 'critical' health education as the major driver and distinctive voice of health promotion.

INTRODUCTION

The primary concern of this book is to provide insight into the factors that contribute to the effective and efficient design of health promotion programmes. The way in which health is conceptualized has major implications for planning, implementing and evaluating programmes. Equally, the approach adopted at each of these stages will be influenced by the values of those working to promote health.

HEALTH AS A CONTESTED CONCEPT

Developing clear goals will depend on how health is defined. Yet it is widely acknowledged that health is, as Gallie (1955) famously described, an essentially contested concept. Its many, often conflicting, meanings are socially constructed. Lowell S. Levin likened the task of defining health to shovelling smoke. It is difficult, to say the very least, to provide precise definitions, largely because health is one of those abstract words, like love and beauty, that mean different things to different people. However, we can confidently say that health is, and apparently always has been, a significant value in people's lives. If we do not acknowledge the contentious nature of health and have a sound understanding of the determinants of our preferred conceptualization, it is unlikely that we will be able to develop incisive strategies for promoting it.

Defining health: contrasting and conflicting conceptualizations

A number of tensions emerge in defining health. These include the relative emphasis on:

- disease or wellbeing
- holistic or atomistic interpretations
- the individual or the collective
- lay or professional perspectives
- subjective or objective interpretations.

One of the most persistent distinctions between definitions of health has been whether the focus is on wellness or on the absence of disease. This is encapsulated in the classical myth of Hygeia and Asclepius (see box), but continues to have relevance to contemporary debates about the nature of health and the purpose of health promotion.

The confrontation of Hygeia and Asclepius

Hygeia was a goddess who symbolized the virtues of wise living and wellbeing; Asclepius was a physician who lived in the twelfth century BC and came to represent the medical view of health. As Dubos noted:

> The myths of Hygeia and Asclepius symbolize the never-ending oscillation between two different points of view … For the worshippers of Hygeia, health is the natural order of things, a positive attribute to which men [sic] are entitled if they govern their lives wisely. According to them, the most important function of medicine is to discover and teach the natural laws which will ensure to man a healthy mind in a healthy body. More sceptical or wiser in the ways of the world, the followers of Asclepius believe that the chief role of the physician is to treat disease, to restore health by correcting any imperfection caused by the accidents of birth or of life.

(Continued)

(Continued)

> While Asclepius is in Luther's words only 'God's body patcher', the serene loveliness of Hygeia in the Greek marble symbolizes man's lost hope that he can some day achieve a state of harmony within himself and with the surrounding world. (1979: 131,134)

Probably the best known definition of health comes from the Constitution of the World Health Organization (1946, 2006): 'Health is a state of complete physical, mental and social well-being and not merely the absence of disease or infirmity.' While this definition has been criticized because of its utopian nature, it extended the boundaries of health beyond the absence of disease to include positive wellbeing and firmly acknowledged the multidimensional, holistic nature of health. The Constitution further asserts that:

> The enjoyment of the highest attainable standard of health is one of the fundamental rights of every human being without distinction of race, religion, political belief, economic or social condition.

This assertion, also enshrined in numerous UN human rights treaties such as the International Covenant on Economic, Social and Cultural Rights (OHCHR, 1966) and the Universal Declaration on Human Rights (United Nations, 1948), politicizes health and places pressure on governments to create the conditions supportive of health (WHO, 2007d). Furthermore, this emphasis on health as a fundamental human right focuses the attention of those seeking to promote health on equity and empowerment.

Saracci (1997) argues that definitions of health, such as the WHO definition, couched in terms of total wellbeing, essentially equate health with happiness. This potentially makes the limits to health boundless, leading to all problems becoming 'health' problems and potentially unleashing unlimited demands for health services. It therefore undermines health and human rights arguments. Doll refers to the limited practical utility of the WHO definition:

> a fine and inspiring concept and its pursuit guarantees health professionals unlimited opportunities for work in the future, but it is not of much practical use for specialists in public health medicine ... (1992: 933)

He proposes a more objective interpretation:

> I shall therefore use the term health in the limited sense of a state distinguished by the absence of disease or of physical or mental defect, that is, the absence of conditions that detract from functional capacity whose incidence can be measured objectively. (1992: 933)

In contrast, the Scottish Government's National Programme for Improving Mental Health and Wellbeing emphasizes the important contribution of mental wellbeing to a 'healthier, wealthier and fairer, smarter, greener and safer Scotland'. It defines mental wellbeing as having:

three main dimensions – emotional, social and psychological wellbeing. This includes our ability to cope with life's problems and make the most of life's opportunities, to cope in the face of adversity and to flourish in all our environments; to feel good and function well, both individually and collectively. (2007: 2)

Lay interpretations of health

Notwithstanding the undoubted difficulties associated with measurement, from a health promotion perspective, the subjective element – health as it is experienced within people's lives – is of central importance. Potvin and McQueen (2007) argue that this requires a 'realignment' of our knowledge base – first, integration of knowledge across a range of social sciences and, secondly, recognition of the legitimacy of lay knowledge. Buchanan, who has defined health as synonymous with the 'good life' (2000) emphasizes the importance of subjective, autonomous interpretations:

> ... we should shift the emphasis in the field from the rather narrow focus on producing specimens of physical fitness, to a broader concern for human wellbeing, here understood in terms of enhancing moral judgment, promoting greater self-understanding, liberating people from scientistic assumptions (perpetuating the belief that human behavior is determined by antecedent causes that only highly trained scientists can divine), advancing the cause of social justice, and promoting respect for the diversity of understandings of the good life for human beings. (2006: 302)

This draws attention to lay interpretations of health which will be considered more fully in Chapter 2. However, for now it is relevant to observe that lay interpretations are complex and multidimensional. The absence of disease is central to lay views, but resilience – the ability to cope with life – and functional capacity are also important. Social class differences have also been noted (Blaxter, 1990; Calnan, 1987), with a greater emphasis on the ability to function in lower social classes and a more multidimensional conceptualization including positive wellbeing in higher. While lay interpretations are often taken to be different from more systematized 'professional' accounts, commonalities do exist. Lay accounts – particularly public as opposed to private accounts – tend to incorporate biomedical interpretations (Cornwell, 1984; Stainton Rogers, 1991).

Adaptation, actualization, ends and means

Utopian visions of health, while aspirational and even inspirational, are ultimately unattainable. Humanity rarely, if ever, achieves stasis. People are constantly engaged in an often problematic process of adaptation to their environments – to their physical, material, economic and social circumstances. The dynamic interaction between individuals and their environments is recognized within definitions of health promotion as enabling people to gain control over their lives and their health (WHO, 1984). The central tenet of Dubos' influential perspective on health is that positive health is a mirage – it is evanescent and unattainable, but worth pursuing. If health means anything, it resides in the pursuit, in engaging with these constantly changing and typically unpredictable environmental forces.

Aspects of Maslow's (1970) notion of self-actualization resonate with Dubos' perspective on the nature of health. Maslow defines it as follows:

> Self-actualization ... refers to man's desire for self-fulfilment, namely, to the tendency for him to become actualized in what he is potentially. This tendency might be phrased as the desire to become more and more what one idiosyncratically is, to become everything that one is capable of becoming ... In other words, 'What a man *can* be, he *must* be.' (1970: 46)

Apart from providing a useful operational definition of psychological health and his emphasis on the importance of self-esteem, Maslow's work has considerable relevance for the empowerment imperative of health promotion. Furthermore, it raises the issue of whether health is an end in itself – a terminal value – or whether it is instrumental for the achievement of other valued goals. The latter interpretation is encapsulated in the Ottawa Charter conceptualization of health as a 'resource for everyday life, not the objective of living' (WHO, 1986) and in the Declaration of Alma Ata (WHO, 1978) as a means of achieving a 'socially and economically productive life'. Whether desired goals in this context are defined by individuals themselves or by society generates further questions about the respective emphasis on self-actualization or collective responsibility.

The way health is conceptualized clearly has implications for practice as illustrated in the box.

Concepts of health in practice: exercise on prescription

Exercise on prescription schemes are currently receiving considerable attention. However, different conceptualizations of health may be evident in the way they are developed and implemented.

An emphasis on the **absence of disease** would lead to a focus on achieving optimal body mass index, blood pressure, cholesterol levels and so on. In contrast, attention to **physical wellbeing** would include cardiovascular fitness even if it is at the expense of mental and social wellbeing. Alternatively, a more **holistic** interpretation of health would include attention to the effects on mental and social health. Similarly, an **empowerment** view would involve enabling people to take control of their physical activity rather than merely conforming with a prescribed regimen.

Coherence, commitment and control: health as empowerment

In an article published posthumously, Antonovsky (1996) declared his concern about the dominant paradigm common to both medicine and health promotion. This, he argued, is based on the dichotomous classification of people into those who have succumbed to disease, as a result of exposure to risk factors, and those who have not. He urged health promoters to move away from this obsession with risk factors and adopt a 'salutogenic model' which views health and disease as a continuum and focuses on the conditions leading to wellness.

'Salutogenesis' is a key concept that focuses on the 'salutary' – that is, health enhancing – rather than 'pathogenic' – that is, disease causing aspects of health. It incorporates Antonovsky's main theory about the factors that determine the extent to which people become healthy and experience wellbeing. Central to this theory is the challenge posed by coping with 'the inherent stressors of human existence' (1996: 15) – encapsulated in the notion of 'entropy' which refers to the level of disorder within systems. At a psychological level, it refers to *perceptions* that disorder exists. People's worlds may be more or less chaotic. Such 'chaos' is held to be undesirable whether it exists in reality or only in people's perceptions. The salutogenic approach is, therefore, designed to reduce entropy and perceptions of entropy and, in so doing, generate a sense of coherence, which it identifies as a central attribute of a healthy person.

Antonovsky defines coherence as:

> ... a global orientation that expresses the extent to which one has a pervasive, enduring though dynamic feeling of confidence that one's internal and external environments are predictable and that there is a high probability that things will work out as well as can reasonably be expected. (1979: 123)

The three main elements are comprehensibility, manageability and meaningfulness.

Health and empowerment

The concept of empowerment will receive further consideration throughout this book. For now, we will confine discussion to the relationship between empowerment and health. If we accept that having control is central to definitions of health, a number of alternatives follow. First, empowerment could be seen as synonymous with (positive) health. In other words, to be healthy is to be empowered! Alternatively, empowerment could be seen as instrumental – that is, as a means to achieving (positive) health. A third conceptualization is also possible. Empowerment could be viewed as both a terminal and an instrumental value. The standpoint here is that empowerment will necessarily be a key component of positive health as an end. At the same time, it will be a means, if not the most important means, of achieving disease prevention and management goals which are components of holistic interpretations of health.

The Commission on Social Determinants of Health (2007) emphasizes the importance of empowerment as a means of achieving health equity. It identifies three key dimensions of empowerment – material, psycho-social and political – and focuses attention on the structural factors necessary for empowerment. It notes particularly the disadvantaged position of women.

We might make two further observations on empowerment in the context of salutogenesis. First, two of the three key requisites of a sense of coherence – notably comprehensibility and manageability – are concerned with beliefs about control and these also figure prominently in conceptualizations of empowerment. Secondly, there is potential conflict between empowerment and the sense of meaningfulness, which is the third element of a sense of coherence. In short, while the feeling that 'all is for the best in the best of all possible worlds' will doubtless make people feel better, and that life, from a salutogenic perspective, is more meaningful, it may well be delusory and hence disempowering.

HEALTH: A WORKING MODEL

As may be seen from Figure 1.1, for all practical purposes, health is defined as having both positive and negative aspects. The term 'wellbeing' is used as shorthand for the positive dimension. Rather than seeing wellbeing and disease as opposite ends of a single spectrum, they are represented as coexisting. Furthermore, although each may influence the other, they can vary independently. For example, although wellbeing may be affected by the presence of negative disease states, it is possible, even desirable, to have high levels of wellbeing regardless of disease being present. Conversely, there may be high or low states of wellbeing in the absence of disease. We are quite clear that preventing and managing disease and disability is a laudable goal in its own right and a central concern of those who are professionally involved in healthcare and health promotion. On the other hand, it is equally clear that the more positive dimensions must also figure prominently in the formulation of a satisfactory definition of health. In the first place, those involved in public health and health promotion cannot ignore its importance. But also, those measures that result in the achievement of positive goals are frequently more effective in achieving preventive outcomes than the more limited tactics employed by espousing a narrow disease prevention model.

Being all that you can be

The three components that make up WHO's holistic conception of health are featured in the model. Following Maslowian self-actualization principles, it is tempting to argue that maximal health status involves 'being all that you can be'. Healthy individuals would thus be those who had fulfilled their mental, physical and social potential. As we have argued, the attainment of complete mental, physical and social health is logically and practically impossible. Furthermore, it would be feasible to achieve high levels of potential in relation to one component of health at the expense of others. For example, the degree of commitment required to achieve maximal physical fitness might not only militate against social health and, possibly, be inconsistent with cultural norms, it might also be viewed as evidence of obsessional neurosis! Equally, a lifestyle characterized by sloth and self-abuse might lead to considerable happiness and a very successful social life, but result in an early death.

Accordingly, health must involve some kind of balance between mental, physical and social components. How, though, is such a balance to be determined? Do individuals themselves make the decision or should society decide for them? As the second option is inconsistent with the principles of empowerment (which are intrinsically healthy), only the first option is a serious contender. We will, however, emphasize later in this book the importance of healthy individuals being guided by commitment to a considerate way of life. Thus, individuals should be in a sufficiently empowered position to enable them to choose a course of action, provided only that the rights of other people are not damaged and, ideally, take action to support those who may be disadvantaged.

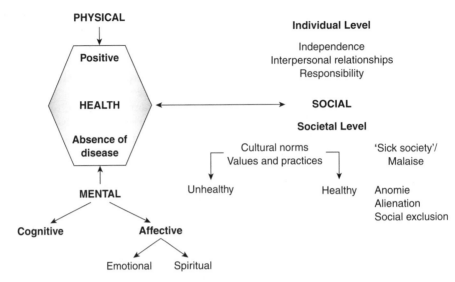

Figure 1.1   A working model of health

Mental, social and spiritual health

The definition of physical health is comparatively straightforward. On the one hand, it is associated with minimizing disease and disability; on the other hand, it may involve having a sufficient level of fitness necessary for achieving other (more important) life goals or/and the experience of high-level wellness or, more realistically, the feelings of wellbeing (allegedly) associated with a high degree of physical fitness. Wellbeing may thus be associated with fitness, but is by no means an identical dimension of health. A person might, for example, exhibit high levels of fitness, but limited feelings of wellbeing or, alternatively, high levels of wellbeing but minimal fitness!

Defining mental health is rather more complicated and problematic. We will confine current discussion to making just two observations. First, it is useful to consider mental health as having both cognitive and affective dimensions. The affective dimension includes emotions and feelings and most discourse on mental health centres on this aspect. The cognitive dimension rarely features in definitions of mental health, but might be incorporated in a holistic model. 'Being all you can be' in cognitive terms refers to the extent to which individuals fulfil their intellectual potential. The reasons for failure to fulfil intellectual potential have been a source of considerable study and evidence of inequity in this regard has provoked concern. It is thus intimately associated with broad-based health promotion initiatives designed to address general social inequalities and break cycles of deprivation, as exemplified by SureStart, the UK Government programme 'designed to deliver the best start in life for every child' (SureStart, 2005). Second, many people have asserted that any serious consideration of positive health must include the spiritual dimension. This is itself open to several interpretations, but features in Figure 1.1 in the context of mental health and wellbeing. It has both a cognitive element, consisting of the doctrinal aspects of, for instance, a religious system, and the emotional commitment associated, in this case, with the value system central to the notion of faith – that has been referred to as '… an illogical belief in the occurrence of the improbable' (an observation attributed to the American journalist H.L. Mencken). Notwithstanding such scepticism, faith can be integral to meaningfulness and the sense of coherence which is central to salutogenesis. Furthermore, religious values can underpin personal health choices and a sense of responsibility towards upholding the rights of others to health.

Social health: individual and society

The social dimension of health is equally complex. As can be seen from Figure 1.1, there are two categories. The first of these refers to the social health of the individual; the second is concerned with the health of society itself. Three main aspects of individual social health have been identified.

- **Independence**: a socially mature individual acts with greater independence and autonomy than a relatively immature individual.
- **Interpersonal relationships**: a socially healthy individual is characterized by the capacity to relate to a number of significant others and cooperate with them.
- **Responsibility**: a person who is socially mature accepts responsibility for others.

The distinction between the social health of individuals and the health of society is recognized in everyday parlance with references to 'sick societies' and 'social malaise'. We will make further reference to this dimension of social health later in this chapter and at a number of points in this book when we consider health promotion's concerns with powerlessness, meaninglessness, normlessness, isolation and self-estrangement which are characteristic of 'sick societies' and contribute to social exclusion.

PROMOTING HEALTH: COMPETING IDEOLOGIES

> No science is immune to the infection of politics and the corruption of power.
>
> Dr Jacob Bronowski, *The Ascent of Man*, BBC2, 1973

Defining health promotion

A key issue in defining health promotion is whether it is viewed as an umbrella term, covering the activities of a range of disciplines committed to improving the health of the population, or as a discipline in its own right. Bunton and Macdonald (1992: 6) suggest that 'recent changes in the knowledge base and the practice of health promotion are characteristic of paradigmatic and disciplinary development'. They take a discipline to involve an ordered field of study embracing associated theories, perspectives and methods. A discipline would be expected to have its own ideology that would also inform standards of professional practice. Prior to our analysis of the ideology of health promotion and the values integral to different models, we will briefly clarify the distinction between health education and health promotion.

Although the generic use of the term 'health promotion' to describe any activity that improves health status can be traced back earlier, Terris (1996) noted that in 1945 Henry Sigerist described the four tasks of medicine as the promotion of health, prevention of illness, restoration and rehabilitation of the sick (cited by French, 2000). However, it was not until the late 1970s that this term began to be applied in a more specific way to a concept, movement, discipline and, indeed, profession. While a systematic account of the history of health promotion is beyond the scope of this text, we should note that the roots of contemporary health promotion are in health education.

The earliest examples of health education in the context of public health would now be described as health propaganda. This typically took the form of pamphleteering, which was intended to generate political change in support of a variety of environmental health measures designed to combat squalor and provide clean water supplies. Early health education was thus seen as an adjunct to public health efforts. Indeed, Naidoo and Wills (1994: 63) note that, by the 1920s, health education had become associated with 'diarrhoea, dirt, spitting and venereal disease!' With this increasing focus on personal rather than public health, health educators continued their adjuvant role in support of the medical profession. Their activity during this period essentially involved giving information and persuading people using mass communication strategies.

The dominant themes in the early health education journals of the 1950s and 1960s centred on methods of delivering information in ways that would attract attention and interest people in the substantive content of health messages. The primary concern was very much with the technicalities of delivering information. The assumption was that if people were given the 'right' knowledge, they would act appropriately. As we will see in Chapter 3, this grossly underestimated the complexity of the task.

Two broad paths can be traced in the subsequent development of health education. One – the *preventive approach* – sought evermore sophisticated ways of achieving behaviour change by means of the application of psychological theory. The other, which was more in tune with progressive educational philosophy, was concerned with enabling people to make informed choices – the so-called *educational approach*.

In the period following the Lalonde report (1974), a renewed interest in the importance of the social and environmental influences on health status – both directly and indirectly by shaping behaviour – brought health education under fierce critical scrutiny (see for example Navarro, 1976; Ryan, 1976). Of particular concern were the emphasis on individual responsibility and the failure to recognize constraints on individuals' behaviour – most notably their economic and material circumstances. Health education was accused of 'victim-blaming' – a term attributed to Ryan. The essence of victim-blaming lies in attempts to persuade individuals to take responsibility for their own health while ignoring the fact that they are victims of social and environmental circumstances. Accordingly, Ryan argued that the fundamental factors governing health were power and money.

Being poor is stressful. Being poor is worrisome; one is anxious about the next meal, the next dollar, the next day. Being poor is nerve-wracking, upsetting. When you're poor it's easy to despair and it's easy to lose your temper. And all of this is because you're poor. Not because your mother let you go around with your diapers full of bowel movement until you were four; or shackled you to the potty chair before you could walk. Not because she broke your bottle on your first birthday or breastfed you until you could cut your own steak. But because you don't have any money. (1976: 157)

The emergence of health promotion was in response to the need to address the environmental as well as the behavioural determinants of health – the so-called upstream determinants. In effect, it marked a shift from being concerned with healthy choices to making 'the healthy choice the easy choice'.

Health promotion includes efforts to tackle the social and environmental determinants of health by means of healthy public policy. The scope of health promotion can therefore be summed up in a simple formula:

health promotion = health education × healthy public policy

We will review different models of health promotion later in this chapter. At this point, we will consider the influence of WHO on the development of health promotion.

The contribution of the World Health Organization (WHO) to the definition of health promotion

The evolution of health promotion has been accompanied by considerable debate about its nature and purpose – debate that has exposed its core underlying values. WHO has been a major voice in shaping the development of health promotion. Not only have its documents been a source of reference for health promotion practice, they have also been assimilated into professional training courses – that is, they have become part of the doctrine of health promotion.

As mentioned above, WHO has taken a holistic view of health from its inception. The 'Health for All' movement was launched at the Thirtieth World Health Assembly in 1977. The following year saw the *Declaration of Alma Ata* (WHO, 1978), which identified primary healthcare (PHC) as the principal means of attaining 'Health for All' targets. Primary healthcare – as distinct from primary medical care – was envisaged as embracing all the services that impact on health, including, for example, education, housing and agriculture.

A number of key issues in the *Declaration* have informed subsequent thinking. In addition to emphasizing the importance of a holistic view of health, the following assertions figure in many WHO publications and declarations:

- health as a fundamental right
- the unacceptability of inequality in health within and between nations
- health as a major social goal
- the reciprocal relationship between health and social development
- the need to involve a number of different sectors in working towards health
- the rights and duties of individuals to participate individually and collectively in their own healthcare
- education as the means of developing communities' capacity to participate.

In January 1984, WHO set up a new programme on 'health promotion'. A discussion document on health promotion (WHO, 1984) saw it as a 'unifying concept', bringing together 'those who recognize the need for change in the ways and conditions of living, in order to promote health'. It defined health promotion as 'the process of enabling people to increase control over, and to improve, their health'.

Income, shelter and food were acknowledged to be primary requisites for health. Importance was also attached to the provision of information and life skills, the creation of supportive environments providing opportunities for making healthy choices and the creation of health-enhancing conditions in the economic, physical, social and cultural environments.

The document outlined the key principles of health promotion as:

- the involvement of the whole population in the context of their everyday life and enabling people to take control of, and have responsibility for, their health
- tackling the determinants of health – that is, an upstream approach, which demands the cooperative efforts of a number of different sectors at all levels, from national to local
- utilizing a range of different, but complementary, methods and approaches – from legislation and fiscal measures, organizational change and community development to education and communication
- effective public participation, which may require the development of individual and community capacity
- the role of health professionals in education and advocacy for health (WHO, 1984).

Action was therefore seen to require an integrated effort to encourage individual and community responsibility for health along with the development of a health-enhancing environment. The document reflected a commitment to voluntarism and formally acknowledged the risk of dictating how individuals should behave. This has been referred to as 'healthism' – a notion that we will return to later. Other potential problems included an overemphasis on individual behaviour rather than the social and economic determinants of behaviour and the possibility of increasing social inequality if the varying capacity of different social groups to exercise control over their health was not tackled. A further concern was that health promotion might be appropriated by particular professional groups to the exclusion of others and lay people.

A series of major international conferences followed. The Ottawa Charter, developed at the First International Conference on Health Promotion (WHO, 1986), built on many of the key principles set out in the WHO discussion document and has been a constant source of reference. It identified three broad strategies for working to promote health:

- **advocacy** to ensure the creation of conditions favourable to health
- **enabling** by creating a supportive environment, but also by giving people the information and skills that they need to make healthy choices
- **mediation** between different groups to ensure the pursuit of health.

The Ottawa Charter listed five main action areas that have been central to the conceptual framework of health promotion:

- build healthy public policy
- create supportive environments
- strengthen community action
- develop personal skills
- reorient health services.

There is potentially some tension between individual and societal responsibility for health, between individual and collective responsibility, and between voluntarism and control. The Ottawa Charter handled this by seeing individuals as having responsibility for their own health, but also a collective concern for the health of others. However, there is an overriding societal responsibility to create the conditions that enable people to take control of their health. Recognition that health is created where people 'learn, work, play and love' heralded the 'settings approach' to health promotion.

The Second International Conference on Health Promotion in Adelaide (WHO, 1988) focused on healthy public policy as a means of creating supportive environments that would be health-enhancing in themselves and would also – in the words of the much-used phrase – contribute to making the healthy choice the easy choice. In particular, it acknowledged the importance of addressing the needs of underprivileged and disadvantaged groups and emphasized the responsibility of developed countries to ensure that their own policies impacted positively on developing countries. It saw healthy public policy as 'characterized by an explicit concern for health and equity in all areas of policy and an accountability for health impact'. The Adelaide Conference identified the need for strong advocates and also saw community action as a major driving force.

The Sundsvall Conference (WHO, 1991) addressed the issue of supportive environments for health. In addition to the physical environment, it recognized the importance of the social environment and the influence of social norms and culture on behaviour. It also noted the challenge to traditional values arising from changing lifestyles, increasing social isolation and lack of a sense of coherence. The need for action at all levels and across sectors was recognized and, in particular, the capacity for community action. The key elements of a 'democratic health promotion approach' were seen to be empowerment and community participation. The importance of education as a means of bringing about political, economic and social changes was recognized as well as its being a basic human right.

The Jakarta Declaration on Leading Health Promotion into the 21st Century (WHO, 1997) was developed at the Fourth International Conference on Health Promotion. It viewed health both as a right and as instrumental to social and economic development. It envisaged the 'ultimate goal' of health promotion as increasing health expectancy by means of action directed at the determinants of health in order to:

- create the greatest health gain
- contribute to reduction in inequities
- further human rights
- build social capital.

The Jakarta Declaration built on the commitments of the previous documents and provided clear endorsement of the value of comprehensive approaches and involving families and communities. It called for strong partnerships to promote health including – for the first time – the involvement of the private sector.

Overall, the priorities set out for the twenty-first century were to:

- promote social responsibility for health
- increase investments for health development

- consolidate and expand partnerships for health
- increase community capacity and empower the individual
- secure an infrastructure for health promotion.

The first resolution on health promotion, which was passed at the Fifty-First World Health Assembly in May 1998 (WHO, 1998c), incorporated the thinking of the Jakarta Declaration.

As it moved into the twenty-first century, WHO (1998e) identified the following key values underpinning the 'Health for All' movement:

- providing the highest attainable standard of health as a fundamental human right
- strengthening the application of ethics to health policy, research and service provision
- equity-orientated policies and strategies that emphasize solidarity
- incorporating a gender perspective into health policies and strategies. (1998e: v)

The Fifth Global Conference on Health Promotion held in Mexico in 2000 focused on 'bridging the equity gap'. It issued a Ministerial Statement signed by some 87 countries, including the United Kingdom (WHO, 2000a), that acknowledged that 'the promotion of health and social development is a central duty and responsibility of governments that all sectors of society share' and concluded that 'health promotion must be a fundamental component of public policies and programmes in all countries in the pursuit of equity and health for all'. The Mexico conference emphasized the need to 'work with and through existing political systems and structures to ensure healthy public policy, adequate investment in health, and facilitation of an infrastructure for health promotion' (WHO, 2000b: 21).

The Bangkok Charter for Health Promotion in a Globalized World (WHO, 2005) responded to emerging global issues by focusing attention on increasing inequalities between countries, commercialization and new patterns of consumption and communication, and also global environmental change and urbanization. It identified the following required actions:

- **advocate** for health based on human rights and solidarity
- **invest** in sustainable policies, actions and infrastructure to address the determinants of health
- **build capacity** for policy development, leadership, health promotion practice, knowledge transfer and research, and health literacy
- **regulate and legislate** to ensure a high level of protection from harm and enable equal opportunity for health and wellbeing for all people
- **partner and build alliances** with public, private, non-governmental and international organizations and civil society to create sustainable actions.

It further demanded four key commitments to make health promotion:

- central to the global development agenda
- a core responsibility for all of government
- a key focus for communities and civil society
- a requirement for good corporate practice.

While the primary concern of these documents has been with identifying appropriate action, they are underpinned by clear values. Indeed, it could be said that unless activity is consistent with these values, it should not be regarded as 'health promotion'. These values include equity and empowerment – the twin pillars of health promotion – along with health as a right, voluntarism, autonomy, participation, partnerships and social justice. Consideration of rights and responsibilities, power and control generates some interesting paradoxes in relation to health education and policy interventions, which we discuss more fully below.

Ideology, social construction and competing discourses

Defining ideology

The original meaning of 'ideology' was merely the scientific study of human ideas. It has been transformed over time into a concept that includes cognitive, affective and action dimensions. Although ideologies are value laden – and it is not unusual for the term to be used synonymously with value systems – the contemporary construction of the word ideology is much more complex.

De Kadt, discussing the ideological dimensions involved in implementing WHO's 'Health for All' agenda, states that ideologies are an amalgam of fact and unsubstantiated assertion. He observes that, 'comprehensive ideologies (as opposed to partial ideologies) are commitment-demanding views about societies, their past history and present operation, which contain a strong evaluative element and hence provide goals for the future' (De Kadt, 1982a: 742).

In order to clarify the central meaning of 'ideology', Eagleton contrasts the emotionally charged nature of ideology, which has a 'partial and biased view of the world', with an 'empirical' or 'pragmatic' approach. There is, of course, a tendency for those espousing political causes to describe their 'pragmatic' construction of reality as rational and based on common sense whereas opponents' views are characterized by ideological zealotry involving, as Eagleton notes, their:

> ... judging a particular issue through some rigid framework of preconceived ideas which distorts their understanding. I view things as they really are; you squint at them through a tunnel vision imposed by some extraneous system of doctrine. There is usually a suggestion that this involves an oversimplifying view of the world — that to speak or judge 'ideologically' is to do so schematically, stereotypically, and perhaps with the faintest hint of fanaticism. (1991: 3)

Eagleton (1991: 4) provides a sardonic illustration of alternative constructions of political events which could equally be applied to contemporary happenings:

> What this comes down to is that the Soviet Union is in the grip of ideology while the United States sees things as they really are ... to seek some humble, pragmatic political goal, such as bringing down the democratically elected government of Chile, is a question of adapting oneself realistically to the facts; to send one's tanks into Czechoslovakia is an instance of ideological fanaticism.

Ideology, values and ethics

Belief systems and doctrine are major parts of the territory of ideology. However, values and value systems feature with equal prominence. Rokeach defines values as 'an enduring belief that a specific mode of conduct or endstate of existence is personally or socially preferable to an opposite or converse mode of conduct or endstate of existence' (1973: 10). Following Guttman's (2000) review, the major ethical values assumed to underpin health promotion (or, more specifically, 'public health communication interventions') are:

- beneficence, or, 'doing good'
- non-maleficence, or, 'doing no harm'
- respect for personal autonomy
- justice or fairness
- utility and the public good
- (possibly) community involvement and participation.

As we will see, the extent to which these values are actually central to the ideology of health promotion will depend on the preferred model. At this point, it is interesting to note the remarkable degree of resonance between the empowerment model of health promotion and the stewardship model (see box) developed by The Nuffield Council on Bioethics. It sets out the ethical principles which should underpin the development of healthy public policy and achieve balance between individual and government responsibility.

The stewardship model

Acceptable public health goals include:

- reducing the risks of ill health that result from other people's actions, such as drinking and smoking in public places;
- reducing causes of ill health relating to environmental conditions, for instance provision of clean drinking water and setting housing standards;
- protecting and promoting the health of children and other vulnerable people;
- helping people to overcome addictions that are harmful to health or helping them to avoid unhealthy behaviours;
- ensuring that it is easy for people to lead a healthy life, for example by providing convenient and safe opportunities for exercise;
- ensuring that people have appropriate access to medical services; and
- reducing unfair health inequalities.

At the same time, public health programmes should:

- not attempt to coerce adults to lead healthy lives;
- minimise the use of measures that are implemented without consulting people [either individually or using democratic procedures]; and
- minimise measures that are very intrusive or conflict with important aspects of personal life, such as privacy.

(Nuffield Council on Bioethics, 2007)

The centrality of power

Given the emphasis on empowerment in this book, it is axiomatic that individual and community power are pivotal issues in the ideology of health promotion and central to the design of health promotion programmes. Questions of power feature prominently in discussions of ideology. Giddens is quite explicit about this:

> Ideologies are found in all societies in which there are systematic and engrained inequalities between groups. The concept of ideology connects closely with that of *power*, since ideological systems serve to legitimize the differential power which groups hold. (1989: 727)

In Fairclough's laconic phrase, ideology is, in fact, 'meaning in the service of power' (1995: 18).

Eagleton provides a comprehensive account of the mechanisms whereby a dominant group exerts its power and creates 'false consciousness':

> A dominant power may legitimate itself by *promoting* beliefs and values congenial to it; *naturalizing* and *universalizing* such beliefs so as to render them self-evident and apparently inevitable; *denigrating* ideas which might challenge it; *excluding* rival forms of thought, perhaps by some unspoken but systematic logic; and *obscuring* social reality in ways convenient to itself. (1991: 5–6) [our emphasis]

The relevance of ideology is not only measured in terms of the ways in which the power of dominant social groups is legitimized. More significant for health promotion are the ways in which subordinate groups are 'de-powered' by dominant groups. Indeed, the radical ideology underpinning the model of health promotion proposed in this book is substantially concerned with empowering subordinate and oppressed social groups. Pursuing the matter of false consciousness, Eagleton reminds us of the subtle and potentially insidious ways in which people may be de-powered:

> The most efficient oppressor is the one who persuades his underlings to love, desire and identify with his power; and any practice of political emancipation thus involves that most difficult of all forms of liberation, freeing ourselves from ourselves. (1991: xiii)

He does, however, caution against exaggerating the power of this 'hegemonic' process and optimistically notes that nobody is ever wholly mystified. Despite a capacity for self-delusion, human beings are at least moderately rational and, unless the process of domination provides sufficient gratification over time, the dominated will rebel. If this were not true, health promotion's emancipatory strategies for critical consciousness raising would be seriously compromised.

Ideology, discourse and narrative

'Discourse' is 'a pattern of talking and writing about or visually representing an event, object, issue, individual or group' (Lupton and Chapman, 1994: 38). The notion of discourse has its roots in linguistics. It is more than mere language, rather the thought underlying language. Accordingly, 'discourse analysis' involves penetrating beneath the surface of language or images and seeking out subtexts and meanings relating to wider beliefs and value systems – often their social and political contexts.

Discourse analysis has relevance for health promotion by providing insight into the way people's ideas about health – or indeed health promotion messages – are constructed, along with their underpinning values and motivations. It can equally be applied to professional discourse to identify the underlying ideology.

Scott-Samuel and Springett draw attention to the interrelationship between discourse and power. Increase in the prominence of discourse may increase the power of groups which it represents and conversely power relations among different groups may shape the level of influence of discourse. They assert that the dominance of public health medicine has influenced the public health discourse and led to 'hegemonic suppression of the radical element within the public health agenda' (2007: 212).

Critical discourse analysis focuses on power and dominant ideologies and the way these are both reflected in and perpetuated by language (Lupton, 1992). Fairclough has referred to it as 'discourse analysis "with an attitude"' (Fairclough, 2001 cited by Porter, 2006). Porter (2006) examined the Ottawa and Bangkok Charters using critical discourse analysis. She identified a shift from a '"new social movements" discourse of ecosocial justice in Ottawa to a "new capitalism" discourse of law and economics in Bangkok' (2006: 75). She also contends that while the Bangkok Charter proposes actions to tackle the problems of a globalized world, its discourse may serve to perpetuate the structural determinants of those very problems.

Medical discourse and the preventive model

The history of health promotion has been marked by a struggle to distance itself from the medical model that has dominated twentieth-century discourse on health and illness. Some would contend that this break is more evident in the rhetoric than in the practice of health promotion (Kelly and Charlton, 1995). Although the medical model has been alluded to earlier, it is worthwhile considering – in the context of our discussion about ideology, power and control – the nature of the model and the origins of concern about its applicability to health promotion. The key features of the medical model have been variously seen as including:

- a mechanistic view of the body
- mind–body dualism
- disease as the product of disordered functioning of the body or a part of it
- a focus on pathogenesis – that is, the causes of disease
- the pursuit of the causal sequences of disease and an emphasis on micro-causality
- specific diseases having specific causes.

The medical model is therefore very much in tune with modernist rational thought and characterized by a reductionist view of the causes of ill health, together with a mechanistic focus on micro-causality.

The medical model is inextricably linked with medical practice and, more generally, biomedicine. It shares common ideological origins and has acquired added authority as a result of its association with the power and authority of the medical profession. The dominance of medicine has itself been the subject of an extensive sociological critique – for example, its role in supporting a capitalist value system (Navarro, 1976; Doyal and Pennell, 1979); the monopolization of healthcare (De Kadt, 1982a); the comodification of health and appropriation of authority over the areas that influence health (Illich, 1976); and maintaining gendered power structures in society (Doyal and Pennell, 1979; Ehrenreich and English, 1979).

The medical model belongs to a group that Rawson has termed 'iconic models' – that is, 'simplified descriptions of some aspect of known reality, portraying a literal or isomorphic image of nature' (1992: 210). It is possible, in principle, to identify a number of different models within medical practice and, equally, the medical model can be recognized within a range of different types of professional practice. It is also worth noting, in passing, that the ascendancy of high-tech medicine in the twentieth century and marginalization of preventive medicine has not gone unchallenged within medicine itself. The work of McKeown is well known in this regard (see, for example, McKeown, 1979). The emergence of 'The New Public Health' has been an attempt to retreat from an emphasis on individual responsibility for health and health actions and refocus on the factors that collectively influence health status. However, critics such as Petersen and Lupton (1996) contend that 'The New Public Health' has not entirely freed itself from the ethic of individual responsibility. Nor has it mounted an effective challenge to the increasing disparity in wealth and power within many societies.

Application of the medical model to health promotion leads to an emphasis on prevention. This association with prevention effectively 'rebadges' the medical model as the preventive model.

The dominant concept is that of risk, whether viewed as a 'property of individuals or as an external threat' (Petersen and Lupton, 1996: 174). Furthermore, the conceptualization of risk is often narrow, ignoring the wider social and environmental determinants of health. The emphasis is on individual responsibility, which – as noted above in our comments on 'victim-blaming' – places the onus on individuals to reduce their exposure to risk by avoiding risky behaviour and contact with risks in the environment. O'Brien notes that the focus on risk leads to health being:

> constructed as a series of encounters with risk factors in diet and behaviour, at work and at play, in public and private networks, factors that can be monitored and correlated, channelled and controlled, prioritized and targeted. (1995: 196)

Attempts to improve health primarily take the form of health education interventions to persuade individuals to adopt healthy behaviours and lifestyles.

The preventive model has a number of consequences. As we noted above, it results in an essentially 'victim-blaming' approach in its disregard for the social, environmental and political factors that shape and, indeed, constrain behavioural choices.

Illich's (1976) critique of the extension of medical control beyond legitimate concern with disease to include ordinary aspects of human experience – so-called 'social iatrogenesis' or medicalization of life – is well known. Including exposure to risk within the medical remit and, along with it, a whole range of behavioural and lifestyle factors, extends the notion of medicalization even further and brings substantial areas of life under expert, rather than autonomous, control. Kelleher, Gabe and Williams note that, along with the decline in organized religion, this has led to:

doctors being cast more and more in the role of secular priests whose expertise encompassed not only the treatment of bodily ills but also advice on how to live the good life, and judgements on right and wrong behaviour. (1994: xii)

Moreover, the acknowledgement of expert authority over areas of life normally managed by individuals, families and communities erodes confidence in their own capacity to take responsibility for their health. By undermining self-reliance, communities and cultures are disempowered. Illich refers to this as 'cultural iatrogenesis', which he sees as: 'destroy[ing] the potential of people to deal with their human weaknesses, vulnerability, and uniqueness in a personal and autonomous way' (1976: 42).

Horrobin's (1978) riposte to Illich accepts the existence of some undue dependence on the medical profession in matters of sickness, but notes the remarkable resistance of the healthy to accept medical advice and over-exaggeration of the power of medicine to influence people. He quotes John Owen's sixteenth-century verse:

God and the doctor we like and adore
But only when in danger, not before;
The danger o'er, both are alike requited,
God is forgotten, and the doctor slighted.
(1978: 25)

Furthermore, he contends that Illich's portrayal of society as 'an ignorant and unwilling victim of medical imperialism' (1976: 29) is a misrepresentation. Similarly, O'Neill's (2002) thought-provoking Reith Lectures draw attention to the lack of trust in contemporary society and suggest that the acceptance of treatment or advice cannot be taken as indicative of trust when no effective alternatives are available to people.

Notwithstanding these arguments, medicine is still accorded considerable expert power. Deference to such authority provides further legitimation. It reinforces the dominance of the medical model and, ipso facto, the preventive model, even when the view espoused is at odds with the experiences of individuals.

What, then, is the source of this medical authority? De Kadt suggests that:

Expertise and the 'life and death' responsibilities of the physician are used to provide ideological justification for physician dominance in the doctor-patient (healing) context. (1982a: 746)

Parsons' (1958) concept of the 'sick role' throws further light on the doctor–patient interaction. When people are ill, they are unable to fulfil their normal social roles and everyday activities. Diagnosis will medically legitimate their adoption of the sick role which exempts them from their normal social obligations. However, there is a concomitant obligation to attempt to get better, by seeking and complying with medical advice. The sick role therefore requires submission to medical authority and compliance with a therapeutic regimen.

Formalization of the 'at risk' role within the preventive model makes equivalent demands in terms of an obligation to modify behaviour and exposure to risk (Baric, 1969). Individuals are held responsible for their exposure to risk and failure to act accordingly may be attributed to ignorance at best or deliberate fecklessness at worst. Unlike the sick role, the at risk role does not confer any rights. The outcome of this is twofold. On the one hand, it labels as deviant those who cannot or choose not to comply with admonitions on how to live their life, and holds them responsible for the consequences. The categorization of more and more areas of life as healthy or unhealthy effectively creates its own dogma about ways of living, coupled with the associated moral sanction of disapproval if unhealthy options are chosen. As Petersen and Lupton note:

> The idealization of the 'normal', 'healthy' subject as one endowed with certain 'natural' capacities and inclinations fails to recognize the multiplicity of possible subject positions, and can serve to coerce, marginalize, stigmatize and discriminate against those who do not or cannot conform with the ideal. This ideal denies difference – whether this is based on social class, gender, sexuality, 'race' ethnicity, physical ability, or age – and the kinds of personal commitments and demands that are required of those who are called upon to conform to it. (1996: 178)

On the other hand, it creates a remorseless pressure to improve health:

> The contemporary citizen is increasingly attributed with responsibilities to ceaselessly maintain and improve her or his own health by using a whole range of measures. To do this she or he is increasingly expected to take note of and act upon the recommendations of a whole range of 'experts' and 'advisers' located in a range of diffuse institutional and cultural sites. (Bunton and Burrows, 1995: 208)

An overemphasis on keeping healthy has been referred to as 'healthism' – a term attributed to Crawford who defines it as:

> the preoccupation with personal health as a primary – often the primary – focus for the definition and achievement of wellbeing; a goal which is to be attained primarily through the modification of lifestyles, with or without therapeutic help. (1980: 368)

Despite healthism's emphasis on positive health, its focus on individual responsibility can be seen to have some parallels with victim-blaming. The no fault principle enshrined in the notion of the sick role does not apply and is replaced by a 'your fault dogma'. Those, therefore, who fail, or refuse, to seek health-promoting ways of life become 'near pariahs' (Crawford, 1980: 379) – see the box for an illustration of this. Furthermore, preoccupation with health elevates it in status to a super value – health becomes an end in itself rather than a means of achieving other values and positive health behaviour acts as a hallmark of good living.

Discrimination and the obese

There is evidence that children and adolescents who are overweight or obese are more likely to be bullied (see for example Janssen et al., 2004; Lucy et al., 2004; Robinson, 2006)

Adults also experience discrimination. A British woman was refused immigration into New Zealand because she was overweight. Her partner managed to slim to reach the BMI requirements (Williams, 2007).

A literature review also found that among nurses there were some negative attitudes towards overweight patients (Brown, 2006).

Reference to our earlier discussion of health promotion will indicate that the preventive model and healthism are both inconsistent with the two central tenets of health promotion – equity and empowerment. The emphasis on individualism and lack of attention to the social and environmental factors that impinge on health – both directly and indirectly as a result of their influence on behaviour – could, in fact, increase rather than reduce the health gap in society. Health gains will inevitably be greatest in those who are most able to make changes by virtue of their relatively advantaged position.

However, even though we have argued that a preventive model is inconsistent with the values position of health promotion, we should finish on a word of caution. Rejection of the preventive model does not necessarily imply rejection of the need for biomedical knowledge or appropriate preventive action. Horrobin (1978) argues that it is inadequate knowledge and insufficiently rigorous criteria that have been responsible for the unnecessary use of screening procedures rather than the inexorable spread of medical knowledge cited by Illich (1976). Furthermore, evidence about cause is necessary to much health promotion practice – indeed, any attempts to influence behaviour in the absence of evidence that this will be beneficial would be unethical. The problem lies not so much with a biomedical interpretation per se, but with too exclusive a reliance on it and dismissal of other perspectives – that is, with the imbalance of power and the dominance of medical expert authority. Our discussion of empowerment in Chapter 3 also draws attention to the importance of knowledge and the ability to access and interpret accurate knowledge as key components of empowerment. Such knowledge and understanding can give people greater control over their own lives. It also enables them to enter into a circle of shared understanding with professionals, thereby breaking down power structures and facilitating dialogue.

Education and the discourse of voluntarism

Health education is a key component of health promotion. We propose the following 'empirical' definition, which centres on the process of learning:

> health education is any planned activity designed to produce health- or illness-related learning.

'Learning' has frequently been defined as a relatively permanent change in capability or disposition – that is, the change produced is not transitory and, after the educational intervention, people are capable of achieving what they were not capable of achieving before the intervention and/or feel differently about ideas, people or events. Accordingly, effective health education may result in the development of cognitive capabilities such as the acquisition of factual information, understanding and insights. It may also provide skills in problem solving and decision making and the formation or development of beliefs. It might also result in the clarification of existing values and the creation of new values – and, quite frequently, in attitude change. Health education also aims to foster the acquisition of health-related psychomotor or social interaction skills. It may even bring about changes in behaviour or lifestyle or create the conditions for the adoption of healthy public policy.

One of the most important and enduring sources of ideological argument centres on the question of rationality and voluntarism. For example, Hirst (1969) asserted unequivocally that the central purpose of *all* education should be rationality. The educational philosopher Baelz contrasts education with manipulation and with indoctrination:

> The educator encourages his [*sic*] pupil to develop the capacity to think for himself, while the indoctrinator wishes to make it impossible for his pupil ever to question the doctrine that he has been taught. (1979: 32)

The concept of doctrine is equated with the notion of dogma and typically refers to some creed or body of religious, political or philosophical thought that is offered for acceptance as truth. The purpose of indoctrination is, therefore, to present a body of ideas in an appealing way such that the ideas are accepted. The distinction between indoctrination and education is therefore fundamental.

Health education, voluntarism and choices for health

For many health educators, voluntarism is an ideological sine qua non. Note, for instance, Green and Kreuter's influential definition:

> Health education is any combination of learning experiences designed to facilitate *voluntary* actions conducive to health ... *Voluntary* means *without coercion* and with the full understanding and acceptance of the purposes of the action. (1999: 27) [our emphasis]

Faden and Faden (1978) made the point even more forcibly in their discussion of the ethics of health education. They cited the Society of Public Health Educators' (SOPHE) *Code of Ethics* (1976), noting its affirmation of the importance of voluntary consumer participation:

> Health educators value privacy, dignity, and the worth of the individual, and use skills consistent with these values. Health educators observe the principle of informed consent with respect to individuals and groups served. Health educators support change by choice, not by coercion.

According to the educational model of health education, coercive strategies and techniques are, therefore, unacceptable. Coercion occurs when an individual's or group's freedom of action is constrained. Faden and Faden (1978) cite Warwick and Kelman (1973), who defined coercion as a process forcing individuals to act or refrain from acting under the threat of severe deprivation – and clearly involving the application of power to reward or punish. It frequently results from externally imposed sanctions or other barriers.

It is important, then, to recognize the existence of two varieties of coercion. The first of these is externally imposed. For instance, it involves the implementation of policy measures imposing a potentially wide range of restrictive regulations, in the form of legislation, fiscal measures and environmental engineering. Examples of such 'healthy public policies' would include banning smoking in public areas; redesigning roadways and traffic calming measures; the inclusion of vitamins in popular food products;

regulation of the food industry to reduce the fat content of products; increase in the price of alcohol; and so on. An interesting example of Japanese health legislation was the banning of the Pill in order to promote the use of condoms as a device to control the spread of HIV (Jitsukawa and Djerassi, 1994). The attraction of these various coercive strategies is doubtless self-evident, but McKinlay summarized it succinctly as follows:

> One stroke of effective health legislation is equal to many separate health intervention endeavours and the cumulative efforts of innumerable health workers over long periods of time. (1975: 13, in Guttman, 2000: 85)

The second form of coercion is perhaps less obvious and may be designated as psychological rather than environmental manipulation. It involves the use of certain techniques to create a particular kind of learning that lacks the element of genuine informed choice that characterizes the principle of voluntarism. Figure 1.2 locates these techniques on a continuum ranging from high degrees of coercion to maximal potential for facilitating 'free' choice. Accordingly, 'brainwashing' is seen as highly coercive while 'facilitation' is, by definition, seeking to assist learners to achieve their own goals. 'Persuasion' is generally viewed as an intervention concerned with achieving the goals of the persuader rather than helping the persuadees to make up their own minds.

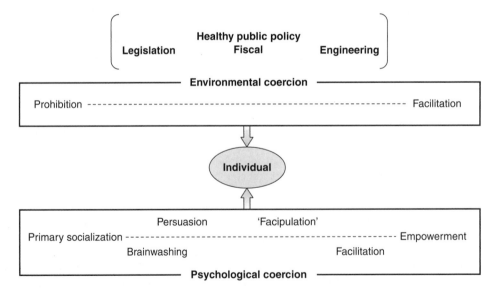

Figure 1.2   A spectrum of coercion

In the case of psychological coercion or 'persuasion', personal choice is modified in some way without the knowledge of the person in question. Faden and Faden (1978) in proposing this latter description had in mind Warwick and Kelman's (1973) definition of persuasion as a 'form of interpersonal influence, in which one person tries to change the attitudes or behaviour of another by means of argument, reasoning, or, in certain cases, structured listening'. In fact, it is somewhat misleading to define coercion of this kind solely in terms of the persuadee's lack of knowledge of what is going on. 'Insight' might be a better term as it is clear that, in many instances, individuals are well aware that someone is trying to influence them. Indeed, the most blatant form of psychological coercion, brainwashing, leaves the unfortunate recipient under no illusion that some fairly dramatic coercive techniques are being applied!

It may at first glance seem surprising that brainwashing has been partnered with primary socialization. This represents both an expression of doubt about the power of brainwashing to fundamentally affect firmly grounded values and, at the same time, seeks to acknowledge the potentially greater power of the processes of 'shaping', conditioning and modelling that are part and parcel of the childrearing experience.

At a more mundane level, people exposed to persuasive advertising also know that the advertiser is seeking to influence them. They may, however, lack insight into the influence process – for instance, why the advertiser is manipulating certain images or using certain presenters. This lack of insight into the psychodynamics of the attempt to influence militates against the principle of voluntarism, albeit in a rather more subtle way than the deliberate presentation of misleading information or the partial presentation of evidence supporting the attitude or behaviour change the persuader is seeking to induce.

Warwick and Kelman (1973) use the term 'structured listening' to refer to a type of interpersonal encounter that, at first glance, does not seem to involve coercion. It is particularly interesting as it serves as a reminder of the way in which a technique, that would be considered eminently educational – non-directive counselling – may, with a few apparently minor modifications, be employed as a persuasive tool. Effective counselling depends on the deployment of such social skills as active listening, empathy, appropriate self-disclosure and the constant supply of unconditional positive regard. Janis (1975) has noted how the replacement of the ethically unex-ceptionable unconditional positive regard with what he terms 'quasi unconditional positive regard' can be a compelling device for influencing attitude and behaviour change – in a nonvoluntaristic way. This technique involves implying that the highly rewarding positive strokes supplied by the health educator will be rationed and made contingent on the client adopting certain healthy practices. This apparently benevolent method will presumably be all the more powerful as it is difficult to detect the overt attempt to influence.

Rather like structured listening, the coined term 'facipulation' has been used for a persuasive method cosmetically concealed under a cloak of educational respectability (Constantino-David, 1982). Essentially, it refers to the subtle process whereby 'leaders' actually manage to manipulate their clients under the guise of 'facilitation' with the intention, conscious or otherwise, of promoting the leaders' own political and ideological agenda.

Facilitation would usually be viewed as fundamentally voluntaristic and therefore ethical. After all, its concern is, by definition, to help people achieve the objectives that they have set for themselves. However, voluntaristic choice is not necessarily consonant with the ethics of health promotion. For instance, the term 'facilitation' might reasonably describe any enabling process, irrespective of its goals. Training individuals to achieve their felt needs to become better terrorists might be appropriate to certain revolutionary ideologies, but is certainly inconsistent with the aims of health promotion! As we will note later, freedom to choose applies only to those objectives that do not militate against the key values of health promotion.

Limits to freedom of choice

One of the avowed aims of an empowerment model of health promotion is to remove obstacles to rational decision making and freedom of choice. In some instances, overcoming such barriers is relatively simple – for example, the barrier created by ignorance. Others are more substantial – consider, for example, the case of addiction or other compulsive behaviours that sap freedom of choice. As McKeown pointed out:

> it is said that the individual must be free to choose [whether he wishes to smoke]. But he is not free; with a drug of addiction the option is open only at the beginning. (1979: 125)

Environmental barriers to voluntaristic action have received considerable recognition in recent years and, in part, have contributed to the formulation of the contemporary ideology of health promotion. Indeed, probably the greatest progress in health promotion in recent years has been acknowledgement of the fact that material, social and cultural environments can both damage health and limit people's capacity to take action to promote their own health and the health of their communities. It is quite apparent that various natural disasters, such as famine and war, may damage health both directly and indirectly by removing the possibility of making empowered health-related decisions. Climate change and environmental degradation also pose major challenges (WHO, 2007b) and their effects are likely to be experienced disproportionately by the most disadvantaged in society.

Poverty and social inequality damage individuals' and communities' capacity for action and are now recognized as being major determinants of public health. On a smaller scale, lack of access to affordable healthy food will largely nullify the effects of health education initiatives about the importance of a healthy diet. Less obviously, the complementary effects of culture and childrearing may effectively block choice and genuine decision making. For instance, in the process of socialization, cultural values may result in certain foods being classified as 'taboo', thus creating a moral imperative against consumption, regardless of the nutritional value of the food in question.

In the face of these many and varied psychological and environmental obstacles to the achievement of health, the emphasis on 'healthy public policy' is hardly surprising. Policy measures typically involve fiscal, economic and legislative measures and associated environmental change. On the one hand, they can create the conditions which support health and individual health choices. On the other hand, as is apparent from Figure 1.2, other more draconian measures that have been proposed can militate against freedom of choice. The Nuffield Council on Bioethics suggests that individual consent may not be required if measures are not 'very intrusive' or 'prevent significant harm to others'. Further, collective approval through democratic processes can replace individual consent when there is only limited interference with individuals' liberty (2007, paras 2.22–2.26). Although it is argued that healthy public policy makes the healthy choice the easy choice, it may effectively make the healthy choice the only choice! How can such attacks on freedom be reconciled with the discourse of voluntarism, which characterizes an 'educational model'?

The fact is, of course, that unbridled freedom is only the prerogative of the despot and, possibly to a lesser extent, of certain privileged groups. There are inevitably and appropriately limitations on freedom of choice. It could well be argued that 'true' education should encourage people to think in a systematic way about what is of most importance to them in their lives so that they might consistently act in accordance with the values they have clarified. It is also important that educated individuals should be helped to make decisions rather than uncritically absorb dogma. There are, however, obvious limitations to freedom of choice. As noted elsewhere (Tones, 1987), all values are not equally acceptable in a given society: antisocial behaviour would not normally be considered acceptable.

Health promotion would certainly not subscribe to unfettered freedom of choice. It is avowedly committed to certain major values to which most nations subscribe (or to which they at least pay lip-service) and which have been incorporated into the various doctrines and discourse propagated by WHO. This position is, or should be, non-negotiable. While cultural sensitivity is part of a concern for people in general, where cultural practices are inconsistent with the overriding values of health promotion, they must be challenged – take for example the issue of female genital mutilation. In the context of the principles of voluntarism, we must therefore observe two major qualifying principles. People should have a right to self-fulfilment, provided that this does not impede others' right to fulfilment and/or otherwise damage the wellbeing of the community at large. A good deal of consideration has, in fact, been given to the question of imposing limitations on liberty. The resulting ideological principles are most usefully expressed in terms of utilitarianism and paternalism. These principles provide support for the occasional overriding of personal liberty, either for the greater good or because some people seem incapable of exercising choice.

Utilitarianism, paternalism and the justification of coercion

There are two broad approaches to defining the ethics of interventions. One of these supports the principle that the integrity of a moral principle should be of prime consideration, whatever the consequences. For example, it is always wrong to deliberately provide inaccurate information, even if this might seem to be in the interests of the recipient of that information. The alternative view is that it is the results of actions that are most important (Guttman, 2000). This latter moral principle is generally described as utilitarianism.

There is an obvious and generally acceptable rationale underpinning actions based on the principle of utilitarianism. In short, people's freedom of action should be respected, so long as it does not interfere with the general good (for example, Mappes and Zembary, 1991). Indeed, it provides a simple baseline value for health education that legitimately espouses the imperative of self-actualization. However, personal gratification should not limit others' equal right to self-actualization.

It follows logically, therefore, that it is quite legitimate to use many of the varieties of coercion identified in Figure 1.2 where individuals' actions can be shown to damage others. The restriction on smoking in public places, for example, is therefore entirely justifiable in that smoking is not merely a public nuisance, but puts non-smokers at risk as a result of passive smoking.

Less clear-cut perhaps is the argument that seeks to restrain self-destructive behaviour on the grounds that the prudent in society should not have to pay for the excesses of the imprudent. More generally, economic arguments have indicated how self-inflicted illness damages the economy in terms of reduced productivity due to working days lost and increases the burden on already hard-pressed health services. Legislation can, therefore, be justified. For instance, in the UK, legislation enforcing seatbelt use and the wearing of protective headgear by motorcyclists has been in place for some time and is demonstrably effective. The situation regarding smoking is more equivocal. Certainly, many arguments have been used to demonstrate that smokers cover the cost of their morbidity and early mortality as a result of the finances levied by taxation and should actually be treated as social benefactors, just as the fictitious civil servant Sir Humphrey Appleby pointed out to the Prime Minister seeking to introduce legislation to ban all advertising of cigarettes in an episode of the television series *Yes, Prime Minister* (see box).

Lies, damned lies and statistics?

Prime Minister:

Cholera killed 30,000 people in 1837 and we had the Public Health Act. Smog killed 2500 in 1952 and we had the Clean Air Act. Certain drugs kill half a dozen people and they are withdrawn from sale. Cigarettes kill 100,000 people a year and what do we get?

Sir Humphrey:

Four billion pounds a year, 35,000 jobs in the tobacco industry, a flourishing cigarette export business helping our balance of trade, 250,000 jobs related to tobacco – newsagents, packing, transport ...

Prime Minister:

They're just guesses!

Sir Humphrey:

No, they're facts!

Prime Minister:

So your statistics are facts and my facts are statistics? ... Humphrey, we're talking about 100,000 deaths a year.

(Continued)

(Continued)

Sir Humphrey:

Yes, but cigarette taxes pay for one third of the cost of the National Health Service. We're saving many more lives than we otherwise could – because of those smokers who voluntarily lay down their lives for their friends ... they are national benefactors!

Yes, Prime Minister, 1990

The cost–benefit analysis of smoking is a matter for health economics and so will not be debated here. However, a serious point is frequently made that those indulging in high-risk activities should be allowed to do so, providing that this does not damage the wellbeing of others and that possible social and medical costs are covered by insurance. The financial argument would not, of course, apply to those who impose a financial burden on the state because of illness for which they cannot be blamed. Wikler, however, compares diabetics (who cannot be blamed for their illness) with smokers and suggests that the distinction is by no means clear-cut. Smokers could only be blamed for their condition if their actions were truly deliberate and voluntary.

> If the smoker's behaviour is less than voluntary, if it is the result of irresistible commercial or societal conditioning or of psychological need, then the smoker is, morally speaking, in the same position as the diabetic. His need becomes deserving, and the resulting burden is not especially unfair. (1978: 234)

The principle of utilitarianism, then, does not prove as unambiguous as it first appears. The question of limitations to free choice again proves problematic and leads us to consider the second principle, which may justify coercive methods. If people are not really responsible for their actions, then society must make decisions on their behalf, for their own good. These decisions will inevitably involve the restriction of liberties and involve some degree of coercion. This principle of paternalism (Nikku, 1997), though, proves even more difficult to justify than the appeal to utilitarianism. Beauchamp cites John Stuart Mill's (1961) treatise on liberty and his assertion that utilitarianism is the only justification for coercion:

> The only purpose for which power can be rightfully exercised over any member of a civilized community, against his will, is to prevent harm to others. His own good, either physical or moral is not a sufficient warrant. He cannot rightfully be compelled to do or forbear because it will be better for him to do so, because it will make him happier, because in the opinion of others, to do so would be wise, or even right. These are good reasons for remonstrating with him, or reasoning with him or persuading him or entreating him, but not for compelling him. (1978: 244)

However, as Daniels indicates:

> Even a view that holds the individual to be the best architect of his ends and judge of his interests rests on important assumptions about the information available to the

agent, the competency of the agent to make these decisions rationally, and the voluntariness of the decisions he makes. It is because these assumptions are not always met that we require a theory of justifiable paternalism. (1985: 157, in Guttman, 2000: 52)

Pollard and Brennan (1978), in discussing the basis for governmental intervention in cases of self-regarding behaviour – that is, behaviour affecting only the individual but not others – cite Dworkin's justification of paternalistic behaviour on the grounds that some adults may not be capable of rational thought because 'at some point in the future the individual will see the wisdom of the paternalistic intervention, even though at present he or she is not aware of its value' (1972: 71).

The intervention thus, in some way, protects the 'real' will of the individual. At first glance, such a proposition looks distinctly dubious. However, it is undoubtedly true that most societies routinely take responsibility for certain categories of individual. For instance, the very young, the insane and those having a substantial degree of mental impairment would routinely be protected in many societies. Again, the notion of protecting someone's real will is not as Machiavellian as it might appear. For instance, it would seem fairly clear that a substantial majority of smokers would prefer not to smoke and it is appropriate to recall McKeown's observation that 'the critical decision to smoke is taken not by consenting adults but by children below the age of consent' (1979: 125). Paternalistic intervention to limit people's freedom to choose to smoke might make some sense ethically. Furthermore, even if suicide were legal, a depressed person might be legitimately prevented from taking his or her life on the reasonable supposition that, when no longer depressed, (s)he would not wish to do so.

Wikler poses the question, 'Is there, then, a case for paternalist coercion for health?' and answers it as follows:

It depends on whether the behaviour slated for change is involuntary or not, whether there exists a practical, non-intrusive way to find out if it is voluntary or not, whether actual policies and programmes can be made subtle enough to distinguish in practice between voluntary and involuntary behaviour; and whether pressure can be applied to specific behaviours without the need to take on whole cultures. It also depends on whether those making and executing policy in this area can distinguish between involuntary actions and actions which are merely different from their own; whether they can restrain themselves from enforcing their views in subjects on which they are not expert; whether the coercive methods they use inflict greater intrusions and privations than the behaviours they attempt to eradicate; and whether allowing health professionals to exercise paternalistic power within these strict limits will lead inexorably to abuses and unjustified restrictions on liberty. These questions are empirical, not philosophical, and those who would want to justify coercive lifestyle reform programmes on paternalist grounds would do well to engage in the research needed for answers. (1978: 232)

Beauchamp (1978) critically appraises the argument advanced by his namesake Dan Beauchamp (1976) that the state should adopt a paternalistic stance, then rejects it! The notion, however, merits some further consideration. It relates to the general concept of 'distributive justice'. Distributive justice is about the ways in which both social goods and burdens are distributed – for example, healthcare and the taxation needed to pay for it. Dan Beauchamp advocates social justice, asserting that all people have an *entitlement* to health protection and minimum standards of income – a position equivalent to WHO's association of health with human rights. It is worth noting at this point the view expressed in the World Health Report that it is 'not sufficient to protect or improve the average health of the population, if – at the same time – inequality worsens or remains high because the gain accrues disproportionately to those already enjoying better health' (2000c: 26).

The question of choice versus coercion in the interest of public health is very real. On the one hand, the principle of voluntarism urges freedom of choice unless good reason can be provided for coercive measures on the basis of utilitarianism, paternalism or 'social justice'. On the other hand, it seems particularly difficult to reach consensus about when, where and to what extent these principles can be used to justify coercive interventions in the interest of public health. Those of a left-wing orientation might object to any infringement of liberty of disadvantaged people, but wholeheartedly support paternalistic (or should it be 'maternalistic'?) measures by the nanny state on the grounds of social justice and equity. Equally, the more tough-minded advocates of market forces would object vocally to interventions that restricted their own freedom of action, but might well subscribe to utilitarian restriction of the liberty of people of a different political persuasion! Public attitudes about individual versus government responsibility were explored by the Kings Fund (see box).

Public attitudes to public health policy: individual responsibility and control

- Most of the people surveyed (89%) agree with the statement that individuals are responsible for their own health and 93% agree that parents have greater responsibility for their children's health than anyone else. However, more than 60% think tackling poverty would be the most effective way of preventing illness.
- More than 40% agree with the statement that there are too many factors outside individual control to hold people responsible for their own health.
- A higher proportion of those in socio-economic group DE feel that health is beyond individual control than those in socio-economic group AB and that tackling poverty is the best way of preventing illness.

A large majority of those surveyed say the Government should intervene to prevent illness by:

- providing information and advice (86%);
- encouraging employers to promote health at work (82%);
- preventing actions that put others' health at risk (77%); and
- actively discouraging people from putting their own health at risk (75%).

Kings Fund, 2004: 2

The stewardship model described in the box on p. 22 provides a framework for considering the balance between individual freedom and state responsibility in relation to public health. We may be able move some way towards resolving the dilemma by promoting self-empowerment. However, we should take account of Beauchamp's noteworthy observation that 'Public health should – at least ideally – be suspicious of behavioural paradigms for viewing public health problems since they tend to "blame the victim" and unfairly protect majorities and powerful interests from the burdens of prevention' (Beauchamp, 1976, reprinted in Beachamp and Steinbock, 1999: 106). Accordingly, our later analysis and discussion of empowerment will emphasize the importance of *community* participation and *community* empowerment.

Health promotion and the discourse of empowerment

The assertion that health promotion's main concern should be that of empowerment is becoming increasingly acceptable, although this acceptance often takes the form of lip service rather than practice and policy! Certainly, as noted above, most of the key documents published by WHO since the inception of 'Health for All by the Year 2000' have placed emphasis on individuals gaining control over their lives and their health and on the importance of active participating communities. In his Harveian Oration, Marmot (2006: 2081–2) recognized the central importance of the social environment and empowerment asserting that: 'Failing to meet the fundamental human needs of autonomy, empowerment and human freedom is a potent cause of ill health.'

It is axiomatic from our earlier discussion that empowerment is based on the principles of voluntarism. The key issue for health promotion is how people who lack power can become more powerful and actually gain a reasonable degree of control over their lives. How can they compete with, and resist coercion by, those who already have power?

Further reflections on power

Empowerment, by definition, has to do with people acquiring a degree of power and control. Self-empowerment describes the extent to which individuals have power and control over their interactions with their physical and social environment. Further, an empowered community is an identifiable group of people which also possesses power and control. It is a matter of some importance to understand the different circumstances under which people acquire power, wield it and yield to it.

Definitions of power and related concepts

The notion of power may manifest itself at macro, meso and micro levels. All three levels have some degree of relevance for health promotion. Studies of power at the micro level are concerned with influences on, and exerted by, individuals or small groups; meso-level power might refer to the power exerted by organizations or communities; the influence of national policy would be a macro-level influence – as would the kinds of ideological controls discussed above.

The classic Weberian analysis identifies three forms of power:

- **social power** based on such factors as prestige, family status, lifestyle and patterns of consumption
- **economic power** based on a group's relationship to the mode of production, its position in the labour market and general life chances
- **political power** based on affiliation to parties, bureaucracy and legal structure.

Naturally, there are a number of different ideas associated with power. For instance, concepts such as 'control', 'authority' and 'influence' may be used almost interchangeably with power. Corwin (1978), for instance, defines 'authority' as legitimized institutionalized power (and uses the term 'coercion' to refer to the illegitimate use of power). He posits a continuum of control ranging from a situation in which there is a capacity for applying a high level of sanction through to an opposite in which control is limited to minimal sanction capability delivered in relatively informal circumstances. Corwin employs the term 'influence' to describe this latter circumstance. He also identifies a further kind of authority, which he calls 'consensual authority', which is when power and control depend on the outcome of negotiation based on the differential possession of resources. Corwin also refers to the notion of 'social power':

> Social power is the probability that a person or group can realize its will against opposition. Since power pervades most social relationships, it can be observed when armies fight, corporations bribe politicians, employers direct their employees, a political candidate sways voters, teachers evaluate their students, prison guards shoot rebellious prisoners, parents set examples for their children, and unions negotiate with management. (1978: 65)

Bachrach and Baratz (1970) acknowledge the variations in the nomenclature and meaning of these various terms and offer a useful typology of influence (see box).

A typology of influence

Force	The individual or group is obliged to comply by removing all choice.
Coercion	Compliance is achieved by the threat of deprivation where conflict exists regarding values or courses of action.
Manipulation	This is a 'subconcept' of force. Compliance results in the absence of recognition by those who comply or the source of nature of the demand made.
Influence	This term is used when an individual or organization succeeds in causing others to change their intended actions, but without overt or tacit threat of deprivation.
Authority	This form of power operates when people comply because they accept that commands are reasonable in terms of their own values or because an appropriate and acceptable procedure has been adopted.

Bachrach and Baratz, 1970: 28

Lukes (1974) reminds us that dominant groups shape people's needs and wants – by means of mass media, 'indoctrination' at school or, more powerfully, by socialization. Lukes' analysis is clearly consistent with our earlier discussion of the often subtle means whereby dominant ideologies are perpetuated, including the creation of false consciousness. These observations are not only relevant to our discussion of ideologies in general, but, as we noted earlier in this chapter, more particularly to questions of utilitarianism and paternalism. They also have an important bearing on our later examination of the assessment of health needs. Moreover, these two notions underpin thinking about empowerment, bearing in mind Kindervatter's definition of empowerment as: 'People gaining an understanding of and control over social, economic and/or political forces in order to improve their standing in society' (1979: 62). A clear understanding of the different constructions of power also has special significance in, for example, determining the success or failure of lobbying and advocacy for the implementation of healthy public policy at macro and meso levels.

Notwithstanding the relevance of these macro- and meso-level influences on the development of healthy public policy, at this juncture we will focus on the individualistic perspective and the micro-level exercise of power. After all, continuing pressure is placed on individuals from a variety of sources, both explicitly and implicitly, to modify their behaviours in ways which may – or equally may not – be healthy.

Five varieties of power: an individual perspective

One of the classic, and still valid, analyses of power at the micro level was provided by French and Raven (1959), who distinguished five varieties of power. This scheme (which has similarities to Weber's analysis of charismatic, traditional and rational–legal power) is frequently used to illuminate interactions when analysing small group dynamics and discussing leadership functions. Their analysis comprises the following five varieties of power.

- **Legitimate power**: authority is derived from legitimate status formally bestowed by a given social system.
- **Expert power**: authority derives from the actual and perceived expertise of the individual in question. It may or may not be associated with legitimate authority or be an informal adjunct of referent power (see below).
- **Reward power**: authority derives from the individual's capacity for providing rewards.
- **Coercive power**: authority derives from the individual's capacity to sanction.
- **Referent power**: authority derives from the referent's individual characteristics, which, for some reason, are valued by the person who is influenced.

Stardom and charisma

Alberoni (1962, in McQuail, 1972) also discusses the characteristics of individuals who, despite lacking legitimate authority, nonetheless can exert quite a powerful influence over other people. He describes this 'powerless "élite"' as 'stars'. Their 'institutional power is very limited or nonexistent, but [their] doings and way of life arouse a considerable and sometimes even a maximum degree of interest'. He likens their personal characteristics to Weber's notion of charisma:

By charisma we mean a quality regarded as extraordinary and attributed to a person ... The latter is believed to be endowed with powers and properties which are super-natural and superhuman, or at least exceptional even where accessible to others; or again as sent by God, or as if adorned with exemplary value and thus worthy to be a leader. (Weber, 1968: 241)

It is sometimes said, with a degree of acrimony, that many celebrities in contemporary society are 'famous for being famous'! It is certainly the case that these charismatic characters may well exert a quite dramatic degree of influence on people. They may influence taste and preferences and act as models. This phenomenon will be revisited in Chapter 7 when we consider the influence of source credibility and attractiveness in persuading individuals to adopt healthy or unhealthy courses of action.

The concept of referent power also merits some further comment. The individual's influence is bestowed on him or her by 'followers' on account of that person's perceived expertise or reward value. The concept has some points in common with the notion of charismatic leadership. It also relates to opinion leadership and the principle of 'homophily', both of which feature in the communication of innovations theory, which will be considered in Chapter 3.

French and Raven's conceptual scheme provides a bridge between the broader sociological perspective on power and the meso- and micro-level perspectives of social psychology and attitude change theory. It is, for example, consistent with the 'Yale Hovland' approach that guided research into the relative effects of source, message, audience and channel on the recipients of persuasive communications (Hovland et al., 1953). In short, the source of a communication may play a significant part in determining the beliefs, attitudes and even behaviour of its recipients. Of more direct relevance to the study of empowerment are those investigations that have examined the effect of message source on an individual's compliance and conformity. Perhaps the best known – and most alarming – of such studies is the work of Milgram, who demonstrated that, under the influence of an authority figure, 65 per cent of a group of 'ordinary' people were prepared to administer a 450-volt electric shock to an experimental subject. Many of them did this even while experiencing obvious concern and conflict (Milgram, 1963). As Higbee and Jensen point out:

people find it extremely difficult to refuse any request by an experimenter. In experimental settings people have tried to balance a marble on a steel ball and eat a large number of dry soda crackers, dump out cans of garbage and sort it into piles of similar material, add adjacent numbers on sheets containing random digits, tearing up each sheet after completing it, and continuing for five and a half hours until the experimenter gives up, and pick up a poisonous snake, put their hands into nitric acid, and throw acid into an assistant's face (the people thought they were doing these things). (1978: 27)

We might legitimately conclude that empowered individuals would be more able and willing to resist pressure and not submit to unreasonable demands, particularly those that run counter to their existing values.

While analyses such as French and Raven's are undoubtedly useful in designing health promotion programmes, it is essential to ask how someone comes to wield legitimate authority, how they are in a position to reward, how they acquire the power to coerce, how they acquire expert authority or come to be treated as referents by their communities. As we noted earlier, power does not rely only on the crude application of force and coercion, but can also be exerted by the ideological control of culture and the hegemony of political and state institutions.

Self-empowerment, community empowerment and reciprocal determinism

Earlier in this chapter, we emphasized the dramatic effects an oppressive environment can have on individuals' health and their capacity to make choices. It is therefore self-evident that empowerment – people's opportunities to make genuinely free choices – is not possible unless physical, socio-economic and cultural circumstances are favourable. Thus, it is imperative that empowerment policy and the ensuing strategies must engage with the thorny question of environmental change. On the other hand, it is clear that individuals are, in many situations, capable in principle of making choices even when the environment is not especially conducive to individual action. Three different perspectives on human agency can be identified (see Figure 1.3).

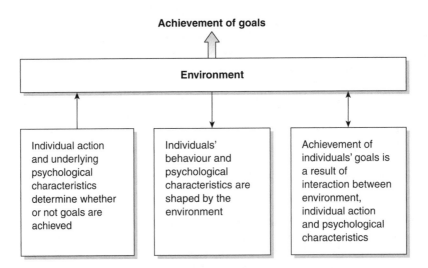

Figure 1.3   Three perspectives on human agency

In the first situation, the focus of attention is centred on individuals and those characteristics that explain their behaviour. The theorist may be interested only in psychological phenomena or even be effectively blind to the existence of the environment. Some forms of counselling may be characterized by this approach. In the second instance, individuals are viewed as being largely controlled by their circumstances – directly or indirectly.

The third formulation of human agency asserts that humans (and animals) interact with their environments. They are, on the one hand, affected by environmental forces but, on the other, typically capable of having at least some impact on the various physical, socio-economic and cultural factors that influence them. The ideology and practice of empowerment ultimately derives from this last standpoint and has been a central feature of social learning theory. Its major exponent and advocate is Bandura (1986) who described the interactive process as 'reciprocal determinism' and contrasted it with the Skinnerian assertion that 'A person does not act upon the world, the world acts upon him' (Skinner, 1971: 211). Bandura argues that a process of 'triadic reciprocality' operates when humans engage with life. In short, there is an often complicated system of interaction between psychological factors (such as beliefs and attitudes), behaviour and the environment. A more comprehensive account of this system is given, and discussed, in Chapter 3.

We should also note that this archetypal psychological analysis of human agency is by no means inconsistent with the broader perspectives of sociology. For instance, Giddens (1991: 204) observes that 'actors are at the same time creators of social systems yet created by them'.

Individual and community dimensions of empowerment

The logic of reciprocal determinism for an empowerment model of health promotion is inescapable. If empowerment is about facilitating voluntaristic decision making and achieving free choices (or those that are consistent with moral imperatives), then it must operate at both the level of the environment and at the level of the individual. Furthermore, it is important to recognize that the environment itself has many levels – from macro to meso, from the level of national policy to the level of regional organizations and institutions, down to the level of the neighbourhood or village. At each level, individuals exist within a web of social systems. At the neighbourhood level, the community is a social system which has particular significance for health promotion. Figure 1.4 gives an indication of this complexity within the context of commenting on both individual and community empowerment.

As may be seen from Figure 1.4, the community may mediate individual agency in relation to the general physical, socio-economic and cultural environment. The community is an especially important social system within the lexicon of empowerment and health promotion. Following the doctrine of the Ottawa Charter, an active, empowered community is perhaps seen as the most important of the desirable empowerment outcomes of health promotion activities. In short, it enables people to take an active part in influencing policy. Three key features of an empowered community are also shown, namely: a sense of community – that is, a therapeutic feeling of identification with fellow community members; an active commitment to achieve community goals; and what is increasingly termed 'social capital' (see Chapter 2 for more about this).

Individual or self-empowerment, on the other hand, comprises a cluster of attributes related to a personal capacity for voluntaristic action.

Self-empowerment is a state in which an individual possesses a relatively high degree of actual power — that is, a *genuine* potential for making choices. Self-empowerment

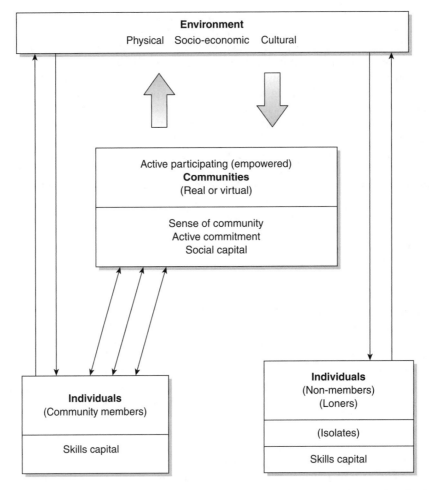

Figure 1.4 Reciprocal determinism and empowerment of communities and individuals

is associated with a number of beliefs about causality and the nature of control that are health promoting. It is also associated with a relatively high level of realistically based self-esteem together with a repertoire of *life skills* that contribute to the exercise of power over the individual's life and health. (Tones and Tilford, 2001: 40)

Clearly, a community is composed of its membership – and it is arguable whether or not a community is more than the sum of the individuals making up this membership. In all events, a community is generally considered to be beneficial for its individual members, and the characteristics and capabilities of these individuals will contribute to the power of the community as a whole.

Figure 1.4 makes a distinction between 'real' and 'virtual' communities. The former represents a traditional idea of community as a group of people within a relatively small geographical area having a sense of identity and a network of relationships.

A virtual community may lack the narrow geographical dimension of a real one, but otherwise has a shared identity. For instance, we can realistically talk about the gay community. What may be lacking, however, are interpersonal relationships. On the other hand, a virtual community may actually have more power at its disposal than a real community and, moreover, with the advent of technology such as the Internet, may benefit from different kinds of interaction.

Although often ignored in discussions of communities, Figure 1.4 reminds us that some individuals may not be part of any community – real or virtual. We have labelled as 'non-members' individuals who exist in relative isolation because no community exists. By contrast, and borrowing terminology from the domain of sociometry, we have used the term 'loner' to distinguish people who do not wish to belong to a community from those whose felt need is to belong, but who are not accepted or rejected – so-called isolates. Figure 1.4 also notes that individuals are affected by, and in turn affect, their environments at different levels without the mediation of community groups.

We might also note that environments do not exert their effects in a unidimensional way. It is more realistic to consider any given environment as exerting both facilitative and inhibitory influences of different strengths on communities and individuals. The sum total of both positive and negative pressures might be described in terms of these macro or meso influences 'making the healthy choice the easy choice' or, alternatively, being fundamentally oppressive. The specific, technical, detailed aspects of both community and individual empowerment will be explored at some length in Chapter 3.

One of the factors most closely associated with empowerment – with respect to both ideological and technical aspects – is that of participation. WHO has frequently commented on the importance of an active, participating community and the desirability of individual involvement in decision making is virtually taken for granted as a healthy development. We will also note in Chapter 5 the centrality of participation to the needs assessment process. How does participation actually contribute to empowerment? It is almost a matter of common sense! A community that takes action – that is, participates in action to influence policy or practice at local or national level – feels that it has actually achieved something, even if the outcome is not dramatic. Similarly, individuals who are actively involved are likely to experience at least some degree of control. Obviously, there are many different degrees of involvement and Figure 1.5 indicates an assumed relationship between degrees of participation/involvement and empowerment. It draws on the classic analyses of Arnstein (1971) and Brager and Specht (1973).

It should be noted that Figure 1.5 applies equally not only to communities but also settings such as health-promoting hospitals and health-promoting schools and, at the micro level, interactions between individuals, such as doctor and patient.

An empowerment model of health promotion

We have considered the medical discourse associated with public health and a preventive model of health promotion or, rather, health education. We have also explored ideas related to the discourse of voluntarism, which might be said to give rise to an educational model of health promotion. Both of these models are limited in that they are inconsistent with the ideological thrust of health promotion. They are also technically

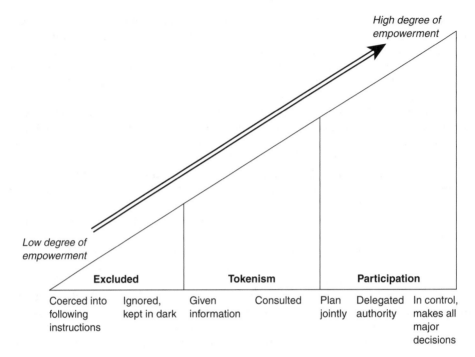

Figure 1.5 Participation and the empowerment gradient

limited in their capacity to explain what would be involved in achieving the empowerment goals of health promotion. Figure 1.6 sets out the main components of an empowerment model of health promotion and their interrelationships.

The central dynamic of the empowerment model is the interplay of education and healthy public policy. The development and implementation of policy is the essential precursor to the creation of health-promoting environmental influences. The relationship is multiplicative, as we noted earlier in the 'formula' health promotion = health education × healthy public policy. The empowering function of education not only strengthens individual capabilities for health-related action, but also makes a major contribution to the establishment of healthy public policy.

Action to achieve healthy public policy

We discussed the five action areas of the Ottawa Charter earlier in this chapter, including the imperative to reorientate health services. Accordingly, Figure 1.6 shows how policy initiatives are necessary to improve service provision to meet the health needs of particular populations. More importantly, it identifies the importance of policy initiatives to address physical, socio-economic and cultural circumstances. The focus is more on reframing than reorientation. In tune with modern multidisciplinary public health, it recognizes the contribution to health of a range of services whose primary *raison d'être* may not be health in any formal sense, for example transport, housing, economic development. However, all of these have a major impact on health and, indeed, on disease.

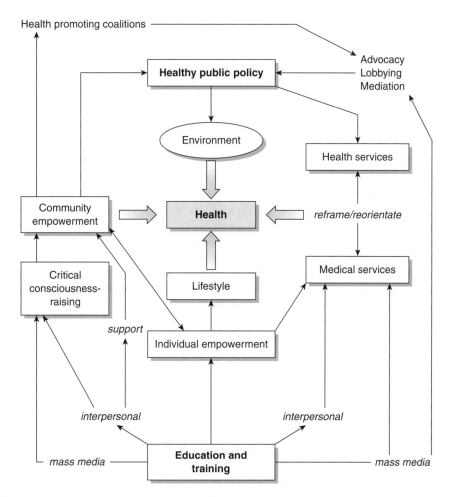

Figure 1.6   An empowerment model of health promotion

Two major action strategies are included in the model. One is the traditional means of seeking to influence policy, such as lobbying. Advocacy is defined here as lobbying of those who exercise power by those who have power but who are doing so on behalf of the relatively powerless. The term 'mediation', which was incorporated within the Ottawa Charter list of major actions, refers to the process of mediating between competing interests. By way of illustration, we might consider the different concerns of the owners and producers of mass media programmes and health professionals. The main goal of the former is to entertain the public and advertise products in order to make profits. The interests of the health promoters, on the other hand, are to control advertising and any representation of health issues in ways that are considered to be damaging to the public health.

The second – ultimately the most powerful – means of producing policy change is to create a sufficient level of public pressure so that decision makers and politicians at national or local level feel obliged to change. Within a democracy, this might, in the last analysis, result in change by means of the ballot box.

The catalyst for change is health education, but emphatically not the variety of health education that has been tarred with the brush of victim blaming! Rather, following the precepts of critical theory, it might usefully be called 'critical health education' and its purpose is radical and political. Again, the nature of education and its technology will be reviewed in Chapters 7 and 8 and particular attention will be devoted to its radical and critical manifestations.

Health education and individual empowerment

Figure 1.6 includes an analysis of the essential contribution made by education to individual action. A training function has also been included in the model to demonstrate the continuing importance of providing skills – not only to communities, but also to the professionals who work in the various services to which reference was made above. This training would include awareness-raising of the health-promoting role of the organizations, as well as making available the competences needed to communicate with clients and the general public, providing appropriate education and analysing the impact of policy on health – and making appropriate adjustments in the interest of effectiveness and efficiency.

We earlier reviewed the traditional health education function. We noted that its purpose was to persuade individuals to adopt behaviours that would result in the prevention of disease, both with regard to lifestyle and making proper use of medical services. The role of critical health education is not primarily that of persuasion (which is both ethically dubious and of limited effectiveness), but one of empowerment and support. Empowered individuals are more likely to make an effective contribution to community action, which, in turn, contributes to their empowerment, as we mentioned earlier. They are also more likely to engage with the various services contributing to health in an assertive and productive fashion. They are almost certainly more likely to adopt a lifestyle conducive to achieving the objectives of preventive medicine than if they were not empowered! Indeed, one of our more forceful assertions here is that the successful adoption of an empowerment model of health promotion is not only more likely to achieve positive health outcomes in an ethical fashion, but also to be more efficient in attaining the important outcomes associated with the prevention and management of disease and disability.

The empowerment model: critiques and reservations

The empowerment model of health promotion is not without its critics. For instance, some might reasonably argue that empowerment is a fashionable term distinguished by its lack of clarity in conceptualization and use (the same criticism could, of course, be levelled at health promotion itself and even the notion of public health). A second objection derives from the assertion that empowerment lacks a theoretical base. This assertion is fundamentally incorrect, as we are in the process of demonstrating!

What is undoubtedly more problematic is translating the rhetoric into action. For instance, Mayo and Craig (1995: 2) cite the Bruntland Commission's conviction that the prerequisite for sustainable development is securing the effective participation of citizens, the World Bank's inclusion of empowerment as a main objective of community participation and the Human Development report definition of participation in terms of people having constant 'access to decision-making and power'. They also remind us that functionalist sociologists such as Parsons (1967) considered that power in society was a 'variable sum' and thus 'the powerless could be empowered, and could then share in the fruits of development, alongside those who had already achieved power'. Mayo and Craig argue that an alternative, and perhaps more convincing, viewpoint is that power is a 'zero sum'. Accordingly, the powerful will be reluctant to yield their power in the interest of empowering the powerless and will utilize the various ideological devices discussed earlier to keep the powerless in their place!

Croft and Beresford observe that participation is at the heart of social policy and political debate, but 'generates enthusiasm and hostility in equal proportion' (1992: 20) and is frequently handled in both a 'superficial' and 'depoliticized' way. It needs very careful scrutiny. Grace (1991) considered that empowerment in general has 'major problematic contradictions and inconsistencies' and, critically reviewing the discourse of empowerment, argued that it was not dissimilar to the discourse of marketing! De Kadt adopted a similarly sceptical note when he contrasted WHO's rhetoric about participation with the reality at grass-roots level. He referred to Werner's review of 40 rural health programmes in Latin America, which concluded that genuine community participation was a rare event. On the other hand, there were many examples of 'handouts, paternalism and superimposed, initiative destroying norms' (Werner, 1980: 94 cited by De Kadt, 1982b).

The superficial concern demonstrated by oligarchy is, of course, well recognized in the failure of 'trickle-down' theories of wealth creation. It is also apparent in the neoliberal, New Right attack on welfare and the nanny state, with its emphasis on the efficiency of the private market and the illusory freedom of the individual from the state that such measures allegedly create. A lack of true empowerment can also characterize the self-help movement, despite its several benefits. Although self-help initiatives may well be empowering in their contribution to demedicalization, they may also minimize the need to look for radical solutions to health problems by reducing state expenditure.

It should hopefully be clear from the observations made in this chapter that power and politics are central to health promotion. It would be a mistake to underestimate the difficulties of challenging power structures. Nonetheless, we believe that sophisticated analysis grounded in sound theory can result in the development of empowering strategies that can achieve results. The empowerment model of health promotion is advocated here on grounds of both ideological soundness and practical effectiveness. Moreover, it stands up well to ethical scrutiny.

PUBLIC HEALTH, HEALTH PROMOTION AND HEALTH EDUCATION

Health promotion and modern multidisciplinary public health

We have considered at some length the ideology of health promotion and have argued in favour of an empowerment model which recognizes the primacy of the broader social, cultural, economic and environmental determinants of health. To conclude this chapter, we will briefly examine the relationship between health promotion and modern multidisciplinary public health and the position of health promotion as a profession. We will also consider the future role of health education.

For some, there is no distinction between health promotion and public health. Kickbush (2007) reminds us of the subtitle to the Ottawa Charter for Health Promotion – *the move towards a new public health.* Indeed, the Ottawa Charter has been hailed as heralding the third public health revolution. Potvin and McQueen (2007) have characterized revolutionary change as affecting three fundamental dimensions of systems:

- the direction or finality of the system – the target, objectives and goals
- knowledge base – including the conditions that support the production of knowledge as well as substantive knowledge itself
- actions – including design, implementation and evaluation.

Terris (1983) identified the first public health revolution as concerned with tackling communicable disease and the second with noncommunicable disease. Breslow (1999, 2004, 2006) puts the case that the emphasis on health as a resource for living constitutes the third revolution.

However, for some authors, health promotion and public health are not synonymous, although related. Raeburn and MacFarlane refer to some governments seeing public health as health protection plus health promotion, where health protection comprises 'the more regulatory, centralized and reactive aspects of public health' (2003: 245) and health promotion is more self-determined, community based and developmental. In this interpretation, public health is the umbrella term and health promotion a defined sphere of activity within it.

The Bangkok Charter refers to health promotion as a 'core function of public health' (WHO, 2005). Potvin and McQueen see health promotion as 'a strategy for public health that reflects modernity' (2007: 14). They note that subsequent to its emergence in the 1970s and more formal adoption in the 1980s, health promotion rapidly spread through public health organizations and institutions internationally. However, latterly, while the principles and strategies remain relevant, the term health promotion appears to be becoming 'outmoded' in some parts of the world. There were certainly signs of this happening in the UK in the early 'noughties' when policy documents tended to refer to modern multidisciplinary public health rather than health promotion.

Potvin and McQueen argue that while some countries may have a cadre of health promotion professionals, health promotion activity involves a wide range of groups, including lay people, and that health promotion is 'not a discipline, nor an institution, nor a profession' (2007: 16). They see health promotion as embracing a 'structured discourse and a set of practices' and identify its two characteristic features as 'a distinctive perspective on health; and a critical orientation towards action' (2007: 16).

However, our position, set out earlier in this chapter, is that health promotion is a discipline with its own ideology and we will at later points in this book identify the theories, perspective and methods that characterize it as an 'ordered field of study'. A study of the views of key informants in the UK by Tilford et al. (2003) found that they associated health promotion with a clear set of values as well as a set of activities. These included instrumental values associated with ways of working as well as terminal values, notably a holistic conceptualization of health, equity, empowerment, autonomy/self-determination and justice/fairness. While there was felt to be some degree of consensus between the values of public health and health promotion, there was a much stronger emphasis for health promotion on empowerment and autonomy with the associated instrumental values of involvement and participation. Prevention and protection featured more prominently in relation to public health along with a clear population focus and greater attention to 'ends'. In contrast, health promotion was more concerned about means and had a broader focus which included individuals as well as communities. Tilford et al. conclude that within the context of the move to multidisciplinary public health, health promotion makes a distinctive contribution through its core values (see box). By virtue of its more radical orientation, health promotion has in the past been described as the militant wing of public health. The emphasis on attention to process might also lead to it being seen as the critical conscience of public health.

Values at work

Values influence the ways that health issues are understood, the ways that knowledge and theoretical bases are developed and the nature of strategies identified for health improvement. Values also influence the selection of activities that are undertaken to promote health and the priorities accorded to actions, the balance between activities at individual and population levels, the relationships with individuals and communities who participate in initiatives, the goals which are being sought, and decisions about means and ends in achieving goals.

Tilford et al., 2003: 120

As we noted above, the early emergence of health promotion was characterized by a struggle to distance itself from public health, held to be associated with the preventive medical model of health. Furthermore, it also sought a separate identity from health education – viewed as the 'handmaiden of public health' and tainted by association with approaches deemed to be victim-blaming in orientation. The move towards the 'New Public Health', which subscribed to a social model of health, brought about greater alignment with health promotion. Most of those who claim to be 'health promoters' would see commonalities with the broad statement of purpose used for public health:

- to improve health and wellbeing in the population
- to prevent disease and minimize its consequences
- to prolong valued life
- to reduce inequalities in health. (Skills for Health and Public Health Resource Unit, 2009)

Within the UK, the origins of modern multidisciplinary public health can be traced back to the Acheson Report (Department of Health, 1988) which defined public health as: '… the science and art of preventing disease, prolonging life and promoting health through the organized efforts of society.' The report also recognized that public health:

> ... works through partnerships that cut across disciplinary, professional and organizational boundaries and exploits this diversity in collaboration, to bring evidence and research based policies to *all areas* which impact on the health and well being of populations.

Clearly, health promotion is an integral part of this wider view of public health, but what is the effect of assimilation under the multidisciplinary public health umbrella on the professional identity of those engaged in health promotion? A brief summary of recent developments in the UK with particular reference to England and Wales provides a useful example. The inclusive view of public health referred to above was reflected in the English CMO's Project to Strengthen the Public Health Function (Department of Health, 2001a) which identified three main groups of workers.

1 **Wider public health workforce**: those who make a positive contribution to public health through their work although their primary role may not necessarily be public health, for example teachers, social workers (see box also);
2 **Public health practitioners**: those who spend a major part of their time involved in public health practice, for example health visitors, environmental health officers;
3 **Public health specialists**: those who work at a strategic or senior level.

The breadth of the public health workforce

The introduction of personal travel advisers in England as part of the Government's Sustainable Transport Strategy announced in 2007 was intended to reduce traffic congestion. Notwithstanding their primary aim, they will also have an incidental influence on health through their impact on physical activity, reduction in traffic volume and associated noise and stress, and potentially on rates of injury and lower pollution levels.

Towards a competent health promotion workforce

Where does health promotion feature in this? Should health promotion have a separate identity and should there be distinct career pathways for those engaged in health promotion? Towards the end of the old millennium, the term health promotion started to be used less frequently in both policy documents and job titles, despite the fact that the sphere of activity which had hitherto been described as health promotion was receiving more attention. Scott-Samuel and Springett (2007: 212) refer to this as the 'semantic eclipse of health promotion'. Further, health promotion courses began to disappear from universities' portfolios of provision to be replaced by a variety of titles including Public Health and Public Health Promotion (Scriven, 2007). In many instances, this was merely a re-badging exercise rather than a significant change in content, but still generated concerns about the future of health promotion as a discipline and a profession. A review of specialist health promotion practice in England and Wales conducted by Griffiths and Dark concluded that 'Specialised health promotion is a discipline integral to public health' but 'has been eroded in recent years' (2005: 6). They recommended that the specialist health promotion workforce requires recognition and advocacy along with systematic skills and competency development. A collaborative programme, 'Shaping the Future of Health Promotion', was set up in 2006 to implement these recommendations and:

- achieve recognition and identity for specialized health promotion
- develop an agreed career pathway for specialized health promotion staff.

Specification of core competencies and systems for professional registration can serve to define areas of professional practice and ensure standards. The UK Voluntary Register of Public Health introduced in 2003 set up a system of registration for public health specialists. Since 2006, a defined specialist arm has provided opportunity for health promotion specialists to register. While creating some opportunity for registration, it is important to note that the criteria for this have been shaped by the discourse of public health rather than health promotion. A public health skills and career framework has also been developed in the UK (Skills for Health and Public Health Resource Unit, 2009) to include the whole of the public health workforce, from initial entry through to the most senior levels. The framework identifies a number of core competencies operationalized for each level as well as five defined areas of competence (see box). The use of the term 'health improvement' rather than 'health promotion' is noteworthy.

Public health skills and career framework

Core areas

1 Surveillance and assessment of the population's health and wellbeing
2 Assessing the evidence of effectiveness of interventions, programmes and services to improve population health and wellbeing
3 Policy and strategy development and implementation for population health and wellbeing
4 Leadership and collaborative working for population health and wellbeing.

Non-core (defined) areas

5 Health improvement
6 Health protection
7 Public health intelligence
8 Academic public health
9 Health and social care quality.

Skills for Health and Public Health Resource Unit, 2009

There is some debate about the use of a competency based system. Naidoo and Wills (2005), for example, have argued that the narrow mechanistic focus of competencies is not an adequate basis for assessing professional practice because it overlooks not only the theoretical base but, importantly, the values which underpin critical reflective practice.

There are also dissenting views about maintaining a separate identity for health promotion. Ashton, for example, is concerned that it is inconsistent with 'an inclusive, holistic and integrated approach to public health practice' and risks 'health promotion apartheid' (2007: 207). The alternative position is that 'health promotion has been the subject of hegemonic absorption by an increasingly individualistic public health discourse' (Scott-Samuel and Springett, 2007: 211). The consequence of not acknowledging the distinctive contribution of health promotion will be failure to nurture – and risk losing – the specific set of skills and values which it brings to modern multidisciplinary public health. It will also result in suppression of what has long been regarded as the more radical and militant wing of public health. Responding to contemporary challenges to health, both nationally and internationally, has never before put so much emphasis on the importance of health promotion. For many, it is seen as an idea whose time has come (Scriven, 2007). Rising to this challenge requires recognition of the distinctive contribution of health promotion; the development of proper career pathways; and support for the professional development of a specialist cadre of health promotion staff – i.e. those who see their role as entirely concerned with health promotion.

A statement on priorities for action issued by the International Union for Health Promotion and Education (IUHPE) and the Canadian Consortium for Health Promotion Research (see box) identified a specialist health promotion role as well as the need for a multisectoral response. It emphasized the importance of building a competent health promotion workforce. A number of countries have developed their own competency standards (see, for example, the account by Shilton et al. (2008) of updating the Australian competencies). However, the IUHPE has proposed transnational agreements on core competencies 'to further define the field and provide common direction for curriculum development' (2007: 5). The Galway Consensus Conference (SOPHE, 2008) aimed to encourage 'global exchange and understanding concerning domains of core competency in the professional preparation and practice of health promotion and health education specialists'. The identification of core competencies, standards and quality assurance systems was seen to be essential for developing and strengthening the capacity to improve public health in the twenty-first century. Eight domains of core competency were identified:

- Catalyzing change
- Leadership
- Assessment
- Planning
- Implementation
- Evaluation
- Advocacy
- Partnerships.

St Leger (2001) draws attention to the fact that we need to consider more than just the technical ability of practitioners, which is not necessarily matched by an understanding of the *raison d'être* of health promotion. Mittelmark's discussion of Calderwood's work on professional communities for social justice notes that professions are characterized by 'specialised bodies of knowledge, a client base, self-regulated accountability and strict guidelines for membership' (2008: 3). The notion of community adds the important element of shared values – in this instance, commitment to social justice. He argues that health promotion is a professional community for social justice. Sindall (2002) points out that health promotion should not take its own moral credentials for granted, but that a moral framework for practice is needed – an issue we will return to throughout this book. It will be clear from our earlier discussion that defining a competent health promotion workforce should go beyond skills to include the values and ethical principles integral to health promotion – in short, it must be shaped by the discourse of health promotion and more specifically by an empowerment model of health promotion.

Priorities for action

- Putting healthy public policy into practice
- Strengthening structures and processes in all sectors
- Towards knowledge-based practice
- Building a competent health promotion workforce
- Empowering communities

IUHPE and Canadian Consortium for Health Promotion Research, 2007

The 'new' critical health education

We have touched on health education at a number of points in this chapter. To bring the chapter to a close, we will briefly summarize our position on the role of health education vis-à-vis health promotion. The emergence of health promotion effectively marginalized health education by shifting attention towards the broader determinants of health and the need for a policy response. Yet this begs the question of how change is to be instigated and what processes should be put in place to improve the health of populations and, indeed, individuals. Our contention here is that the primary driver has to be health education. While it is acknowledged that health education requires a supportive environment to achieve its goals, the converse is all too often overlooked. The development of healthy public policy to create a supportive environment is dependent on health education. As Figure 1.6 makes clear, the development of healthy public policy requires some form of learning – and *ipso facto* education – be it among policy makers themselves, advocates or communities seeking change.

Critiques of health education have centred on its individualistic, victim-blaming orientation. However, what the critics are actually attacking is the preventive medical model of health education. Alternative, coexisting models of health education – especially the more radical, empowering models – are overlooked, effectively discarding the health education baby with the victim-blaming bathwater. Health education has a key role in tackling the structural determinants of health. Even at the individual and community level, health education can have an empowering and emancipatory function. It can also facilitate the voluntary adoption of health-enhancing behaviour. The review by Tilford et al. of the values of health promotion supports the continued relevance of health education that is empowering and in tune with the precepts of critical theory:

> We have also concluded that health education, especially using a critical empowerment model, still has an important part to play in health promotion and public health. (2003: 120)

Health education can thus be a major driver within an empowerment model of health promotion – shedding its behaviourist, victim-blaming associations. To emphasize the distinction, we refer to health education that incorporates this wider vision as the 'New Health Education'. Subsequent chapters, which address planning and strategies for health promotion in more detail, will provide opportunity to examine its potential more fully.

KEY POINTS

○ There are alternative conceptualizations of health. A working model is proposed which includes physical, mental, social and spiritual health and incorporates positive wellbeing as well as the absence of disease.

○ Although health is influenced by human agency, structural factors have a major influence on health and health-related behaviour.

○ Health promotion is a discipline with its own ideology and core values. These include equity and empowerment along with health as a right, social justice, voluntarism, autonomy, participation and partnerships.

○ Ethical health promotion practice requires attention to these core principles along with the more general principles of beneficence, non-maleficence and the pursuit of the public good.

○ Power is a key factor in relation to individuals' health behaviour and health choices. Power also shapes discourse about health and health promotion.

○ While different models of health promotion exist, the case is put forward for an empowerment model.

○ Health promotion should generally uphold the principle of voluntarism, but the use of more coercive methods may exceptionally be justified on the grounds of utilitarianism, paternalism or social justice.

○ Health promotion has a specialist role within a wider, multidisciplinary response to improving public health.

○ Critical and empowering, the 'New' Health Education is a major driver within health promotion.

2

ASSESSING HEALTH AND ITS DETERMINANTS

In questions of science, the authority of a thousand is not worth the humble reasoning of a single individual.

Galileo Galilei (1564–1642)

OVERVIEW

This chapter considers approaches to assessing the health of communities and identifying the range of factors which impact on health and health inequalities. It will:

- identify the contribution of epidemiology to understanding health and its determinants
- establish the need for alternative perspectives including the lay perspective
- consider salutogenic as opposed to pathogenic explanations of health and ill health
- consider lifestyle and environment as determinants of health
- focus on inequality, social capital and social exclusion, with particular reference to issues of definition and measurement.

INTRODUCTION

Green and Kreuter (1991) trace their initial motivation to develop a planning model for health education to their observation that, in practice, they could frequently discern no apparent reason for choosing the health issue to be addressed, nor the target population to be reached. Furthermore, the intervention strategy selected was also often simply a preferred method of working rather than the most strategic option to achieve defined outcomes. They assert that 'The systematic and critical analysis of priorities and presumed cause–effect relationships can start the planner on the right foot in health promotion today' (1991: 25). What is required, therefore, is:

1 an analysis of health issues/problems
2 prioritization
3 analysis of the determinants.

We are said to be living in an increasingly target-driven culture. It is paramount, therefore, that we remain critically aware of how targets are defined and, indeed, given our earlier discussion of ideology, whether they are appropriate. Health promotion, as noted in Chapter 1, is characterized by its multisectoral nature and the involvement of a variety of different professional groups. Furthermore, a central tenet of health promotion is the importance of involving individuals and communities. The differing ideological positions and values among various professional and lay groups will inevitably influence the way in which the determinants of health and causal factors are defined, the evidence that is accepted to support their existence and the ways in which priorities are identified and framed. We will begin by looking at epidemiological perspectives before considering alternative or complementary approaches.

EPIDEMIOLOGICAL PERSPECTIVES

Epidemiology has been viewed as a 'primary feeder discipline' for health promotion by virtue of its contribution to setting the agenda and its role in driving the system (Tannahill, 1992: 97). As we shall see, there is considerable criticism of over-reliance on epidemiological perspectives, which are often equated with a biomedical interpretation of health. However, for now, we will confine discussion to consideration of its scope and potential contribution.

Epidemiology has typically been defined as 'the study of the distribution and determinants of disease in human populations' (Barker and Rose, 1984: v). While this draws attention to the focus of epidemiology on populations rather than individuals, it will be immediately apparent that this interpretation conforms to a negative model of health. More recent definitions signal some move towards including a positive dimension – for example, 'the study of the distribution and determinants of health-related states or events in specified populations, and the application of this study to control of health problems' (Last, 1988, in Beaglehole et al., 1993: 3). This particular example also emphasizes the action-orientated role of epidemiology.

Unwin et al. (1997) identify three categories of information needed as a basis for planning interventions to improve the health of populations and communities:

• basic demographic information
• the health status of communities
• determinants of health in the community.

Kroeger (1997) further lists nine key epidemiological questions that can inform the planning process. These can be organized under four headings, as shown in the box.

Nine epidemiological questions

Identification

1   What are the main health problems?

Magnitude and distribution

2   How common are they?
3   When do they generally occur?
4   Where do they occur?
5   Who is affected?

Analysis

6   Why does the problem occur?

Action and evaluation

7   What measures could be (were) taken to deal with the problem?
8   What results were anticipated (achieved)?
9   What else could be done?

Derived from Kroeger, 1997

Descriptive epidemiology

As we demonstrated in Chapter 1, health is both a contested concept and a subjective state. It is not without difficulty, then, that epidemiology seeks to measure health objectively. Basch (1990) asserts that some composite indicator of health status is desirable but, ultimately, unattainable and a best estimate is therefore obtained by looking at levels of ill health. Descriptive epidemiology is essentially concerned with charting the disease burden of communities, together with the patterns of distribution of diseases – classically in relation to time, place and persons. There is frequently a heavy reliance on the use of routinely collected official health data, such as mortality and morbidity statistics, together with basic population data.

Mortality rates

The collection of data on vital events has its origins in the civil registration of births, marriages and deaths. Registration in England and Wales began in 1837, subsequent to the Births and Deaths Registration Act of 1836. Prior to this, the only records were in parish registers.

Because of the legal requirement to register deaths, mortality data are regarded as providing a complete representation. Deaths are recorded by underlying cause – confirmed either by a medical practitioner or an inquest. The death certificate requires identification of the immediate cause of death together with any underlying cause, defined as 'the disease or injury which initiated the train of events leading to death' (Unwin et al., 1997: 12). Other significant conditions contributing to death can also be recorded. The production of mortality statistics is based on coding of the underlying cause of death according to the International Classification of Disease (ICD) (see WHO, 2007c). Distinguishing between the immediate cause of death and underlying cause can be a source of error. Death rates are expressed in a number of different ways, as summarized in the box.

Mortality rates

Actual rates	
Crude mortality rate	number of deaths per thousand people.
Age-specific mortality rate	number of deaths per thousand people in a specific age group.
Infant mortality rate	number of deaths in the first year of life per thousand live births.
Under-five mortality rate	number of deaths in the first five years of life per thousand live births.
Sex-specific rates	number of deaths per thousand women/men.
Cause-specific rates	numbers of deaths from a specific cause per thousand people.
Constructed rates	
Age standardized mortality rates	the death rate that would exist in a population if it had the same age structure as a standard population (for example, national population, European standard population, Segi World Population, WHO World Standard Population (Ahmad et al., 2001)). A direct method of standardization.
Standardized mortality ratio (SMR)	the ratio of the actual number of deaths in a population to the number of deaths that would be expected if that population had the same levels of mortality as a reference population. The ratio is multiplied by 100. A SMR greater than 100 indicates a level of mortality higher than the reference population. An indirect method of standardization.

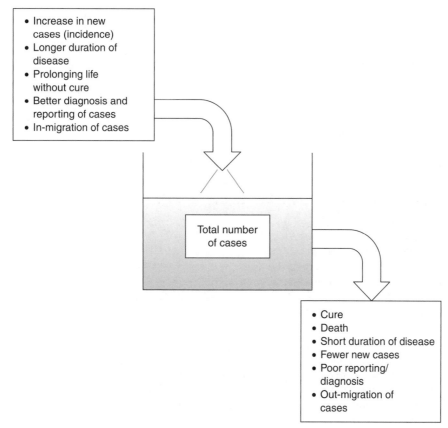

Figure 2.1   The prevalence pool

Clearly, each of the various mortality rates will create a different overall picture. The actual rates provide insight into the burden of mortality, but, given that the level of mortality is influenced by the age structure of the population, they are of little use when comparing populations with different age structures. The standardized rates, although artificial constructs, compensate for variations in age structure and can be used for comparative purposes. It is important, therefore, that appropriate rates are selected according to the intended purpose.

Morbidity rates

An important distinction in morbidity rates – and indeed health-related behaviour – is between incidence and prevalence. *Incidence* represents the number of new cases within a particular time period. *Prevalence*, in contrast, includes all the cases – either at a point in time (point prevalence) or over a defined period in time (period prevalence). Prevalence is often depicted as a pool, its overall magnitude being determined by the balance between factors filling and emptying the pool, as shown in Figure 2.1.

Morbidity data, unlike mortality data, are not complete in the sense that only those who come into contact with the health services will be routinely recorded. They are regarded as representing the tip of the clinical iceberg (Last, 1963) and below the surface are those who are self-medicating, using alternative therapy, with subclinical symptoms or just putting up with their symptoms. The volume under the surface is likely to be greater the less serious – and, *ipso facto*, the more common – the condition. It will also be influenced by the availability of services and cultural factors associated with their usage. The main sources of routinely collected morbidity data are summarized in the box.

Routine morbidity data in the UK

- Hospital activity data
- General practice data
- Cancer registrations
- Notification of infectious disease
- Sexually transmitted diseases
- HIV/AIDS
- Congenital anomalies.

Given that the majority of day-to-day illnesses never bring people into contact with the health service, they will go un- or under-reported. Figure 2.2 applies the notion of the clinical iceberg to the availability of data and their completeness in what might be referred to as a 'data iceberg'.

Relatively little routine information is available on minor illnesses, states of wellbeing or health-related behaviour. Obtaining data on these is, therefore, usually dependent on surveys. In Great Britain, the General Household Survey, for example, asks each year about:

- long-standing illness, disability or infirmity and the extent to which this limits activities
- acute sickness or restricted activity during the preceding two weeks
- use of health services
- general health during the preceding year.

It also includes questions about health-related behaviour such as smoking and drinking and other issues on a more occasional basis (see ONS, 2005).

Population data

Beaglehole et al. (1993) note that the central tool of epidemiology is the comparison of rates.

Rate = number of events in a population (numerator) ÷ size of the population (denominator)

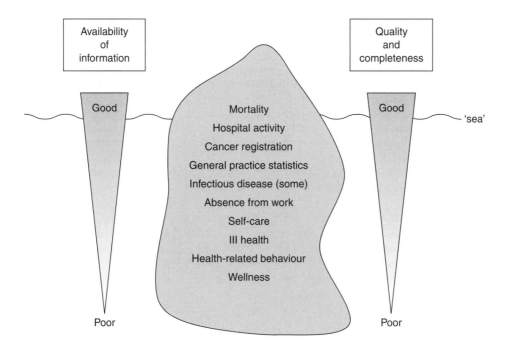

Figure 2.2   The data iceberg

In order to calculate rates, it is essential to know the size of the population and, for comparative purposes, the characteristics of that population. Such information is typically obtained by a census, which has been defined as 'a complete count or enumeration of a population conducted under the auspices of some governmental authority' (Ginn Daugherty and Kammeyer, 1995: 293). The United Nations Statistics Division also notes that national population and housing censuses provide valuable information on vulnerable groups, such as those affected by gender issues, children, youth, the elderly, those with an impairment or disability, and the homeless and migrant populations (United Nations Statistics Division, 2002).

The first complete modern census was carried out in Sweden in 1749 (Ginn Daugherty and Kammeyer, 1995). The UK census dates back to 1801 and has been conducted every ten years since then, with the exception of 1941. The nature of a census is such that it attempts to count the entire population. It therefore provides the denominator information required for the calculation of rates. Despite attempting to obtain complete coverage, it has been estimated that there was, in fact, only 98 per cent coverage in the 1991 UK census (National Statistics, undated a) – omitting the so-called 'missing million'. The census also provides the opportunity to collect additional information on a range of demographic and socio-economic factors – those selected tend to vary over time and between countries. For example, a question on long-term illness was introduced into the UK census in 1991. The United Nations Economic Commission for Europe and the Statistical Office of the European

Communities (undated: 7) suggest that the topics included in a census should result from a balanced consideration of:

- the needs of the country, national as well as local, to be served by the census data
- the achievement of the maximum degree of international comparability, both within regions and on a worldwide basis
- acceptability of questions to respondents and their ability to provide the required information without an undue burden being placed on them
- the technical competence of the enumerators (if any) to obtain information on the topics by direct observation
- the total national resources available for enumeration, processing, tabulation and publication, which will determine the overall feasible scope of the census.

A list of the areas included in the UK's 2001 census is provided in the box. Kerrison and Macfarlane (2000) draw attention to two potential limitations of health data obtained by the census. First, the precise wording of the questions is important in relation to the response elicited. Second, it relies on the accuracy of self-reporting, which will be subject to a whole range of potentially contaminating or distorting factors.

Areas included in the UK Census 2001

- Household accommodation and car ownership.
- Demographic characteristics (age, sex, marital status).
- Health/long-term illness/provision of care.
- Qualifications.
- Household relationships.
- Cultural characteristics (such as ethnic group).
- Migration.
- Employment.
- Workplace and journey to work.

National Statistics, undated b

Life expectancy, HALE, DALYs and QALYs

Life expectancy is frequently used as a general indicator of a population's health status. It is the average number of years individuals of different ages can be expected to live if current mortality rates apply (Beaglehole et al., 1993). It is included as a measure in the Health Profile for England – life expectancy at birth is currently 76.9 years for men and 81.2 years for women. However, not all those years are likely to be lived in full health (Department of Health, 2007c). The notion of healthy life expectancy (HALE) makes allowance for this. It is the 'average number of years that a person can expect to live in "full health"' and takes into account those years 'lived in less than full health due to disease and/or injury' (WHOSIS, 2007). Table 2.1 provides a comparison of life expectancy, healthy life expectancy and early life mortality rates in three countries.

Table 2.1 Comparison of life expectancies and early mortality in selected countries

Indicator	Value (year)		
	UK	**Sierra Leone**	**Japan**
Life expectancy at birth (years) males	77.0 (2005)	37.0 (2005)	79.0 (2005)
Life expectancy at birth (years) females	81.0 (2005)	40.0 (2005)	86.0 (2005)
Healthy life expectancy (HALE) at birth (years) males	69.0 (2002)	27.0 (2002)	72.0 (2002)
Healthy life expectancy (HALE) at birth (years) females	72.0 (2002)	30.0 (2002)	78.0 (2002)
Probability of dying (per 1000 live births) under five years of age (under-5 mortality rate)	6 (2005)	282 (2005)	4 (2005)
Infant mortality rate (per 1000 live births)	5.0 (2005)	165.0 (2005)	3.0 (2005)

Source: derived from WHO Statistics, 2006

Mortality can be considered premature if individuals do not survive to an expected age and this shortfall can be regarded as years of life lost. The total number of premature years of life lost (PYLL) due to different causes of mortality can be calculated. The use of PYLL as a measure of disease burden and for comparative purposes clearly attaches more weight to deaths occurring in younger age groups.

The concept of PYLL is extended and refined by the notion of disability adjusted life years (DALY) which, in addition to premature loss of life, includes loss of healthy life, broadly referred to as disability. 'DALYs for a disease are the sum of the years of life lost due to premature mortality (YLL) in the population and the years lost due to disability (YLD)' (WHO, 2007a). The severity of the disability is graded on a scale from 0 (perfect health) to 1 (dead).

DALY = YLL + YLD

The DALY was introduced in the World Development Report 1993 (World Bank, 1993) as a means of measuring the global burden of disease. Effectively, it is a measure of the health gap between the current situation and the ideal in which everyone lives to an old age in full health. Whereas assessing disease burden had formerly been overly reliant on mortality statistics, the DALY provided a broader view of disease burden by including conditions which affect health status. The use of DALYs, for example, has revealed the magnitude of the contribution of neuropsychiatric conditions to the global disease burden – an issue that had been overlooked by analyses of mortality statistics (WHO, 1999a). The World Health Report 2003 (WHO, 2003) noted that mental, neurological and substance use disorders contribute 13 per cent of overall disability adjusted life years (DALYs) globally and 33 per cent of overall years lived with disability (YLDs). See also Table 2.2.

The well-known health promotion maxim of adding life to years not just years to life draws attention to the issue of *quality* of life. Although, in principle, quality of life embraces 'emotional, social and physical wellbeing, and ability to function in the ordinary tasks of living' (Donald, 2001), quality of life measures tend to focus on disease states. The notion of quality adjusted life year (QALY) was developed as

Table 2.2   Leading causes of disease burden (DALYs) for males and females aged 15 years and older, worldwide, 2002

Males	% DALYs	Females	% DALYs
1 HIV/AIDS	7.4	1 Unipolar depressive disorders	8.4
2 Ischaemic heart disease	6.8	2 HIV/AIDS	7.2
3 Cerebrovascular disease	5.0	3 Ischaemic heart disease	5.3
4 Unipolar depressive disorders	4.8	4 Cerebrovascular disease	5.2
5 Road traffic injuries	4.3	5 Cataracts	3.1
6 Tuberculosis	4.2	6 Hearing loss, adult onset	2.8
7 Alcohol use disorders	3.4	7 Chronic obstructive pulmonary disease	2.7
8 Violence	3.3	8 Tuberculosis	2.6
9 Chronic obstructive pulmonary disease	3.1	9 Osteoarthritis	2.0
10 Hearing loss, adult onset	2.7	10 Diabetes mellitus	1.9

Source: WHO, 2003

a means of assessing the benefits of interventions in terms of the number and quality of years gained. The QALY was primarily developed to provide a utility rating to compare the health benefits of different interventions. It is a way of assigning a numerical value to a health state, based on the premise that, if a year of good-quality life expectancy is given the value of one, then a year of poor-quality or unhealthy life must be worth less than one. It therefore combines the length and quality of life into a single index (Bowling, 1997a).

Quality in this context is generally taken to be the absence of negative health states (i.e. disease and disability) rather than positive wellbeing which we discuss below. The EuroQol Group has developed the EQ-5D as a standardized instrument for measuring health outcome (EuroQol, undated). It uses five dimensions of health (mobility, self-care, usual activities, pain/discomfort, anxiety/depression) and each dimension comprises three levels (some, moderate or extreme problems). Given the subjective nature of quality of life and the various philosophical interpretations of health and wellbeing referred to in Chapter 1, it will come as no surprise that there is considerable debate about attempts to measure these factors objectively.

This use of QALYs has been much criticized. The criticisms are both technical, on account of their method of construction, and ethical (for a full analysis, see Edgar et al., 1998). The use of QALYs as a means of prioritization of healthcare has been viewed as unjust because it is essentially ageist – systematically favouring interventions that improve the health status of the young by virtue of their longer life expectancy. It also arbitrates on the basis of capacity to benefit rather than on the basis of actual need – a point we will return to in Chapter 5. However, arguments in defence of QALYs refer to the need for a single index of health with which to compare the outcomes of different interventions in order to deploy limited resources to achieve maximum benefits for the community (Williams and Kind, 1992). Kelly (2006: 183) confirmed that evidence about cost-effectiveness based on cost per QALY will form an 'integral part' of the development of National Institute for Health and Clinical Excellence (NICE) guidance about public health. The Wanless Report (2002), for example, compared the cost-effectiveness of smoking cessation estimated between £212 and £873 per QALY with £4000 to £8000 per QALY for statins (drugs that reduce cholesterol). The second Wanless Report (2004) used Type 2 diabetes as a case study and identified a number of interventions below £20,000 per quality adjusted life year, the level at which NICE criteria used for making judgements about cost-effectiveness become more stringent (see box).

Interventions for Type 2 diabetes that are cost-effective using a threshold of £20,000 per QALY

- tight control of blood glucose and blood pressure for all diabetics
- ACE inhibitors for diabetics with one other risk factor not otherwise quantified (e.g. for tight control of blood pressure)
- retinopathy screening for all diabetics
- foot screening for those at high risk
- screening obese for impaired glucose tolerance (IGT) and relevant treatment
- multiple risk factor management
- self-care including patient education
- reduction of obesity and physical inactivity in high risk groups.

Wanless, 2004: 144

The allocation of resources based on DALYs is surrounded by similar arguments to those about QALYs. In addition, the greater value attached to adult life as opposed to that of children or the elderly in the construction of DALYS, attracts particular criticism (Abbasi, 1999).

Positive health

Much of the foregoing has focused on mortality and morbidity. The application of this information to the assessment of health is predicated on the assumption that the absence of disease is indicative of health. Yet, we noted in Chapter 1 that health is more than just the absence of disease. Catford's (1983) early attempt to identify positive health indicators provides examples of individual behaviour and health knowledge, socio-economic conditions and aspects of the physical environment. However, the analysis is still located within a disease causation continuum. The factors identified can only be deemed healthy by virtue of their contribution to prevention of disease and do not, of themselves, constitute positive wellbeing. Surveys such as the Health Survey for England (Department of Health, 2007d) collect data about the nation's health and exposure to selected risk factors. The survey was established in 1991 to monitor trends and progress towards national health targets (MIMAS, 2001). It includes a questionnaire as well as objective measures such as physical measurements and the analysis of blood samples. The survey has a 'core' which is repeated annually plus additional modules on topics of special interest such as cardiovascular disease and accidents. The core topics included in the survey are listed in the box.

Core topics included in the Health Survey for England

- general health and psycho-social indicators
- smoking
- alcohol
- demographic and socio-economic indicators
- use of health services and prescribed medicines (focus may vary)
- blood pressure
- measurements of height, weight and blood pressure.

Department of Health, 2007d

Kemm (1993) notes the relative ease of defining negative rather than positive health states and the greater success of epidemiology in handling the former rather than the latter. Bowling (1997a: 5) suggests that positive health:

> implies 'completeness' and 'full functioning' or 'efficiency' of mind and body and social adjustment. Beyond this there is no one accepted definition. Positive health could be described as the ability to cope with stressful situations, the maintenance of a strong social support system, integration in the community, high morale and life satisfaction, psychological wellbeing, and even levels of physical fitness as well as physical health.

Both authors are in agreement that the components of wellbeing require both precise definition and the formulation of criteria. A key issue is whether positive and negative states are opposite ends of the same dimension with some neutral midpoint or, as argued by Downie et al. (1996), they occupy different dimensions. These alternative conceptualizations are shown in Figure 2.3. Kemm (1993) asserts that there is little evidence to support positive health being viewed as a distinct dimension, although there may be theoretical reasons for doing so. Furthermore, positive and negative health may occupy the same dimension for some aspects, such as objective physical health, but different dimensions for subjective health.

A number of different scales exist for assessing aspects of quality of life and wellbeing. These include:

- SF-36
- Nottingham Health Profile
- Health Assessment Questionnaire
- Sickness Impact Profile
- Missoula-VITAS Quality of Life Index.

There is considerable variation in the conceptual underpinnings of the various instruments and their validity and reliability. (For a more detailed discussion, see Bowling, 1997a, 1997b; Edgar et al., 1998; and Donald, 2001.) Some of these scales derive from professional perspectives; some – such as the Nottingham Health Profile – have incorporated lay views in their development.

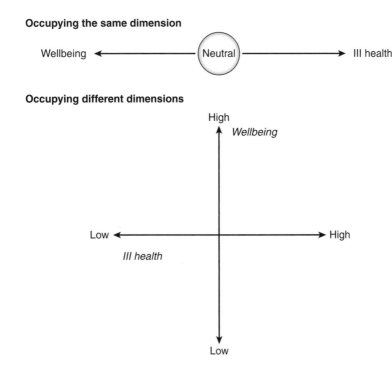

Occupying the same dimension

Wellbeing ⟵——————— Neutral ———————⟶ Ill health

Occupying different dimensions

High
Wellbeing

Low ⟵——————————————⟶ High

Ill health

Low

Figure 2.3   Dimensions of wellbeing and ill health (derived from Kemm, 1993 and Downie et al., 1996)

Analytic epidemiology

While the patterns of distribution of disease revealed by descriptive epidemiology may generate tentative hypotheses about causation, analytic epidemiology focuses specifically on exploring cause-and-effect relationships. One of the best-known early examples is the work of John Snow, who, by meticulously mapping cholera outbreaks in London during 1848–49 and 1853–54, was able to demonstrate that cholera was spread by contaminated water (Chave, 1958). Although derided by the miasmatists, who favoured the view that such diseases were caused by the miasma emanating from filth and putrefying material, and well in advance of Koch's discovery of the micro-organism that causes cholera in 1884, Snow's work provided evidence to support the general introduction of public health measures, such as improved water and sanitation – over and above the renowned removal of the handle of the Broad Street water pump to halt an outbreak of cholera in the vicinity.

The evidence for causality is subject to epistemological debate. Furthermore, many contemporary health problems are not the product of simple cause-and-effect relationships. Analysis is often concerned with multiple causes and, in some instances, multiple effects. Frequently, the focus is, therefore, on complex multifactorial webs. Moon and Gould (2000) identify three main conditions that must be present if observed associations are to be judged as causally linked. First, do the levels of exposure and disease vary in the same way – that is, co-variation? Second, does cause precede the effect – that is, temporal precedence? Third, have other possible explanations and confounding factors been eliminated?

A number of different types of epidemiological studies are used to explore causality. These range from observational studies, such as ecological and cross-sectional studies, which are regarded as relatively weak in their capacity to demonstrate causality, to the more robust case control and cohort studies. Intervention or experimental studies are more able to control for confounding variables and may take the form of randomized controlled, field or community trials. Beaglehole et al. (1993) provide a useful set of guidelines for assessing causality and these are listed in the box.

Guidelines for causality

Temporal relation	Does the cause precede the effect?
Plausibility	Does it make sense in the light of existing knowledge and mechanisms of action?
Consistency	Do other studies produce similar findings?
Strength	Is there a strong association?
Dose–response relationship	Does increase in exposure produce increased effect?
Reversibility	Does the risk decrease when the possible cause is removed?
Study design	Is the evidence robust and derived from strong studies?
Judging the evidence	How many lines of evidence lead to the conclusion?

Derived from Beaglehole et al., 1993

We will give further consideration to the complexity of causal relationships in health promotion programmes when we discuss evaluation in Chapter 11. However, returning to the subject of disease causation, Beaglehole et al. (1993: 71) define the cause of a disease as:

an event, condition, characteristic or a combination of these factors which plays an important role in producing the disease. Logically a cause must precede a disease. A cause is termed *sufficient* when it inevitably produces or initiates a disease and is termed *necessary* if a disease cannot develop in its absence. [Our emphasis]

It therefore follows that, in many instances, well-recognized causal factors are neither necessary nor sufficient. Take smoking, for example. Some people who have never smoked will develop lung cancer, so smoking cannot be seen as necessary, and some people who smoke do not develop lung cancer, hence smoking is not sufficient. There is, however, indisputable evidence that smoking is an important causal factor that increases the probability of developing lung cancer and, conversely, that this will be reduced by smoking cessation. Thus, it becomes important to think in terms of probability and risk. The term 'risk factor' is applied to those factors that are associated with the development of a disease, but not sufficient in themselves to cause it – often with the underlying intent of identifying factors that can be modified to prevent disease occurring. 'Relative risk' is the ratio of the rate of the disease in those exposed to a particular factor to the rate in those not exposed (see the box on risk). It indicates the number of times *more likely* it is that an individual exposed to the factor will develop the disease. It is useful in establishing the strength of the association and also in graphically encapsulating the levels of additional risk incurred by individuals.

In contrast, the notion of 'attributable risk' acknowledges the fact that many diseases develop independently of exposure to risk factors. In order to assess the amount of disease that is actually attributable to exposure, the rate in those not exposed to the risk factor (that is, those who would have developed the disease regardless of exposure) is subtracted from the rate in those exposed (see box for formula).

A related concept is the 'population attributable risk' (see box). This indicates the amount of disease that would be avoided in a population if exposure to the risk factor was completely eliminated. Reference to Table 2.3 (derived from Doll et al., 1994) shows that although the relative risk among heavy smokers for lung cancer is much higher than for heart disease, indicative of a stronger causal relationship, more actual deaths from heart disease can be attributed to smoking.

Assessment of risk

Relative risk (x)	= rate of the disease in those exposed to the risk factor ÷ rate of the disease in those not exposed
Attributable risk (rate)	= rate of the disease in those exposed to the risk factor – rate of the disease in those not exposed
Population attributable risk	= attributable risk x proportion of the population exposed to the risk factor

Table 2.3   Relative and attributable risk of smoking

Cause of mortality	Non-smoker	Annual mortality rate per 100,000 men			Relative risk of smokers 25+ per day	Attributable risk per 100,000 for smokers 25+ per day
		Current smokers				
		1–14 per day	15–24 per day	25+ per day		
Lung cancer	14	105	208	355	355/14 = 25.4	355–14 = 341
Bladder cancer	13	29	29	37	37/13 = 2.8	37–13 = 24
Ischaemic heart disease	572	802	892	1025	1025/572 = 1.8	1025–572 = 453
Cerebral thrombosis	93	93	150	143	143/93 = 1.5	143–93 = 50

Source: Data derived from Doll et al., 1994

Establishing the potential and feasibility for prevention rests on the capacity to identify modifiable risk factors. Conventionally, different levels of prevention are distinguished:

- **primary prevention** is concerned with preventing the development of disease by reducing exposure to risk factors – environmental and behavioural
- **secondary prevention** in contrast, focuses on early diagnosis – for example, by screening – to improve the prospects of treatment
- **tertiary prevention** includes measures to reduce the consequences of illness and is often seen as integral to a rehabilitation programme.

A fourth level of prevention has also been recognized (Beaglehole et al., 1993):

- **primordial prevention** aims to prevent the emergence of social, economic and cultural patterns known to be associated with disease in cultures that already have healthy traditional ways of life.

A further issue is whether it is preferable to target preventive interventions at the population in general or high-risk groups (Rose, 1992). Arguments in favour of the high-risk approach include its greater cost-effectiveness and the fact that people who are known to be at high risk may be more motivated to change. However, it presupposes that it is both possible to identify those at risk and that the disease will not occur in those who do not fall within this category. Nor would such an approach contribute to changing general norms, so it might be more difficult for individuals to make changes. Furthermore, health and health behaviour are influenced by a broad range of social and environmental factors that can only be tackled at the population level. Even when focusing on specific behaviour, the whole population approach has the capacity to achieve a significant reduction in disease. Although major change may be achieved at the population level, it requires many individuals to make changes and relatively few of them will gain any personal benefit – referred to by Rose (1992) as the 'prevention paradox'. Charlton notes that a population-wide approach potentially labels the whole population as being at risk. It also creates the new category of the 'worried-well'. As Illich (1976: 97) cautioned, this can also lead to undue dependence on the medical profession and the medicalization of life – so-called social iatrogenesis:

> The concept of morbidity has been enlarged to cover prognosticated risks ... People are turned into patients without being sick. The medicalization of prevention thus becomes another major symptom of social iatrogenesis.

THE NEED FOR ALTERNATIVE PERSPECTIVES

Two key questions are often asked when assessing the utility of health information.

- Is it necessary?
- Is it sufficient?

Both are pertinent to the selection of information to identify priority health issues and assess health needs. Furthermore, the answers to both will be influenced by issues of ideology, epistemology (concerned with the nature of knowledge and how it is acquired) and, not least, practicality.

Epidemiological approaches to assessing health status and identifying the determinants of health are consistent with a modernist emphasis on rationality and faith in the scientific method. De Kadt (1982a) suggests that perspectives on health are informed by the dominant conceptions of medicine. Of particular relevance are its mechanistic nature, together with its focus on micro-causality. As a consequence, attention is directed towards individuals who become sick and, by inference, their unhealthy lifestyles rather than the social, economic and environmental factors that are responsible for these lifestyles. Krieger (2001) states that the early epidemiology and public health of the mid-to late-nineteenth century clearly recognized that population health is shaped by both social and biological processes. However, increased interest in personal preventive measures in the late nineteenth and early twentieth centuries signalled a shift in emphasis for mainstream modern epidemiology. Criticism of this shift has come from within epidemiology itself as well as from other fields, such as sociology and anthropology. Moon and Gould (2000: 143) draw on an editorial in the *Lancet* (Anonymous, 1994) to suggest that:

> the discipline's focus is now so far 'downstream' that it has lost sight of what is going on up river. The result is an exclusion of the *contexts* in which disease happens unless they are immediately measurable and the *voices* of those people whose social conditions threaten their health ...

They are critical of the way in which modern epidemiology is consistent with, and upholds, dominant value systems. Furthermore, they challenge the methodological assumptions associated with its positivist methodological position – particularly its reductionist principles and the lack of attention to context. While accepting that there is some value in identifying causal factors, they assert that they reveal little about the structural factors that influence people's lives.

The emergence of 'social epidemiology' in the 1950s was distinguished by its explicit focus on the *social* determinants of health – a position reflected in the 'new public health' movement. 'Critical epidemiology', furthermore, 'places an emphasis on the social and power relations that shape disease definition and disease causation' (Moon and Gould, 2000: 7).

Issues of micro-causality are undoubtedly relevant to understanding the factors that impact on health status, such as is the case with exposure to the tubercle bacillus and the development of tuberculosis. However, they are not sufficient. They need to be understood within the context of the social and environmental factors – such as overcrowding, social class, poverty and urbanization – that are also associated with the development of the disease. Furthermore, Kelly and Charlton (1995) caution against reification of the social system and a simple deterministic view of the relationship between social factors and ill health, which merely replicates the type of thinking integral to a biomedical approach – albeit further upstream. They note the tension in health promotion discourse between free will and determinism – that is, between *agency* and *structure* – and call for an understanding of the reciprocal relationship between the two.

The application of science and rationality to the analysis of the determinants of ill health, or even positive health states, assumes that there is an objective reality. A postmodern understanding, in contrast, views reality as both contextual and contingent. Rather than one objective reality, there are multiple perspectives and interpretations of reality. Graham's work on smoking provides a useful example. Smoking is strongly linked to social disadvantage. An 'outsider's' view of mothers in low-income households sees smoking as irrational by virtue of the cost and health risks incurred. However, an 'inside view' is that, for the mothers themselves, smoking can be part of their coping strategy. Graham's (1987) study revealed that, from the mothers' perspective, smoking was associated with breaks from their caring role, which enabled them to recharge, and was also a means of coping when things got too much. Looking at the issue from the perspective of the mothers transforms apparently irrational behaviour into a rational response to their situation.

Furthermore, contrary to the customary view that science and the scientific method are concerned with the objective pursuit of truth, in fact, science itself is socially constructed – both in its focus and its methods. The breadth of scientific enquiry is restricted by the limits of current paradigms (Kuhn, 1970). The construction of problems – the ways in which they are framed and the determinants explored – are all socially shaped (Petersen and Lupton, 1996). How far upstream will, or should, the quest for determinants go? What risk factors are regarded as legitimate areas of enquiry? What evidence will be accepted?

Official statistics form the basis of much epidemiological and, indeed, sociological enquiry. It is appropriate at this point to consider the nature of official data.

Official health data – reality or myth?

The characteristics of official health statistics are that they generally include large data sets that have been collected regularly by official agencies over long periods of time. It is a truism that data do not exist in their own right, but are constructed. There are clearly issues concerning the technicalities of data collection, its representativeness and completeness. As we have already noted, official health data will only include those who have come into contact with services, registered vital events or been included in official surveys. Consulting a doctor or taking time off work will inevitably be influenced by a range of social and cultural factors. The collection of some official data – such as mortality and census data – attempts to include all cases, whereas surveys will only involve a sample.

The way in which data are classified and categorized is also socially constructed. For example, in relation to certification of death, 'old age', which featured prominently as a cause of death in the late-nineteenth century, becomes an inadequate descriptor in our more biomedically enlightened times – more specific causal explanations are required. There is a well-known tendency towards under-reporting of emotionally charged issues, such as suicide and AIDS. Furthermore, at what point in the temporal sequence of causality do we identify a single cause? For a child dying in one of the least-developed parts of the world, is it measles, malnutrition or poverty? For a man dying prematurely in a rundown inner-city area, is it lung cancer or smoking or unemployment? Interestingly, the tenth revision of the *International*

Classification of Disease introduced a set of codes for factors that influence health status and contact with health services. When even ostensibly objective issues such as mortality and morbidity can be seen to be socially constructed, assessing 'quality of life' becomes even more problematic. Classifying people by gender, ethnic group and socio-economic status provides further evidence of social construction.

Official data, then, are not facts in their own right, but are constructed. The ways in which they are constructed will be influenced by both technical and ideological issues. The Radical Statistics Health Group lists a series of questions to consider when assessing the quality of official health data (see the box).

Confronting the statistics

- How were the data collected?
- How were the data coded and classified?
- How were the data tabulated and analysed?
- How were the statistics selected and interpreted?
- What has been left out or ignored?
- It can't be true – my experience was different. (Is it atypical?)

Radical Statistics Health Group, 1987: 188–9

May (1993) identifies three schools of thought in relation to official statistics:

- **realist** considers official statistics to be objective indicators of phenomena
- **institutionalist** sees official statistics as artificial constructs revealing more about an institution's priorities in collecting data than the phenomena they purport to represent
- **radical** extends the institutionalist view to include discretionary practices embedded within and replicating the power structure and dynamics of society.

By way of example, let us take the use of waiting lists for hip replacement surgery as an indicator of prevalence and need. A realist interpretation would presuppose that individuals have equal access to general practitioners, who would refer them to hospital for treatment and the length of the waiting lists would simply be the product of the number of individuals requiring treatment and the period required for throughput. An institutionalist view would question the way in which the hospital constructed the waiting list for treatment. For example, have treatment waiting lists been kept short by having a long waiting period prior to consultation? A radical view would locate this last question within the context of any national imperative to reduce waiting lists and political pressure to demonstrate more efficient services. Changes in these contextual factors would inevitably influence the comparability of data over time.

Conspiracy theorists would subscribe to the view that statistics are deliberately manipulated to suit an agenda rather than being the unconsciously biased products of systems and practices. Huff's delightfully subversive *How to Lie with Statistics* (1979) identifies a number of tactics. These include:

- using a sample with an in-built bias, such as self-selected respondents
- choosing the 'right' average – if a distribution is skewed, the median will be less affected than the mean, so, for example, a few high-earners would raise the mean earnings but not the median
- using very small samples
- manipulating graphs:
  - numbered axes
  - plotting means to obscure highs and lows
  - changing the vertical scale or cutting off the bottom of graphs to exaggerate trends
  - using pictorial representation
- tacitly implying associations when none have been proved
- assumptions about causality.

The danger in seeing official data merely as social constructs is that it can lead us to reject them as having no inherent value. We then have a limited capacity to assess health status and identify problem issues. The evidence that initially exposed, and continues to document, the effects of social inequality, for example, drew substantially on official health data. Without this insight, it would have been difficult to mount an argument in favour of tackling social inequality. What is needed is the *critical* use of health data that takes full account of the ways in which they have been constructed. This is aptly summed up by Roberts (1990: 13):

> An over-reverent approach to figures supports the empiricist fallacy that figures are merely given objective facts, a proper understanding of which compels one conclusion and one only. An over-sceptical approach sustains the equally erroneous belief that statistics are mere mystification, a way of obscuring truth and legitimizing error, that they are born in deception and formed of quantified ideology.

The lay perspective

The lay perspective introduces a completely different dimension. Lay knowledge is rooted in the direct and vicarious experience of individuals and communities and their cultural understandings. It is interpreted within the context of people's real lives and day-to-day experiences. The earlier reference to the 'clinical iceberg' would indicate that most of our individual and collective experiences of ill health and health occur below the surface. There, it is effectively hidden from the reaches of routine data-collection systems and, hence, does not feature in most official accounts of health.

Faith in the value of lay knowledge about health and ill health has been central to the development of the self-help movement – a movement that challenged medical, and, indeed, expert hegemony. Furthermore, community activists have used their own insights, derived by means of what has been termed popular or lay epidemiology, to mount campaigns to tackle what they perceive to be the cause of local health problems. Williams and Popay (1994) provide a number of high-profile examples, such as tackling the problems of toxic waste and environmental pollution, but, equally, lay epidemiology can support the case for local measures, such as improved housing and traffic-calming measures.

Frankel et al. (1991) see lay epidemiology as being concerned with the interpretation of health risks by lay people as a result of observation and discussion within their own personal networks and the public arena, as well as information derived through the media. Moon and Gould (2000: 7) note that, although critics have challenged this approach as being 'anecdotal, uninformed and even dangerous', it provides direct insight into the ways in which health and ill health are commonly experienced, understood and managed. Roberts' (1998) work on injury prevention provides a useful example of this. Participatory research involving children and families revealed how they manage to successfully negotiate what are intrinsically dangerous environments and the expense that this incurs in relation to children's loss of freedom and parental anxiety. It also enabled the antecedents of accidents and near accidents to be identified rather than the sequelae that feature in routinely collected data based on hospital admissions. Clearly, the former has much greater relevance for planning preventive health promotion interventions. A more recent example is provided by UNICEF's (2007a) report on the views of young people who have experienced conflict (see box).

The voice of young people living in conflict zones

We all have one thing in common: Our lives have been affected by armed conflict. That is why, even though we come from different places and our problems are not always the same, we speak with one voice.

We have not given up all hope yet. We still want to go to school and play with our friends. We want to help build peace in our societies and make this world a better place. We still have big dreams.

For some of us, getting together for the sake of this report gave us a rare opportunity to sit with our friends and share our stories. It has also been an opportunity to finally tell you what we feel and think.

But talking is not enough. Will we see any change after you meet to talk about us? Will you hear our voices and act on what we tell you?

UNICEF, 2007a

Lay interpretations of health are complex and multidimensional. Far from being trivial, they demonstrate coherent and sophisticated understandings. A number of major studies have explored these understandings (for example, Herzlich, 1973; Blaxter and Patterson, 1982; Williams, 1983; and Cornwell, 1984) and the following key dimensions can be identified:

- the absence of disease, illness, pain
- a reserve for coping with stress and illness
- the functional ability to allow tasks to be performed
- an ideal state, including positive wellbeing.

Basch (1990) adds to this list:

- conformity with expected norms.

Lay recognition of the absence of disease, illness and pain as integral to health is noteworthy as the professional discourse on wellbeing does not always explicitly address this issue.

There is some interplay between professional and lay accounts of health, though. For example, the germ theory is fully integrated into most Western lay interpretations of disease. It is interesting to note, however, that lay accounts might include such reductionist explanations, but they also go further, addressing issues associated with meaning, such as 'Why me?' and 'Why now?' (Williams and Popay, 1994). A full understanding of health and ill health will necessarily seek to incorporate these hitherto often private accounts.

The premise underpinning our earlier discussion of risk was that, from an epidemiological perspective, it can be measured objectively. In the same way that health and illness are not simple biological states, but are socially constructed, lay interpretations and perceptions of risk are also complex. As we will explore more fully in Chapter 3, they derive from the interplay of a plethora of psycho-social and cultural factors.

Frankel et al. (1991) note that lay perceptions of risk are often in tune with mainstream epidemiological analyses. For example, with regard to coronary heart disease, there is lay understanding of an association with both hereditary factors and adverse social circumstances – issues that rarely feature in health education campaigns. Frankel et al. raise the interesting question as to why there was a rapid and dramatic reduction in egg consumption in the UK in the late 1980s in response to concerns about salmonella infection when years of warning about the harmful effects of the cholesterol content of eggs brought about little change. They propose that there are different lay conceptualizations of risk. At one end of the spectrum, the risk is both immediate and easily imagined and therefore to be avoided – encapsulated as 'bad/poisonous behaviour'. At the other end of the spectrum, risks are perceived to be less immediate and less specific. Some behaviours associated with this type of risk, such as smoking, are acknowledged to be harmful, but may also have desirable aspects – hence, they are termed 'bad/desirable behaviour'. They suggest that the advertising industry attempts to keep behaviour away from the bad/poisonous end of the spectrum by emphasizing the desirable elements. Individuals may also use humour to the same effect – for example, 'naughty but nice' and 'what's your poison?'

The biomedical model has often been criticized because of its expert-led, top-down orientation. However, even interpretive approaches – which purport to provide greater insight into the experiences of lay people – may still remain an essentially expert-led analysis of that experience. A true commitment to including the lay perspective involves going beyond seeing people merely as research subjects. It requires an egalitarian approach to seeking their active involvement at all stages of the research process – not least in formulating the priority issues to address.

Pathogenesis or salutogenesis

Regardless of whether or not they conform to a reductionist, biomedical or more interpretive position, the majority of studies of the determinants of health and ill health are located within a pathogenic paradigm. As Kelly and Charlton (1995: 82) note:

The social model of health is, in this regard, no different to the medical model. In the medical model the pathogens are microbes, viruses or malfunctioning cellular reproduction. In the social model they are poor housing, unemployment and power-lessness. The discourse may be different but the epistemology is the same. The social model is not, in our view, an alternative to the discredited medical model. It is a partner in crime and a very close modernist relative.

Antonovsky (1984) asserts that the fundamental assumption of this paradigm is that individuals are in a state of balance or homeostasis and that when this state is challenged by microbial, physical or chemical factors or psycho-social stressors, regulatory mechanisms come into play to restore homeostasis. He identifies a number of consequences of this thinking:

- the tendency to think dichotomously about people, classifying them as healthy or diseased
- a focus on disease states or risk factors
- the search for cause or multifactorial causes
- the assumption that stressors are bad
- mounting wars against specific diseases
- ignoring the factors associated with wellness.

In proposing a salutogenic paradigm, Antonovsky advocates a radical change in perspective concerning what is involved in staying healthy. This shifts the focus away from specific diseases and towards those general factors involved in health, and in moving along what he terms the 'health-ease/dis-ease continuum' (Antonovsky, 1984: 117). He does not, however, totally abandon the pathogenic paradigm, but offers salutogenesis as an *additional* perspective.

I am not proposing that the pathogenic paradigm be abandoned, theoretically or institutionally. It has immense achievement and power for good to its credit. I have attempted to point to its limitations, to the blinders involved in any paradigm.

Salutogenesis focuses on the factors associated with successful coping, which are envisaged as buffers mitigating the effects of stressors. While there are numerous individual coping variables, Antonovsky (1987: 19) proposes the 'sense of coherence' (SOC) as an overarching explanatory variable.

The sense of coherence is a global orientation that expresses the extent to which one has a pervasive, enduring, though dynamic feeling of confidence that:

1 the stimuli deriving from one's internal and external environments in the course of living are structured, predictable and explicable
2 the resources are available to one to meet the demands posed by these stimuli and
3 these demands are challenges, worthy of investment and engagement.

These three components of the SOC are called comprehensibility, manageability and meaningfulness.

In considering how a strong SOC helps people to cope with stressors, Antonovsky (1984) attempts to identify generalized and specific resistance resources. The features that such resistance resources have in common are:

- **consistency** – the greater the consistency of life experiences, the more they will be comprehensible and predictable
- **underload–overload balance** – demand is appropriate to capability
- **participation in decision making** – the emphasis here is on active participation rather than control.

Early formulations of the SOC suggested that it was the product of early life experiences and that, by adulthood, it was more or less a fixed part of a person's makeup. Such a view offers little to those seeking to improve health. However, Antonovsky subsequently accepted that movement along the SOC can occur even in adulthood, albeit within fairly narrow limits. While he still subscribes to the view that macrosocial change is the only way to achieve substantial change in SOC for most people, he accepts that changes in everyday life can make some difference (Antonovsky, 1984).

Whose voice counts?

The validity of different accounts of health is the subject of debate, caught up in epistemological questions concerning ways of knowing and what constitutes truth. Beattie (1993) provides a useful analysis of 'different ways of knowing' based on modes of thought and the focus of attention. Modes of thought are seen as ranging from 'hard' mechanistic approaches consistent with the natural sciences to 'soft' humanistic approaches associated with sociological enquiry. Similarly, lay perspectives are often

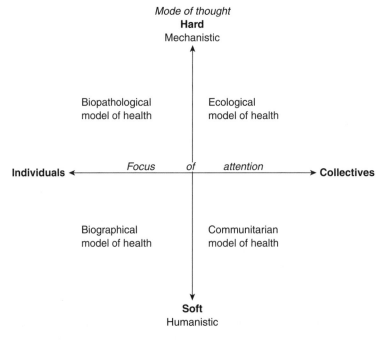

Figure 2.4   Accounts of health (Beattie, 1993)

regarded as prerational and trivial in contrast to the rational, and therefore supposedly serious, view of the so-called experts. The focus of attention ranges from individuals to collectives. Figure 2.4 provides an overview of the relationship between these and identifies four models.

Beattie equates each model with different sociopolitical philosophies and attempts to identify cultural bias within the various accounts of health as summarized in Table 2.4.

One of the characteristic features of health promotion is its concern with holism – a view of health that includes positive wellbeing in addition to the absence of disease, a broad conceptualization of the determinants of health and an emphasis on participation. Its information needs, therefore, are necessarily broad and include a range of different professional interpretations deriving from different disciplinary bases and including the lay perspective.

Table 2.4   Accounts of health – sociopolitical philosophies and cultural bias

Account of health	Sociopolitical philosophy	Cultural bias
Biopathological	Conservative	Subordination
Biographical	Libertarian	Individualism
Ecological	Reformist	Control
Communitarian	Radical pluralist	Cooperation

Source: Beattie, 1993

Much of the literature on lay perspectives draws on a discourse of conflict, couched in such terms as 'mounting a challenge' to biomedical interpretations and 'struggle over meaning'. Sociological accounts are also frequently expressed in this vein. Debate about the relative merits of the contributions of different research disciplines and perspectives is helpful in so far as it exposes the strengths and limitations of the various approaches and their respective utility – particularly when this results in positive attempts to redress shortcomings by seeking complementary approaches. It becomes damaging when it is merely a contest between different epistemological positions and methodologies in laying claims to the truth and different accounts of health are afforded different status.

A narrow and partial analysis of health problems cannot provide a secure basis for identifying priority issues and their determinants. Green and Kreuter (1991: 50) suggest that priorities are 'generally based on an analysis of data indicating the pervasiveness of the problems and their human and economic cost'. Mainstream epidemiological diagnoses, as we have noted, are concerned with objectively assessing the magnitude and distribution of diseases and health states together with the factors that contribute to them. Green and Kreuter argue strongly that a wider view is needed and problems should be defined from the outset in broad social terms. They offer two main reasons for this. Involving communities helps to ensure that their priority social and quality of life concerns are addressed and so avoids missing the mark in relation to social targets. It also contributes to encouraging community participation. They see the relationship between social and epidemiological diagnoses as complementary, operating in what they term either a 'reductionist' or an 'expansionist' way. Starting with an analysis of social problems, a reductionist approach would analyse the health and non-health factors that contribute to, or cause, the problem. The expansionist approach, in contrast, starts with an epidemiologically defined issue and works towards identifying the way this 'fits' into the larger social context. Green and Kreuter suggest that this avoids any tendency towards oversimplification.

While recognizing its contribution, Tannahill (1992) also cautions against an overemphasis on epidemiology as a driver in health promotion programme planning. He suggests that it neglects methodological issues by focusing on 'what to' rather than 'how to', creates an incomplete view of health, takes a narrow view of outcomes and leads to unsound programme planning. Of particular concern is the translation of single-issue problems into single-issue programmes, which ignores, on the one hand, the broader determinants and, on the other, that there may be factors common to a number of different conditions. For example, tobacco would be a common issue in relation to coronary heart disease, cancers and addiction, and all three are influenced by socio-economic status. Programmes that address single issues in isolation – so-called 'vertical programmes' – therefore risk duplication of messages and inefficiency. Our position is that we need multiple complementary perspectives to identify priority health issues and their determinants, as encapsulated in The Leeds Declaration (see the box).

The Leeds Declaration – Principles for Action

- There is an urgent need to refocus upstream, to move away from focusing predominantly on individual risks towards the social structures and processes within which ill health originates.
- Research is needed to explore factors that keep some people healthy despite living in the most adverse circumstances.
- Lay people are experts and experts are lay people – lay knowledge about health needs, health service priorities and health outcomes should be central to public health research.
- The experimental model is an inadequate gold standard for guiding research into public health problems.
- Not all health data can be represented in numbers – qualitative data have an important role to play in public health research.
- There is nothing inherently 'soft' about qualitative methods or 'hard' about quantitative methods – both require rigorous application in appropriate contexts and hard thinking about difficult problems.
- An openness to the value of different methods means an openness to the contributions of a variety of disciplines.
- Public health problems will only be solved through a commitment to the application of research findings to policy and practice.
- Research funding should address the new directions that follow from these principles.

Nuffield Institute for Health, 1993

DETERMINANTS OF HEALTH

Major improvements in health in the latter part of the nineteenth century have been attributed to improvements in the environment and general living and working conditions. The development of the germ theory and the improved possibility for immunization towards the end of the nineteenth century shifted the emphasis towards personal preventive services. The introduction of insulin and sulphonamide drugs in the 1930s heralded the dawn of the therapeutic era (Ashton and Seymour, 1988). The numerous subsequent technological developments in the biomedical field and faith in their capacity to improve health led to the rise of high-tech medicine. An increasingly technological view of health resulted in a shift in emphasis away from public health and community-based services and towards hospitals – so-called 'disease palaces'. Green (1996) noted that, in North America, towards the end of the twentieth century, over 90 per cent of expenditure on health was on medical care and less than 10 per cent on promoting healthy behaviour, lifestyles and environments, even though these accounted for between 50 and 71 per cent of all preventable premature mortality before the age of 75.

The Lalonde Report (1974) is frequently cited as the seminal document challenging the narrow, technically focused emphasis on disease and advocating a broader, social model. It recognized the need for a simple conceptual framework to bring order to the many and various factors influencing health:

> to organize the thousands of pieces into an orderly pattern that was both intellectually acceptable and sufficiently simple to permit a quick location, in the pattern, of almost any idea, problem or activity related to health; a sort of map of the health territory. (Lalonde, 1974: 31)

This was achieved using the 'health field concept', which identified four main elements – human biology, environment, lifestyle and healthcare organization (see the box).

Elements of the 'Health Field Concept'

- **Human biology** includes all those aspects of health, both physical and mental, which are developed within the human body as a consequence of the basic biology of man [sic] and the organic makeup of the individual.
- **The environment** includes all those matters related to health which are external to the human body and over which the individual has little or no control.
- **Lifestyle** consists of the aggregation of decisions by individuals which affect their health and over which they more or less have control.
- **Healthcare organization** consists of the quantity, quality, arrangement, nature and relationships of people and resources in the provision of healthcare.

Lalonde, 1974: 31–2

The health field concept therefore marked a radical break from the increasing emphasis on high-tech medicine, elevating the other three categories to equal standing.

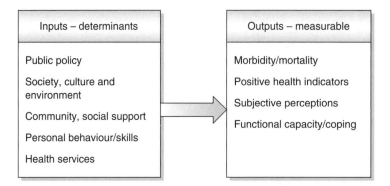

Figure 2.5   The expanded health field concept (derived from Raeburn and Rootman, 1989)

The concept itself is both simple and comprehensive. It was designed to provide insight into the factors associated with sickness and death and identify courses of action to improve health. The health field concept was also expected to encourage an analysis of any health problem in relation to all four categories. It could therefore be used to identify areas for research and guide policy and planning.

Some fifteen years after the publication of the health field concept, Raeburn and Rootman (1989) noted that the development of health promotion within this framework had focused particularly on lifestyle with insufficient attention being given to the influence of the environment. They also suggested that it was implicitly concerned with reduction of morbidity and mortality. To address these limitations, they proposed an expanded model that includes both inputs and explicit outputs (see Figure 2.5). The output side moves beyond morbidity and mortality to include functional capacity, positive health indicators and subjective perceptions. The input side is derived from the five action areas of the Ottawa Charter. With the exception of human biology, the other elements of the original health field concept are present. The reasons offered for its omission are that it is both a 'given' and an issue that falls under the aegis of health services rather than within the wider domain of policy, planning and research to promote over-all health and wellbeing.

Lifestyle and environment

The relative importance of lifestyle and environment as determinants of health has been the subject of much debate – a debate that has contributed to defining health promotion as a discipline.

Lifestyle

The recognition of chronic diseases as the major cause of death in the more highly developed parts of the world in the mid-twentieth century – against a backdrop of escalating healthcare costs – brought renewed interest in the role of prevention. In the UK, documents such as *Prevention and Health: Everybody's Business* (Department of Health and Social Security, 1976) identified lifestyle as a key factor in improving health status. Green et al. (1997) acknowledge the importance of lifestyle, too, when they contend that, in developed nations, a large proportion of deaths are associated with a relatively small number of behavioural risk factors. In the United States, for example, the ten leading causes of death have been causally related to one of three main behavioural risk factors, namely smoking, dietary practices and alcohol use.

Despite widespread recognition of the importance of lifestyle factors, there is little agreement about the meaning of the term. The WHO Health Education Unit (1993) identifies the following different interpretations:

- patterns of consumption and general living relevant to health
- freely chosen habits and behaviour
- a general way of living – the product of living conditions and individual patterns of behaviour determined by sociocultural factors and personal characteristics (O'Brien, 1995).

The way in which the construct has become blurred over the years is succinctly encapsulated by Sobel (1981: 1, in O'Brien, 1995: 197): 'If the 1970s are an indication of things to come, the word lifestyle will soon include everything and mean nothing, all at the same time.' O'Brien's analysis of the appropriation of 'lifestyle' identifies three major influences:

- new systems of product marketing that segment the population into groups on the basis of lifestyle characteristics and consumption patterns (see the box for examples)
- counterculture movements and alternative lifestyles as markers of ideological commitments
- critiques of modernization and a reemphasis on self-determination.

Green and Kreuter (1991: 12) draw on anthropological, sociological and psychological interpretations to define lifestyle as:

> patterns of behaviour that have an enduring consistency and are based in some combination of cultural heritage, social relationships, geographic and socio-economic circumstances, and personality.

They are critical of the widespread and erroneous use of the word 'lifestyle' for any kind of behaviour and note that it has even been applied to temporary behaviour or single acts. Antonovsky (1996) also notes that an examination of the literature on lifestyle and health reveals little more than a list of behavioural risk factors. One example of an attempt to classify different categories of lifestyle is provided in the box.

Examples of lifestyle categories

Superprofiles use census and other data to distinguish ten lifestyles. The categorization was principally developed for marketing purposes but has also been used within the context of health inequality.

(Continued)

(Continued)

- affluent achievers
- thriving greys
- settled suburbans
- nest-builders
- urban venturers
- country life
- senior citizens
- producers
- hard-pressed families
- have-nots
- unclassified.

See Local Government Data Unit – Wales, 2003; Carr-Hill and Chalmers-Dixon, 2005

Green and Kreuter (1991: 13) suggest that the term 'lifestyle' should be used only to describe 'a complex of related practices and behavioural patterns, in a person or group, that are maintained with some consistency over time'. They argue that greater precision in the distinction between behaviour and lifestyle supports a more holistic and comprehensive approach to promoting health. If behaviour is understood within the context of the complex web that makes up a lifestyle, it immediately becomes evident that attempts to change that behaviour will need to have regard for the social, environmental and cultural circumstances that sustain that lifestyle. Furthermore, it demands sensitivity to possible knock-on effects for other aspects of the lifestyle. They also suggest that the use of the terms 'behaviour', 'action' or 'practice' to describe targets signals greater realism than the more aspirational term 'lifestyle', which is notoriously difficult to influence independently of the wider environmental context. This raises the issue of the relationship between lifestyle and environment, which we will explore more fully along with a consideration of environmental factors.

Much of the literature on lifestyle is located within a pathogenic paradigm and focuses on the association between risk behaviours and disease (Antonovsky, 1996). In contrast, the focus within a salutogenic paradigm would be on the identification of those aspects of lifestyle that actively promote health – so-called 'salutary factors' – rather than the absence of risk factors. The recent interest in 'social capital' makes some move towards incorporating this salutogenic perspective.

Environment

The health field concept's interpretation of 'environment' placed considerable emphasis on the *physical* aspects of the environment with only passing reference being made to the *social* environment. Its central defining criteria for environmental factors are that they are external to the body and outside our immediate control. More recently, there has been much greater emphasis on social, cultural and economic aspects, particularly in the context of inequality.

Environmental factors can influence health either directly or indirectly. Simple examples of direct effects include exposure to toxic materials, shortage of food, lack of safe drinking water and overcrowding. Others factors will operate in a more indirect way. For example, lack of facilities for exercise in the environment will be associated with lower levels of physical activity and poorer heart health, while poor access to health services will be associated with low levels of uptake and so on.

Health and neighbourhood renewal

Poor health is both a symptom of living in a poorer neighbourhood and a cause of its continuing decline. Socio-economic factors such as income, educational attainment, housing, environment, crime, fear of crime and social support networks greatly influence the health of individuals – from before birth right through life. Also, in deprived areas, these problems can be compounded by poor access to health services, but also by poor day-to-day access to healthy, affordable food, safe leisure and recreation and affordable, convenient public transport.

The neighbourhood renewal agenda emphasizes the importance of joining up between different policy areas, service providers and communities themselves.

NRU, 2003

Environmental factors may also interact – in some instances creating vicious circle effects (see box). Poverty is associated with poor housing, diet, education and healthcare, for example, leading to fewer life chances overall. Even ostensibly random occurrences, such as natural disasters, disproportionately affect poorer communities. It is estimated that, of the 80,000 deaths that occur each year because of natural disasters, 95 per cent occur in poorer countries (WHO, 2001). Equally, global warming – itself the product of atmospheric pollution – is predicted to affect water supplies and food production, resulting in population displacement as well as causing changes in some disease patterns. Again, the major effects are anticipated to be felt to the greatest extent by the world's most vulnerable populations. WHO predicts that over and above natural disasters, climate warming will increase vector borne disease such as malaria and dengue fever along with food and water borne diarrhoeal diseases. Climate change that has occurred since the baseline period of 1961–90 is estimated to have caused '150,000 deaths and 5.5 million DALYS in the year 2000' (WHO, UNEP and WMO, 2003: 31). For these reasons, health promotion and public health have been under pressure to make links with initiatives to support sustainable development and Agenda 21 (Rogers and Whyms, 1995).

Our earlier discussion of the term 'lifestyle' indicated that it is heavily influenced by the environment. The Lalonde Report discusses the validity of using free choice as the basis for distinguishing between lifestyle and environmental factors in the health field concept. The premise is that individuals can make choices about their lifestyle, but can do little about the environment. The Lalonde Report (1974: 36), while accepting that the environment does affect lifestyle, concludes that: '… the deterministic view must

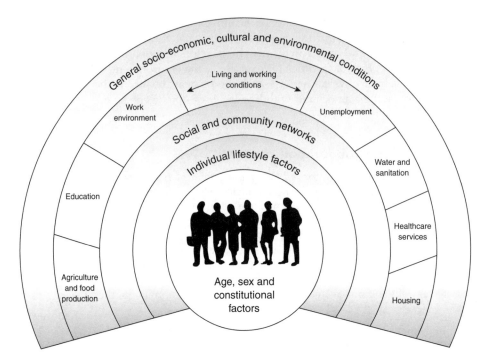

Figure 2.6   The main determinants of health (Dahlgren and Whitehead, 1991)

be put aside in favour of faith in the power of free will, hobbled as this power may be at times by environment and addiction.' However, there has been increasing doubt about whether or not behaviour can legitimately be seen to be under autonomous control. Green and Kreuter (1991: 12) see it as 'socially conditioned, culturally embedded and economically constrained'.

O'Brien (1995: 192) draws on earlier sociological interpretations of lifestyle to identify two main elements in its construction – political, economic and cultural resources and the psycho-social characteristics of the individual or groups – that is, a combination of environmental and personal factors, with the former having the major influence: '"Lifestyle" implied "choice" within a constrained context and the contexts were held to be more important than the choices.'

There is clearly tension between recognizing humans as autonomous free agents and taking a deterministic view of environmental factors. This tension between agency and structure is also evident in decisions about the relative merits of environmental or lifestyle approaches to health promotion. Clearly, the two are inextricably linked. The PRECEDE planning model (Green and Kreuter, 1991) recognizes the interrelationship between behaviours and environment. It identifies factors in the environment and conditions of living that facilitate actions by individuals or organizations – 'enabling factors'.

Diagrammatic representation of the health field concept – which has typically shown the four elements of lifestyle, environment, human biology and healthcare organization as discrete entities – has perhaps reinforced the tendency to see them as

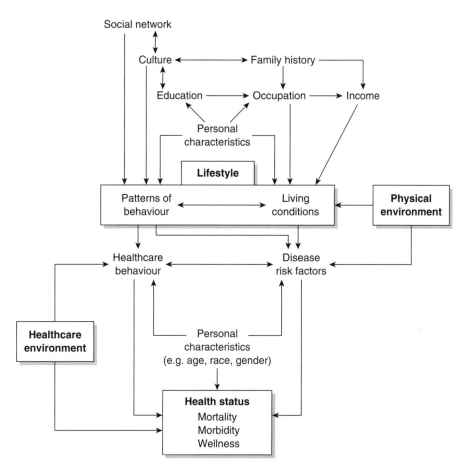

Figure 2.7   Some interrelations in the complex system of lifestyle, environment and health status (Green et al., 1997)

independent variables. Nesting the main determinants within each other, as depicted by Dahlgren and Whitehead (1991), is more indicative of their broad interrelation-ships and the respective positioning of macro and micro determinants, as shown in Figure 2.6. Green et al. (1997) provide a more detailed analysis of the complex inter-relationships, as shown in Figure 2.7.

An alternative approach acknowledges the relative importance of the various major determinants of health at different stages of the lifespan – for example, the powerful early influence of primary socialization. This conceptualization is central to the notion of the 'health career', which charts individuals' progress through the lifespan and the ways in which different factors come into play over time (Tones and Tilford, 2001). The focus is on individuals and their cumulative experience rather than a more general overview of determinants. Figure 2.8 represents the health career as a coaxial cable, with the central core being made up of an individual's values, attitudes and beliefs. The

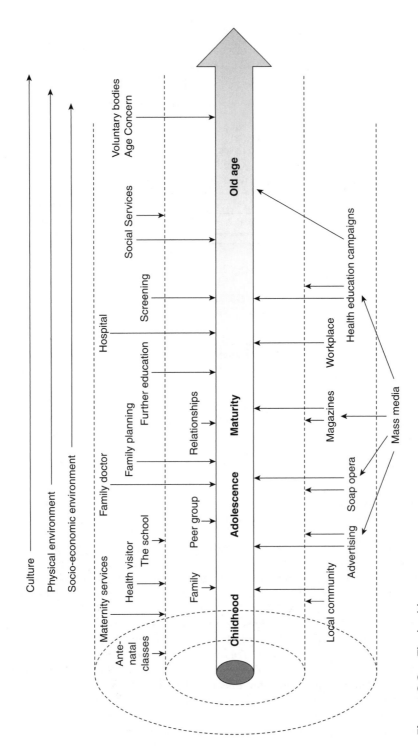

Figure 2.8 The health career

health career analysis can assist in ascertaining the key influences on individuals at different stages in their life and also in identifying opportunities for intervention.

Social capital

There is an increasing body of evidence suggesting that social relationships and social support are protective against ill health, while social isolation and exclusion are associated with higher levels of ill health – indeed, some 100 articles per year were cited in the Current Contents journal abstracting service from 1989–91 (Gottlieb and McLeroy, 1992). The box provides examples of some of the major early prospective studies to have demonstrated the association. Similarly, Mittelmark (1999a) cites Schwartzer and Leppin's (1992) meta analysis of 80 studies, which demonstrated the negative association between social integration/social support and morbidity/mortality.

Major early studies demonstrating the effect of social support on mortality

Alameda County Study, Berkman and Syme (1979)
Tecumseh Study, House et al. (1982)
Durham County Study, Blazer (1982)
North Karelia Study, Kaplan et al. (1988)
Kuopio Study, Kaplan et al. (1994)
In Sweden, Welin et al. (1985) and Orth-Gomér and Johnson (1987)
In relation to mortality from cardiovascular disease, accident and suicide, Kawachi et al. (1996)

Derived from Stansfield, 1999

Stansfield (1999) makes the important distinction between social networks and the functional aspects of support. A measure of social networks would include the number and frequency of contacts – taking account of the closeness of the contacts – and the density of the network. The quality of the support would include positive emotional and practical support and also any negative, undermining aspects of close relationships. Over and above offering direct support and encouraging health-enhancing behaviour, social connectedness, in itself, has been shown to have a positive effect on health status, possibly by acting as a buffer for stressors.

Mittelmark (1999a: 447) suggests that the anticipated benefits of strengthening social ties are 'better-functioning individuals, families, neighbourhoods and work groups, and improved physical and mental health'. He also summarizes the various pathways that have been proposed to explain how social ties affect health. These include:

- sources of information to help avoid high-risk or stressful situations
- positive role models
- increased feelings of self-esteem, self-identity and control over the environment
- social regulation, social control and normative influences
- sources of tangible support
- sources of emotional support
- perceptions that support is available
- buffering actions of others during times of stress.

The conceptual model developed by Berkman et al. (2000) locates social networks within the upstream social and cultural context which shapes them. It then identifies four primary pathways through which social networks operate downstream at the behavioural level:

1   provision of social support
2   social influence
3   social engagement and attachment
4   access to resources and material goods.

While the emphasis in the literature is on the health-enhancing consequences of social ties, Mittelmark draws attention to the emerging evidence (spearheaded by fields such as gerontology) that they may also be a source of social strain. Such strain would derive from actions by persons in an individual's social network, such as excessive demands, criticism, invasion of privacy and meddling, that, 'intended [or] unintended, cause a person to experience adverse psychological or physiological reactions' (Mittelmark, 1999: 448).

Furthermore, he contends that social support and social strain are not opposite ends of the same continuum – and so not mutually exclusive – but separate constructs. It follows, then, that there can be four permutations – high support/high strain, high support/low strain and so on.

The notion of 'social capital' has been applied to the social resources within a community and is currently enjoying a good deal of popularity. The concept was first explored by Bourdieu (1980) and further developed by other authors such as Coleman (1988, 1990) and Fukuyama (1999). However, the term is particularly associated with Putnam and his early work on local government in Italy (Putnam, 1993). For Putnam (1995: 67), social capital:

> refers to features of social organization such as networks, norms and social trust that facilitate coordination and cooperation for mutual benefit ... life is easier in communities blessed with a substantial stock of social capital ... networks of civic engagement foster sturdy norms of generalized reciprocity and encourage the emergence of social trust. [They] facilitate coordination and communication ... and allow dilemmas of collective action to be resolved. Finally, dense networks of interaction probably broaden the participants' sense of self, developing the 'I' into the 'we' ...

This interpretation encompasses more than just the existence of community networks and the resources available. It also includes the social norms of trust and reciprocity, a sense of belonging and willingness to engage in civic activity. While the density of networks is of general relevance to social capital, the notion has been extended to include different forms based on the characteristics of networks:

- **Bonding social capital** – refers to the ties between people in closely linked similar situations such as families or closely knit neighbourhoods
- **Bridging social capital** – refers to looser connections between people which may cross-cut boundaries, for example workmates and wider friendships
- **Linking social capital** – refers to links between people occupying different hierarchical and power positions, i.e. those who are not on an equal footing. (Woolcock, 2001; National Statistics, 2003; Performance and Innovation Unit, 2002)

Fukuyama (1999) – writing from the perspective of an economist – provides an interesting interpretation of social capital. He notes that the usual definitions of social capital actually refer to *manifestations* of social capital rather than to its basic constructs. Thus, his (1999: 1–2) definition is as follows:

> social capital is an instantiated informal norm that promotes cooperation between two or more individuals. The norms that constitute social capital can range from a norm of reciprocity between two friends, all the way up to complex and elaborately articulated doctrines like Christianity or Confucianism. They must be instantiated in an actual human relationship: the norm of reciprocity exists *in potentia* in my dealings with all people, but is actualized only in my dealings with *my* friends. By this definition, trust, networks, civil society, and the like which have been associated with social capital are all epiphenomenal, arising as a result of social capital but not constituting social capital itself.

According to Fukuyama (1999: 2), the norms that constitute social capital are 'related to traditional virtues like honesty, the keeping of commitments, reliable performance of duties, reciprocity, and the like'. Notwithstanding the potential for cooperation, which can extend beyond the immediate group, social capital can have negative effects (just as 'physical capital can take the form of assault rifles or tasteless entertainment, human capital can be used to devise new ways of torturing people'). Moreover, a group's internal cohesion may be achieved by treating outsiders with suspicion, hostility or even hatred. According to the author, organizations such as the Ku Klux Klan and the Mafia, because they have shared norms and cooperate, actually have social capital, but they produce 'abundant negative externalities for the larger society'. 'Good' social capital results in 'positive externalities' – that is, it will be beneficial to external individuals and groups. Furthermore, if a group's social capital produces positive externalities, the 'radius of trust' will extend beyond the group itself. Fukuyama sees modern society as a series of overlapping radii of trust – from friends, family and cliques up to large organizations and religious groups. Small radii of trust and within-group solidarity reduce the capacity for cooperation with outsiders and may be typical of more traditional social groupings. C. Campbell et al. (1999: 97) refer to the warning by Pahl (1995) that:

romanticized views of past community life in England serve to conceal the fact that these idealized cohesive communities were often organized around socially exclusive and repressive hierarchies characterized by, among other things, greater repression of women.

The large variety of overlapping social groups in modern societies may make it easier to transmit information, have greater resources and be readier to innovate than was the case in the past. Fukuyama asserts that social capital is an important feature of modern economies and underpins modern liberal democracy.

There has been considerable recent interest in the notion of social capital as a means of improving health prospects and particularly as a response to the adverse effects of social exclusion, which we will discuss below. For example, Hyyppä and Mäki (2001) used the concept of social capital to account for differences in active life and mortality between groups in an area of Finland. The Swedish-speaking minority has a longer active life than the Finnish-speaking majority, yet the two groups have similar profiles of socio-demographic variables, socio-economic circumstances and availability of healthcare – and similar exposure to conventional risk factors. The better health prospects of the Swedish-speaking community were attributed to higher levels of social cohesion due to its small size, strong institutional network, cultural activity and geographic stability.

In France, Jusot et al. (2007) found an association between subjective perception of social capital (trust and civic engagement, social support, sense of control and self-esteem) and health. Sense of control at work was the major determinant, but civic engagement and social support were also important.

Social capital is viewed as a prerequisite for an active participating community. Gottlieb and McLeroy (1992) make related points in their examination of the meaning of social health, which for them includes social integration or involvement (quantity and quality of relationships), social support (functional content of relationships, such as emotional support) and social networks (the structure of relationships with other people within a social system).

Assessing levels of social capital is challenging because of the nebulous nature of the concept and its cultural sensitivity (Babb, 2005). C. Campbell et al. (1999) describe an exploratory qualitative study in the UK to assess the applicability of Putnam's conceptualization of social capital to the UK context as well as the variations in social capital between different communities with comparable socio-economic status but different health experiences. They conclude that:

- the social capital constructs of trust and civic engagement may be particularly relevant to health status
- sources of social capital may cross the geographically defined boundaries of communities
- some network types (diverse and geographically dispersed) might be more health-enhancing than others
- Putnam's typology of social networks needs to be expanded to include informal networks
- the provision of community facilities does not constitute social capital – the processes by which such facilities are established and run require consideration

- Putnam's notion of community cohesion should be reconsidered in the light of the high levels of mobility and plural nature of contemporary communities
- there are major differences within communities in the ways in which social capital is created, sustained and accessed.

Commonly used measures of social capital are the levels of civic participation and social trust (Cooper et al., 1999). For example, Kawachi (1997) reports high levels of trust being associated with both lower mortality rates and higher levels of reported good health in the United States. Furthermore, bowling league membership (used by Putnam (1995) as indicative of levels of social participation) also correlates with lower mortality rates.

Fukuyama (1999) distinguishes two broad approaches to measuring social capital:

- a census of the groups and group membership in a given society
- a survey of levels of trust and civic engagement.

Putnam, for example, draws on group membership (derived from the number of groups, bowling leagues, sports clubs, political groups and the membership of groups) as an indicator of the level of civic engagement and social capital in society. He is sceptical about the contribution of 'mailing list' organizations to social connectedness on the grounds that the members do not actually meet and their ties are to a common ideology rather than to each other (Putnam, 1996), and he is cautious about the impact of the Internet:

> I think strong social capital has to have a physical reality — a purely virtual tie is a pretty thin reed on which to build anything; it's highly vulnerable to anonymity and spoofing and very difficult to build trust. (Putnam interviewed by Bunting, 2007)

Nonetheless, the increased role of virtual communities in contemporary society is beginning to receive attention.

Fukuyama identifies a number of additional relevant variables:

- the internal cohesion of groups
- the radius of trust and the extent to which this encompasses the whole group plus or minus outsiders
- group affiliation and the extent to which this engenders distrust of outsiders.

Coulthard et al. (2002: 1) suggest that the main indicators of social capital are:

- social relationships and social support
- formal and informal social networks
- group memberships
- community and civic engagement
- norms and values
- reciprocal activities, such as childcare arrangements
- levels of trust in others.

Examples of some of the key variables are provided in the box.

Neighbourhood and community involvement

View of the local area:

- 87 per cent enjoyed living in the local area
- 60 per cent felt very safe walking during the daytime
- 33 per cent felt fairly safe walking during the daytime
- 26 per cent felt a bit unsafe or very unsafe walking after dark
- 20 per cent never went out alone after dark
- 15 per cent had been victims of crime in the last year.

Civic engagement:

- 59 per cent felt well informed about local affairs
- 56 per cent felt that communities could influence decisions in the area
- 26 per cent felt that they personally could influence decisions in the area
- 21 per cent were involved in a local organization
- 27 per cent had been involved in action to solve a local problem
- 18 per cent felt civically engaged
- 16 per cent were not civically engaged.

Neighbourliness:

- 27 per cent spoke to neighbours daily
- 19 per cent spoke to neighbours once a week
- 46 per cent knew most or many people in their neighbourhood
- 48 per cent knew a few people in their neighbourhood
- 6 per cent knew nobody
- 58 per cent felt that they could trust most or many people in their neighbourhood.

Social networks:

- 27 per cent spoke to relatives daily
- 82 per cent spoke to relatives at least once a week
- 30 per cent had at least five close friends living close by
- 27 per cent had no close friends living in their local area
- 44 per cent had no relatives they felt close to living close by
- 66 per cent had a satisfactory friendship network
- 52 per cent had a satisfactory relatives network
- 20 per cent had neither.

Social support:

- 97 per cent could get help if they were ill in bed
- 93 per cent could get a lift if they needed to be somewhere
- 86 per cent could borrow £100 if in financial difficulty
- 58 per cent had at least five people they could turn to in a serious personal crisis
- 18 per cent had at least three people they could turn to in a serious personal crisis
- 2 per cent had nobody.

Derived from Coulthard et al., 2002

Within the UK, there has been considerable interest in developing a harmonized approach to measuring social capital in official surveys. For this purpose, the definition adopted by National Statistics was: 'networks together with shared norms, values and understandings that facilitate cooperation within or among groups' (Cote and Healy, 2001, cited by Babb, 2005). The following five key constructs were identified and modules of questions developed for each (available at www.statistics. gov.uk/socialcapital):

- civic participation
- social networks and support
- social participation
- reciprocity and trust
- views about the local area.

However, it is acknowledged that cultural specificity and national characteristics may limit its use for international comparison (Babb, 2005). Furthermore, the way social capital has been conceptualized may fail fully or adequately to address the experience of specific groups such as young people who tend to have more informal social networks and less involvement in political and civic activity (Deviren and Babb, 2005).

INEQUALITY AND SOCIAL EXCLUSION

Exposure to a plethora of different determinants throughout the course of life will inevitably result in some variations in health experience. A central concern of health promotion – one that is driven by a vision of health as a basic human right, together with a commitment to the fundamental value of social justice – has been to reduce inequality in health, both within and between nations (see box for examples). There is a vast body of literature on inequality which addresses the key issues of social class, gender, ethnicity, age, disability and unemployment – many of which are interrelated and mediated through poverty and social exclusion. However, we will confine ourselves here to key definitional issues.

Selected key facts on health inequalities in England and Wales

- There are great differences in life expectancy, for example males in Blackpool have a life expectancy eight years less than males in Kensington and Chelsea.
- The incidence of lung cancer among men and women in the most deprived areas is around twice that in the most affluent areas, and death rates are about two and a half times higher.
- Infant mortality has fallen faster in higher social groups than in 'routine and manual' groups resulting in a widening of the relative health inequalities gap since 1997–99. However, the latest data for 2002–04 show no further widening.
- Babies born to mothers who live in Birmingham are over six times more likely to die in their first year of life than babies born to mothers in Eastleigh, Hants.

(Continued)

(Continued)

- In England and Wales, babies of mothers who were themselves born in Pakistan have a death rate that is almost double the overall infant mortality rate.
- Women in routine and semi-routine occupations are one and a half times as likely to be obese as women in managerial and professional occupations.
- In England, the proportion of Bangladeshi men who smoke is over 60 per cent higher than the national average, and the proportion of Indian men who smoke is 20 per cent lower.

Derived from Department of Health, 2006b

While some variation in health experience is unavoidable, much of it can be attributed to unequal opportunities – that is, social inequality. The use of the term 'equity' introduces greater precision here. Whitehead (1990: 5) makes the important distinction between *inequality*, which can simply apply to any variation, and *inequity*, which is applied to variations deemed to be both avoidable and unjust:

> The term 'inequity' has a moral and ethical dimension. It refers to differences which are unnecessary and avoidable but, in addition, are also considered unfair and unjust. So, in order to describe a certain situation as inequitable, the cause has to be examined and judged to be unfair in the context of what is going on in the rest of society.

The box below provides a simple checklist for assessing which differences in health are inequitable. However, in many industrialized countries, the term 'inequalities in health' is often taken to be synonymous with inequity (Leon et al., 2001).

Which health differences are inequitable?

Determinant of differentials	Potentially avoidable?	Commonly viewed as unacceptable?
Natural biological variation	No	No
Health-damaging behaviour if freely chosen	Yes	No
Transient health advantage of groups who take up health-promoting behaviour first (if other groups can easily catch up)	Yes	No
Health-damaging behaviour where choice of lifestyle is restricted by socio-economic factors	Yes	Yes

(Continued)

(Continued)

Exposure to excessive health hazards in the physical and social environment	Yes	Yes
Restricted access to essential healthcare	Yes	Yes
Health-related downward social mobility (sick people move down social scale)	Low income – yes	Low income – yes

Whitehead, 1992: 4

There is considerable evidence that social class is a key determinant of health status. Within the UK, such evidence has accumulated throughout the twentieth century – from the early work of Rowntree at its dawn to the Acheson report (1998) at its close (see Table 2.5).

Table 2.5   All cause death rate[1]: by social class and sex in England and Wales (Rate per 100,000 people)

	1986–92	1993–96	1997–99
Males			
Professional, managerial & technical	460	379	347
Skilled non-manual	480	437	417
Skilled manual	617	538	512
Skilled, semi-skilled & unskilled manual	776	648	606
Non-manual	466	396	371
Manual	674	577	546
Females			
Professional, managerial & technical	274	262	237
Skilled non-manual	310	262	253
Skilled manual	350	324	327
Skilled, semi-skilled & unskilled manual	422	378	335
Non-manual	289	257	246
Manual	379	344	330

[1] Data have been directly age standardized using the European standard population.
Source: Babb et al., 2004: 82

Social class has typically been measured as occupational class. The main government classification system – the social class based on occupation (Registrar General's Social Class) – was based on grouping occupations according to the levels of skill involved. Using this system, the population could be divided into six classes, as shown in the box below. This broad pattern of categorization was introduced in 1921 and, apart from subdividing class III into manual and non-manual in 1971, has remained substantially unchanged.

A new social classification system was introduced in 2001 to reflect the changing patterns of work – the National Statistics Socio-economic Classification (NS-SEC) – see the box. Although still based on occupation, it focuses on employment conditions and, particularly, the amount of control people have over their own and other people's work rather than on skill. It also includes a category for the long-term unemployed and those who have never had paid work.

Socio-economic classifications

Social class based on occupation

I   Professional occupations
II   Managerial and technical occupations
III Skilled occupations:
     (N) non-manual
     (M) manual
IV   Partly skilled occupations
V   Unskilled occupations

National Statistics Socio-economic Classification (NS-SEC)

1	Higher managerial and professional occupations	
1.1	Large employers and higher managerial occupations	Professional and managerial
1.2	Higher professional occupations	
2	Lower managerial and professional occupations	
3	Intermediate occupations	Intermediate
4	Small employers and own account workers	
5	Lower supervisory and technical occupations	Routine and manual
6	Semi-routine occupations	
7	Routine occupations	
8	Never worked and long-term unemployed	

Derived from National Statistics, 2007 and Babb et al., 2004

Much of the evidence on health inequality is based on occupational class. However, there has been some debate about its relevance for groups such as women, the unemployed, the elderly and children, and concern that occupational class may not fully reflect their circumstances. For example, married women have often been classified by their husband's occupation. This conceals their own employment status and may fail to fully recognize the effects of paid employment and working conditions on women's health. It also overlooks their contribution to the family's standard of living (Whitehead, 1987). Sacker et al. (2000) note that, using the NS-SEC, occupational class emerged as the most important influence on mortality for men, but was less sensitive to variation in mortality for women, even when allocated by their own occupation.

A further issue concerns what occupational class actually measures. Family members are usually classed according to the occupation of the head of the household and, although they may not be directly exposed to occupation-linked factors, share the variation in health associated with social class – childhood injuries, for example, show a marked social gradient (Roberts and Power, 1996). Occupational class, therefore, clearly encompasses a whole constellation of factors over and above different occupational conditions. These would include levels of income, housing, area of residence, education and lifestyle. Nichols (1979) also notes that occupational class incorporates a cultural element and reflects status within the community. The landmark Black Report analysed possible explanations for variation in health status with social class and concluded that, although genetic and cultural factors might make some contribution, the major underlying factor was material inequality and deprivation (Department of Health and Social Security, 1980).

Income has frequently been identified as a key determinant of social variation in mortality. Dorling et al. (2007) distinguish different levels of income (see box). They note that over the last 15 years there are more poor households in Britain, but fewer very poor and that there has been increased polarization between areas – wealthy areas have become wealthier and poor areas poorer.

Levels of income

- *Core poor*: people who are income poor, materially deprived and subjectively poor.
- *Breadline poor*: people living below a relative poverty line, and as such excluded from participating in the norms of society.
- *Non-poor, non-wealthy*: the remainder of the population classified as neither poor nor wealthy.
- *Asset wealthy*: estimated using the relationship between housing wealth and the contemporary Inheritance Tax threshold.
- *Exclusive wealthy*: people with sufficient wealth to exclude themselves from the norms of society.

Dorling et al., 2007

Absolute and relative poverty

Poverty influences physical health as it limits access to good-quality nutrition and housing, but also has an effect on mental health (Shaw et al., 1999). Yet, against a backdrop of overall improvement in general prosperity and health status, differentials seem to be widening – a pattern not untypical of industrialized nations. A key factor would seem to be income inequality (Davey Smith, 1996). Indeed, Wilkinson (1994) states that life expectancy has increased most in industrialized nations where income differences have narrowed and mortality is more closely related to income inequality *within* countries than absolute differences in income *between* countries (Wilkinson, 1997).

This raises the issue of absolute and relative poverty. *Absolute* poverty exists when insufficient resources are available to provide the basic essentials of life, such as food and shelter. The World Bank, for example, has used the notional 1 dollar per day as an absolute minimum survival budget. However, this measure of extreme poverty has little meaning in the context of advanced industrialized societies. Some countries, such as the United States, have defined an official poverty line based on the cost of a basic food basket. The Canadian Council on Social Development (2001) provides an analysis of different ways of defining poverty and notes the debate over which items should be regarded as necessities. A key issue concerns whether a poverty line should be set in relation to a basic survival budget or a level of income that would enable people to participate in society.

Relative poverty, in contrast, involves comparing individuals or groups with some notional norm (Calman, 1997) and focuses on comparative conditions of living.

> Adam Smith himself closely embraced a relative definition of poverty, arguing that to be poor was to have to go without what was needed to be a 'creditable' member of society. (Canadian Council on Social Development, 2001)

An article by Frank (2000) in the *New York Times Magazine* drew attention to the importance of relative poverty/affluence in people's lives:

> Consider a choice between the two scenarios:
>
> World A: You earn $110,000 per year and others earn $200,000.
>
> World B: You earn $100,000 per year and others earn $85,000.
>
> The figures for income represent real purchasing power. Although in absolute terms individuals would be better off in Scenario A, a majority of Americans chose Scenario B.

There are several different ways of establishing relative poverty levels – for example, the proportion of income needed to cover the basic necessities of life, the proportional relationship to the median income and measures based on 'market baskets', which would include items in line with community norms. The South East Public Health Observatory has developed an online tool that provides support in relation to methodologies for assessing inequality and deprivation (Carr-Hill and Chalmers-Dixon-, 2005).

A national survey of poverty and social exclusion in Britain published by the Joseph Rowntree Foundation (Gordon et al., 2000) used a variety of measures of poverty. These included not being able to afford what are generally perceived to be 'necessities'. The box gives a list of items that over 75 per cent of the adult population regard as necessities. It is clear that the interpretation of what constitutes a necessity goes beyond the basic survival needs of subsistence diet, shelter, clothing and fuel to include participating in social customs, fulfilling obligations and taking part in activities.

Items perceived as necessities

Item	% considering item 'necessary'
Beds and bedding for everyone	95
Heating to warm living areas of the home	94
Damp-free home	93
Visiting friends or family in hospital	92
Two meals a day	91
Medicines prescribed by doctor	90
Refrigerator	89
Fresh fruit and vegetables daily	86
Warm, waterproof coat	85
Replace or repair broken electrical goods	85
Visits to friends or family	84
Celebrations on special occasions such as Christmas	83
Money to keep home in decent state of decoration	82
Visits to school, such as sports day	81
Attending weddings, funerals	80
Meat, fish or vegetarian equivalent every other day	79
Insurance of contents of dwelling	79
Hobby or leisure activity	78
Washing machine	76
Collecting children from school	75

Derived from Joseph Rowntree Foundation, 2000

There has been no tradition of routinely collecting official data on poverty in the UK – partly due to the difficulties of defining levels of poverty. The receipt of social security benefits has been used as a proxy indicator. However, there have been moves to redress this (for a detailed discussion, see Kerrison and Macfarlane, 2000). Since 1999, the Department for Work and Pensions has reported annually on progress in relation to tackling poverty and social exclusion using a series of indicators, including income, organized around stages of the lifecycle (see, for example, Department for Work and Pensions, 2007b). The New Policy Institute also reports regularly on a series of 50 indicators of poverty and social exclusion. Setting a level for income poverty is challenging not only in an absolute sense, but also in terms of whether this is done at the individual or family level and before or after considering housing costs. The New Policy Institute (undated) has set out a number of principles for choosing low income thresholds. It supports:

- using household rather than individual income
- a main threshold related to changes in levels of income
- having fixed as well as relative thresholds to provide a fuller picture
- monitoring persistency of low income
- considering income after making allowance for housing costs because of considerable regional variation
- the widely accepted primary threshold of income poverty as 60 per cent of median income.

The Joseph Rowntree Foundation has attempted to develop a Minimum Income Standard for Britain. This goes further than thresholds based on relative income, measures of deprivation or budget standards calculated on baskets of goods and services to establish a level of income which is sufficient to support 'having what you need in order to have the opportunities and choices necessary to participate in society' (2008: 1).

The UNDP, recognizing the complex relationship between economic indicators such as per capita income and human wellbeing, uses the Human Development Index (HDI) for international comparison. This incorporates three dimensions of human development: 'living a long and healthy life (measured by life expectancy), being educated (measured by adult literacy and enrolment at the primary, secondary and tertiary level) and having a decent standard of living (measured by purchasing power parity (PPP) income)' (UNDP, 2008) (see box).

Human Development Index

For illustration, Table 2.6 shows the overall Human Development Index (HDI) and its three components for Gambia. The number of the country indicates its position in the ranking of all countries for which there is data and this ranges from 1 to 177. The HDI for Gambia is 0.502, which gives the country an overall rank of 155 although it ranks higher at 138 for life expectancy. For comparative purposes, the two countries above and below for each dimension are also identified in the table along with the highest and lowest ranking countries.

Table 2.6   Human development indices

HDI value	Life expectancy at birth (years)	Combined primary, secondary and tertiary gross enrolment ratio (%)	GDP per capita (PPP US$)
1. Iceland (0.968)	1. Japan (82.3)	1. Australia (113.0) (60,228)	1. Luxembourg (60,228)
153. Yemen (0.508)	136. Haiti (59.5)	147. Benin (50.7)	142. Comoros (1,993)
154. Uganda (0.505)	137. Ghana (59.1)	148. Tanzania (United Republic of) (50.4)	143. Kyrgyzstan (1,927)
155. Gambia (0.502)	138. Gambia (58.8)	149. Gambia (50.1)	144. Gambia (1,921)
156. Senegal (0.499)	139. Madagascar (58.4)	150. Myanmar (49.5)	145. Senegal (1,792)
157. Eritrea (0.483)	140. Cambodia (58.0)	151. Solomon Islands (47.6)	146. Haiti (1,663)
177. Sierra Leone (0.336)	177. Zambia (40.5)	172. Niger (22.7)	174. Malawi (667)

Source: UNDP, 2008

Whereas absolute poverty is a central issue in the developing world, poverty in urban, industrialized countries has been defined (Supplementary Benefits Commission, 1979, cited in Dahlgren and Whitehead, 1991) as:

> a standard of living so low that it excludes and isolates people from the rest of the community. To keep out of poverty they must have an income which enables them to participate in the life of the community.

This definition focuses attention on social exclusion, which is currently receiving considerable attention. The concept of social exclusion encompasses material deprivation and relative poverty, but also includes the process of marginalization of some individuals and groups from social and community life (Shaw et al., 1999). This process is not solely restricted to economic factors, but would also include other forms of cultural and social discrimination. Major groups of socially excluded people are the unemployed, ethnic minorities, refugees, the elderly, lone parents and their children and those, especially children, with disability.

A report by the Terence Higgins Trust (2001) notes that the groups primarily affected by HIV in the UK are those marginalized or socially excluded by society. They attribute this to low self-esteem among those excluded, which is associated with risk-taking and social exclusion, making sexual health a low priority. Furthermore, people with HIV may experience further exclusion on account of their HIV status and this may influence the way in which they access appropriate care.

Clearly, social exclusion exerts a powerful psycho-social influence and there are obvious links with the notion of social capital. Kawachi (1997) demonstrates lower levels of social trust in states with a higher 'Robin Hood Index' – a measure of income inequality based on the proportion of aggregate income that would have to be redistributed to level up earnings. Similar findings are obtained for participation in voluntary associations. However, Lynch et al.'s (2000) analysis of income inequality and mortality cautions against an exclusive emphasis on psycho-social effects and the lack of social cohesion, which, they allege, is akin to victim-blaming at the community level. They propose that the main causes of health inequality are material – including access to both private and social resources, such as education, healthcare, social welfare and work. Raphael's (2001a: 30) analysis of social inequality and heart disease in Canada provides a concise summary of the interaction between these various elements.

> Social exclusion is a process by which people are denied the opportunity to participate in civil society; denied an acceptable supply of goods or services; are unable to contribute to society, and are unable to acquire the normal commodities expected of citizens. All of these elements occur in tandem with material deprivation, excessive psycho-social stress, and adoption of health-threatening behaviours shown to be related to the onset of, and death from, cardiovascular disease.

Composite indicators of deprivation

The concept of deprivation can apply both to individuals and areas and includes material and social elements (Krieger, 2001). There is some evidence that, independently of an individual's level of deprivation, living in a deprived area has an adverse effect on health (Shaw et al., 1999).

There are composite indicators of deprivation that can be used to assess the overall levels of deprivation within different areas. The Jarman and Townsend indices have been used widely in the UK and draw on census data (see the box). The Jarman index has been much criticized – both on account of its method of construction and also because it is biased towards classifying areas in London as being deprived rather than those in the North (Talbot, 1991). This has been attributed to the skewed distribution of single-parent families and highly mobile populations, for example, which tend to be more concentrated in the inner London area.

The Jarman and Townsend Indices of Deprivation

Jarman underprivileged area score (UPA)

Derived from GPs' views about factors that influence their workload.

- Percentage of children under five
- Percentage of unemployment
- Percentage of ethnic minorities
- Percentage of single-parent households
- Percentage of elderly living alone
- Overcrowding factor
- Percentage of lower social classes
- Percentage of highly mobile people
- Percentage of unmarried couple families
- Poor housing factor

The above ten items were originally included in the Jarman UPA score, but the last two are omitted from the Jarman UPA8 score.

Townsend combined deprivation indicator

- Percentage of economically active residents aged 16–59/64 who are unemployed
- Percentage of private households that do not possess a car
- Percentage of private households that are not owner occupied
- Percentage of private households with more than one person per room

Derived from Whitehead, 1987

Attempts to measure levels of deprivation on a large geographic scale often obscure smaller pockets of deprivation. There is considerable interest, therefore, in small area analysis. The Department of the Environment, Transport and Regions (DETR) developed an Index of Multiple Deprivation (DETR, 2000) later updated by the Neighbourhood Renewal Unit to include seven different domains (NRU, 2004):

- income deprivation
- employment
- health deprivation and disability
- education, skills and training deprivation
- barriers to housing and services

- crime
- living environment and deprivation.

Each domain is assessed using a series of indicators and the weighted domains are combined to produce an overall index of multiple deprivation for each electoral ward.

Carr-Hill and Chalmers-Dixon (2002) emphasize that these various indices are artificial constructs and only partial or proxy measures of phenomena such as deprivation. They caution against reification, which can occur when operational constructs used as approximate measures become substituted for the actual meaning of the concepts they purport to measure. While their argument focuses on the measurement of deprivation, it would apply equally to other indicators of health status.

Childhood poverty

Childhood poverty, particularly when persistent over a number of years, is of concern not only because of its immediate effects on this vulnerable group but also because of longer-term effects and its contribution to sustaining cycles of deprivation. Within the UK, the government had pledged to reduce child poverty by half by 2010 and eliminate it by 2020. Nonetheless, in 2005–06, 2.8 million children (22 per cent of all children) were in households with an income below the poverty threshold of 60 per cent median income before deduction of housing costs and 3.8 million (30 per cent of all children) after deduction of housing costs (Child Poverty Action Group, 2007; Department for Work and Pensions, 2007a).

International comparison clearly presents challenges in terms of selection and comparability of indicators. UNICEF's (2007b) comparison of children's material wellbeing among 21 industrialized nations (see box for indicators used) ranked Sweden the highest and Poland the lowest, with the UK in 18th place. The report provided a more comprehensive assessment of young people's wellbeing by including a number of other relevant dimensions – health and safety, educational wellbeing, family and peer relationships, behaviours and risks and subjective wellbeing (see Table 2.7).

Material wellbeing

Components	Indicators
Relative income poverty	– percentage of children living in homes with equivalent incomes below 50% of the national median
Households without jobs	– percentage of children in families without an employed adult
Reported deprivation	– percentage of children reporting low family affluence – percentage of children reporting few educational resources – percentage of children reporting fewer than 10 books in the home

UNICEF, 2007b

Table 2.7 Comparison of children's wellbeing

Dimensions of child well being	Average ranking position (for all 6 dimensions)	Material wellbeing	Health and safety	Educational wellbeing	Family and peer relationships	Behaviors and risks	Subjective wellbeing
Netherlands	4.2	10	2	6	3	3	1
Sweden	5.0	1	1	5	15	1	7
Denmark	7.2	4	4	8	9	6	12
Finland	7.5	3	3	4	17	7	11
Spain	8.0	12	6	15	8	5	2
Switzerland	8.3	5	9	14	4	12	6
Norway	8.7	2	8	11	10	13	8
Italy	10.0	14	5	20	1	10	10
Ireland	10.2	19	19	7	7	4	5
Belgium	10.7	7	16	1	5	19	16
Germany	11.2	13	11	10	13	11	9
Canada	11.8	6	13	2	18	17	15
Greece	11.8	15	18	16	11	8	3
Poland	12.3	21	15	3	14	2	19
Czech Republic	12.5	11	10	9	19	9	17
France	13.0	9	7	18	12	14	18
Portugal	13.7	16	14	21	2	15	14
Austria	13.8	8	20	19	16	16	4
Hungary	14.5	20	17	13	6	18	13
United States	18.0	17	21	12	20	20	–
United Kingdom	18.2	18	12	17	21	21	20

Source: UNICEF, 2007b: 2

Tackling inequality

Measuring inequality within and between nations is not an abstract exercise, but serves to expose social injustice and highlight the need for action (see, for example, Acheson, 1998). Marmot (2005: 1099) drew attention to the inequitable 'spread of life expectancy of 48 years among countries and 20 years or more within countries' in his call for political action to address inequality. The need to measure and understand the problem was recognized in the priorities for action set out in the final report of the Commission on Social Determinants of Health (CSDH, 2008) – see box.

Principles of action for closing the health gap

1 Improve the conditions of daily life – the circumstances in which people are born, grow, live, work and age.
2 Tackle the inequitable distribution of power, money and resources – the structural drivers of those conditions of daily life – globally, nationally and locally.

(Continued)

Health Promotion

THE CONTR

It is axiom
of the cu
consid
Ra
in

110

(Continued)

3 Measure the problem, evaluate action, ex
  workforce that is trained in the social de
  awareness about the social determinants

An effective policy response clearly de
While the extreme effect of poverty and
emphasizes the importance of underst
inequalities – which he refers to as the
(2008) notes the need to tackle the unequal distri
resources.

Looking at inequality within countries, Wilkinson and Marmot (2003) iden
following key areas:

- the social gradient
- stress
- early life
- social exclusion
- work
- unemployment
- social support
- addiction
- food
- transport.

Graham and Kelly (2004: 1) also recognize a 'number of axes of social differentiation' over and above social class. These include ethnicity, gender, sexuality, age, area, community and religion which are mediated by dimensions such as socio-economic disadvantage and discrimination. They propose *social position* as the lynchpin in the causal chain of factors affecting health status through its influence on access to societal resources as well as exposure to risk. They emphasize the distinction between the determinants of health and determinants of health inequality.

The fact that the overall health status is improving in industrialized countries such as the UK yet inequalities persist – or even increase – raises fundamental questions about the relationship between efforts to improve health and efforts to tackle health inequality. There are two broad options for tackling inequality (Graham and Kelly, 2004):

- focusing on the poorest and most socially excluded who experience poorest health
- recognizing the whole social gradient, including those who could not be regarded as socially excluded, yet are still disadvantaged in health terms because of their social position.

Clearly, to be effective, any efforts must be based on an understanding of the *unequal distribution* of the determinants of health.

...tic that planning interventions to promote health requires understanding ...rent health status of populations and the factors that influence it. We have ...red different approaches to assessing health and its determinants.

...ther than engage in sterile debate about the relative superiority of biomedical or ...erpretivist approaches, we would contend that they offer complementary insights. ...ension arises from the unequal power positions of those subscribing to different methodologies and the dominance of biomedicine. This has been challenged from both professional and lay quarters. In that health is essentially a subjective experience, the lay perspective is particularly relevant. Furthermore, understanding a complex multidimensional concept such as health necessarily needs to draw on multiple perspectives – including salutogenic as well as pathogenic perspectives.

The emergence of health promotion as a discipline placed emphasis on environmental influences on health – both directly and in terms of shaping behaviour and lifestyle. Notwithstanding the debate about the primacy of agency or structure, it is clear that there is a reciprocal relationship between the two elements. The complexity of the interrelationship has become more evident as our conceptualization of the environment has broadened. While the contribution of social and socio-economic aspects of the environment has been recognized for some time, the recent resurgence in interest in social capital focuses attention on social connectedness and opportunities for civic engagement.

The measurement of health and quality of life and their determinants is undoubtedly challenging. To conclude this chapter, we should note that the capacity to assess the health of communities and identify key determinants underpins rational planning processes. Clearly, the way such assessment is approached should reflect the ideology and values of health promotion and pay particular attention to factors associated with health inequalities.

KEY POINTS

○ Measuring health and its determinants is of fundamental importance to efforts to improve health.

○ Epidemiological measures contribute to our understanding of health and its determinants – particularly in relation to mortality and morbidity.

○ Multiple perspectives, including the lay perspective, are needed for a more complete understanding of health, including positive wellbeing.

○ Salutogenic explanations of health should be considered as well as pathogenic.

○ Both environment and lifestyle factors influence health and are themselves interrelated.

○ Social aspects of the environment, including social connectedness and social capital, have an impact on health status.

○ Poverty and material deprivation are major causes of health inequality.

○ Understanding the wider social determinants of health inequality and social exclusion are of central importance in developing initiatives to tackle inequality.

3

THE DETERMINANTS OF HEALTH ACTIONS

The truth is rarely pure and never simple.

Oscar Wilde (1854–1900), *The Importance of Being Ernest*

OVERVIEW

The purpose of this chapter is to consider the factors that influence the adoption of health-related behaviour. More specifically, it will:

- consider the factors influencing the adoption of health behaviours at the community level
- identify the major influences on individual health decisions using the Health Action Model as a framework
- examine the factors which affect whether health intentions are put into practice
- analyse those factors which contribute to control and empowerment.

INTRODUCTION

The emphasis of this chapter is on understanding at the individual, or micro, level how various factors interplay to influence behaviour by drawing on explanatory theory. Given the central importance of empowerment to health promotion, particular attention will be given to the dynamics of empowerment. These various influences on individuals are nested within, and are themselves the product of, meso- and macro-level social systems. Detailed discussion of social change is beyond the scope of this chapter. However, we will begin by locating our discussion of individual change in the context of the adoption of innovations within social systems using a theoretical analysis that has been frequently applied to the adoption of health innovations – Diffusion of Innovations Theory.

THE ADOPTION OF INNOVATIONS WITHIN SOCIAL SYSTEMS

Diffusion of Innovations Theory

Diffusion of Innovations Theory was originally known as Communication of Innovations Theory (Rogers and Shoemaker, 1971) and has subsequently been developed and regularly updated. The latest version was published in 2003 (Rogers, 2003). Diffusion theory is concerned with the factors relating to the adoption of innovations within social systems. An 'innovation' is defined as 'an idea, practice or object perceived as new by an individual or other unit of adoption' (Rogers, 2003: 12). The theory can be applied to organizations as well as individuals, but for the purpose of this chapter we will focus on the latter. Adoption is 'the decision to make full use of the innovation as the best course of action available' (Rogers, 1995: 21). The core principle of the theory is that the adoption of innovations by individuals within a relatively fixed social system follows a consistent pattern. There is a slow initial rate of adoption, the *lag* phase. The process then gathers momentum (*take-off* phase) to involve the majority and then tails off as *saturation* is reached. Cumulative adoption therefore follows an S-shaped curve as shown in Figure 3.1.

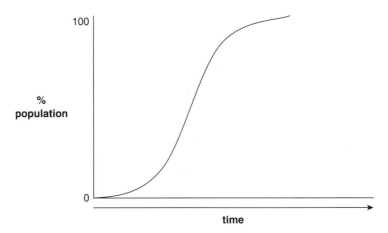

Figure 3.1   The classic 'S' shaped curve

The overall shape remains the same regardless of the intervention. However, the gradient of the slope will be steeper for innovations that are relatively 'attractive' and taken up rapidly. The various adopter categories and their typical characteristics are:

Initiators (2.5%)	venturesome
Early adopters (13.5%)	opinion leaders, successful, respected within their social circle
Early majority (34%)	deliberate before adopting new ideas
Late majority (34%)	cautious and sceptical
Laggards (16%)	traditional

It is estimated that when between ten and twenty per cent are involved, a 'critical mass' is reached when diffusion becomes self-sustaining through social networks.

The theory identifies the pathway leading to adoption. Initial *awareness* is followed by *interest* and seeking more information. Then *evaluation* involves mentally applying the intervention and deciding whether or not to try out. This may lead to a *trial* involving full use of the innovation and the ultimate decision about whether to continue, i.e. *adoption*.

The innovation–decision process itself has five stages (Rogers, 2003):

1 Knowledge — development of awareness and understanding
2 Persuasion — the formation of an attitude to the innovation
3 Decision — engagement in activities leading to choice, possibly including trying out the innovation
4 Implementation — putting the innovation into practice
5 Confirmation — reinforcement based on experience of the outcomes.

From a health promotion perspective, identifying the factors associated with the uptake of practices conducive to health is essential for effective programme planning. Furthermore, attention also needs to be given to the final stage if initial adoption is to be sustained. The classical diffusion model identifies four key elements associated with uptake:

- the characteristics of the innovation
- communication channels
- time
- the social system.

The characteristics of the innovation

It is well recognized, and indeed common sense, that people's perceptions about the nature and implications of the innovation they are being asked to adopt will be a highly significant factor in determining whether or not they are willing to try it out. Adoption is influenced by the following key features:

- relative advantage – offered by the innovation compared with current practice
- compatibility – with values, previous experience and current needs
- complexity – the extent to which the innovation is felt to be difficult to understand or implement
- trialability – the possibility of testing out before making a more permanent commitment
- observability – the extent to which the results are visible to others.

Communication channels

According to Rogers (2003), the main elements of the communication process are held to be the innovation, an individual (or unit) that knows about the innovation or has experience of it, an individual (or unit) without such knowledge and a channel of communication between the two. It might be assumed that communities having extensive and sophisticated mass media would be inclined to change more rapidly than those without (witness, for instance, the inroads made by global marketing and the appearance of Coca-Cola and McDonalds in the most unlikely places!). Certainly, mass media offer potential as the most rapid means of creating awareness, but, on the other hand, interpersonal influence is known to be more effective in changing attitudes and developing skills.

The role of the change agent is of importance to the diffusion process. Change agents frequently differ from the population in general because of greater technical competence and other characteristics such as education and social status, i.e. they are heterophilous. Leadership characteristics will parallel our earlier comments on power in Chapter 1 and, in particular, French and Raven's (1959) analysis on page (40). They also relate to the notion of credibility of the source, to which further reference will be made in later discussions about attitude change theory.

The powerful principle of 'homophily' suggests that people are more likely to be influenced by those with whom they identify. Rogers and Shoemaker (1971: 14) define it as follows:

> Homophily is the degree to which pairs of individuals who interact are similar in certain attributes, such as beliefs, values, education, social status and the like. A further refinement of this proposition includes the concept of empathy ... the ability of an individual to project himself into the role of another.

Rogers (2003) notes that individuals depend to a great extent on the experience of 'near peers' in making decisions and that this is at the heart of the diffusion process. Ideally, then, change agents would collaborate with opinion leaders, who share characteristics more closely with the community and act as referents and models.

Time

The time factor is an important element of the diffusion process and reflected in the relative steepness of the diffusion curve. Rogers (2003) specifies its relevance to three areas: the innovation–decision process, the innovativeness of the individual and the rate of adoption within the system. The level of innovativeness will vary between the various adopter categories identified above – indeed it is the basis of their classification. Innovators, for example, will be quick to adopt and can cope with higher levels of uncertainty about the innovation. At an aggregate level, however, the rate of adoption is concerned with the proportion of individuals in a social system who take up the innovation.

The social system

The social system influences diffusion in a number of ways – first through the type of relationships including both the more formal elements of social structure and the informal (and more homophilous) interpersonal relationships; and, secondly, through the norms and level of resistance to new ideas. Rogers (2003) notes that the most innovative members of a social system may be perceived as 'deviant' and therefore have limited capacity to influence others. Opinion leaders on the other hand are, by definition, accepted and respected.

> The most striking characteristic of opinion leaders is their unique and influential position in their system's communication structure: they are at the center of inter-personal communication networks. (Rogers, 2003: 30)

Typically, they are more exposed than their peers to external communication, have higher socio-economic status and tend to be more innovative.

A further factor in the adoption of an innovation is of especial importance – not least because of its centrality to the ideological commitments of health promotion. In short, it concerns the extent to which the community is involved in defining its own needs (a point to which we will return in the context of needs assessment) and in identifying ways of meeting those needs. Figure 3.2 sets out the relationship between this degree of participation and the anticipated rate of adoption of a given innovation.

Further explication of the application of diffusion of innovations theory and, indeed, other models of social system change is beyond the scope of this chapter (for more information, see Parcel et al., 1990; Goodman et al., 1997; Oldenburg et al., 1997; and Bartholomew et al., 2001). Our concern now is to shift focus from the macro to the micro level, to examine influences on individual health actions.

Level of community participation	Anticipated rate of adoption of the innovation
Community spontaneously recognizes it has a problem Community identifies solution to problem	Very rapid change
External agency considers that community has a problem External agency prescribes solution	Very slow – or never!

Figure 3.2 Participation by rate of adoption

CHANGE AT THE INDIVIDUAL LEVEL – INFLUENCES ON INDIVIDUAL HEALTH INTENTIONS

A thorough understanding of broader social and environmental influences on health and illness-related behaviours is, of course, essential. However, in the last analysis, it is individuals who make decisions and the sum total of their decision making that ultimately determines social action. For instance, why exactly might people be motivated to adopt an innovation once they have become aware of its existence? What does it mean when we say that adoption is influenced by people's perceptions of the innovation's characteristics? Are we really talking about perceptions or would 'beliefs' be a more accurate description? What are the psycho-social dynamics involved in an individual ultimately making a decision to adopt and then either maintain the new practice or reject it?

It is the purpose of this next part of the chapter to provide a detailed examination of the various psychological, social and environmental determinants of health or illness-related choices and behaviour.

The Health Action Model

A plethora of models and theories is available to those wishing to understand individual decision making. While they have many features in common – even though the terminology may differ – they vary in emphasis and their own particular orientations. Many were developed for general use, but have been found to have special relevance for health behaviour, while others were constructed with health education, health promotion and public health in mind. They include:

- the health belief model
- the theory of reasoned action
- the theory of planned behaviour
- the transtheoretical model of change
- the social learning theory
- the protection motivation theory.

(For further details, see Bennett and Murphy, 1997; Nutbeam and Harris, 2004; Conner and Norman, 2005.) A number of texts on patient education also utilize a psychological approach (for example, Rankin and Stallings, 2001).

It is not possible here to review all the models listed above. Accordingly, one particular model will be used to identify the constructs that are central to understanding health and illness-related behaviour and particularly relevant to planning health promotion programmes. The model in question is the 'health action model' (HAM) which was initially devised by Tones in the early 1970s to provide a theoretical base for the emerging specialist professional practice of health education (Tones, 1979, 1981). It was subsequently modified to take account of the shift in emphasis that took place with the emergence of health promotion (with its emphasis on healthy public policy and related macro influences). As will be apparent, it draws eclectically, pragmatically (and unashamedly!) on a number of key models and theories. It is reproduced as Figure 3.3. The health action model (HAM) identifies key psychological, social and environmental influences on individuals adopting and sustaining health- or illness-related actions. It comprises two major sections – the systems that contribute to 'behavioural intention' and the factors that determine the likelihood of that behavioural intention being translated into practice.

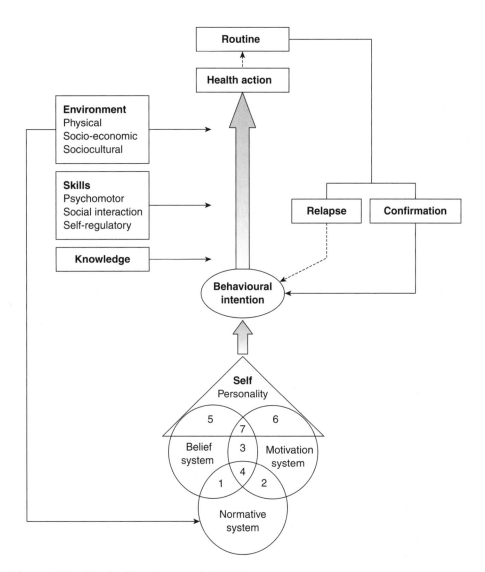

Figure 3.3   The health action model (HAM)

In short, four interacting systems – concerned with beliefs, motivation, normative influences and the self – all determine the likelihood of an individual developing an *intention* to adopt a particular course of health- or illness-related action. Whether this happens or not will depend on a number of enabling or facilitating factors, including the knowledge and skills necessary to adopt the health action. Of special importance – as should now be apparent – is the availability of a supportive environment that 'makes the healthy choice the easy choice'. An alternative way of expressing the importance of these enabling factors is to assert that health promotion is charged with removing those psychological, behavioural and environmental barriers that militate against people making healthy choices.

The health actions in question may include actions related to positive health outcomes and/or actions designed to prevent disease. In both cases, the actions are not necessarily confined to individual health, but may also contribute to the health of the community – for instance, by empowering individuals to undertake political actions that contribute to healthy public policy. HAM acknowledges the difference between single time, discrete health actions and routines. A discrete health action might be involved when, for example, only one visit is necessary to a clinic to have a child immunized or a potential political activist writes a letter of complaint to a Member of Parliament. Usually, though, benefits only accrue when health actions become part of a routine – for instance, when individuals routinely build exercise into their lifestyle or the political activist continues to stir up public indignation at breaches of human rights.

When a single-time choice has been made or, more commonly, when a routine has been established, two outcomes are possible. The first is that the health action in question is not problematical and results in confirmation of the behavioural intention. Alternatively, the innovation may be rejected and the individual relapses. The notion of relapse is traditionally associated with addictive or quasi-addictive behaviour, such as giving up smoking or other drugs. However, it could equally be applied to those actions that involve discomfort or inconvenience. The transtheoretical model, which we will consider more fully later, is especially concerned with questions of maintenance and relapse. Usefully, it notes how those who initially relapse will frequently try again (and even again and again!) before finally being confirmed in a healthy way of life (Prochaska and DiClimente, 1984; Prochaska et al., 1997).

The belief system

The K-A-P formula   One of the simplest attempts to explain the adoption of partic-ular behaviour is encapsulated in the K-A-P 'formula'. It is based on the reasonable assertion that knowledge alone does not lead to behaviour – it is usually necessary, but rarely sufficient. Accordingly, the provision of knowledge (K) has to be supple-mented by persuasive techniques designed to bring about a change in attitude(s) (A) before the target person or population will adopt appropriate practices (P).

The model is, of course, amazingly naïve, but so-called KAP surveys are still in evidence. They might, for example, ask about the sexual practices of a community, check whether sexually active people are aware of associated risks, for example in relation to HIV/AIDS, and ascertain their attitudes to unsafe or safer sexual practices.

As will be apparent from Figure 3.3, a much more sophisticated analysis involving a constellation of constructs is necessary if behaviour is to be understood and influenced. One of the most important of these is the concept of belief, which in HAM is presented as part of a belief system – that is, a complex of interacting elements.

Beliefs defined   To understand how beliefs operate, it is essential to make some conceptual distinctions, particularly in relation to knowledge, beliefs and attitude. As with knowledge, beliefs are cognitive constructs, whereas attitudes are affective – that is, they refer to a person's evaluation of some object, person or activity. Attitudes, therefore, refer to feelings in favour of or against the object in question – be it exercise, smoking, sun exposure or immunization. Fishbein (1976) classically defined a belief as:

> a probability judgement that links some object or concept to some attribute. The terms 'object' and 'attribute' are used in a generic sense and both terms may refer to any discriminable aspect of an individual's world. For example, I may believe that Pill A (an object) is a depressant (an attribute). The content of the belief is defined by the object and attribute in question, and the strength of the belief is defined by the person's subjective probability that the object-attribute relationship exists (or is true).

In relation to attitudes, Fishbein (1976: 103) notes:

> An attitude is a bipolar evaluative judgement of the object. It is essentially a sub-jective judgement that I like or dislike the object, that it is good or bad, that I'm favourable or unfavourable towards it. [The term 'object'] ... is used in a generic sense. Thus I may have attitudes towards people, institutions, events, behaviours, out-comes, etc.

Beliefs are, thus, subjective probabilities and will frequently operate in parallel with objective probabilities. By way of example, epidemiological data might suggest that cancer is a major cause of mortality – a statistical observation mirrored by individu-als' beliefs about seriousness. On the other hand, subjective and objective interpreta-tions might operate independently. For example, there may be no objective/scientific evidence that the fumes from a local industrial site contribute to lung disease in an adjacent neighbourhood. Moreover, statistical analysis might also reveal that the prevalence of lung disease in the neighbourhood is neither more nor less than in the population at large. The members of the community, on the other hand, are convinced that they have a real problem of 'chesty coughs' (their non-specific lay version of lung disease) and consider it is self-evident that these are due to the fumes from the incin-erators in the factory.

The health belief model   The health belief model (HBM) is probably the most fre-quently used model of all those purporting to explain health-related decision making. Originated by Hochbaum (1958), based on pioneering work by Lewin (1951) and developed by Rosenstock (1966, 1974), the model was devised to explain variations in the utilization of preventive medical services.

In its early manifestation, it was essentially a model of the expectancy–value/value–expectancy variety. In other words, it argues that decision making depends on individuals believing that a particular course of action will result in the likelihood of a valued outcome being achieved. While it is not possible to provide a full review of this model (see Becker, 1984 and Scheeran and Abraham, 1996 for more detail), it is useful to specify the four major beliefs which it identifies:

- belief in personal susceptibility to a negative event
- belief that the event is serious

- belief that the recommended preventive measure will be effective in reducing the threat of the negative event
- belief that the recommended measure will not entail too heavy a cost.

The formulation is eminently logical as common sense suggests that individuals would not take action to avoid an unpleasant event if they did not believe it was likely to happen to them or, if it did, it would be insignificant. Again, it might well be assumed that people would not follow advice if they did not believe it would work and if the disadvantages outweighed the benefits.

Two further elements were subsequently added to the model:

- cues to action
- health motivation.

The originators of the model considered that the four beliefs alone might need some additional trigger to jolt into action those who were already predisposed to certain courses of action by their beliefs. A general factor – health motivation – was included in a later version of the model. It was considered that the explanatory value of the HBM might be improved if a measure of people's general health motivation were to be included.

As Scheeran and Abraham (1996: 51) rightly observe in their thorough analysis of the model:

> The HBM has provided a useful theoretical framework for investigators of the cognitive determinants of a wide range of behaviours for more than thirty years. Its commonsense constructs are easy for non-psychologists to assimilate and apply and it can be readily and inexpensively operationalized. It has focused researchers' and health-care professionals' attention on modifiable psychological prerequisites of behaviour and provided a basis for practical interventions across a range of behaviours.

How effective are the HBM beliefs in explaining health-related behaviour? A completely comprehensive model that incorporates every social, psychological and environmental influence on health choices would account for 100 per cent of the difference in people's health actions (the variance). The evidence suggests that HBM explains *some* of the variance, but not a lot!

Belief hierarchies and the notion of salience

One of the particularly useful formulations in Fishbein and Ajzen's (1975) seminal work is the demonstration that beliefs may be either 'salient' or 'latent'. The phenomenon of salience is relevant for health education strategies. Translating latent beliefs into salient beliefs, say in the course of group discussion or face-to-face interaction, might alter the belief–attitude dynamic, reduce uncertainty and result in commitment to adopting a healthy course of action. Figure 3.4 provides an example of a typical hierarchy of beliefs associated with stopping smoking. These beliefs may be salient or latent.

There are several lessons for health promotion. For instance, it is inefficient, even pointless, addressing higher-order beliefs without first ensuring that necessary precursor

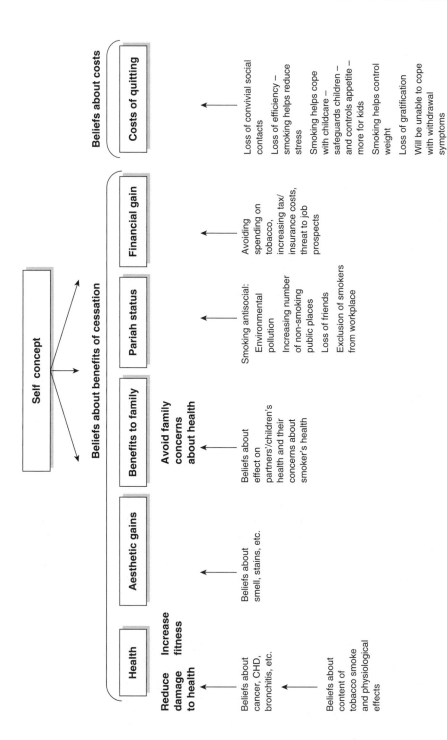

Figure 3.4 Example of a belief system concerning stopping smoking

concepts and subordinate beliefs have already been acquired. It is also apparent that a kind of mental balance sheet is operating and that the outcome will depend on the ultimate balance and relative strengths of the beliefs about the positive and negative outcomes of giving up smoking. This will reflect the relative strengths of the various motivational forces that determine action.

The motivation system

Whereas the belief system is cognitive, the motivation system is affective – it is concerned with feelings. 'Motivation' refers to goal-directed behaviour and its psychological underpinning. It defines the push and pull forces that impel individuals towards the achievement of pleasure and away from undesirable outcomes.

Different kinds of motivation can be identified and operate at different levels. Four kinds are distinguished in the HAM motivation system: values, attitudes, drives and emotional states.

The values dimension   There is a reasonably clear consensus in psychology about the definition of values and their origin. The doyen of research in this area is Rokeach (1973: 3) who makes five assertions about the nature of human values:

- the total number of values is relatively small
- everyone possesses the same values to different degrees
- values are organized into value systems
- values are created and influenced by culture, society and its institutions and personality
- values play a part in virtually all phenomena investigated by the social sciences – psychology, sociology, anthropology, psychiatry, political science, education, economics and history.

In relation to other psychological and social constructs – all of which are of importance in explaining health- and illness-related decisions – values have a transcendental quality, in so far as they energize attitudes and underpin behaviour. In Rokeach's words, 'values are guides and determinants of social attitudes and ideologies on the one hand and of social behaviour on the other (1973: 13).

As with beliefs, values typically occupy hierarchies having superordinate and subordinate levels. Rokeach, for example, usefully distinguishes 'terminal values' from 'instrumental values'. Moreover, he (1973: 14) links these with self-esteem – that major, higher-order value that has special prominence in empowerment theory and health promotion generally.

Terminal values are motivating because they represent the supergoals beyond immediate, biologically urgent goals. Unlike the more immediate goals, these supergoals do not seem ... to satiate – we seem to be forever doomed to strive for these ultimate goals without quite ever reaching them ... there is another reason why values can be said to be motivating. They are in the final analysis the conceptual tools and weapons that we all employ in order to maintain and enhance self-esteem. They are in the service of what McDougall (1926) has called the master sentiment – sentiment of self-regard.

There are also two kinds of instrumental values: moral values and competence values. Interestingly, one of the examples of an intrapersonal competence value that figures prominently in Rokeach's discussion has to do with self-actualization, which, as we noted earlier, can be viewed as a healthy state in its own right or as the peak of a hierarchical motivational structure.

The attitude dimension   The concept of attitude is central to social psychology. Reference was made earlier to Fishbein's definition of attitude, but a number of alternative and influential formulae, can also be found. Perhaps the most common of these makes reference to disposition or readiness for action. Occasionally, the term is used to describe a psychological construct having not only affective but also cognitive and conative elements. The cognitive dimension involves 'beliefs', the affective dimension is concerned with feelings and the conative aspect with the action implications of a given attitude. In HAM, we follow Fishbein and Ajzen in limiting the conative element to 'behavioural intention'. As we will see, this is viewed as the product of the belief, motivation and normative systems and, depending on the availability of 'empowering' knowledge, skills and environment, may or may not be translated into actual behavioural outcomes or health actions.

Again, attitudes operate within a hierarchical system based on values and may be more or less salient or latent. Figure 3.5 provides a review of the values associated with stopping smoking and thus complements the belief hierarchy presented in Figure 3.4 above.

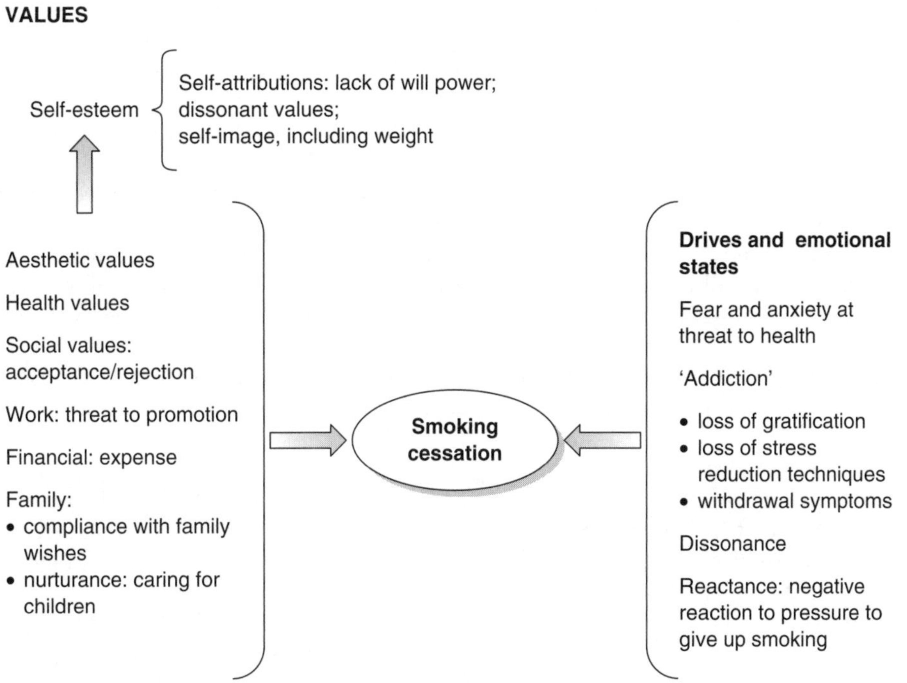

VALUES

Figure 3.5   Motivations and smoking cessation

Inspection of Figures 3.4 and 3.5, however, reveals that the combined force of values and beliefs ought to generate an overwhelmingly negative attitude to smoking and a resoundingly positive attitude to stopping. The fact that this does not always happen is due to the third key element in the motivation system – that cluster of often primitive feelings that are here variously described as drives and emotional states.

Drives, acquired drives and emotional states   In addition to values and attitudes, a third motivational category is identified in HAM. This includes the concepts of drive and emotional state. At the risk of being simplistic, we could sum up the term 'drive' as a kind of primary motivation that is considered to be innate or instinctive. It energizes readily recognized behaviour that frequently has survival value. The most instinctive of these are hunger, thirst, sex and the avoidance of pain.

It is assumed that drives typically exert a greater influence over behaviour than motivation derived from values and attitudes. Indeed, Maslow's (1954) pyramid viewed physiological needs for 'air, food, water, sleep, etc.' as providing a foundation for his motivational hierarchy. Although self-actualization and the achievement of various values were located at the top of the hierarchy, the physiological needs required satisfying before higher-order needs could be fully achieved.

Whereas there is clearly evidence that the achievement of valued goals might, for some people, override the need for food or sex, it would be unwise to rely on this! As WHO has observed, the need for peace, safety and security must be satisfied before people consider adopting behaviour that will improve their health.

The term 'acquired drive' is used to refer to what are normally termed addictions. Again, we must avoid oversimplification, but the power of dependence on various substances generally has more in common with the traditionally defined innate drives than it does with values.

The term 'emotional state' cannot be accorded a precise definition. For instance, while fear is undoubtedly an emotional state, it could equally qualify as a drive, both in respect of its innate qualities and its effects on the individual experiencing it. On the other hand, anxiety would not normally be considered a drive, though it has been defined as a 'fractionated fear response' – that is, a watered-down version of pure fear. In all events, emotional state can exert a powerful effect on decision making and behaviour and should be considered as qualitatively different from a value.

Consider, for example, the case of breastfeeding. Factor analytic research typically reveals two major value-related factors that influence the decision to breastfeed or use bottles. They are the value associated with health and the value associated with social convenience. Furthermore, 'embarrassment' is a factor associated with the rejection of breastfeeding (see, for instance, Wilson and Colquhoun, 1998). The definition of 'embarrassment' is by no means clear and this emotional state may vary in its strength from slight modesty at the prospect of breastfeeding in public to an almost neurotic anxiety about being seen by even close relatives.

Perceptions about the threat posed by actions (or, indeed, failure to act) coupled with beliefs about personal vulnerability may well generate some degree of autonomic arousal ranging from mild concern to panic. Such perceptions may be the product of the individual's own thought processes or, alternatively, be externally induced by shock-horror attempts to influence behaviour. Regardless of their origin, the resulting emotional state will be a factor in determining an individual's response.

One final example of an emotional state that frequently contributes to intention to act is that of 'cognitive dissonance' (Festinger, 1957). It is best described as a state of unease that results from simultaneously holding two or more cognitions (beliefs) that are psychologically inconsistent. The theory posits that individuals experiencing the uncomfortable emotional state of dissonance will be motivated to act to remove it. The dissonance phenomenon has been extensively researched and some further comments will be made in our discussion of attitude change in Chapter 7. However, the position adopted here is that dissonance is but one of many different emotional states that may contribute to behavioural intentions. Its impact can be demonstrated in laboratory situations, but, in real-life situations, it will typically compete with a highly complicated system of drives and values in its effect on behavioural intention. One such competitor is encapsulated in the notion of social pressure, to which we now turn.

The normative system

The normative system describes the network of social pressures that might be brought to bear on an individual's intention to adopt or reject health actions. As may be seen from Figure 3.6, it is conceived as a hierarchical set of influences ranging from the proximal impact of close family and friends to the increasingly distal effects of community and the further reaches of the social system. It is assumed that the effect of significant individuals, close family and friends will typically be more powerful than community pressure, which, in turn, will have more influence than national norms.

Interpersonal influences   The potential power of interpersonal pressure exerted face to face needs little further explication here. Those individuals who exert a direct effect are commonly described as 'significant others'. In addition to close friends or partners, individual professionals might well play an important part in influencing attitudes and behaviour (our earlier discussion of the nature of leadership has already suggested the characteristics that might result in the 'other' being considered 'significant'). The relative importance of family and significant friends will, of course, depend on the nature of existing relationships. However, at the levels of both research and anecdote, the impact of a passionately antismoking partner is well documented!

Peer pressure   While the peer group is generally held to exert an influence on its members, this effect is often portrayed as being disproportionately powerful in the case of adolescents and young people. Furthermore, because this influence is also typically assumed to be negative or unhealthy, it supports the view that young people need to be provided with an armamentarium of skills that will enable them to resist this social pressure. However, there is evidence that the peer effect is more complex (see, for example, Coggans and McKellar, 1994; Michell and West, 1996; Michell, 1997). Young people recognize a number of different groups among their peers and tend to align themselves with friends on the basis of shared interests and behaviour. This raises the question of whether individuals may actively prefer to conform with, rather

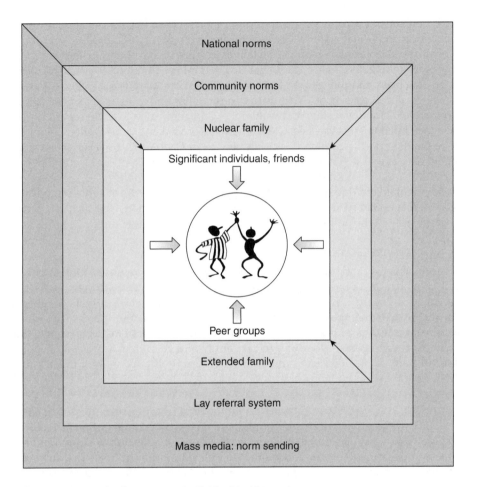

Figure 3.6   Social influences on individual health actions

than resist, the persuasive influence of their peers. Furthermore, it is important to recognize that peers can have a positive influence both directly and by providing a group identity and protection for those who feel they differ from other groups. Indeed, harnessing this positive potential is integral to peer education which will be discussed more fully in Chapter 7.

Social norms and the community   As noted above, the assumption reflected in Figure 3.6 is that the influence of norms will be greater the more proximal groups are to the individual. Nonetheless, the more distal national and community norms will have some effect – both directly and by shaping the norms of families and peer groups. As we comment elsewhere, a genuine community, by definition, has common norms and a network of contacts and relationships, which traditionally include extended families. Where such a community exists, the extent of its social influence will be substantially greater than in a social system characterized by anomie (normlessness).

Due to the effects of socialization, it is likely that community norms will be reinforced by families and adopted by individuals. In fact, following earlier observations about the subtle and powerful effect of dominant ideologies and following the assumptions inherent in the notion of false consciousness, normative pressures may reinforce the status quo and, thus, the social power structure.

The lay referral system and pressure to comply   Over and above their norm setting function, communities and the various groups within them are a repository of lay knowledge which individuals may draw on. The notion of a lay referral system (LRS) has its origins in sociological analyses of the factors associated with compliance with medical advice and the appropriate use of health services. It has been influential in providing insight into the effects of community norms on the adoption of 'appropriate' health- and illness-related behaviour. Freidson (1961: 146–7) writes:

> the process of seeking help involves a network of potential consultants from the intimate and informal confines of the nuclear family through successively more select, distant and authoritative lay-men [*sic*] until the 'professional' is reached. This network of consultants which is part of the structure of the local lay community, and which imposes form on the seeking of help, might be called the 'lay referral structure'. Taken together with the cultural understandings involved in the process we may speak of it as the 'lay referral system'.

While the lay referral system is, by definition, distinct from formal health provision, the box provides an example of an initiative which taps into the LRS using so-called Health Trainers:

> In touch with the realities of the lives of the people they work with and with a shared stake in improving the health of the communities they live in, health trainers will be friendly, approachable, understanding and supportive. Offering practical advice and good connections into the services and support locally, they will become an essential common sense resource in the community to help out with health choices. (Department of Health, 2004: 103)

NHS Health Trainer Programme

Health trainers:

- either identify, or have referred to them, appropriate 'clients' drawn from hard to reach, disadvantaged groups – clients can self-refer too
- work with those clients 1:1 to assess their lifestyle and wellbeing and identify any areas they wish to work on
- work with the client to set goals, agree an action plan and provide individual support where necessary, focusing on behaviour change
- monitor and review their clients' progress and revise the plan where necessary to meet the clients' goals.

Department of Health, 2008b

Label and libel – the nature of stigma   It is appropriate at this point to refer to a particularly important effect of social pressure on individual health – the question of stigma.

One of the major barriers preventing individuals seeking available help for curable and preventable conditions is the cultural conceptualization of particular diseases and the emotional reactions to these. To the extent that diseases are associated with culpable or antisocial actions or are considered to be due to the intervention of supernatural forces, anticipated public disgrace – which may even take the form of violence – may militate against help-seeking behaviour. Such diseases as leprosy, TB and AIDS will immediately spring to mind in this regard. Following the observations about the power of social pressure discussed above, the existence of a close-knit community will increase the perceived threat of disclosure.

A comment by a respondent to a survey on TB in Nepal (Pool, 1992: 108) provides a flavour of the anticipated effects of stigma:

> 'If it is discovered in my district … they would make me separate from the commu-nity as if I had leprosy. Where I live there isn't anywhere nearby to get good treat-ment and so leprosy people whatever they've touched isn't eaten, in fact anything they've touched or used is not touched or used by other people.' (a student from the remote district of Mugu where there are few medical services)

Mass media pressures   More detailed analysis of the nature and effectiveness of mass media will be provided in Chapter 8. For the present, we will merely assert that the impact of the mediated norms of the larger culture transmitted in this way are likely to be considerably less effective than the other social influences discussed above.

Beliefs, motivations and normative pressures – interaction effects

Reference to Figure 3.3 (see page 117) indicates that several points of overlap exist between these separate systems and that the nature of the interaction is signalled by the various 'segments' numbered from 1 to 7.

Normative beliefs and motivation to comply   There is a point of distinction between the actual norms within communities and an individual's perception of those norms based on their subjective assessment. The normative system discussed above actually exerts its effect on behavioural intention via the mediation of both the belief and motivation systems. HAM follows the practice adopted by Fishbein and Ajzen (1975) as it is both theoretically satisfying and practically useful to separately identify beliefs about normative pressures and motivation to conform to those pressures. According to Fishbein, individuals have a set of (salient and latent) beliefs about the likely reactions of key individuals to their intentions to act. However, this anticipated approval or disapproval by significant others will only affect their intention to act if they are also concerned about their reaction. If the others are not actually significant, they will have no influence. Segment 1 indicates beliefs about the reactions of others and segment 2 indicates motivation to comply.

In HAM, Fishbein and Ajzen's formulation has been extended to the remaining potential influences included in the motivation system. Accordingly, beliefs about the likely reactions of peer groups, awareness and beliefs about the nature of social norms and national norms transmitted by mass media will also contribute to intention to act, provided that the individual in question is also motivated to conform to these various social pressures.

According to the 'pressure gradient', the motivational effect of mass media norm sending is unlikely to be as powerful as interpersonal pressures, and any effect is likely to result from the individual's evaluation of the information content of the message.

Interaction of belief and motivation systems   The above discussion of the normative system describes a *particular* case of the mutual effects of beliefs and motivation. The belief and motivation systems in general routinely interact as a two-way influence process. As we emphasized earlier, beliefs represent subjective probabilities. These internalized probabilities may then trigger emotional states or generate attitudes to particular courses of action as a result of becoming 'affectively charged' by personal values. The strength of the ensuing intention to act will depend on the combined strength of beliefs and motivations that interact in a multiplicative fashion.

The most common health education interventions probably operate in a manner designed to influence people's beliefs in order to generate a level of motivation that will result in some approved action or actions. However, it is important to recall that, although beliefs influence motivation, motivation also influences beliefs. In short, people frequently engage in autistic thinking – that is, they typically believe what it is comfortable to believe. When faced with uncomfortable facts and experiences, they may well selectively attend to information that confirms their prejudices or is otherwise less threatening. They may reinterpret and distort messages or indulge in defensive avoidance and denial. In relation to dissonance, discussed above, people may resort to autistic thinking in order to reduce the discomfort experienced when beliefs about self and behaviour are in conflict. Marcel Proust's observation (cited by Sutherland, 1987) provides an excellent example of the impermeability of human defences to unpalatable facts:

> The facts of life do not reach the place where our beliefs are to be found; nor do they bring them into existence; they cannot destroy them; they can inflict on them the continual violence of contradiction but they cannot weaken them; a family assaulted by successive avalanches of misery and sickness will not lose its faith either in the clemency of its God or in the skill of its physician.

We should also note that individuals may not only hold beliefs that *generate* motivation, but may actually have beliefs *about* motivation. This phenomenon is represented by segment 3 in Figure 3.3 above. For instance, in Marsh and Matheson's (1983) classic survey of adult smoking attitudes and behaviour, one of the most important factors determining whether or not smokers intended to quit smoking in the future was the belief they held about the unpleasant withdrawal symptoms they expected to experience and their anticipated loss of gratification. Thus, beliefs about effects significantly reduced their intention to act.

Segment 4 in Figure 3.3 also refers to individuals' beliefs about affect. In this case, it indicates their beliefs about the level of their motivation to comply with (or resist) normative pressures – for example, the degree of discomfort they expect to experience if they do not comply with a partner's wishes or choose to confront the smoking norms of their workmates.

Segments 5 and 6 indicate the relationships of belief and motivation systems respectively with the self. Segment 5 refers to what is normally described as the 'self concept' – that is, the sum total of individuals' beliefs about themselves as persons interacting with other persons and living in a given environment. Segment 6 describes what elsewhere we term 'self sentiment', which is the sum total of feelings individuals might have about themselves as people. This key motivational component is more commonly described as self-esteem. As we will see, it plays a central part in the principles and practice of health promotion.

The final segment – segment 7 – acknowledges the fact that individuals will typically be able to articulate their beliefs about the feelings they have about themselves – for example, acknowledging that their self-esteem is unrealistically low.

The triangle in Figure 3.3 describes the totality of the individual self, including objectively defined elements of personality as well as the more subjective beliefs and values about self already referred to. This final influence on individual intentions to act will now be subjected to scrutiny in the context of consideration of empowerment.

EMPOWERMENT: A CRITICAL REVIEW OF THE DYNAMICS

In Chapter 1, we discussed ideological issues underpinning the definition and practice of health promotion. We examined the discourse of empowerment and argued that an empowerment model of health promotion should govern theory and practice. We now consider what might be involved in operationalizing empowerment so that we understand how philosophy might be translated into practice. Therefore, we will focus on what could be called the anatomy and dynamics of empowerment. We will do so within the framework of HAM, which locates self-empowerment within the interlocking systems of beliefs, motivations and normative influence. Recognizing the facilitating or inhibiting effects of the physical, social and economic environment, our focus then shifts on to the systems that determine whether or not 'empowered' intentions can be translated into practice.

However, before considering the various constructs of empowerment in detail, reference to Figure 3.7 will indicate how they interact.

Defining the self concept

As we observed above, segment 5 in Figure 3.3 refers to the self concept. A number of beliefs about self have especial significance for health status. For instance, body image can influence the self both positively and negatively. Moreover, low self-esteem may result in mental and physical illnesses, such as those associated with eating disorders. On the other hand, mental illness may create low self-esteem. Other beliefs contribute indirectly to health and our emphasis here will be on beliefs about susceptibility to negative outcomes and, more particularly, on beliefs about control, which are central to the process and state of empowerment. Nonetheless, given the importance of the

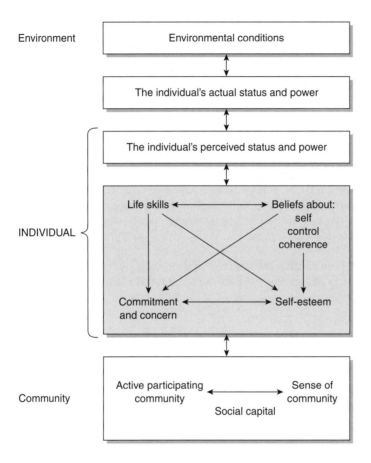

Figure 3.7 Elements of empowerment

notion of the self and the considerable amount of research, past and present, it is appropriate to give further consideration to this construct.

Defining the self

It is important to make the distinction between the self as perceived by the individual and that perceived by an external observer or delineated in more objective fashion by a psychometric test. Segment 5 in Figure 3.3 refers to the former and represents the personal formulation of self.

From the perspective of health promotion theory and practice, there are two key issues. The first of these is the extent to which the self concept is a global construct rather than comprising an aggregate of different component parts (such as sexual attractiveness or intelligence). The second issue concerns the relationship between the self concept and self-esteem – including the possible tension between the formulation of an ideal self and an actual, perceived self.

The increased interest in the self concept in recent years – and the varieties of subordinate concepts – are revealed by the number of instruments designed to measure these. For instance, Keith and Bracken's (1996) review of instrumentation identifies some 20 scales and instruments in current use. In all events, the contemporary view is that the self concept has a structure that is derived from the substantial body of information that people have accumulated about themselves. This structure is multidimensional and hierarchical. It becomes increasingly differentiated over time as a result of age and experience. Shavelson and Marsh (1986), Song and Hattie (1984) and Hattie (1992) have produced influential taxonomies that illustrate both the differentiation and the hierarchical structure. Figure 3.8 summarizes this structure and, in relation to the 'academic' category, emphasizes, not only the importance of school-related achievement, but also general intellectual competence and skills. It also indicates the importance of the interpersonal context (note, for instance, our earlier observations about peer group influence) and, of course, the prime importance of body image and the associated attributes of confidence and self-esteem. It is doubtless self-evident that taxonomies of this kind are essentially culturally constructed and, because of the origins of most of the research, tend to reflect North American values and ideals.

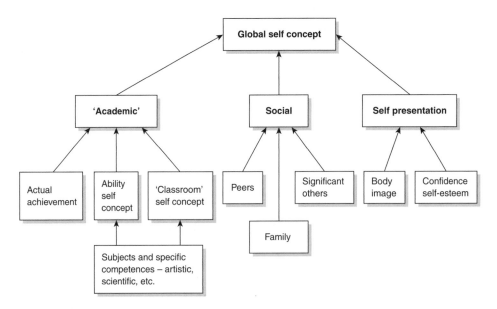

Figure 3.8   A taxonomy of self

The self concept, susceptibility and risk taking

As mentioned earlier, beliefs about susceptibility to disease are a key feature of the HBM. Beliefs about susceptibility when associated with beliefs about the seriousness of disease generate a level of perceived threat (in HAM terms, an emotional state associated with the fear drive). This, in turn, is anticipated to lead to preventive action, provided beliefs about the benefits of that action are considered to outweigh the costs. Perception of susceptibility thus signals a specific belief about the self. The belief in question relates to risk. However, as with other beliefs, it reflects – and, quite frequently, may distort – objective reality. Accordingly, the unthinking use of this belief about vulnerability to predict cautious, preventive decision making may very well lead to dramatically inappropriate conclusions. First of all, a substantial amount of productive research effort has been devoted to the description of *objective* risk – that is, to the use of statistical techniques to accurately record the probabilities of particular activities and circumstances resulting in negative consequences. Second, it is clear from equally sound research that individuals' perceptions of risks and beliefs about vulnerability are only imperfectly related to objective risk. For instance, there is a clearly demonstrated tendency to overestimate the likelihood of the unlikely and underestimate the real frequency of relatively common threats (Lichtenstein et al., 1978; Slovic et al., 1982; Weinstein, 1982, 1984; and Kasperson et al., 1988). One broad set of factors contributing to these misperceptions of threat has to do with faulty information processing and a lack of decision-making skills (Janis and Mann, 1977). For instance, the so-called 'availability heuristic' results in risk appraisal being biased by frequently reported, but not necessarily frequently occurring, events.

Again, affective factors often influence the interpretation of risk. The intuitive observation that young people consider themselves immortal is supported by academic research demonstrating that there is a tendency for people to underestimate the extent of their personal vulnerability to harm – what Weinstein (1982) termed 'unrealistic optimism' – a phenomenon often closely related to wish fulfilment!

By contrast, when frequent reporting of dangerous situations and disasters is accompanied by, for example, extensive media coverage in full and gory Technicolor, the availability heuristic can introduce the dread factor into beliefs about personal vulnerability. A further discussion of the inflation of perceptions of risk and associated feelings of threat is to be found in 'social amplification of risk' theory (Kasperson et al., 1988).

An additional problem with a naïve interpretation of susceptibility is the fact that some individuals actively pursue risk. They would, by definition, not pursue it unless they believed that they were susceptible to some negative outcome. There are various explanations of the motivation for deliberate risk seeking. One suggestion is that some individuals enjoy the physiological effects. To put it somewhat crudely, it would seem that they become addicted to these. Note, for instance, Delk's (1980: 134) reference to high-risk behaviour as 'a form of tension-reduction behaviour with addictive qualities related to the build-up of intoxicating stress hormones'. This might well explain the attractions of theme park and fairground rides which produce adrenaline arousal accompanied by a belief that there is no real danger. However, it would not account for other circumstances where risks are taken only when there is genuine danger. Lyng (1990) offers an interesting explanation of this phenomenon – one that is of particular interest in the context of our discussion of empowerment and control. He employs the term 'edgework', which is seen as a way of handling 'the problem of negotiating the boundary between chaos and order'.

Lyng's analysis could be said to have a certain authority as it is based on participant observation as a jump pilot! He (1990: 856) asserts that all edgework involves:

a clearly observable threat to one's physical or mental wellbeing or one's sense of an ordered existence. The archetypal edgework experience is one in which the individual's failure to meet the challenge at hand will result in death or, at the very least, debilitating injury.

He also argues that many features of drugtaking and even binge drinking do not involve self-destructive behaviour as such but, rather, an attempt to demonstrate mastery and control – both concepts that are central to the notion of empowerment, as we will demonstrate later.

The psychological analysis of susceptibility and risk taking described above poses a serious challenge for the HBM. It may also create a dilemma for those who espouse a narrow preventive model of public health. The paradoxical pursuit of control in hazardous circumstances can result in serious casualties, even when a damage-limitation approach is used and individuals are taught about safety procedures, including how to use drugs 'safely' and deal with an overdose. It poses no difficulty for an empowerment model, provided that there is evidence that risktakers are making empowered decisions. Clearly, if the casualty rate is so high as to impose too heavy a burden on society or risktakers put other people at risk, then, following the principle of utilitarianism, coercive measures may prove necessary. However, in the vast majority of circumstances, empowerment is healthy – both in positive and preventive terms.

Empowerment and health

Self-esteem and health

As we noted above, self-esteem is the affective counterpart of the self concept in the HAM. Indeed, a number of instruments to which reference was made in the discussion of the self concept above focus on self-esteem, such as Coopersmith's self-esteem inventories, the culture-free self-esteem inventories and Rosenberg's self-esteem scale.

It is axiomatic that self-esteem has a significant effect on health – both directly and indirectly. For instance, self-esteem is typically considered a key feature of mental health and therefore worth pursuing in its own right. It may also have an indirect influence through its contribution to intentions to undertake healthy or unhealthy actions. For instance, at a commonsense level, individuals who respect and value themselves will, other things being equal, seek to look after themselves by adopting courses of action that prevent disease. Less obviously perhaps, and pursuing earlier observations about cognitive dissonance, there is strong evidence that people enjoying high self-esteem are less willing to tolerate dissonance and more likely to take rational action to reduce that dissonance, by, for example, rejecting unhealthy behaviour (Aronson and Mettee, 1968). Again, those having low self-esteem are more likely to conform to interpersonal pressures than those enjoying high self-esteem (Aronson, 1976) with unfortunate consequences when such social pressure results in 'unhealthy behaviour'. In terms of empowerment, though, any unthinking yielding to social pressure would be considered unhealthy!

It is also worth noting that various aspects of the self concept contribute differentially to self-esteem. It is generally considered that a discrepancy between the ideal self and actual self is likely to generate low self-esteem (unless, of course, the individual has a sufficient belief in his or her capability to remedy that discrepancy – in which case, successfully bridging the gap will actually enhance self-esteem).

The relationship between body image and self-esteem is well recognized. Although Hoge and McScheffrey (1991) and Marsh and Holmes (1990) found that children's self-esteem was more strongly related to social acceptance than physical appearance, Harter (1985; 1993) found the reverse to be true. Indeed, she reported that students' scores on global self-worth correlated above 0.60 with their perceived physical appearance, compared with 0.45 with their perceived social acceptance. This is not surprising given the widespread dissatisfaction with body image – particularly among young women – and its relationship with eating disorders and the use of cigarette smoking to achieve and maintain a level of slimness bordering on anorexia. However, such discrepancies are not surprising as self-esteem must reflect prevailing personal and cultural values and norms. For a more detailed discussion of social acceptance and the 'social self concept', see Berndt and Burgy (1996).

Self-esteem, then, can be influenced in various ways, one of the most important of which is a belief about being in control.

The case of learned helplessness and hopelessness

The phenomenon of learned helplessness was demonstrated by Seligman (1975: 9). 'Helplessness is the psychological state that frequently results when events are uncontrollable.' Even if something pleasurable happens to an individual, the sense of uncontrollability and the consequent helplessness will result if this 'reward' is not contingent on an individual's own actions.

> Organisms, when exposed to uncontrollable events, learn that responding is futile. Such learning undermines the incentive to respond, and so it produces profound interference with the motivation of instrumental behaviour. It also proactively interferes with learning that responding works when events become uncontrollable, and so produces cognitive distortions. The fear of an organism faced with trauma is reduced if it learns that responding controls trauma; fear persists if the organism remains uncertain about whether trauma is controllable; if the organism learns that trauma is uncontrollable, fear gives way to depressions. (Seligman, 1975: 74)

Lack of control therefore has three main effects:

- **cognitive** – it disrupts the ability to learn
- **conative** – it saps the motivation to take action
- **affective** – it produces emotional disturbance.

Seligman speculated on the physiological mechanisms affected by learned helplessness. At the time, this speculation seemed somewhat fanciful, but more recently interest has grown in the notion of 'biological transition'. For instance, Brunner (in Blane et al., 1996) argued for a quite direct link between the lack of control experienced by the lower grades of civil servants in the second Whitehall Study and specific physiological effects, postulating the existence of a pathway linking:

the chronic stress response of the hypothalamic pituitary adrenal system with result-ing elevated levels of corticosteroids to central obesity, insulin resistance, poor lipid profile and increased tendency for the blood to clot. (Marmot in Brunner, 1996: 290)

Again, Karasek and Theorell's (1990) 'job demand–control model' argues that a com-bination of heavy demands and limited decision latitude to moderate these demands results in 'job strain', which, in turn, creates various negative health consequences, including the dramatic and peculiarly Japanese *Karoshi* – stress death from overwork!

In all events, the general notion of helplessness is convincing. However, its original formulation was criticized, largely on the grounds that, clearly, individuals do not always subside into helplessness when they experience uncontrollability, even after frequent exposure to circumstances in which there is little consistency in the relationship between behaviour and the outcomes of that behaviour. Accordingly, a modification of the theory was suggested by Seligman and other researchers (Abramson et al., 1978; Miller and Norman, 1979). The modification involved an emphasis on an individual's 'attribution of causality' – that is, their beliefs about what causes particular outcomes.

The above comments relate in general to individual health. However, as will be apparent from the reference above to false consciousness, the pathological effects of disempowerment can be applied to notions of social health and, conversely, to social malaise. We will therefore return to this theme in the context of later discussions of *community* empowerment.

Indirect effects of empowerment on health – beliefs about control

As we have noted before, empowerment can be viewed as a health state in its own right – for both individuals and communities. A lack of empowerment can be seen as unhealthy and/or have direct negative physiological effects. More commonly, how-ever, empowerment is considered to have an indirect effect on health by influencing individual and community action. In this context, it is viewed as involving both *actual* possession of power and *beliefs* about having power. Different kinds and levels of beliefs have been identified (see, for instance, Lewis, 1987 and Sarafino, 1990). The hierarchy below exemplifies these different levels.

- **Informational control** refers to the possession of information necessary for taking action.
- **Cognitive control**, according to Lewis, relates to the acquisition of information that allows the intellectual management of an event and, thus, possibly reduces its threaten-ing properties. In Sarafino's (1990: 113) words, it is:

the ability to use thought processes or strategies to modify the impact of a stressor. These strategies can include thinking about the event differently or focusing on a pleasant or neutral thought or sensation. While giving birth, for instance, the mother might think about the event differently by going over in her mind the positive meanings the baby will give to her life.

- **Decisional control** refers to having opportunities to make decisions.
- **Behavioural control** indicates the possession of skills necessary for translating decisions into action. It can also be applied to the possession of skills to enhance 'cognitive control'.

- **Existential control**, a term employed by Lewis in the context of patient education, refers to a belief about the meaningfulness of circumstances rather than control proper.
- **Contingency control** refers to individuals' beliefs that the outcomes of decision making and action are actually under their own control – that is, are contingent on their decision making. This approximates to the concepts of 'locus of control' and 'self-efficacy'.
- **Locus of control** is perhaps the best-known and most influential conceptualization of control. It was developed by Rotter (1966) in the context of social learning theory. He named it 'perceived locus of control' (PLC) to emphasize the fact that it referred to a *subjective* probability rather than the *actual* degree of control possessed by individuals.

The purpose of empowerment strategies is, of course, to foster internality. Perhaps the most important aspect of this notion is the fact that beliefs or expectancies are generalized: they refer to a general tendency to believe that one is in charge of one's life (internal PLC) or, by contrast, generally powerless (external PLC). We should also note that there are two varieties of externality – first, a belief that one is controlled by chance, luck or fate and, second, that one's life is controlled by 'powerful others'.

Health locus of control

Of particular interest to health promotion is a variant on the notion of PLC in the form of 'health locus of control' (HLC). This originated with the work of Kirscht (1972), who developed measures of PLC specifically orientated towards health, and Wallston et al. (1976), who subsequently developed a more sophisticated version in the form of the 'multidimensional health locus of control scale (MHLC)'. Parcel and Meyer (1978) also produced a special version of MHLC for children.

The concept of perceived locus of control has been subjected to considerable scrutiny and, in 1982, Wallston and Wallston reported that, at the time of writing, there had been over 1000 published papers, in addition to 'a myriad of unpublished theses, dissertations and studies investigating the construct'. Researchers have examined the relationship between PLC and HLC and a range of health-related topics (such as health knowledge, smoking, birth control, weight loss, information-seeking and compliance, seatbelt use and so on). Some results were encouraging, though Wallston and Wallston considered that their (1982) review of *health* locus of control was disappointing.

A thorough review by Norman and Bennett (1996) also concluded that the predictive power of HLC is weak. Wallston concurs with this opinion, but, with a touch of irritation, voices the opinion that critics 'do not properly understand or appreciate the theoretical underpinnings of the construct' (1991: 251). Wallston makes the very important point that it is essential to consider HLC together with individuals' health values and other important constructs in any prediction equation, such as specific measures for 'self-efficacy', for example. In short, 'An individual's health behaviour is multidetermined; there is no sense kidding oneself that HLC is the most important determinant'.

Self-efficacy – specific beliefs about control

The concept of self-efficacy is one of the most useful, and applicable, notions in social psychology. It is attributed primarily to Bandura (1977, 1982, 1986, 1992). Its relevance can be appreciated from Bandura's (1982: 122–3) own definition:

> Perceived self-efficacy is concerned with judgements of how well one can execute courses of action required to deal with prospective situations ... Self-percepts of efficacy are not simply inert estimates of future action. Self-appraisals of operative capabilities function as one set of proximal determinants of how people behave, their thought patterns, and the emotional reactions they experience in taxing situations. In their daily lives people continuously make decisions about what course of action to pursue and how long to continue those they have undertaken. Because acting on misjudgements of personal efficacy can produce adverse consequences, accurate appraisal of one's own capabilities has considerable functional value. Self-efficacy judgements, whether accurate or faulty, influence choice of activities and environmental settings. People avoid activities that they believe exceed their coping capabilities, but they undertake and perform assuredly those that they judge themselves capable of managing.

Self-efficacy is one of the most valuable and practical features of social cognitive theory (SCT) – an extension and elaboration of social learning theory. Its importance is reflected in the fact that it has been added to Fishbein and Ajzen's theory of reasoned action as a kind of bolt-on extra. Their revised model was rebranded as the *Theory of Planned Behaviour* (Ajzen, 1991; Conner and Sparks, 1996). Self-efficacy also forms a key part of the so-called 'ASE' (attitude social norm efficacy) model devised by researchers in the Netherlands (Kok et al., 1992).

As noted earlier, SLT/SCT offers a simple but effective model of successful human agency. It includes the formula: action is the product of response efficacy and self-efficacy where response efficacy is the belief that a particular course or courses of action will result in the achievement of some desired outcome. It follows that self-efficacy refers to the individual's conviction that he or she is actually capable of undertaking the actions necessary to achieve the outcome. Self-efficacy, like PLC, is therefore what was described earlier as a contingency belief, though self-efficacy differs from PLC in its specificity. Perhaps due to this specificity, it is clear that single measures of self-efficacy can correlate substantially with behavioural outcomes. For instance, de Vries (1989) demonstrated a correlation of 0.71 with smoking outcomes. Self-efficacy is also useful in predicting outcomes in the field of rehabilitation. For example, Ewart (1992: 287) stated that interventions to improve self-efficacy enabled patients 'to cope more effectively with the many challenges posed by heart attack'. Holman and Lorig (1992: 305) asserted that 'perceived self-efficacy to cope with the consequences of chronic disease is an essential contributor to developing self-management capabilities'.

The notion of 'reciprocal determinism' is also central to the formulation. In other words, there is a reciprocal relationship between the environment and the individual – each influences the other and outcomes depend on the results of that interaction. The interaction is expressed diagrammatically in Figure 3.9.

In addition to having beliefs about the nature of a health action and the likelihood of being able to perform it, individuals also have beliefs about the extent to which they possess the skills and capabilities they need to achieve the health action goals. Self-efficacy beliefs can be influenced by, and also create, emotional states, such as shame or anxiety at the prospect of failure or failing to take any action because of lack of confidence.

As we mentioned above, response efficacy is also an affective factor related to an acceptance that the health action is a worthwhile goal. Active goal setting will occur to the extent that individuals believe they are capable of achieving those goals. Furthermore,

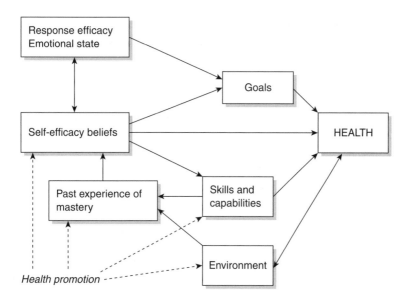

Figure 3.9   Self-efficacy and reciprocal determinism

they will have beliefs about the relationship between the environment and the health action. They must accept that there is a reasonable probability of their being able to overcome any environmental barriers before they commit themselves to action. Typically, it will be necessary to have certain capabilities and skills related to the attainment of the desired outcome, including decision-making skills. If individuals do not believe that they possess these competences, their commitment to change will be reduced.

Self-efficacy beliefs will depend substantially on past experience of mastery – of success or failure. The role of health promotion is threefold. First, it aims to influence efficacy beliefs directly. Second, it aims to exercise an indirect influence by providing the competences and skills needed to carry out a health action and/or cope with environmental barriers. Third, it aims to remove those environmental barriers that militate against the formation of efficacy beliefs.

Self efficacy – implications for health promotion

Bandura argues that there are four general factors influencing self-efficacy beliefs. They are (in descending order of power) direct experience, vicarious experience, verbal persuasion and physiological state. These are listed in Table 3.1 in conjunction with implications for health promotion.

Personality and behavioural intention

Personality is included in the portrayal of 'self' in the HAM. It is considered to be one of the factors contributing to behavioural intention. Personality differs from other psychological constructs in that it refers to the relatively fixed and enduring attributes of

Table 3.1   Influences on self-efficacy – implications for health promotion

Influences on self-efficacy	Examples of implications for health promotion
Direct experience	Provide experience through role play
Physiological state 'people rely partly on information from their physiological state in judging their capabilities. ... Fear reactions generate further fear through anticipatory self-arousal. By conjuring up fear-provoking thoughts about their ineptitude, people can rouse themselves to elevated levels of distress that produce the very dysfunctions they fear'	Anticipatory guidance Stress management techniques
Verbal persuasion 'to try to talk people into believing they possess capabilities that will enable them to achieve what they seek'	Various, well-recognized attitude change techniques, such as using credible sources, appropriate message style, right level of emotional arousal, minimizing reactance. *Beware:* changes may be short-lived and this strategy is not empowering and of dubious ethicality!
Vicarious efficacy information 'information conveyed by modelled events ... People judge their capabilities partly by comparing their performances with those of others'	Observation of credible/'homophilous' models achieving success

Source: Quotations are from Bandura, 1986: 399ff.

the individual. These attributes may be described in terms of 'traits', which may be further classified into 'types' and 'profiles'. Despite some earlier dalliance with attempts to link personality with health-related behaviour, traditional analyses of personality have not been considered to be particularly useful in health promotion.

We will make some reference to the use of 'depth psychology' in advertising in our discussion of mass media in Chapter 8, but for now will limit ourselves to noting four instances where aspects of personality do seem to affect intentions and action to a greater or lesser extent.

Coherence, hardiness and resilience

The existence of a 'hardy personality' has been identified (for example, Kobasa, 1979) and it is of interest to our present discussion as its three major characteristics have special relevance to our discussion of empowerment and, in its reference to 'challenge', to radical health promotion. Hardiness has three main features:

- a sense of **personal control** – to all intents and purposes identical to locus of control
- **commitment** – a sense of purpose and involvement with community and life in general
- **challenge** – change is viewed as opportunity.

In addition to its similarity to Antonovsky's 'sense of coherence' (SOC, to which reference was made in Chapter 1), it is also virtually synonymous with the notion of 'resilience', used by Garmezy (1983) to describe children who grow up to be competent and well-adjusted adults despite adverse circumstances. Studies of resilient children have recorded, with some surprise, a tendency for them to recover rapidly from adversity, be well adjusted, have good social skills and, above all, a sense of personal control and relatively high self-esteem – all this despite experiencing horrific circumstances, including being raised by dysfunctional families, being abused and even growing up in concentration camps (see, for instance, Werner, 1987). It is difficult to account for such phenomena when they are so inconsistent with the received wisdom of theories of learned helplessness. To the extent that such characteristics do reflect personality, it would seem necessary to have recourse to explanation in terms of inherited, 'temperamental' traits.

Type A and B personalities

The personality types which have received greatest attention in relation to health are so-called Type A and Type B. The former has been characterized as 'an excess of free-floating hostility, competitiveness, and time urgency' (Bennett and Murphy, 1997: 20). In contrast, Type B is more relaxed and easy going. Interest in the association with health derives from research (by Friedman and Rosenman, 1974) which demonstrated that Type As carried twice the risk for heart disease as Type Bs, after controlling for other risk factors such as smoking. A mixed profile has also been recognized, referred to as Type A/B or Type X. Clearly, from a health promotion perspective, it is not possible to change enduring traits such as personality. Nonetheless, the associated behaviours are amenable to modification.

The sensation-seeking personality

Another psychological construct having pretensions to a personality trait or type – and of relevance for health promotion – is the concept of 'sensation seeking'. Individuals vary in the extent to which they actively seek sensations and Zuckerman (1990) developed a sensation-seeking scale (SSS). Bearing in mind earlier observations about risk taking and phenomena such as edgework, the reality of this personality characteristic is of some importance to health promoters (and creates still more tension for the HBM's notion of susceptibility). Table 3.2 provides a flavour of the operationalization of sensation seeking.

Thuen assessed the relationship between a modified sensation-seeking scale and injury-related behaviour and concluded that there was indeed a strong relationship, 'well above … the typical correlations between personality trait and behaviours' (1994: 471).

Radicalism v. conservatism and related social characteristics

One final example of personality traits relevant to health promotion relates to social values. It is not that relevant to the individual adoption of preventive health actions, but, rather, to the ideological values that underpin policy development and implementation and social change.

Cattell (1966) identified 16 personality traits, two of which might predispose individuals towards particular models of health promotion. The first – 'openness to

Table 3.2   Sample items from the sensation-seeking scale (SSS)

Categories of sensation-seeking	Examples
Thrill and adventure seeking	*'I would like to try parachute jumping'*
Experience seeking	*'I like to try new foods I have never tried before'*
Disinhibition	*'I often like to get high (drinking liquor or smoking marijuana)'*
Boredom susceptibility	*'I like people who are sharp and witty, even if they do sometimes insult others'*

Source: Thuen, 1994

change' – juxtaposes radicalism with conservatism. The second – 'sensitivity' – ranges from 'tough-minded' to 'tender-minded' (rather esoterically termed *Premsia* v. *Harria*!)

Eysenck (1960) incorporated these traits into a two-dimensional model that he argued would help explain political orientation. For instance, a tough-minded radical would favour communism, while tough-minded conservatism would characterize a fascist tendency. Readers might care to experiment with applying this typology to professional colleagues of their acquaintance!

TRANSLATING INTENTION INTO PRACTICE: REMOVING BARRIERS AND EMPOWERING COMMUNITIES

The discussion so far has centred on self-empowerment and examined various psychological characteristics associated with those personal capabilities and characteristics that help an individual gain control over his or her life and health. However, bearing in mind the paramount importance of reciprocal determinism, it is not possible to seek to facilitate individuals' empowerment without paying due attention to the nature of the environment. Indeed, to do so is merely to engage in a more sophisticated form of victim-blaming. Accordingly, we will now consider what is involved in translating behavioural intentions into action.

Assuming that the complex of multiple influences between self, belief, motivation and normative systems have resulted in an intention to act, it is imperative to consider what more is needed to maximize the chances of individuals achieving the goals they have set for themselves. However, let us not forget – and taking account of the principles of self-efficacy – that an individual's beliefs about the nature and strength of environmental barriers and deficits may cause the intention to act to be aborted. Returning to HAM (shown in Figure 3.3 on page 117), it will be seen that three kinds of facilitating factors may be necessary before intention is translated into practice (or, conversely, three kinds of barriers may need to be removed). These will now be reviewed.

Facilitating health actions – knowledge and skills

The contribution of knowledge

In terms of HAM, it is important to clarify the two different contributions made to health choices by knowledge. The first concerns the acquisition of information that may influence the formation of beliefs – this may, ultimately, contribute to an intention to act.

The second of these merely involves providing the information that people who are already committed to taking action need to help them translate their intention to act into practice.

With regard to the first of these two contributions made by knowledge, it is important to remember that knowledge alone, although necessary, will very rarely be *sufficient* to lead to behaviour. As we noted earlier, knowledge rarely leads to practice without, at the very least, a shift in attitude. We might also observe that, frequently, a positive attitude to making a particular health choice may lead to a search for knowledge to clarify and support the tentative intention to act. In such a case, it would not be a K-A-P progression, but, rather, an A-K-I-P progression (from attitude to knowledge to intention to practice!). It is often said that knowledge is power, but this is true only up to a point. For example, while it is true that knowing about the existence of family planning clinics offering contraceptive advice might be essential to the routine adoption of condom use, social skills would also be necessary to interact confidently and assertively with professional staff – and, more importantly, to negotiate condom use with a partner. Knowledge thus has only a contributory role in empowering progress from intention to action. But, conversely, lack of knowledge can be totally depowering.

The importance of skills

There is no precise definition of skills in general – apart from an implication that they are goal-directed and would be applied to some practical purpose. However, a number of specific skills can be precisely identified, together with the conditions needed to acquire proficiency. The box contains a summary of the key skills of concern to health promotion.

Skills for empowerment

(May be referred to as health skills if applied to specific health scenarios)

Cognitive skills

- **Literacy** – the ability to read and write is intrinsically empowering.
- **Decision-making skills** – competences associated with cognitive problem-solving, such as assessing the costs and benefits of particular courses of action.

Psycho-motor skills

- Skills involving the integration of perception and movement, such as the hand–eye coordination involved in the correct use of a condom.

Social interaction skills

- **Life skills** – the use of skilled responses to a range of social situations. Although 'life skills' also incorporates applied knowledge and understanding, its emphasis is on the acquisition and practice of skills and particularly social interaction skills, such as how to deal with housing officials or how to work in groups and organize for radical social action.
- **Assertiveness** – a valuable package of the knowledge and skills needed to achieve desired goals while, at the same time, recognizing other people's needs and rights.

The vexed question of health literacy

Health literacy has been proposed as a set of skills which is critical to achieving a state of empowerment (Nutbeam, 1998b). It has its origins in the USA in relation to the development of patient literacy and the ability to comply with treatment regimens. While notions of compliance may seem at odds with empowerment, the converse position – not being able to understand what is needed – is totally de-powering. The concept has now been applied to health more generally. For example, Nutbeam (1998b: 357) defines it as:

> the cognitive and social skills which determine the motivation and ability of individuals to gain access to, understand, and use information in ways which promote and maintain good health.

Abel (2007: 59) also makes the point that 'adequate health literacy not only supports personal health management, but also increases the chances of changing health-relevant living conditions'.

Nutbeam (2000b) distinguishes three levels of health literacy:

- **functional health literacy** – concerned with knowledge about risks and health services and the adoption of prescribed actions
- **interactive health literacy** – additionally includes personal and social skills and the motivation and self-confidence required to take personal action
- **critical health literacy** – having the knowledge and skills that enhance individual resilience to adverse circumstances, and support effective social and political action as well as individual action.

It should be evident that health literacy incorporates the same constructs as empowerment. Indeed, in a scathing critique, Tones (2002) argued that health literacy is merely a re-branding of empowerment. Nonetheless, it continues to gain currency. While its focus on the development of knowledge and skills may offer some potential in enabling individuals to influence their environment, health literacy – in contrast to comprehensive models of empowerment – pays scant attention to the reciprocal effect of the environment on their capacity to do so. We now turn our attention to this dimension.

Empowerment – the role of the environment

The significance of environmental factors in determining health status has been emphasized throughout this book and will, therefore, receive only brief attention here as a factor influencing the translation of intention into action. Clearly, failure to address physical, social, economic and cultural circumstances is to unwittingly blame the victim whose health suffers from those circumstances and whose scope for action is dramatically impeded by them. This is acknowledged by the NICE Guidance on behaviour change which recommends:

> Identify and attempt to remove social, financial and environmental barriers that prevent people from making positive changes in their lives, for example, by tackling poverty, employment or education issues. Although equipping people with necessary

beliefs (predominantly about self) and skills is an essential part of the empowering process, people will not find themselves in control of their lives and health when barriers remain and the environment in which people live and work does not actively conspire 'to make the healthy choice the easy choice'. (NICE, 2007: 4)

The physical environment ranges from the drastic effects of natural and man-made disasters and the debilitating effect of squalor and preventable disease to access to clean water supplies and user-friendly health services, from smoke-free public places to wide availability of condoms – in a machine or (as was the case in certain African workplaces) in the pay packet. As we described earlier at some length, the socio-economic environment is a key factor in health inequalities through the absolute effects of poverty, but also through the more subtle effects of having wide income differentials in society. The sociocultural environment includes those various normative practices that may either be intrinsically healthy or unhealthy and the social networks to which individuals may have recourse.

The empowerment model of health promotion to which we subscribe in this book (described in Chapter 1) is premised on a need for action for self-empowerment, but, importantly for empowerment, directed at social and environmental change. One of the main strategies is the Ottawa Charter principle of the creation of 'active participating communities'. We now consider factors associated with the empowerment of communities and their relationships with the larger social system. First, we will consider the meaning of sick and healthy societies.

Healthy societies and communities

In our discussion of the determinants of health in Chapter 2, reference was made to the popular notion of social capital. As we noted, social capital is typically viewed as a feature of a healthy society, just as financial capital can be considered to contribute to *economic* 'health'. It will doubtless be apparent that, although some difference in emphasis may be discerned, the key features of social capital are virtually synonymous with what has alternatively been described in terms such as sense of community, trust and participation. We will not, therefore, repeat our earlier observations about social capital, but give some thought to the meaning of these parallel ideas and concerns.

At one level, it can be argued that a healthy society or community is an empowered one. Accordingly, it is important to look more closely at what are considered to be the key features of such a community. As it happens, some people might consider that a community is, by definition, healthy – or at least if the standard definition is used, which characterizes a 'genuine' community as a relatively small aggregate of people (probably in a relatively small geographical locality or neighbourhood) that has both a tightly knit network of relationships and a common sense of identity. The reference to a sense of identity is more commonly described as a 'sense of community' and this is frequently seen as highly desirable. However, while a sense of community might well be a feature of an empowered one, the converse is not necessarily true. Indeed, individuals may recognize that they are part of a social group and, for instance, take some comfort from their awareness of sharing a common predicament. This is not necessarily empowering, particularly if we accept the premises of social control by means of false consciousness!

Another paradox related to the apparently healthy effects of a sense of community is illustrated by consideration of religious communities. The phenomenon was revealed by Maton and Rappaport's (1984) investigation into empowerment among members of a 'Christian, non-denominational religious setting'. The members of the community in question clearly demonstrated their access to 'social capital' and were undoubtedly active. They enjoyed the benefits of a sense of coherence in terms of emotional meaningfulness, but, in their dependence on God, it is arguable whether or not they were really empowered, in the sense of being in control of their lives. As Banfield (1958: 109) puts it, 'Where everything depends upon luck or the caprice of a saint ... on divine intervention, there is no point in community action. The community, like the individual, may hope or pray, but it is not likely to take its destiny into its own hands'.

In a more secular context, Kindervatter (1979: 62) emphasizes the key elements of an empowered community as being 'People gaining an understanding of and control over social, economic and/or political forces in order to improve their standing in society'. Rappaport (1987: 130) declared that empowerment was not just an individual attribute but also:

> an organizational, political, sociological, economic, and spiritual [construct]. Our interests in racial and economic justice, in legal rights as well as in human needs, in healthcare and educational justice, in competence as well as in a sense of community, are all captured by the idea of empowerment. The reason we care about fostering a society whose social policies appreciate cultural diversity ... is that we recognize that it is only in such a society that empowerment can be widespread. We are as much concerned with empowered organizations, neighbourhoods, and communities as we are with empowered individuals.

Participation and empowerment

Reference was made earlier to the Ottawa Charter's emphasis on the virtues of empowered, participating communities. The question might legitimately be asked whether empowered communities generate participation or participation creates empowerment – and, ultimately, action. Kieffer (1984: 31) considered that the empowered state consisted of 'an abiding set of commitments and capabilities which can be referred to as participatory competence'. The effects of this were believed to be:

- the development of a positive self concept
- a more critical understanding of the surrounding social and political environment
- the cultivation of individual and collective resources for social and political action.

Additional discussion of empowering communities features in our discussion of community development in Chapter 9.

Empowerment and the avoidance of relapse

It can be seen from HAM that the single time choice of a specific health action is not the end of the story. Although there are instances where they are all that is required – for instance, attendance at a clinic for a one-off vaccination – the more common requirement is that the health action should be sustained and become adopted as a 'routine'.

Once this has happened, the results of that choice may be confirmed. 'Outcome efficacy' may be confirmed and individuals may continue to enjoy the benefits of the health action to which they have committed themselves. Not unusually, though, an individual may discover that the anticipated benefits fail to materialize or actual loss of gratification or discomfort may be experienced. In short, relapse may occur.

Relapse is traditionally associated with various kinds of addiction (a term that, we admit, is open to several interpretations) and it is worth, at this juncture, giving some thought to the applicability of a popular explanatory model – the 'transtheoretical model' (TTM). We will also consider its relationship to the conceptual schema used in HAM.

A useful summary of the model is provided by Prochaska et al. (1997) and its origins are revealing. Prochaska and colleagues carried out detailed analyses of some 300 different theories of psycho-therapeutic interventions and identified ten processes of change. The model scanned these theories and processes (hence, 'trans'), then combined and reformulated them.

While the model can be applied to any behaviour, it has been most frequently applied to those health actions involving the sacrifice of gratification and the experience of discomfort, which create the consequent likelihood of relapse. So, smoking, alcohol and substance misuse, eating problems and obesity feature prominently in research using the model.

A key feature of TTM is its assumption that individuals move through a series of stages (see box) but may relapse at almost any time. However, there is a high level of probability that many will move again from a stage of (temporary) 'precontemplation' and proceed through the various stages once more until, hopefully, they will be successful. The reason for the phrase 'revolving door model' being used as a synonym for TTM is thus, doubtless, apparent.

Transtheoretical model

Stage of change

1	Precontemplation	not even considering change
2	Contemplation	considering making a specific behaviour change
3	Preparation	serious commitment and preparation to change
4	Action	initiation of change
5	Maintenance	sustaining the change
OR		
Relapse		

Prochaska and DiClemente, 1983, 1984

Another point of considerable importance is that interventions designed to achieve behaviour change must be tailored to the individual and, therefore, take account of the particular stage that they have reached in their behaviour change career. Rollnick et al. (1992) provide a good example of such tailoring in their use of the technique 'brief motivational interviewing'.

Prochaska et al. (1997) provide an extensive list of approaches and techniques that have been used to maximize success and minimize the chance of relapse – including not only individual methods, such as 'consciousness-raising' and 'counter-conditioning', but also what they term 'social liberation' – broader, 'primary preventive' social measures to influence social norms that foster unhealthy behaviour.

How does the TTM relate to HAM? Clearly, it relates well to the confirmation/relapse pathway that follows the period of 'trying out' the health action in question. The process of developing a routine – especially where the health action is problematic – may take some time. Following Prochaska's comment about the move from 'maintenance' to 'termination', it may take between six months and five years! On the other hand, as the precontemplation stage describes the state existing prior to the formation of an intention to adopt a healthy course of action, HAM's analysis of the complex of beliefs, motivations, norms and factors associated with self and personality demonstrates that, at this point, the TTM analysis is somewhat superficial!

Returning to our focus on empowerment, one of the empowering approaches to minimize relapse involves attribution theory and, more specifically, reattributing individuals' perceptions of the nature of the barriers to maintaining their avoidance of negative behaviour, such as overeating or other 'addictions'.

As we mentioned earlier, one of the factors influencing adult males' intentions to give up smoking was the belief that they would be unable to cope with the loss of gratification and the side-effects of their dependence on tobacco (Marsh and Matheson, 1983). However, Davies (1992) has suggested (admittedly, a decidedly idiosyncratic point of view!) that it is unhelpful to view behaviour such as substance misuse or overeating in terms of overwhelmingly powerful drive-like states (see box for an example of the tendency to invoke addiction too readily). The title of his book – *The Myth of Addiction* – is revealing. What seems to be necessary is a reattribution of beliefs! Of course, those who believe they are suffering withdrawal symptoms and consider that they crave their chosen substance, would doubt the truth of Davies' view! As we mentioned earlier, our view is that the motivation system comprises qualitatively different motivators, requiring qualitatively different methods to achieve given outcomes.

'Don't blame him, he's just a poor sex addict'

When Valerie Harkess was faced with her toughest question (why *did* you go back and sleep with Alan Clark …) she opted for the twentieth-century equivalent of seeking sanctuary in a holy place. 'I suppose I was addicted to him,' she said. In other words – I need help, not condemnation. I have taken the vows of victimhood. You cannot touch me here …

The general implication is that if you're in the grip of an addiction you are not culpable. What you do might be reprehensible, but the blame for it resides not in you but in your disease … So though Michael Douglas might once have been described as a fornicator and libertine, he now issues a press release stating that he has checked into a clinic to have treatment for sex addiction. Poor thing, we are supposed to think, how brave he is to fight it. Where can we send our donations to help us to stamp out this terrible illness? …

(Continued)

(Continued)

Oddly enough there doesn't seem to be a similar get-out for money – no counsel has *yet* dared to step forward and argue that his client is hopelessly addicted to used notes and is conscientiously attending meetings of Cashaholics Anonymous. This is probably because the compulsive acquisition of money is socially sanctioned anyway, so that moral distinctions are reserved for ways of getting hold of it. But in almost every other sphere of moral action the rule holds good. If you're hooked, you're off the hook.

Sutcliffe, 1994

Empowerment and self control

The adoption of health practices is frequently dependent on having the requisite skills. HAM incorporates one particular class of life or health skills that are similar to some of the intervention measures identified by Prochaska. These are skills derived from a long tradition of work in behaviour modification and are here termed self-regulatory skills.

Empowerment is ultimately concerned with self-determination and, as we have noted, environmental factors may limit the possibility of self-determination. On the other hand, individuals can exercise a good deal of personal control. In short, freedom of will can be a reality. Central to the achievement of personal control are 'self-referent cognitions' – that is, beliefs about oneself – that also include 'meta cognitions' – the uniquely human capacity to think about thought and reflect on reflections.

The paramount importance of Bandura's application of the concept of self-efficacy in understanding how people can successfully interact with their environment doubtless needs no reiteration. Not surprisingly, Bandura (1989: 1182) comments on the importance of self-efficacy beliefs in relation to self-regulation.

Self-generated influences operate deterministically on behaviour the same way as external sources of influence do. Given the same environmental conditions, persons who have developed skills for accomplishing many options and are adept at regulating their own motivation and behaviour are more successful in their pursuits than those who have limited means of personal agency. It is because self-influence operates deterministically on action that some measure of self-directedness and freedom is possible ... Self-regulatory functions are personally constructed from varied experiences not simply environmentally implanted ... Through their capacity to manipulate symbols and to engage in reflective thought, people can generate novel ideas and innovative actions that transcend their past experiences. They bring influence to bear on their motivation and action in efforts to realize valued futures.

With respect to our current discussion, the 'valued futures' mentioned by Bandura above include freedom from addictions. Traditionally, behaviour modification has been employed to deal with these powerful drives. It has its roots in behaviourist attempts (typically in competition with counselling interventions derived from psychoanalysis) to deal with various kinds of mental illness, such as phobias and compulsive behaviour. Following, for example, Skinnerian 'operant conditioning theory', psychologists were concerned to shape unwanted and unhealthy behaviour into that which was acceptable to therapists, their clients (and society as a whole). Many of the methods used – such as counter conditioning by means of electric shock – would seem to be diametrically opposed to the ethics and practice of empowerment. However, more recent developments have switched the emphasis away from 'therapist control' to 'client control'. This was doubtless partly due to the problems of finding enough psychologists to meet clients' needs, but also reflected an acceptance of the importance of self-regulation. In fact, in its review of the morality of health education interventions, the Society of Public Health Education (SOPHE, 1976) agreed that *client contract* behaviour modification (our emphasis) was ethically acceptable along with communication and community development. In short, the DIY version of behaviour modification aimed to put clients in charge of their own 'therapy' and this approach has become integrated into various health-promotion methods concerned with fostering behaviour change.

Kanfer and Karoly (1972) were among the first to address the apparent paradox of employing behaviour modification techniques to achieve voluntaristic outcomes. They pointed out, for instance, how certain tactics that achieved desired behaviour change goals, at least in the short term, did not involve genuine self-control – that is, empowered decision making. They (1972: 408) noted, too, that genuine self-control occurs only when:

> an individual alters or maintains his behavioral chain in the absence of immediate external supports ... Once an obese person has put a lock on the refrigerator or the alcoholic mixed an emetic in his drink [external factors] are sufficient to account for the resulting behaviour.

Returning to observations made in Chapter 1 on voluntarism, it is interesting to note the parallel between these coercive measures at the micro level and the coercive potential of healthy public policy. This may go considerably further than making 'the healthy choice the easy choice' by seeking to make it the only choice!

Before considering the key skills needed to achieve self regulation of behaviour, it is worth recalling that the kinds of behaviour currently under consideration are those where:

- a change in relatively recently adopted health actions occurs as a result of significant reduction in gratification or the experience of significant aversive consequences
- the emergence of a competing motivation of superior strength results in an undesirable behaviour.

An example of the first situation is provided by experience of negative effects after giving up smoking or when vigorous exercise proves painful. The second situation is illustrated by times when the sex drive overrides the motivating force of moral value and/or concern at the prospect of infection in the context of an unanticipated romantic encounter.

Self-regulatory skills – a model

Figure 3.10 seeks to describe key features of self-regulation in the particular context of combating relapse.

An essential feature of many, if not most, situations where people are seeking to change their behaviour is the provision of 'anticipatory guidance'. This term can be

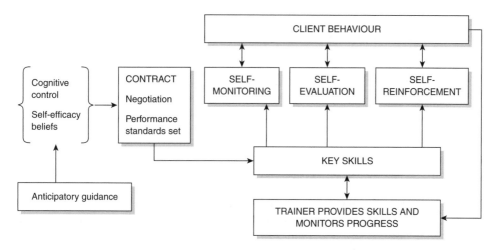

Figure 3.10 Self-regulation of health actions

used to describe the whole package – including the provision of skills. It is used here to refer to providing 'cognitive control' – that is, a degree of empowerment by giving individuals a grasp of what will be involved in the aftermath of choice. More important is the use of methods to generate appropriate self-efficacy beliefs – for example, by using models, those who have successfully moved through the 'maintenance' stage and reached 'termination' (for instance, ex-smokers who have not smoked for more than one year).

A recommended and standard procedure for achieving self-control is the formulation of a contract between trainer and client. As with any contract, there is a process of negotiation and mutual agreement about the responsibilities and commitments of trainer and client, including what the client is prepared to do. The contract might actually be written or merely involve a verbal discussion. The procedure might involve contingency contracting. Examples of this include a cash deposit that will only be refunded once the target behaviour has been attained.

Three key processes are involved in the acquisition of a repertoire of self-regulatory skills:

- self-monitoring
- self-evaluation
- self-reinforcement.

It is generally accepted that, in order, ultimately, to handle motivational problems, clients should first of all be involved in conscious monitoring of behaviour and associated feelings. Monitoring involves paying attention to, and correctly interpreting, external environmental cues and internal, physiological events. For example, clients might ascribe the surge of excitement and gastronomic arousal to the display in the pâtisserie window prior to their succumbing to temptation!

'Proprioception' – the interpretation of internal states – is not only part of acquiring motor skills, it is also important in acquiring self-control skills. The individual learns to become aware of autonomic responses and associated thought processes. In self-monitoring, therefore, feedback is received from external stimuli, one's own behaviour and internal cognitive, affective and autonomic processes.

Self-evaluation consists of comparing self-monitored data with some standard of performance and judging the adequacy of the overall performance. This judgement then serves as a discriminating stimulus for either positive or negative reinforcement. In other words, the performance in the pâtisserie may serve as a cause of self-congratulation or harbinger of guilt!

Perhaps the most problematic of the three processes is that of 'self-reinforcement'. The key task is somehow to override the reinforcing qualities of the unwanted behaviour with some replacement reinforcer. The powerful gratifications delivered by the cream cake must somehow be reduced and/or replaced with a more powerful reinforcer. Unfortunately, it is often difficult to find a really enticing alternative. For instance, some of the suggestions offered in leaflets designed to help smokers quit their habit are distinctly uninspiring, such as, to take your mind off your need for a cigarette, fiddle with a paperclip, suck a mint or take a brisk walk!

Thoresen and Mahoney (1974: 22) identify four major categories of self-reinforcement:

- **Positive self-reward** The self-administration or consumption of a freely available reinforcer only after performance of a specific, positive response, such as treating oneself to a special event after having lost weight
- **Negative self-reward** The avoidance of, or escape from, a freely avoidable aversive stimulus only after performance of a specific, positive response, such as removing an uncomplimentary pig poster from one's dining room whenever a diet is adhered to for a full day
- **Positive self-punishment** The removal of a freely available reinforcer after the performance of a specific, negative response, such as tearing up a dollar bill for every 100 calories in excess of one's daily limit
- **Negative self-punishment** The presentation of a freely avoidable aversive stimulus after the performance of a specific, negative response, such as presenting oneself with a noxious odour after each occurrence of snacking.

Readers may experience doubts about the widespread applicability or acceptability of these tactics and favour less demanding reinforcement schedules such as public praise from peers or even self-satisfaction at meeting goals.

Self-reinforcement will frequently be supplemented by attempts to break the stimulus–response link between situation and gratification. Dieters might be advised not to shop when hungry and smokers might be advised to break habitual links. Some time ago, Roberts (1969) claimed success in reducing smoking by having his clients restrict their smoking to a special 'smoking chair', which is, preferably, located in a rather uninspiring setting such as a chilly outhouse away from family and friends. This stratagem not only breaks the stimulus–response link, but adds a dash of negative reinforcement!

One of the important issues in developing self-regulatory skills is the extent to which a skilled counsellor/trainer should be involved. For instance, as Kok et al. (1992) point out, it is important that attributions *after* failure should not lead to disillusionment. They cite Hospers et al. (1990), who demonstrate that people whose attributions of their failure are 'internal, stable and uncontrollable' are likely to feel that they lack the willpower to lose weight. The task of the trainer would be to change the attribution to 'unstable, internal and controllable' in order to reduce that expectation of failure and the associated guilt or anger that might be felt. Successful counselling would thus create higher persistence, hopefully leading to ultimate success. Attempts have been made to provide mediated help and guidance for individuals via booklets and computers, for example, that are based on targeting individuals and tailoring messages to their apparent needs, often in the context of a 'stages of change' analysis. Success in this endeavour would certainly be cost-effective, but the potential of such approaches must still be treated with a degree of scepticism.

IMPLICATIONS FOR PROGRAMME PLANNING

Our discussion of communication of innovations theory examined in some detail major factors governing the adoption of new practices at the level of social systems. We then paid particular attention to the determinants of health actions at the individual level – especially from an empowerment perspective. It will doubtless be self-evident that any systematic and thoughtful attempts at devising effective interventions and programmes must categorically take account of these various influences on individuals and social systems. Indeed, understanding the determinants of health actions, and the complex interplay between determinants, is essential if we are to develop effective and efficient interventions to influence the factors that govern our health- and illness-related choices. By way of example, the reader may wish to consider which of the various psycho-social determinants of smoking behaviour considered in this chapter will be influenced by the different interventions identified by the guidance on smoking cessation services (NICE, 2008b) listed in the box.

'Proven' smoking cessation interventions:

- Brief interventions – opportunistic advice, discussion, negotiation or encouragement and, where necessary, referral to more intensive treatment
- Individual behavioural counselling – with a trained smoking cessation counsellor
- Group behaviour therapy
- Pharmacotherapies – such as nicotine replacement therapy
- Self-help materials – any manual or structured programme, in written or electronic format, that can be used by individuals
- Telephone counselling and quitlines
- Mass-media campaigns.

NICE, 2008b

This principle does not apply only to individual behaviour change. Indeed, in accordance with our commitment to empowerment, we need to understand which characteristics of individuals and social systems can be influenced in order to enable them to gain control over their environmental and social circumstances.

Empowerment and the principle of reciprocal determinism are central to this endeavour. We are all influenced by our environments at macro and meso levels, and many of us are in a position to reciprocate and exercise power over our physical, social and economic circumstances. Regrettably, too many people have little influence in these areas and react passively to those circumstances. Understanding the determinants of powerlessness is, therefore, of special importance and using that understanding to develop empowering health promotion programmes must constitute our major *raison d'être*.

In the chapters that follow, we will be discussing models that might be used in planning efficient health promotion programmes. In Chapter 5, we seek to demonstrate that it is not only necessary to understand the determinants of health action but also important to use such 'evidence', together with other strategic information, for our programme planning.

KEY POINTS

o   The adoption of new practices within social systems follows a consistent pattern.

o   The rate of adoption is influenced by the characteristics of the innovation, channels of communication, the nature of the social system and time.

o   Individual health intentions are the product of the interplay of beliefs (including beliefs about self), motivations (including self-esteem), normative influences and personality factors.

o   Beliefs about control, both generalized (locus of control) and specific (self-efficacy beliefs), are central to both empowerment and health decisions.

o   The translation of intention into practice is influenced by personal factors such as skills and knowledge together with facilitating environmental factors.

o   Maintenance of new behaviours is influenced by experience and the development of self-regulatory skills can help to avoid relapse when this experience is perceived as negative.

o   Individual empowerment is the product of self-esteem, beliefs about control, a sense of coherence, commitment and concern about others, and possession of a repertoire of appropriate life skills.

o   There is reciprocal interplay between individuals and their environment, but environmental factors will significantly affect the amount of influence individuals have and their actual level of empowerment.

4

HEALTH PROMOTION PLANNING – A SYSTEMATIC APPROACH

The world is divided into people who do things and people who get the credit. Try, if you can, to belong to the first class. There's far less competition.

Dwight Morrow (1873–1931), *Letter to his son*

OVERVIEW

The basic premise of this chapter is that well-planned interventions are more likely to be effective. The chapter will:

- establish the central importance of systematic planning
- introduce a number of planning models
- consider the factors associated with the quality of health promotion programmes
- recognize the need to develop partnerships and identify the characteristics of successful partnerships for health.

INTRODUCTION

Over and above increasing effectiveness, a number of recent developments have emphasized the importance of a systematic approach to health promotion planning. These include the need for greater economic accountability, a target-driven climate and the general move towards evidence-based practice. Furthermore, within the UK, the adoption of market principles for commissioning services introduced by the health service reforms of the early 1990s led to a contract culture that required greater attention to the formal planning and costing of health promotion activity and quality assurance.

Speller et al. (1998) note the central importance of strategic planning to the quality of health promotion programmes, along with programme management and monitoring. There is also an ethical imperative to make explicit the rationale for interventions and the assumptions, values and principles on which they are based.

It will be clear from the earlier chapters that health promotion can involve a wide range of different interventions to achieve health gain, used either on their own or in combination. Green and Kreuter (1991) summarize the purpose of health promotion as intervening to reduce, or prevent an increase in, the proportion of the population engaged in negative health behaviour or exposed to negative health conditions and, conversely, to increase the proportion that exhibits positive health behaviour or is exposed to positive health conditions. Sustainability is achieved by maximizing the conditions that enable individuals or groups to assume control over their health. Such support can range from putting policies in place to changing organizational practices and creating a supportive social climate.

Bartholomew et al. (2001) note that health promotion programmes may be directed at a number of different levels – individual, interpersonal, organizations, community, society and supra-nation. Given the breadth of health promotion and the numerous options concerning possible interventions, the selection of an appropriate course of action can be perplexing and is often influenced either by ideological considerations or custom and practice. However, a number of models exist that provide a guide through the complexity.

This chapter identifies the stages in the process of rational planning and provides examples of planning models. It also considers the issue of quality and health promotion. There is increasing recognition that tackling the complex factors that influence health status is not just the responsibility of the health sector, but requires the coordinated response of a number of different sectors. The participation of communities is also integral to effective health promotion. This chapter concludes by considering intersectoral collaboration and partnership working.

HORIZONTAL AND VERTICAL PROGRAMMES

Before providing an overview of selected planning models, we should note that practitioners are not always in a position to begin with a blank canvas. They may be appointed to a designated programme or required by managerial directives to address particular issues. Such programmes are often defined in terms of disease and are referred to as 'vertical programmes'. The first English national health strategy, *The Health of the Nation* (Department of Health, 1992), set targets for five key areas – coronary heart disease and stroke, cancers, mental illness, HIV/AIDS and sexual health, and accidents. The strategy was criticized on account of its vertical disease orientation. French and Milner (1993: 98), for example, contended:

> it is confined to a set of largely biomedical disease reduction targets and does not address structural influences on poor health or positive wellness, nor the resource commitment necessary to tackle the massed ranks of poverty, poor environment and crumbling social infrastructure ...

Furthermore, it was felt that the emphasis on national targets, although providing a focus for activity, did not encourage the identification of local needs and flexibility in setting local targets (Department of Health, 1998c).

Our earlier discussion of the determinants of health in Chapter 2 and the factors associated with changing behaviour in Chapter 3 would indicate that there are common issues across vertical programmes. Lifestyle factors, such as smoking, would be common to both cancers and cardiovascular disease. Similarly, at a more fundamental level, personal attributes, such as locus of control, self-esteem and life skills, will exert an influence on lifestyle. Furthermore, environmental factors will have an impact on lifestyle, as well as direct effects on health status. There is strong evidence linking poverty with a whole range of vertically defined problems. It is clear that not only are programmes more likely to be effective if they tackle these cross-cutting or *horizontal* issues, but also that reorientation towards a horizontal approach should lead to greater efficiency. Figure 4.1 illustrates how horizontal programmes can be applied to vertically defined problems. It also draws attention to the reciprocal relationship between environment and life skills. The exercise of democratic rights requires appropriate life skills and can be instrumental in achieving healthy (or healthier) public policy. Conversely, public policy will limit individuals' freedom of choice and behaviour and may also determine what opportunities exist to develop life skills.

More recent health strategies have paid greater attention to inequalities and the underlying horizontal influences on health status. For example, *Health Challenge England* (2006c) recognized the contribution of self-confidence, self-esteem and empowerment to health choices and lifestyle. Nonetheless, their orientation is still around either diseases or, more latterly, specific behavioural risk factors. *Saving Lives: Our Healthier Nation* (Department of Health, 1999) focused on cancer, coronary heart disease and stroke, accidents and mental health, while the more recent *Health Challenge England* (Department of Health, 2006c) focused on obesity, physical activity, alcohol consumption, stress, smoking and poor sexual health.

PLANNING MODELS

The overall purpose of systematic planning is to identify goals and the most effective means of achieving them. This involves making strategic decisions about the most appropriate courses of action together with operational decisions about the deployment of resources and ensuring that all the necessary elements are in place. Dignan and Carr (1992: 4) note that:

> Effective planning requires anticipation of what will be needed along the way towards achieving the goal. This statement implies that the goal is defined, as are the necessary steps involved in reaching the goal. Perhaps most importantly, it requires an understanding of the steps and how they interrelate.

We noted in Chapter 1 the wide range of activities that can be included under the health promotion umbrella. It follows that comprehensive health promotion programmes will need to include an appropriate combination of methods and involve a number of different sectors. Programmes are more likely to be successful if planning is

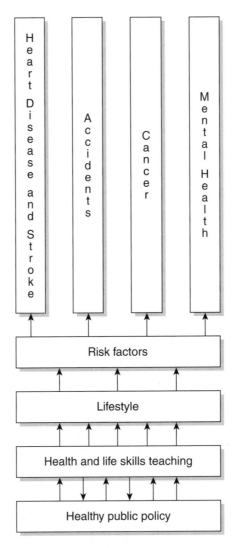

Figure 4.1   Horizontal and vertical programmes

approached in an inclusive way, involving all the major stakeholders. Not only does this create a bigger pool of experience to draw on, but it also establishes collective ownership of the programme. Furthermore, exclusivity runs counter to health promotion's commitment to participation. It is important at the outset, therefore, to identify the stakeholder community.

'Stakeholders' are all those individuals, groups or organizations with an interest in the initiative. They include those affected by the impact of an initiative and those who are in a position to influence its success. The different groups of stakeholders are outlined in the box.

Stakeholders

- **Primary stakeholders** are the potential beneficiaries – those who are directly affected, either positively or negatively, by the initiative.
- **Secondary stakeholders** are those involved in implementing the initiative.
- **Key stakeholders** are those whose support is essential to the continuation of the initiative – for example, fundholders.

The relative power and influence of the different stakeholders should be assessed together with their perceptions of, and willingness to support, the initiative. Such a stakeholder analysis can be instrumental in identifying potential alliances and partners and mobilizing the support required to get initiatives up and running.

The terminology associated with planning tends to be used somewhat loosely and interchangeably within the health promotion literature. In the interests of clarity, we have defined the way we have used the terms here in the box.

Planning terminology

Programme   delineates the area that is being addressed. This is an umbrella term that includes all the activities involved in developing and running, for example, a coronary heart disease programme or a community development programme.

Strategy   the preferred course of action for achieving immediate or longer-term goals. It is selected tactically on the basis of evidence, theory or experience. The term can be used at all levels – for example, an 'overall programme strategy' or an 'implementation strategy'.

Plan   an outline of all the various components and how they relate to each other.

Aim   a broad statement of what is intended to be achieved. Aims can be developed at different levels – for example, overall programme aims, educational aims, policy aims.

Objective   precise and detailed statements of the intended outcomes that will contribute to the overall aim.

Intervention   the activities or collection of activities that will contribute directly to the desired change.

Method   specific approaches or techniques used.

Hubley (1993: 207) poses four questions to guide the planning process:

> Where are we now?
> Where do we want to go?
> How will we get there?
> How will we know when we get there?

These four questions are integral to the planning model proposed by Dignan and Carr (1992) shown in Figure 4.2.

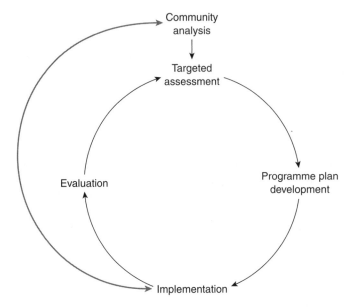

Figure 4.2   Dignan and Carr's planning model (Dignan and Carr, 1992)

The process begins with a needs assessment. This involves a community analysis to identify the programme's focus and the characteristics of the community, followed by a more specific, targeted assessment to identify the determinants of any problems and the key issues that will need to be addressed to achieve change. The goals and objectives for the programme should then be identified, along with resource implications and any potential obstacles. The actual methods to be used in the intervention can then be selected. The logistics of implementation should be considered, and monitoring and evaluation systems put in place.

The apparent simplicity of this model belies the complexity of the decisions required at each stage. There is fuller discussion of these issues at relevant points in this book – indeed, its structure reflects the various stages of the planning process. We have already discussed the determinants of health and health-related decisions in Chapters 2 and 3. Chapter 5 will consider needs assessment in more detail. Chapters 6, 7, 8, 9 and 10 will address different methods and Chapter 11 evaluation. Our purpose in this chapter, however, is to focus on the planning process itself and the adoption of a systematic approach.

There are several different planning models. While conforming to the same broad outline as Figure 4.2, they vary in the level of detail and their relevance for particular purposes. We outline some examples below.

Precede–proceed

One of the best-known planning models is the precede–proceed model (Green and Kreuter, 1991), as shown in Figure 4.3. A particular strength of this model is the attention

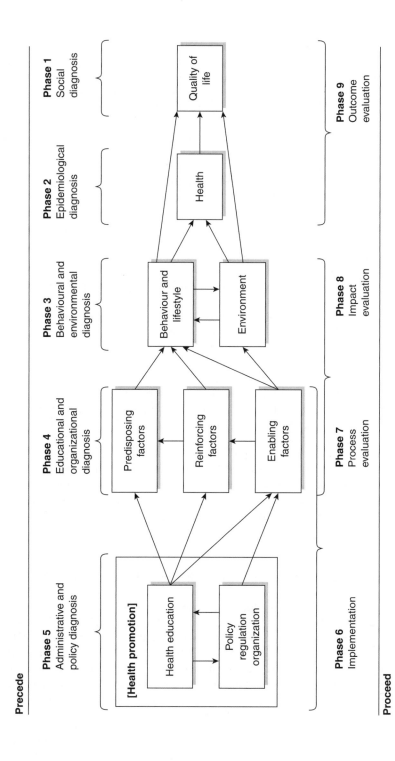

Figure 4.3   Precede–proceed (Green and Kreuter, 1991)

given to identifying the numerous factors that affect health status as a basis for focusing on the subset of factors that need to be addressed by the proposed intervention. Indeed, the model is premised on the view that there are multiple determinants of health and that efforts to improve it require multidimensional and multisectoral action.

The starting point of the model is an assessment of the quality of life and any social problems experienced by the population. It then identifies any specific health problems that contribute to quality of life and establishes which of these should be prioritized. These are then analysed to establish both environmental and behavioural risk factors. The attention given to the environment acknowledges its importance in supporting health-related behaviour as well as its direct influence on health. Further analysis identifies the plethora of factors that influence health behaviour. These are grouped as follows:

- **predisposing factors** – personal factors that influence motivation to change, such as knowledge, beliefs, attitudes, values
- **enabling factors** – factors that support change in behaviour or environment, such as resources and skills, and also any barriers
- **reinforcing factors** – the feedback received from adopting the behaviour.

In essence, these various phases lead to a diagnosis of all contributory factors. Two key considerations influence the selection of factors to focus on in developing an intervention. The extent to which they contribute to the problem is clearly of fundamental importance. However, the resources available and the organization's capacity to deliver health promotion programmes will also be influential.

An appropriate combination of methods can then be selected and the intervention implemented. Evaluation will include process, impact and outcome measures. Although presented as a linear sequence, the evaluation findings should feed back into the earlier stages, creating a more cyclical process.

The various phases of the model draw on a range of different disciplines. Phases 1, 2 and 3, for example, will draw on epidemiological methods and information; phases 3 and 4 on social and behavioural theory; designing interventions will require educational, political and administrative theory; and implementation will draw on political and administrative science and community organization theory.

Logical frameworks

Logical frameworks have their origin in military planning, but were adapted for use by USAID in 1969 and have subsequently been used by other aid programmes in response to demands for more effective planning (Nancholas, 1998). Figure 4.4 provides an overview of the logical framework, or LogFrame, matrix.

The vertical hierarchy corresponds to the stages in developing the LogFrame. It starts with the goal, which is usually expressed in very broad terms, such as reducing teenage pregnancy. The next level is the purpose, which is a statement of the desired achievement of the project. The purpose should make a direct contribution to the goal. Each LogFrame should contain only one goal and one purpose, which are often expressed in behavioural terms. Using the example of teenage pregnancy, the purpose

	Narrative summary	Verifiable indicators	Means of verification	Assumptions
Goal				
Purpose				
Outputs				
Activities				

Figure 4.4 A logical framework 4 x 4 matrix

of a programme might be to increase the proportion of sexually active teenagers who make use of the contraceptive services within a locality.

The outputs are then identified. These are the immediate results, or deliverables, of the programme and could include material factors, organizational change or behavioural change. A number of outputs may be necessary to achieve the purpose – for example, running young people's contraceptive clinics that are user-friendly and scheduled for a time that most suits their needs along with raised awareness among young people of these services.

Finally, the activities that are required to bring about the outputs should be specified. These might include working with clinic managers to persuade them of the need to schedule sessions for young people, running focus groups with young people to establish how clinics could be made user-friendly and what times would be most appropriate for this age group, and providing training for clinic staff to make them aware of the views of young people. Similarly, activities to raise awareness might include developing and pretesting posters, displaying posters in all schools in the locality and so on.

Bell (2001) summarizes the four vertical levels as:

> Why do the thing? (goal)
> What is the thing for? (purpose)
> What are the outcomes of the thing? (outputs)
> How to do the thing? (activities)

The vertical logic should then be verified by working backwards through these various stages and checking out, in principle, *if* one stage is in place, *then* the next will follow, as in Figure 4.5.

Such verification will reveal lapses in logic and identify both omissions and any redundancy. It will also make explicit any assumptions at each level. In our simple illustration, there are several major assumptions – for example, that the contraceptive service provider has both the capacity and resources to run designated young people's clinics, young people are well motivated regarding using contraceptives, schools will be willing to cooperate and display posters, young people will read the posters and so on. Some consideration will need to be given to whether or not the assumptions are well founded or if they expose potentially fatal flaws in the vertical logic and overall design.

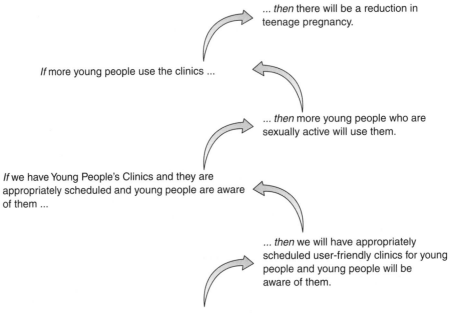

... *then* there will be a reduction in teenage pregnancy.

If more young people use the clinics ...

... *then* more young people who are sexually active will use them.

If we have Young People's Clinics and they are appropriately scheduled and young people are aware of them ...

... *then* we will have appropriately scheduled user-friendly clinics for young people and young people will be aware of them.

If we run focus groups and establish what the needs of young people are and train staff and persuade managers of the need for change and have well-designed posters publicizing the Young People's Clinic and posters are displayed in all schools ...

Start here

Figure 4.5   LogFrames – checking the vertical logical

Returning to our example, if sufficient resources are not available, then, however supportive clinic managers and staff are of the proposed changes, they will be unable to put them into practice. Obtaining funding could be included as an additional output, along with an appropriate cluster of activities. Work may also need to be done to gain the support of those in the position of gatekeeper with regard to displaying posters in schools. If, on the other hand, schools have been actively involved with the development of the project, it may be reasonable to assume that their cooperation will be forthcoming. Nancholas (1998) notes that the process is 'reiterative' and each decision is reviewed and revised as necessary. The value of making explicit all assumptions is that it provides a check that all necessary conditions are in place to ensure the success of the project and that contingency plans exist for any problems that might be anticipated.

At this point, it is worth emphasizing that participatory processes are central to LogFrame planning and decisions should be arrived at by achieving consensus among the stakeholders. Relevant literature and research evidence should also be consulted (Nancholas, 1998). Furthermore, plans should be based on sound preliminary analysis, which would include:

- **stakeholder analysis** to identify the key players, their influence (positive or negative) and level of participation
- **problem analysis** to identify the nature of the problem and its determinants using a 'problem tree' that progressively homes in on the root causes needing to be addressed
- **risk analysis** to identify major obstacles and risks.

Objectively, verifiable indictors (OVIs) need to be specified for each level of the vertical hierarchy and would answer the question 'How will you know that it has been achieved?' These are effectively the objectives of the programme and should be precise, including necessary detail, such as who, how much and when (for example, 80 per cent of school pupils aged 15 to 16 will be able to recall the name, location and opening times of at least one young people's contraceptive clinic in the locality within a month of coming into service). The evidence required to provide objective verification – the means of verification (MOV) – should then be considered. Again, returning to our example, this could be a written questionnaire survey of 15 to 16-year-olds in all schools in the locality. Alternatively, in relation to the goal of reducing teenage pregnancy, an OVI might be a 10 per cent reduction in births to teenage mothers within two years of the introduction of the young people's contraceptive service and the MOV would be routinely collecting data on births. The means of monitoring activities and evaluating outcomes are therefore embedded within the planning process.

The final stages involve operational, management and financial issues. The inputs required for each of the activities should be identified, overall costs estimated and a budget prepared. A time plan, covering implementation of all activities and milestones, will also need to be produced.

Clearly, the preparation of a LogFrame can be demanding in relation to the level of detailed decision making required and the methodology is not without it critics. VSO Netherlands (undated) notes two major criticisms of LogFrames. First, predetermining objectives and indicators leaves no room for recording the often important, yet unanticipated, events that often arise. Second, the emphasis on consensus does not register differing views and diversity of opinion can be the source of innovation.

Broughton (2001) identifies the main weaknesses as being time-consuming, requiring sound understanding of the conventions used to complete LogFrames and, when completed, the danger of becoming 'frozen in time', hence limiting their applicability in rapidly evolving emergency situations. However, he also acknowledges their strength in bringing discipline to clarifying means, ends and assumptions and providing a framework for determining the way in which performance should be measured and for monitoring, evaluation and reporting. Furthermore, they contribute to collaborative working and consensus building.

Nancholas (1998) identifies similar advantages, along with some additional features. LogFrames have the capacity to combine the efficiency of rational planning models with flexibility. They also provide clear and concise summaries of whole programmes, which help to create overall visions of the programmes and communicate these to others.

Daniel and Dearden (2001: 2) note that LogFrames have been viewed as inflexible, restrictive and inappropriate for creative community projects and complex interventions. However, they argue that the approach embraces the key elements of successful projects, notably:

- short- and long-term objectives have to be clarified and coherent
- risks have to be identified and strategies developed to meet them
- indicators for successful intervention need to be agreed at the outset
- methods of collecting and recording evidence of change also have to be set in place.

Daniel and Dearden report on the experience in the UK of using LogFrames for planning Health Action Zone (HAZ) Innovation Fund projects – innovative projects set up to demonstrate new ways of working towards the HAZ inequality and modernization agenda. The advantages of using a LogFrame for planning were identified as being:

- a systematic, logical and thorough approach
- the discipline and structure that it imposes
- the identification of risks and assumptions
- the provision of a framework for monitoring and evaluation
- the encouragement of real partnerships
- flexibility and adaptability.

Conversely, disadvantages of the methodology included:

- conflict with other planning systems in place
- an emphasis on quantitative rather than qualitative indicators
- an assumption that partnerships exist
- its time-consuming nature
- its inflexible and controlling nature
- the use of a lot of jargon
- the requirement of appropriately timed training.

They conclude that 'The logical framework works' in this context and quote one of the trainers:

> LogFrames really do take the mystery out of project planning for local people, they are simple and clear. The problem for professionals is that [working with LogFrames] they have to be transparent – something we have all learnt not to be in order to survive in bureaucracies! Managing that change is the biggest issue, not necessarily managing the LogFrame process ... (Daniel and Dearden, 2001: 6)

While we have shown how LogFrames can guide the whole planning process, others have used them more flexibly. The Health Communication Unit (2001) suggests that they can be used at different stages – for initial 'visioning' and priority setting, for checking out draft goals and objectives to identify gaps and inconsistencies and during implementation in relation to presenting and evaluating the programme. The contribution of logic models to the planning process is summarized as:

- Demonstrating how a program's strategies contribute to the achievement of intended goals and objectives;
- Identifying gaps and inconsistencies within a program, such as objectives that are not being met, or activities that are not contributing to specific objectives;
- Providing an effective communication tool that helps new stakeholders or potential sponsors to understand a program;

- Involving stakeholders in program planning (through the collective development of a logic model); and
- Building a common understanding of what a program is all about and how the parts fit together.

(The Health Communication Unit, 2001: 1)

The PABCAR model

In Chapter 1, we drew attention to the centrality of policy to definitions of health promotion. It follows, then, that development of healthy public policy should be of major concern for health promotion professionals and that advocacy is a legitimate part of their role – issues that will receive further attention in Chapters 6 and 8. Advocacy campaigns are, by their very nature, high profile and Maycock et al. (2001) suggest that there is frequently a dilemma about whether or not to become involved in such campaigns – not only are they time-consuming and costly, organizations risk damaging their reputation if they become publicly aligned with 'inappropriate' causes. Maycock et al. suggest that there is little in the literature to specifically guide decision making about advocacy campaigns. They propose the PABCAR model as a framework for deciding whether or not to support a public health issue. An overview of this model is presented in Figure 4.6.

There are five mains stages:

P   identification of the **p**roblem and its significance for the community
A   assessment of whether or not the problem is **a**menable to change
BC analysis of the overall **b**enefits and **c**osts of intervening, which should be defined broadly and include social impact and ethical considerations, but, clearly, benefits should outweigh costs
A   assessment of the **a**cceptability of intervening to the target group, community, politicians, industry
R   **r**ecommendations for action and monitoring: if there is a high level of acceptability, it may be possible to proceed directly to implementing a public health intervention, but if, in contrast, acceptability is low, then advocacy on behalf of the public health measure will be required (such advocacy should be directed towards those who oppose the intervention as well as ensuring the continued support of those who are in favour of it).

Maycock et al. describe how an analysis using the PABCAR model was supportive of advocacy for the introduction of random breath testing in Western Australia. In short, alcohol-related road injuries were a significant problem. There was evidence that random breath testing offered considerable potential in relation to injury prevention and its sequelae, along with increased freedom for other road users. Over and above the actual cost of implementing random breath testing, other costs included the minor inconvenience of being tested, loss of freedom of the choice to drink and drive, loss of revenue for the alcohol industry and so on. There was a high level of acceptance of random breath testing among the community, but criticism from the alcohol industry, which attempted to gain the support of politicians by framing the argument in terms of the rights and freedom of individuals. Overall, there was a strong case for involvement

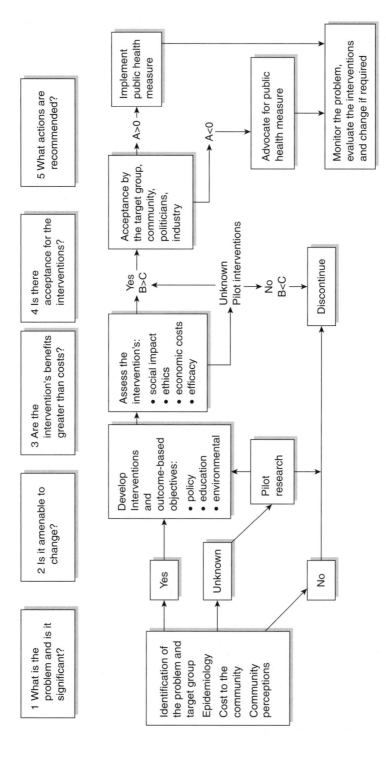

Figure 4.6   Public health decision-making model – PABCAR (after Maycock et al., 2001)

in advocacy on behalf of the issue. Efforts were, in fact, successful, resulting in the introduction of legislation for random breath testing. Using a similar analysis, it was judged to be more feasible to advocate for a 0.05 per cent blood alcohol concentration than 0.0 per cent. Maycock et al. (2001: 64) conclude that the value of the model is that 'its use should help minimize the criticism that can result from advocating for measures that are inappropriate'.

A five-stage community organization model

Systematic planning is often aligned with top-down approaches and held to be inconsistent with community involvement. We would challenge this view and contend that strategies for involving communities are more likely to be effective if they are well planned. The key issue is that the planning process, in this instance, should explicitly address participation and draw on established principles of community development, together with relevant theory. Bracht et al. (1999), for example, describe a five-stage process for community organization, shown in Figure 4.7. Although the various stages are represented as discrete in the model, the authors note that there is some overlap between them.

Stage 1 is concerned with establishing the status quo and setting priorities. It involves:

- defining the community
- constructing a community profile, which includes health and demographic data and information on the community
- assessing the community's capacity by identifying ongoing activities and those organizations, groups or individuals who could offer support – this will also include feasibility and identification of the financial resources required
- assessing any barriers within the community
- assessing readiness for change.

Stage 2 involves designing activities and setting up an organizational structure to mobilize and coordinate community support and involvement. The key components of this stage are:

- setting up a core planning group and identifying a local coordinator
- choosing an organizational structure
- identifying and recruiting members
- defining the goals
- clarifying roles and responsibilities of members
- providing training and recognition.

Stage 3 focuses on implementing activities to achieve goals and includes:

- selecting and prioritizing intervention activities – particularly, assessing whether or not activities are appropriate and sufficiently comprehensive to achieve the goals
- developing a time plan to sequence activities to achieve maximum gains
- generating broader community participation

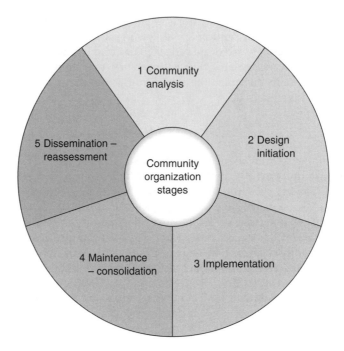

Figure 4.7   Bracht et al.'s community organization model (Bracht et al., 1999)

- planning media coverage
- obtaining financial and other support
- setting up intervention evaluation monitoring and intervention systems.

Stage 4 takes place when the programme is well under way and appraises the current position and future directions. It is concerned with:

- sustainability by virtue of integrating activities into community structures
- establishing a positive organizational climate to encourage the retention of staff and volunteers
- having an ongoing recruitment plan for staff and volunteers
- acknowledging the contribution of volunteers.

Stage 5 involves dissemination and reassessment. Early dissemination of the evaluation findings in an appropriate manner will contribute to maintaining the visibility of the programme and provide a boost for those involved. Formative elements of evaluation will assist in shaping the development of the programme and a final summative evaluation will identify what has been achieved and lessons learned, which should inform future programmes. This stage includes:

- updating the community analysis to identify what changes have been achieved
- assessing the effectiveness of the interventions
- summarizing the findings in a suitable format for different constituencies and developing future plans.

Community empowerment

Empowerment, as we have noted, is a central tenet of health promotion. Yet, Laverack and Labonte (2000) assert that, in practice, although lip service is paid to the discourse of empowerment, top-down programmes maintain unequal power structures in society. Such programmes address issues defined by professionals and empowerment, in this context, becomes a means of achieving predefined goals. This contrasts with bottom-up approaches, which would involve the community in identifying and responding to its own needs. In such instances, empowerment would be a terminal goal – that is, an end in itself rather than a means.

Laverack and Labonte attribute the mismatch between discourse and practice to lack of clarity in how to operationalize empowerment within conventional top-down planning. They suggest that the two can be reconciled without empowerment being used instrumentally to achieve behaviour change goals, but that this requires consideration of empowerment at each stage of the planning process. They propose a model that pursues empowerment goals by means of a parallel track running alongside the conventional programme track, as illustrated in Figure 4.8, although it can also be used for bottom-up community development programmes.

At the design phase, sufficient time should be allowed for the often lengthy process of involving communities in an empowering way. Particular attention should be paid to the needs of marginalized populations who are least able to express their needs. Furthermore, programmes should begin with realistic aims and focus on relatively small-scale, achievable projects to generate early successes and build confidence. Programme planners need to question the ways in which planning processes and programme implementation will contribute to the nine domains of community capacity identified by Labonte and Laverack and listed in the box.

Community capacity domains

1 Community participation
2 Local leadership
3 Empowering organizational structures
4 Problem assessment capacities
5 Ability to ask 'Why?'
6 Resource mobilization
7 Links to others
8 Equitable relationships, outside agents
9 Community control over the programme

Labonte and Laverack, 2001a, 2001b

HEALTH PROMOTION PLANNING – REFLECTIONS

We have presented a number of planning models that differ from each other in relation to the levels of analysis that they include, the extent to which they specify the factors that should be considered at each level and the relative involvement of different

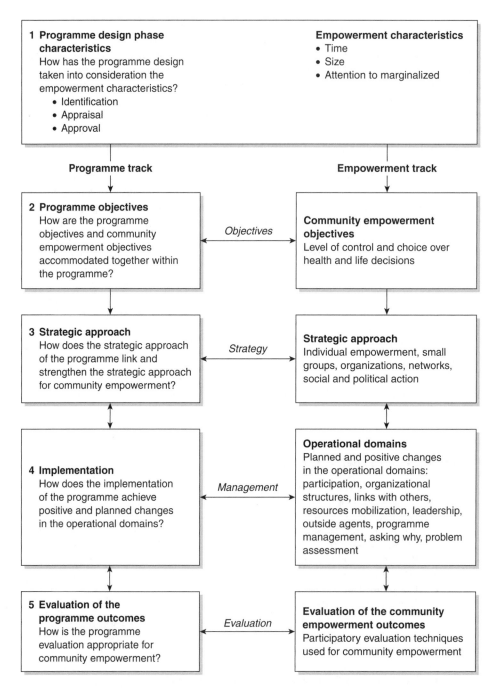

Figure 4.8   A planning framework for incorporating community empowerment into top-down health promotion programmes (Laverack and Labonte, 2000)

stakeholders. Some models are more generic in orientation than others and, hence, applicable to almost any situation or problem, while others, such as the PABCAR model, have been designed to suit more specific purposes. An interesting interchange between two groups of academics on the nature of planning models was sparked by an article by McLeroy et al. which suggested that planning models (such as PATCH, pre-cede–proceed, coalitions/partnerships, lay health adviser approaches, social change models, organizational change models):

> are largely a-theoretical and a-contextual [and further] they are largely indepen-dent of the specific health problem being addressed, they ignore what we know about the social production of disease, they are not connected to the field's collec-tive wisdom about what works, with whom, under what conditions and they may lead to inappropriate interventions for the communities in which they are to be used. (1993: 307)

They called for an ecological planning approach involving three stages:

1 **theory of the problem** which involves analysis of problems and the intrapersonal, interpersonal, organizational, community, cultural and public policy factors that pro-duce and maintain them
2 **theory of intervention** which provides a state-of-the-art view of the relative effective-ness of different interventions
3 **understanding the context of practice** which allows interventions to be matched to the local community or organizational context.

The riposte to this article by Green et al. (1994) highlights some key issues concerning planning models. They put forward a strong argument that they are, in fact, grounded in theory and are consistent with a multilevel, multisector analysis – that is, an ecologi-cal approach to health promotion. Furthermore, we noted above that a precede–proceed analysis should incorporate a range of theoretical perspectives into the various stages.

Green at al. acknowledge that no planning model is immune from misuse, but inappropriate interventions arise from lack of rigour in the detailed application of models rather than from the model itself. Models such as precede–proceed provide a guide through the causal logic underpinning the development of health or health problems and impose a framework for considering all pertinent variables – exposing any omissions and assumptions. Rigorous application of planning models should therefore reduce the probability of interventions being inappropriate. Moreover, some planning models specifically incorporate consideration of contextual factors by means of, for example, a community diagnosis or analysis. Green et al. also suggest that the step-by-step procedure of planning models such as precede–proceed leads to the selection of an appropriate theory to suit both the context and the emergent requirements rather than imposing a theoretical structure at the outset. A sequential approach to planning should, therefore, ensure both relevance and rigour.

MacDonald and Green's (2001) analysis of the process of using a planning model to develop alcohol and drug prevention programmes in schools raises some interesting issues. The project was premised on the view that drug education would be more effective if it were based on local needs and context. Prevention workers were expected to work with schools using the precede–proceed model to guide the planning process. One of the dilemmas facing the workers was achieving a balance between the proactive planning demanded by the project and the tendency of schools to respond to problems in a more reactive way. This raises questions about the suitability of rational planning models where there is a culture of reacting to problems and actions based on common sense and experience rather than analysis. A further issue was the variation in interpretation and application of the model by different workers. Training in the use of models and some assessment of the community's capacity to engage in the planning process will contribute to resolving these issues. However, the question still remains as to whether or not fidelity in implementing the planning model is realistic or possible. MacDonald and Green suggest that successful implementation requires some flexibility to allow adaptation to local circumstances.

An additional consideration is whether or not the complex interplay of factors and alliances associated with health can be addressed by essentially linear planning models. French and Milner (1993) are critical of a simplistic linear view of causality and emphasize the need to consider the many interrelated variables that impact on health behaviour and health status. They also call for realism in relation to what can be achieved and suggest that there can be a number of different starting points from which programmes of work can emerge. For example, the availability of funding for particular streams of work could be the starting point. They suggest that real planning, as illustrated in Figure 4.9, is a systematic, although non-linear, process. Naidoo and Wills (1994: 221) also note that planning is often 'piecemeal or incremental. There is no grand design, but circumstances dictate many small reactive decisions'.

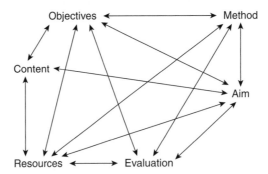

Figure 4.9   French and Milner's view of real planning (after French and Milner, 1993)

Notwithstanding this view, although we have presented the models in this chapter as a linear sequence, in practice it is not essential to start at the beginning – a point acknowledged by Green and Kreuter (1991). The planning process can, in principle, begin at some intermediate point, with the caveat that the preliminary stages should be worked through – as it were, retrospectively – to ensure logical and practical coherence. Furthermore, the possibility of including feedback loops between the various stages in the models provides opportunities for revisiting decisions in the light of emerging issues, thereby enhancing flexibility.

Writing from an evaluation perspective, Judge (2000) also highlights the problem of determining causality in complex social systems. We will provide a fuller discussion in Chapter 11, but this issue is also pertinent to a consideration of the inputs required to achieve change. Judge draws on the work of Pawson and Tilley (1997) to suggest that cause and effect are not 'discrete events', but mechanisms which interact with context to produce outcomes. It is not simply a question of whether or not something works, but more with whom and under what circumstances. The following formula provides a simple summary:

context + mechanism = outcome

The mechanism for change is seen as 'modifying the capacities, resources, constraints and choices facing participants and practitioners' (Judge, 2000: 2). A programme will seek to manipulate these variables to achieve change, but the outcome is also contingent on the context. Therefore, planning appropriate interventions will require a thorough analysis of the context. Judge notes that a 'theory of change approach' (originating from the work of Weiss et al. in the United States (Connell et al., 1995)) can help to clarify exactly how proposed actions are expected to achieve intended outcomes. Using this approach, those involved in planning and implementing initiatives are encouraged to make explicit the ways in which they envisage the links between the various programme components and outcomes – that is, to articulate their theory of change or the assumptive logic underpinning the change that they are trying to achieve. In this context, theory is defined as 'the professional logic that underlies a programme' (Bauld and Judge, 2000).

A systems checklist for health promotion planning

Some years ago, Tones applied a systems approach to planning health education interventions (Tones, 1974). The systems approach had its origins in industrial processes, but, at the time, its relevance to education and programmed learning was receiving considerable attention. The purpose of the systems approach is to identify desired outcomes and all the factors that contribute materially to them. The interrelationships between these factors are then examined so that they can be manipulated to achieve the outcomes with maximum efficiency. The advantages of this approach for education, and specifically health education, are that it demands precision in the formulation of objectives, a clear structure to programmes, the rational selection of methods and specification of the conditions for learning, both within the learner and the learning situation. With the benefit of hindsight, it is questionable whether or not educational processes can, or indeed should, be viewed in quite the same way as production-line manufacturing processes. We have already noted the importance of context and the need for participation and stakeholder support.

There are several concerns about health promotion programme planning being driven by rational processes and governed by formal planning frameworks rather than being allowed to evolve in a more organic way. This is particularly evident in relation to community participation. However, to set rationality and systematic processes against participation, flexibility and context specificity is to impose a false dichotomy. Planning models provide an ordered structure that ensures all relevant variables are considered. The way in which decision-making processes are handled and the information that is brought to bear on this can correspond to a number of different ideological positions. Similarly, goals can be framed in relation to disease prevention, behaviour change, empowerment or community development. The advantages of rational planning may be summarized as:

- making explicit the anticipated causal mechanisms underpinning desired change
- identifying all the necessary conditions for change
- scheduling the various components of an intervention appropriately
- ensuring that all conditions are in place to maximize effectiveness
- providing a forum for bringing together the various stakeholders.

Figure 4.10 provides a checklist of the key issues that need to be considered when developing health promotion programmes. The starting point involves establishing needs and stating the programme's aims or goals. Needs, as we will note in Chapter 5, may be defined in a number of different ways. The ideologies and values of those involved in planning and their conceptualization of health will not only inform the ways in which needs are defined and prioritized, but will also permeate each stage of the planning process. It is worth reiterating that the use of planning models does not in itself impose values on the planning process, but, rather, provides a vehicle for making explicit the values, rationale and assumptions underpinning any decisions. It also exposes those situations where rationality would dictate one course of action and political pressures another (classically demonstrated by the 'Heroin Screws You Up' campaign discussed later in this chapter).

Needs, then, could be professionally or lay defined and focus on positive health states or disease or their various determinants, either environmental or behavioural. Prioritization involves a number of considerations – not least the contextual factors revealed by community profiling. These include the:

- extent and severity of the problem – clearly, life-threatening problems will rate higher than those causing minor inconvenience
- urgency of the problem
- number of people affected
- power and influence of those affected
- possibility of achieving change/improvement
- level of concern, support and commitment among the major groups of stakeholders
- feasibility of taking action in the current context, based on an assessment of the capacity within the organization and/or community
- consistency with the ethics and values of those involved.

If the achievement of equity in health is, as we have argued earlier, a primary goal of health promotion, then some consideration should be given to this in prioritizing needs and the action to be taken to address them. While the *Health Equity Audit* (Department of Health, 2003) was essentially introduced to enable services to be delivered more equitably, its principles are also applicable to the development of health promotion programmes. The *Health Equity Audit* uses 'evidence on inequalities to inform decisions on investment, service planning, commissioning and delivery and to review the impact

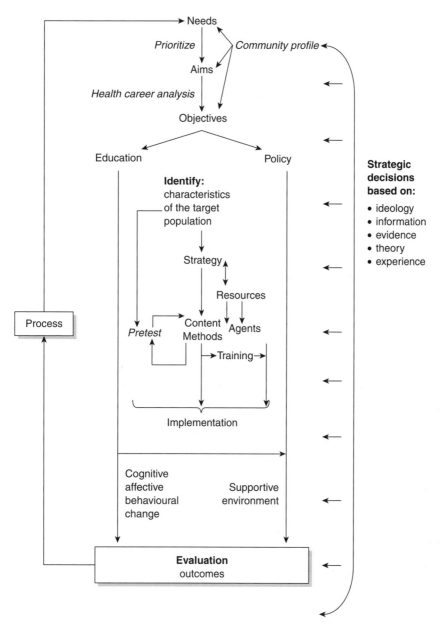

Figure 4.10   A systems checklist for health promotion

of action on inequalities' (Office of the Deputy Prime Minister and Department of Health, 2005: 95). The stages of the Health Equity Audit Cycle are outlined in Figure 4.11. It allows gaps in health status to be identified. Priority can then be given to addressing those needs which would reduce the gap and targeting action appropriately.

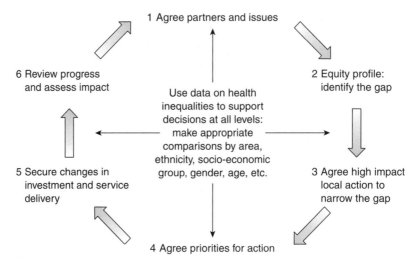

Source: Derived from ODPM and Department of Health, 2005: 94

Figure 4.11   Health Equity Audit Cycle

Aims and objectives

Once priorities have been agreed, then a consensus should be achieved on the overall goal or aim of the programme. Not only does this provide a formal statement of intent as a point of reference to guide future action, but it also ensures that all those involved have a common understanding of what they are trying to achieve. Aims are general, global statements about what the programme intends to achieve (Dignan and Carr, 1992). However, vague, aspirational statements of intent, such as 'improving the quality of life' – while perhaps serving a motivational purpose and acting as a rallying call – offer little in the way of establishing a common purpose. It therefore goes without saying that, although aims are expressed in broad terms, some precision is still required (see box). Aims may be either long- or short-term and framed in a number of different ways, as shown in Table 4.1.

Table 4.1   Examples of aims

Focus	Example
Individual or groups	Increase levels of empowerment among teenage girls in a locality
	Build social capital within a community
Disease	Reduce the level of coronary heart disease within a community
	Reduce the injuries from falls in the over-60s in a locality
Health status	Increase the levels of cardiovascular fitness in the senior citizens in a locality
	Reduce inequalities in health
Health behaviour	Reduce the level of smoking in a community
	Increase the uptake of physical activity within a community
Environment	Improve the safety of the community
Organizations	Introduce a health-promoting school initiative

The importance of clear aims

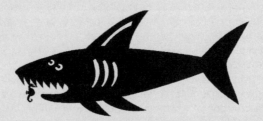

Once upon a time a Sea Horse gathered up his seven pieces of eight and cantered out to find his fortune …
eventually
    … he came upon a Shark, who said, 'Psst. Hey bud. Where ya goin'?'
'I'm going to find my fortune,' replied the Sea Horse.
'You're in luck. If you'll take this short cut,' said the Shark, pointing to his open mouth, 'you'll save yourself a lot of time.'
    'Gee, thanks,' said the Sea Horse, and zoomed off into the interior of the Shark, and was never heard from again.
    The moral of this fable is that if you're not sure where you're going, you're liable to end up someplace else.

Mager, 1975: Preface

Establishing the best way in which to achieve these aims demands a thorough analysis of the determinants of any problem or issue being addressed, along with the context. A health career analysis (referred to in Chapter 2) is a useful device for identifying the major influences on health status and locating possible intervention points. It also helps to identify appropriate target groups and agencies with which to develop collaborative working links. The characteristics of target groups will also need to be assessed.

Consideration of this information, along with relevant theory and empirical evidence of effectiveness, should enable a planning group to establish exactly what change needs to happen to achieve its goal. The broad vision encompassed within the stated aim can then be translated into more precise objectives. Whereas *aims* are, as we have noted, broad and relatively general statements of intent, *objectives* define goals in more specific terms. Thus, one aim may generate a number of subordinate objectives.

Following our earlier discussion of health promotion as the synergistic interaction of policy and education, it should be possible to distinguish *policy* objectives from *educational* objectives. The former would be the specific goals to be attained in the development and implementation of policy, while the latter would be the specific learning outcomes that would result if the health education components of programmes were to be successful (see box for examples).

Examples of objectives from Healthy People 2010

1   Increase the proportion of persons aged 2 years and older who consume at least 2 daily servings of fruit (to 75% from 28% in 1994–6).

2   Increase the proportion of persons aged 2 years and older who consume at least 3 daily servings of vegetables with at least one third being dark green or orange vegetables (to 50% from 3% in 1994–6).

3   Increase the proportion of children and adolescents aged 6–19 years whose intake of meals and snacks at school contributes to good overall dietary quality.

4   Increase the proportion of worksites that offer nutrition or weight management classes or counselling (to 85% from a baseline of 50% in 1998–9).

5   Increase food security among US households and in so doing reduce hunger (to 94% households from a baseline of 88% in 1995).

U.S. Department of Health and Human Services, 2000

The precise formulation of objectives is fundamental to the planning process for a number of different reasons. First, they indicate what strands of activity should be put in place and give structure to the programme. Second, the range of objectives should be sufficiently comprehensive to ensure that all the necessary conditions are achieved in pursuit of the overall aim. Third, as we will note in Chapter 11, they provide a means of evaluating the outcomes of the programme.

There is a recent tendency to use the looser term 'target' in policy documents in the UK consistent with the terminology of public service agreements. For example, *Delivering Choosing Health* (Department of Health, 2005) refers to overarching objectives being underpinned by specific targets. It also identifies 'big wins' – interventions which will have 'the greatest impact on health in the shortest period of time'. In contrast, in the USA, Healthy People 2010 specifies two overarching *goals*. These are to increase the quality and years of healthy life and eliminate health disparities. In pursuit of these, it identifies some 467 specific *objectives*. Notwithstanding the language used, the principle remains the same. It is essential to specify with precision exactly what is to be achieved. For the purpose of this text, we will use the term *objective,* bearing in mind that it is sometimes used synonymously with *target.*

Objectives are highly specific and should be measurable. The acronym SMART is often used to describe the essentials of a clear objective (see the box).

Smart objectives

Specific
Measurable
Achievable
Realistic
Time limited

Objectives should focus on outcomes rather than the process of achieving them. While objectives should be achievable, they should also be sufficiently challenging to attain worthwhile outcomes. The examples of objectives from Healthy People 2010 in the box above specify the levels of outcomes expected in percentage terms. These should not, of course, be arbitrary, but derived from consideration of baseline data and existing time trends. One of the oldest political devices for guaranteeing success is to set objectives that will be achieved automatically if existing time trends continue, independently of any intervention. However, such subterfuge is clearly anathema to the achievement of *worthwhile* goals!

There is typically some variation in the specificity of objectives – the most rigorous objectives are held to be behavioural objectives. Wherever possible, therefore, objectives should be expressed as behavioural objectives that conform to the pattern:

who will be able to do *what* to *what extent* and *when*.

For example, 90 per cent of four-year-olds in locality Z will have been immunized against measles, mumps and rubella within three years of beginning the programme.

Alternatively, if we are focusing on policy and environmental rather than behavioural change, an example would be: Y town council will have introduced traffic-calming measures in 10 per cent of the residential streets in locality X within five years of beginning the programme.

Establishing such objectives presupposes that information is available on the levels of behaviour in question prior to beginning any intervention in order to set achievable, yet challenging, targets. For example, raising the uptake of immunization from 85 to 90 per cent would offer a completely different challenge than from 30 to 90 per cent. Moreover, it is not just a question of the magnitude of the change required. Reference to communication of innovations theory (Rogers and Shoemaker, 1971) in Chapter 3 would indicate that the early introduction of an innovation takes time (and, *ipso facto*, much health promotion effort) as the innovators and, subsequently, the early adopters accept the innovation. There follows a period of more rapid adoption and then the rate of uptake slows considerably as the laggards become involved. Increasing the uptake of behaviour from 5 to 10 per cent is therefore likely to require more effort than from 50 to 55 per cent, and the final 95 to 100 per cent can be particularly problematic as laggards are notoriously difficult to change.

The most rigorous way of expressing behavioural objectives would (in addition to specifying what the learner should be able to do) also define the conditions and acceptable levels of performance. These three components are defined by Mager (1975: 21) as:

1 **Performance** – an objective always says what a learner is able to do.
2 **Conditions** – an objective always describes what the important conditions (if any) are under which the performance is to occur.
3 **Criterion** – wherever possible, an objective describes the criterion of acceptable performance by describing how well the learner must perform in order to be considered acceptable.

While, at first sight, it could appear that behavioural objectives might be more appropriate and easier to formulate when the focus of an intervention explicitly addresses behaviour change, they are readily applied to educational goals. Indeed, their origins are within education and the pursuit of behavioural objectives became a major driving force in the USA in the 1960s and 1970s and the subject of fierce debate (see, for example, Stenhouse, 1975; Popham, 1978). Advocates of behavioural objectives claim that it is possible – and desirable – to develop appropriate behavioural objectives for all cognitive and affective learning outcomes.

One advantage of using behavioural objectives in an educational context is that this acknowledges the active role of the learner. It focuses attention on what we expect the *learner* to be able to do in the specification of outcomes rather than the teacher or health educator. The role of the 'educator' then becomes instrumental and involves putting the conditions in place to *enable* the learner to achieve the behavioural objectives. In that health promotion, by its very nature, is action-orientated, behavioural objectives are particularly relevant. Using behavioural objectives therefore specifies the target group and what we expect them to be able to do, along with how this would contribute to achieving the overall goal. However, we should emphasize that behaviour in this context is merely *indicative* of learning – it should not be taken to imply that the overall goal of the programme is necessarily concerned with behaviour change. For example, in pursuit of a safer environment, an appropriate objective might be: 'A majority of local councillors will vote in favour of the introduction of traffic-calming measures in locality X on date Y.' Achievement of this objective may require a series of subsidiary objectives, such as '90 per cent of local councillors will respond accurately, when interviewed, that locality X has the highest rate of pedestrian injuries in the town within six months of starting the programme.'

Similarly, if participatory approaches are used, a behavioural objective could be phrased thus: 'Using participatory techniques, residents will produce a map identifying the high-risk areas within the locality within three months of starting the programme.'

Although we will return to this at greater length in Chapters 6 and 8, it is worth noting briefly at this point that programmes focusing on policy and environmental change require learning of some sort. This might include greater awareness of an issue, increased motivation to take action or the development of skills in advocacy and lobbying.

Clearly, the overall approach and the relative emphasis on environmental and behavioural factors will be fundamental to shaping objectives. A number of other key decisions will also influence the ways in which they are formulated – whether the programme is horizontal or vertical, the level of operation (individual, family, community, region and so on), the target groups and the timescale.

Listing the programme objectives provides an opportunity to check that consideration has been given to all the necessary elements required for the achievement of the programme's goal and identifies any omissions that may undermine the whole effort. Conversely, in the interests of economy, any overlap or redundancy can also be identified. Furthermore, it encourages articulation of the anticipated mechanism by means of which the change will be achieved – the so-called theory of change referred to above.

From objectives to action

Once programme objectives have been specified, the actual methods to be used – and combinations – can be considered. Clearly, these are many and various and so will be discussed more fully in Chapters 6, 7, 8, 9 and 10. The selection of methods will, again, be based on the intended purpose, local context and characteristics of any target group, theory and evidence of effectiveness – the art of health promotion practice lies in achieving the best fit in relation to all these. Attaching subsidiary objectives to the various activities clarifies their intended purpose. Any preconditions should also be identified. For example, effort may need to be directed towards building a sense of community before community action to improve safety can begin or, alternatively, school staff may need to be trained before a sex education programme can be provided for teenagers. Furthermore, materials and content should be pretested with the target group. Partnerships with other agencies may need to be consolidated and methods of achieving this will also need to be considered.

The so-called 'Penrith Paradox' (Adams and Armstrong, 1995) was born at a symposium to discuss the current state of health promotion theory and practice in the UK. It drew attention to the mismatch that often exists between the type of health promotion practice that might be expected, based on theoretical principles, and the dominant models seen in everyday practice. Of particular concern was the emphasis on individualism in practice when evidence and theory point to the greater effectiveness of community development approaches. The paradox is summed up in the box.

The Penrith Paradox

We talk of a theory–practice gap. Maybe it is more complex and pervasive than this. Some models of health promotion are well supported by theory, quality of theoretical debate and quantity of papers published (e.g. community development/social action). Others (e.g. individualism) are starkly unsupported; in fact greater volume of debate is focused upon criticizing than supporting them. The paradox arises when examining practice in the UK today. The theoretically weak models are dominant in practice whereas theoretically based models to which many practitioners subscribe struggle to be maintained or developed in practice in the UK today.

Adams and Armstrong, 1995: 3

The solution to the paradox was held *not* to involve new models, nor was there a need to test current theories further. What was judged to be needed was a broad disciplinary alliance in both health promotion training and practice and more collaboration between academics and practitioners. There were some moves in this direction in the UK with the development of initiatives such as 'Health Action Zones', 'Healthy Living Centres', 'SureStart' and 'New Deal', together with interest in social capital and urban renewal. There has also been some shift in the political pressures that have influenced practice. The top-down individualist approach that typified Thatcherism (it was Thatcher who famously said 'There is no such thing as Society. There are individual men and women, and there are families.') has given way to a greater emphasis on participation with the New Labour administration. The 'third way' concept at the heart of New Labour health policy involves a combination of state responsibility partnered with greater levels of public participation (Department of

Health, 1997 and 1999). Nonetheless, there are concerns that some of these 'upstream' initiatives which aimed to tackle the root causes of inequality have been short-lived and followed by renewed interest in individual behaviour.

As well as political influences shaping the overall climate within which health promotion activity takes place, political factors can be decisive in the selection of actual methods. The 'Heroin Screws You Up' campaign in the UK was a classic example of flying in the face of expert opinion by allocating considerable resources to funding a high-profile mass media campaign (Tones, 1986). Conventional wisdom – and rational planning – would dictate that drug education for young people should involve a comprehensive programme of personal, social and health education. What the programme did achieve was a demonstration to 'Middle England' that the government was taking action regarding the drug problem, albeit inappropriately.

Returning to the systems checklist (see Figure 4.10 on page 177), at the implementation level, the 5WH formula (outlined in the box) is a well-known acronym for identifying which key issues to address.

5WH

- Who?
- What?
- Where?
- When?
- Why?
- How?

Clearly, with complex, multilevel interventions, all the activities need to be orchestrated so that everything is in the right place at the right time to maximize the effects of the programme and, indeed, minimize the risk of programme failure. Administrative issues such as funding, staffing and deployment need to be managed efficiently. Devices such as Gantt charts are helpful to this end and for detailed operational planning. Gantt charts are essentially bar charts that can be used to visualize the relationships between the various tasks required to achieve the programme's goal. By way of illustration, a brief extract from a Gantt chart is provided in Figure 4.12.

Each task should be specified. Durfee and Chase (1999) suggest that they should also be expressed as an action with a duration. Milestones are important points in the development of the project or programmes and can be marked. They serve as a check that everything is proceeding according to schedule. Beginning some tasks is dependent on the completion of others and this relationship can also be indicated.

The final stages are monitoring and evaluation, which will be discussed at some length in Chapter 11. However, we should note some key points here. First, evaluation should be an integral part of the planning process and considered at all stages. Second, precision in formulating plans and objectives provides a clear focus for monitoring what has been done and evaluating what has been achieved. Finally, plans are not set in stone. Formative evaluation, which would include the pretesting of

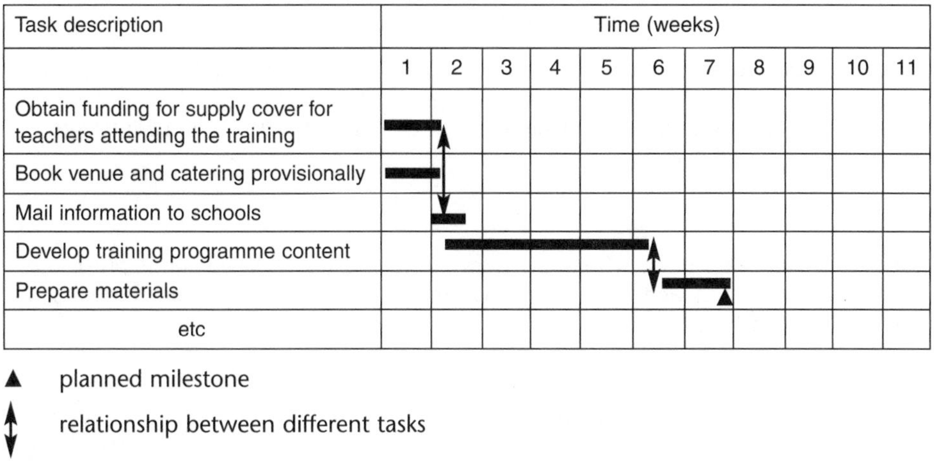

Task description	Time (weeks)										
	1	2	3	4	5	6	7	8	9	10	11
Obtain funding for supply cover for teachers attending the training											
Book venue and catering provisionally											
Mail information to schools											
Develop training programme content											
Prepare materials											
etc											

▲   planned milestone

↕   relationship between different tasks

Figure 4.12 An extract from a Gantt chart for a sex education training programme for school staff

materials, aims to identify what is working well and what is working less well in order to make necessary modifications. Feedback loops in the planning cycle encourage such reflection and adaptation.

QUALITY HEALTH PROMOTION

Generally, the drive for greater efficiency within the health service has placed greater emphasis on value for money and cost improvements, yet the primary concern of the public – and indeed an overriding ethical imperative – is with the effectiveness and quality of the care they receive (Catford, 1993). The target-driven culture of the early twenty-first century has continued to focus on achievement of ends rather than the means of achieving them. Yet, to be consistent with its fundamental values, health promotion should also be concerned with quality and conforming to principles of good practice. The principles of the Ottawa Charter have been a guiding force within the health promotion movement. Evans et al. (1994) suggest that the following core principles should be considered in relation to quality assurance:

• equity
• effectiveness
• efficiency
• accessibility
• appropriateness
• acceptability
• responsiveness.

Catford (1993) also proposes that there should be a common set of criteria to assess performance and quality organized around a number of themes – see the box.

Quality assurance has been defined as:

a systematic process through which achievable and desirable levels of quality are described, the extent to which these levels are achieved is assessed, and action is taken following assessment to enable them to be reached. (Wright and Whittington, in Evans et al., 1994: 20)

and

the work that takes place within any work unit, so as to follow up and improve the unit's own activities and to prevent mistakes or defects from arising. (Berensson et al., 2001: 188)

Themes for assessing quality

- Understanding and responding to people's needs fairly
- Building on sound theoretical principles and understanding
- Demonstrating a sense of direction and coherence
- Collecting, analysing and using information
- Reorientating key decision makers upstream
- Connecting with all sectors and settings
- Using complementary approaches at both individual and environmental levels
- Encouraging participation and ownership
- Providing technical and managerial training and support
- Undertaking specific actions and programmes.

After Catford, 1993

Haglund et al. (1998) note the importance of establishing the purpose of quality assessment and whether it is concerned with checking if standards have been met (that is, providing a borderline between 'good enough' and 'not good enough') or a stimulus for continuous improvement. Speller et al. (1998) describe two main approaches to quality assurance that reflect this distinction: external standards inspection (ESI), where external standards are set in relation to a work process and monitored so that action can be taken if there is any failure to meet standards, and, in contrast, total quality management (TQM), which involves setting internal standards. TQM is also dynamic in approach and is concerned with continuous growth and improvement rather than just ensuring that minimum standards are met, which is typical of the more static approach of ESI. A survey of specialist health promotion services in England (Royle and Speller, 1996) revealed greatest support for internal peer review as being the best way to monitor standards. Opinion was mixed about whether or not there should be a set of national standards and criteria for assuring quality. A 'standard' has been defined as 'a statement that defines an agreed level of excellence' and 'criteria' as 'descriptive statements which are measurable, that relate to a standard' (Evans et al., 1994: 103–4). Speller et al. also distinguish between 'quality assurance programmes', which aim to ensure the quality of all aspects of a service, and 'quality initiatives', in which standards for a particular project or intervention may be agreed.

Quality has been described (British Standards Institute, 1978: BS 4778) as:

the totality of the features and characteristics of a product or service that bear on its ability to satisfy stated or implied needs.

Speller notes that the assessment of the quality of interventions is often based, inappropriately, on outcomes rather than quality criteria. A consensus definition of quality assurance for health promotion was achieved by a European Commission-sponsored project in 1996:

Quality assurance in health promotion is the process of assessment of a programme or intervention in order to ensure performance against agreed standards, which are subject to continuous improvement and set within the framework and principles of the Ottawa Charter. (Speller, 1998: 79)

The principal concern of quality assurance, therefore, is with what is done and whether or not this conforms with agreed standards of practice rather than what is achieved – neatly encapsulated as 'Doing things right is not enough if the right things are not done correctly' (Haglund et al., 1990: 100). The focus is therefore on *inputs* rather than *outcomes*. However, there is inevitably a reciprocal relationship between the two – quality health promotion should draw on evidence of effectiveness and be more effective. The argument that runs through this book is that health promotion should be planned well and that planning should draw on sound evidence at all stages and be informed by principles of good practice. The characteristics of good practice in health promotion are listed in the box.

Characteristics of good practice

- An agreed philosophy
- A clear vision of health
- Decisions based on needs
- A planned approach
- Working in partnerships
- Strategic leadership
- Realistic aims and claims
- Use of effective methods
- Consumer involvement
- Disseminating results
- Reflection
- Motivated and skilled staff.

After Evans et al., 1994

Speller et al. (1998: 145) emphasize that quality assurance can ensure that interventions are 'acceptable, and applicable to the setting, and based on current best evidence'. They contend that only quality-assured programmes should be evaluated and, further, if they prove to be effective, clear guidance on what standards are expected in relation to implementation should be a necessary element of subsequent dissemination. As we will note in Chapter 11, such attention to quality would contribute to avoiding Type 3 errors in evaluation – that is, the inability to detect any effect when interventions were predestined to fail because of poor design and/or implementation.

Haglund et al. (1998) identify a number of tensions in applying models of quality assessment – largely deriving from the commercial and manufacturing sectors – to health promotion. First, quality production standards have generally been developed for routine and repetitive procedures, whereas health promotion interventions are usually unique. Second, quality standards are usually set by the consumer who, in the context of health promotion, may be difficult to define (is it the commissioning agency or the target group?) and also lack a clear voice. Third, health promotion is a multidisciplinary endeavour and views about quality may be influenced by the philosophies to which practitioners subscribe. Furthermore, quality assessment instruments are generally designed for analysing the activities of a single organization and do not adapt well to assessing the cooperation between them.

Some time ago, The Society of Health Promotion Specialists in the UK produced a manual on developing quality in health promotion services. It identified the essential issues to consider, at service level, in relation to quality as:

- guidelines on service provision and practice
- professional development by means of education and training
- recruitment and selection
- principles of professional practice
- measuring and monitoring standards of practice. (Totten, 1992)

Audits are seen as the means of assessing the quality of service provision. Evans et al. (1994: 103) note that the term 'audit' is interpreted in a number of different ways, but that it can be defined as 'the systematic critical analysis of the quality of a health promotion programme' and taken to be synonymous with quality assurance. They propose a quality assurance cycle based on six stages:

- identifying/reviewing key areas for quality assurance
- setting standards
- selecting criteria with which to measure standards
- comparing practice with standards
- taking action
- reviewing the previous stages.

The outcome of the final review stage should feed back into stage one of a new cycle.

Health promotion, by its very nature, is wide-ranging and services are organized in a number of different ways. Speller et al. (1997a) argue that quality assurance should be applied to what might be considered the generic key functions of health promotion. Following a consultation exercise that reflected concern that quality assessment should be grounded in the reality of health promotion practice, they identified six key functions:

- strategic planning
- programme management
- monitoring and evaluation
- education and training
- resources and information
- advice and consultancy.

Strategic planning – particularly intersectoral planning – with a focus on health needs and healthy public policy was seen to be a core function of health promotion. Examples of standards that might be applied to some of these key functions are provided in the box. Alternatively, these could be developed by individual organizations, along with appropriate criteria.

Examples of standards for selected key functions

1 Strategic planning

1.1   There is a group which addresses strategic planning issues in health promotion.
1.2   The health promotion service makes an important contribution to this group.
1.3   A health promotion strategy is produced and/or health promotion figures prominently within other strategy documents.
1.4   The health promotion department's plan relates to the health strategies.

2 Programme management

2.1   A group exists for the planning, implementation and review of each programme area.
2.2   A range of health promotion methods and activities is considered for each programme area in order to determine action plans.

Speller et al., 1997a: 220

Haglund et al. (1990) contend that quality assurance can only be built into the planning phase of interventions. Rather than adopting the flexible TQM approach described above, they focus on the design and planning of interventions to ensure that all the necessary conditions for success are in place. The use of a standardized instrument enables the experiences of local projects to be collected and shared. The 20-item questionnaire used to systematize 'telling the story' of different projects at the Sundsvall Conference (Haglund et al., 1993) was subsequently found to have a role in improving planning. The key issues that were identified for reporting purposes were also the key issues that should inform the development of projects. This interconnectedness should not be altogether surprising. The questionnaire has been revised and now includes six dimensions that relate to the various stages of the supportive environments action model (SESAME) (Haglund et al., 1998), as shown in Figure 4.13.

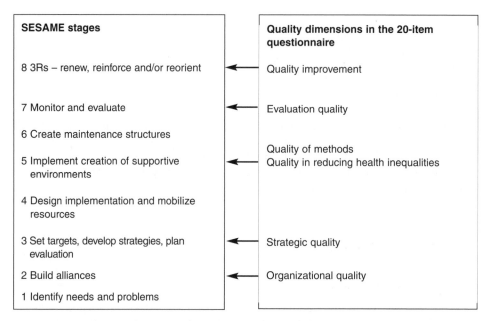

Figure 4.13   Quality dimensions associated with SESAME (After Haglund et al., 1998)

The approach to quality assurance adopted in the Netherlands is similar and aims to improve the effectiveness of programmes by encouraging 'systematic and critical reflection on programmes and projects' (Molleman et al., 2006: 10). A structured instrument is used – the PREFFI (Health Promotion Effectiveness Fostering instrument) now revised as PREFFI2 (Health Promotion Effect Management Instrument). This includes contextual conditions (such as capacity and leadership), analysis of the problem and possible solutions, selection and development of interventions, implementation and evaluation. Quality criteria are specified for each with subsidiary questions about operationalization. In many ways, knowledge is central to the process and we will return to this issue in Chapter 11. Saan and de Haes (undated) see knowledge development as a cycle involving production, sharing/dissemination, critical interpretation and use. Such is its importance that they suggest sharing knowledge should be a quality standard.

In essence, our discussion of quality has come full circle, returning to the assertion that the process of planning is fundamental to the quality of health promotion. Godin et al. (2007) propose that the degree of planning is an indicator of the potential success of programmes. They developed a tool to assess the planning process based on the 19 planning tasks in the 'intervention mapping' framework (Bartholomew et al., 2001). The tool (available at www.msss.gouv.qc.ca/its/outilplanification) was tested using data from 123 projects and the findings are summarized in Table 4.2.

Only 15 per cent of projects properly completed the objective matrix stage and 25 per cent the theory–practice stage. Of particular concern is the lack of attention to objectives and to the selection of theoretical models – identified as a major weakness in project development.

Table 4.2   Proportion (%) of projects that completed tasks, stages and phases

Phase	Stage	Tasks	%
Preparatory phase (89%)		Identify problem	48
		Identify target population	89
		Identify determinants	12
		Analyse environment	97
Operational phases	**Stage 1** Proximal objectives matrices (15%)	Specify population	15
		Overall objective	83
		Performance objectives	41
		Choice of determinants	7
		Learning objectives	6
	Stage 2 Theory–practice (25%)	Choose models	5
		Translate into strategies	23
	Stage 3 Producing the design (68%)	Organizational structure	79
		Content of activities	59
		Producing material	66
	Stage 4 Adoption and implementation (80%)	Support of partners	80
	Stage 5 Evaluation (39%)	Evaluation plan	48
		Process	78
		Impact	8
		Communication	12

After Godin et al., 2007

Haglund et al. (1998) suggest that improving the quality of health promotion rests on three cornerstones:

- user-friendly instruments for practitioners
- quality assessment instruments that reflect the reality of health promotion practice
- professional training for health promoters.

Clearly, quality is dependent on proper financing. Scriven and Speller's (2007) analysis of the global situation based on ten regional field reports reveals 'a chronic shortage of resources, including difficulty associated with workforce capacity and capability for health promotion' (2007: 197). The effects of inadequate funding are summarized in Figure 4.14.

ALLIANCES AND PARTNERSHIPS FOR HEALTH

Recognition that health is determined by a wide range of factors automatically leads to the view that efforts to promote health demand the coordinated action of a number of different sectors and agencies. Hagard (2000: 2) contends that a successful strategy requires:

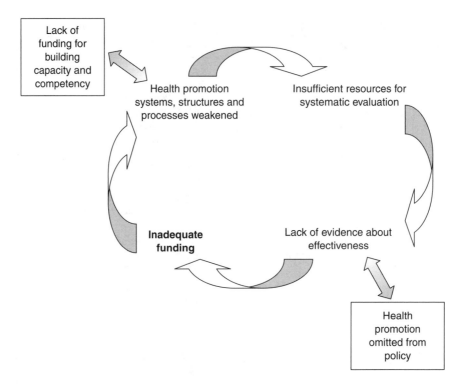

(*Source:* Scriven and Speller, 2007: 196)

Figure 4.14   Consequences of inadequate funding

concerted action by a number of different players, including government at all levels, many sectors of society, such as social services, education, environmental protection and healthcare, the media and nongovernmental organizations, and all public and private bodies that variously contribute to economic activity, social cohesion, justice and human rights.

This notion was recognized by the Ottawa Charter. It has been at the heart of the health promotion and 'Health for All' movements and is integral to settings approaches such as 'Healthy Cities' and the 'Health Promoting School' – indeed, Kickbush has identified partnerships as the 'key to successfully promoting health' (WHO, 1998b). The Jakarta Declaration (WHO, 1997) identified the current challenge as that of releasing the potential for health promotion in different sectors and at all levels of society. Breaking down barriers between sectors and creating partnerships for health were seen as essential. In addition to reaffirming the importance of involving communities and families, the Jakarta Declaration also introduced the issue of investment and public/private partnerships. Overall, the priorities for the twenty-first century were listed as being to:

- promote social responsibility for health
- increase investment in health development

- consolidate and expand partnerships for health
- increase community capacity and empower the individual
- secure an infrastructure for health promotion.

In line with this thinking, the World Health Assembly Resolution on Health Promotion urged all member states to 'consolidate and expand partnerships for health' (WHO, 1998c: 1(3)). Further, the Millenium Development Goals (UNDP, undated) specified the need to develop a global partnership for development (Goal 8) and the achievement of the other seven goals relies on partnerships.

Clearly, at both international and national levels, the development of partnerships will be enhanced by explicit policy support and the development of an appropriate infrastructure. In England, for example, the importance of healthy alliances was recognized in the *Health of the Nation* strategy (Department of Health, 1992) and it is integral to the more recent health strategy *Saving Lives: Our Healthier Nation* (Department of Health, 1999) and the delivery of *Choosing Health* (Department of Health, 2004) and '*Health Challenge England*' (Department of Health, 2006c). The need for the National Health Service to work in partnership and forge stronger links with local authorities was identified by the white paper *The New NHS*: *Modern Dependable* (Department of Health, 1997) with renewed emphasis in *The NHS in England: The Operating Framework for 2008/9* (2007g). Indeed, partnership between government, individuals and local communities is seen as the way forward in improving health and is central to 'Third Way' policies. Government commitment to partnership working as a vehicle for improving local planning also underpinned the development of *Local Strategic Partnerships* (LSPs) (DETR, 2001). These were intended to bring together the various parts of the public, private and voluntary sectors and the community within local government areas to make strategic decisions on issues such as health, education, employment, housing and crime. LSPs give local people a voice in decision making and enable services to be more responsive to the community's needs. They are also a mechanism for developing a coordinated local response to the major issues of social exclusion and neighbourhood renewal. *Local Performance Frameworks* (Communities and Local Government and the Department of Health, 2007) place a duty on local authorities, health authorities and third and independent sectors to work in partnership to undertake joint strategic needs assessment, agree local targets for inclusion in Local Area Agreements and set up local involvement networks (LINks) to ensure local people have a voice.

Over the years, there have been changes in terminology concerning collaborative approaches to working – 'inter-agency working', 'intersectoral working', 'joint working', 'intersectoral collaboration', 'healthy alliances', 'coalitions' and, most recently, 'partnerships'. While it would be easy to dismiss these changes as merely rebadging a familiar concept, they do signal a subtle shift in emphasis – despite the lingering tendency to use them interchangeably. Sindall (1997: 5) notes that 'strategic alliances' are one of the defining characteristics of modern organizational relationships and quotes the Australian Institute of Management's Roundtable definition:

> a long-term partnership involving two or more organizations formed to benefit from the synergy of working together in an environment of trust, sharing information and resources to achieve a common objective.

The move towards using the term partnership is perhaps indicative of a more explicit concern to involve members of the community, rather than assuming their implicit representation as a result of the involvement of organizations. Furthermore, the notion of 'partnership' draws attention to the issue of power and implies participation on an equal footing with the sharing of power. Given the current emphasis on partnerships and alliances, we should consider the implications for planning health promotion before concluding this chapter. We will begin by looking briefly at alliances and intersectoral collaboration before moving on to partnerships.

Delaney (1994b) identifies four key features of organizations that contribute to effective collaboration. Similarity of structure and function is important, but there also needs to be agreement on respective remits and areas of responsibility, along with awareness of interdependence and the collaboration serving to meet needs (see box for a case study).

Case study: interagency collaboration and young people's sexual health

Collaborative initiative involved:

- Teachers
- Community health practitioners
- Health promotion staff
- Youth and community workers

Provision:

- School-based sex education
- Drop-in advice and information facilities
- 'Detached' street work
- Young person's clinic

By working together a comprehensive response to young people's needs was put in place and the work of each agency enhanced.

Bloxham, 1997

Dependence on resources is a further stimulus for collaboration. Delaney (1994b: 219) notes Hudson's (1987) assertion that the 'absence of alternative sources of resources is a "prerequisite" for successful collaboration'. Resources are not necessarily financial – they can include human resources, services and information.

Collaboration is facilitated by formal commitments and structural arrangements for meetings and joint working. Formally ratified strategies and committee structures are a feature of the 'Healthy Cities' initiative. However, networking and the informal working arrangements that develop among people who share the same broad goals are also important. Reticulist (networking) skills that support strategic thinking and crossing boundaries therefore contribute to effective collaboration. Delaney (1994b: 221) cautions against seeing collaboration as 'a purely technical matter to be resolved by the right administrative arrangements' – it also involves negotiation and bargaining. Furthermore, drawing on the work of Lukes (see Chapter 3), she observes that the power relationships within alliances may be unequal and maintained in a variety of subtle ways so that particular organizations and values may come to dominate. At a very basic level, control may be exercised in the ways in which meetings are chaired and agendas constructed. Not only should the interactions within a collaboration be fair in themselves, but they must also be perceived to be fair. The optimal arrangement would appear to be formal structures coupled with informal networking within an overall climate of positive mutual awareness.

Delaney's (1994a) qualitative study of the factors perceived to influence intersectoral collaboration identified the following barriers to success:

- lack of vision and shared commitment
- lack of time
- competition:
  - between individuals and organizations
  - within and between professional networks and dominant or influential professional groups
- conflicting mechanisms and timescales
- different channels of accountability and communication.

In contrast, a summary of the key features of *successful* collaboration is provided in the box. The review of the 'Health of the Nation' strategy (Department of Health, 1998c) also proposed factors external to organizations that would encourage partnerships – notably, a statutory framework that would require local agencies to work together and incentives for developing partnerships for health.

Key features of successful collaboration

Identified by Tones and Delaney (1995: 22)

- Domain awareness and similarity of functions between agencies
- Shared vision
- Compromise and bargaining
- Needs of all parties should be met
- Resources exchange and commitment
- Formal recognition
- Organizational and communication structure, but also flexibility and opportunities to network
- Reticulist skills
- The interpersonal element
- 'Flat', less hierarchical structures rather than authoritarian organizational forms

(Continued)

(Continued)

Identified by Ansari (1998: 18)

- Early vision and understanding
- Clarity of roles, rules, procedures and responsibilities
- Wide representation of stakeholders and a strong membership
- Leadership skills
- Communication between the diverse parties
- Human resource development
- Building on the identified strengths and assets of the partners
- Realistic timeframes and funding cycles

Features of effective partnerships and coalitions identified by Bracht et al. (1999)

- Leadership
- Management
- Communication
- Conflict resolution
- Perception of fairness
- Shared decision making
- Perceived benefits versus costs

Features of successful partnerships (*Saving Lives: Our Healthier Nation*, Department of Health, 1999: 10.13)

Successful partnership working is built on organizations moving together to address common goals; on developing in their staff the skills necessary to work in an entirely new way – across boundaries, in multidisciplinary teams, and in a culture in which learning and good practice are shared. It also means:

- clarifying the common purpose of the partnership
- recognizing and resolving potential areas of conflict
- agreeing a shared approach to partnership
- strong leadership based on a clear vision and drive, with well-developed influencing and networking skills
- continuously adapting to reflect the lessons learned from experience
- promoting awareness and understanding of partner organizations through joint training programmes and incentives to reward effective working across organizational boundaries.

The Department of the Environment, Transport and the Regions (DETR) guidance on good practice in partnership working refers to the stages in the development of a partnership from its initial setting up to maturity, and the need to balance structure and stability in relation to membership, rationale, mode of operation and activities with the opportunity to be flexible and evolve in an organic way in order to respond to specific circumstances internal and external to the partnership (DETR, 2001). The guidance also draws attention to the lack of clarity that often exists in distinguishing between the responsibilities of the partnership and those of individual partners, and also between strategic and operational decision making. Individual partners may hold multiple – and conflicting – roles, for example, as a member of the community, representative of the community, service provider and strategic partner. A clear understanding of roles and responsibilities *vis-à-vis* the partnership is therefore fundamental to success and provides a basis for ensuring accountability. Indeed, the DETR recommends setting up formal systems for monitoring and reporting outcomes and a framework of accountability. Gillies (1998: 101), commenting on a review of the literature on the effectiveness of partnerships, notes that those reported fell into two broad groups:

Micro-level — alliances or partnerships which involve one or more collaborators among individuals or groups or organizations in the public, private or non-governmental sectors in the promotion of health, but which do not seek to affect the underlying systems or structures or architecture for health promotion.

Macro-level — alliances or partnerships which involve one or more collaborators among institutions, organizations or groups in the public, private or non-governmental sector which seek to affect the structural determinants of health.

While the published micro-level studies tended to focus on behavioural outcomes in assessing gains, Gillies notes that they could equally have focused on the wider environmental determinants. What emerged clearly from the review was that the stronger the representation from the community and the higher the level of involvement in practical activities, the greater and more sustainable were the gains. Mechanisms should therefore be put in place to involve local people in planning and practical health promotion activities. Furthermore, lay involvement should be based on power sharing and not mere tokenism. This view endorses that of Labonte (1993), who makes a clear distinction between consultation and participation. Central to participation is shared decision making, negotiated relationships and openness to identifying problems and issues. Furthermore, he suggests that less powerful groups may need support so that they can participate on an equal footing.

A review of the examples of best practice in alliances or partnerships for health collected from around the world (Gillies, 1998: 104) identified the key elements of good partnership to include:

a relevant needs assessment combined with the setting up of committees crossing professional and lay boundaries to steer, guide and account for the activities and programmes implemented.

It was also noted that non-industrialized countries are leading the way in relation to partnerships and community-based health promotion. These examples of good practice placed less emphasis on behavioural outcomes than the published studies and were more concerned with their impact on the broad environmental conditions and process of change. Key outcomes in relation to process (Gillies, 1998: 112) were:

getting agencies to work together; engaging local people; training and supporting volunteers and networks; creating committees; capturing politicians' interest and sustaining political visibility; resource allocation; reorientating organizations and services; promoting flexibility in working practices; and undertaking needs assessment as a way of identifying priorities and galvanizing interest ...

Open communication and trust are essential ingredients of partnership working and are dependent on good networks for sharing information and establishing common values and goals. However, partners may be drawn from diverse professional, cultural and social backgrounds. The management of this diversity will also be integral to success. On the one hand, any conflict that would be a barrier to joint decision making needs to be avoided – especially so when it is associated with an imbalance of power. On the other hand, the DETR (2001) cautions against the 'lowest common denominator' approach, which tends to reduce these differences and stifles creativity and innovation.

Developing partnerships requires:

- leadership
- trust
- learning to continuously improve
- managing for performance.

An interactive tool is available to analyse how partnerships are working in relation to these dimensions. (LGpartnerships – Smarter Partnerships, undated b). Clearly, successful partnerships demand time and commitment, supportive organizational structures and appropriate skills among those involved. Individuals might need to develop their skills in order to engage constructively in partnerships and organizations might need to change their internal ways of working. Capacity building might be required in relation to individuals, communities and organizations before effective partnerships can be established.

It is possible to distinguish a number of stages in the development of partnership (Educe Ltd and GFA Consulting, undated):

1   Forming
2   Frustration
3   Functioning
4   Flying
5   Failure.

Responding appropriately to the stage of development will help to ensure the success of the partnership – for example, at stage 1, developing a common vision will be important; at stage 2, demonstrating 'early wins'; and at stage 4, paying attention to the future relevance of the partnership and sustainability. The characteristics of a 'healthy partnership' identified by LGpartnerships – Smarter Partnerships (undated b) are:

1   Partners can demonstrate real results through collaboration
2   Common interest supersedes partner interest
3   Partners use 'we' when talking about partner matters

4   Partners are mutually accountable for tasks and outcomes
5   Partners share responsibility and rewards
6   Partners strive to develop and maintain trust
7   Partners are willing to change what they do and how they do it
8   Partners seek to improve how the partnership performs.

Notwithstanding the challenges, partnerships offer great potential for developing a coordinated response to the multiple factors that influence health status and achieving health gains. There are also potential gains for partner agencies that might be motivated to enter into such partnerships for reasons not necessarily related to health (see the box).

General benefits of partnership working

- Achievement of organizational objectives and enhanced efficiency and effectiveness
- Improved coordination of policy, programmes and service delivery
- Broadening the scope of influence to include other services and activities
- Greater economy
- Less bureaucracy and regulation
- Business and commercial opportunities
- Access to data and information
- Access to a range of skills and competencies
- Opportunity for innovation and learning
- More involvement of local communities

After DETR, 2001: Annex E

Investment for health

We noted in Chapter 2 that social and economic factors are the single major determinant of health status. Ziglio et al. (2000a) contend that health, as an essential personal and social resource, requires investment and, indeed, health promotion should be considered to be an investment strategy. Clearly, there is an inextricable link between health and social and economic development in that social and economic development leads to health improvement and, conversely, health supports social and economic development. Levin and Ziglio (1997: 363) note that, in many societies, the immediate priorities are 'economic competitiveness and fiscal soundness' rather than health priorities. The 'Investment for Health' (IFH) approach, which received considerable attention towards the turn of the twenty-first century, focused on integrating health promotion into mainstream social and economic development. This raises some questions about ends and means – is the emphasis on the promotion of health or is health merely instrumental to achieving wealth? The expropriation of health to service the needs of capitalist economies has been the subject of fierce criticism by authors such as Doyal and Pennell (1979). However, the IFH approach acknowledges that priority social and economic policy areas, such as education, employment, transport and housing, have a major influence on health. Policy decisions and initiatives by governments – and the private sector – have the potential to improve or harm health. The major concern of IFH, therefore, is to ensure that efforts to improve social and economic standing also improve health status and are equitable, empowering and sustainable (Ziglio et al., 2000b). Kickbush (1997) has identified three key questions that should inform the development of a sound health promotion strategy:

> Where is health promoted and maintained in a given population?
> Which investment strategies produce the largest population health gains?
> Which investment strategies help reduce health inequities and are in line with human rights?

Ziglio et al. (2000b: 4) add a fourth:

> Which investments contribute to economic and social development in an equitable and sustainable manner and result in high health returns for the overall population?

In the post-Ottawa era, there has been widespread acceptance of the importance of environmental influences on health, both directly and via their effect on behavioural choices. Latterly, there has been increased awareness of the complexity of environmental factors and the contribution of social networks, social capital and social inclusion to health. Ziglio et al. (2000a) suggest that, notwithstanding the widespread commitment to a socio-ecological model of health, the health promotion response has been oversimplified. Most change has been 'first-order change', achieving some minor adjustment but without affecting the major determinants of health. They call for a more radical approach in order to achieve 'second-order change' (2000a: 145), which involves new structures and processes – an approach whereby concern for health is interwoven into social systems and the focus is on the creation of health rather than disease prevention.

Organizational policies and activities tend to be sector-based, with little emphasis on intersectoral relationships. Watson et al. (2000: 17) refer to a 'silo model of governance', where different sectors, such as health, education and housing, traditionally have separate structures, funding, channels of accountability and professional 'domains' and there are few opportunities for links. In contrast, 'holistic governance' would be more flexible and involve 'shared objectives, a common understanding of what needs to be done and what others can contribute'. Similar arguments could also be put forward in relation to community involvement.

The issue of partnerships is therefore central to the IFH approach, along with accountability for health impact.

> The IFH approach therefore calls for a new form of partnership. In today's complex world, action for the promotion of health cannot come from the healthcare sector alone. It needs to be built on strong cross-sector alliances between health and healthcare, social development and equitable and sustainable economic development. (Ziglio et al., 2000b: 4)

It also involves policy at all levels, from national to local, and this will be considered more fully in Chapter 6. The core principles of IFH (Ziglio et al., 2001) are:

1   a focus on health
2   full public engagement
3   genuine intersectoral work
4   equity
5   sustainability
6   a broad knowledge base.

Over and above the emphasis on partnerships and policy to address the structural determinants of health, the IFH approach draws attention to the capacity of systems to respond appropriately in order to foster health improvement. Ziglio et al. (2001) refer to the importance of maximizing the health assets in a community as well as identifying and responding to the community's health needs. Indeed, the primary focus of IFH is on strengthening health assets. These assets, they found, include:

- policy investments
- regulatory changes
- the nurturing of non-governmental resources and programme initiatives
- the strengthening of health promotion infrastructures and decision making
- a refocusing on education
- investment in research
- training in the requisite health promotion skills
- environmental improvement.

The principles of IFH offer a means of breaking down traditional barriers to partnership working and spreading accountability for health beyond the narrow confines of the health sector. Hancock (1998) suggests that the involvement of the private sector offers particular challenges, given that the primary motivation is profit and this may well conflict with health interests. He does, however, recognize the potential benefits of working with the private sector, provided partners and their subcontractors meet agreed ethical criteria. The proposed criteria are listed in the box.

Ethical principles for partnership with the private sector

- The activities of the corporation are increasingly environmentally sustainable
- Safe and healthy working conditions are provided for the workforce
- Pay is fair with reasonable benefits, there is a right to collective bargaining and lay-offs are minimized
- Taxes are paid fairly and economic activities do not increase poverty
- Their activities do not pose a danger to consumers or the communities in which they operate and the public is fully informed about any potential hazards
- There is respect for human rights

After Hancock, 1998

HEALTH PROMOTION PLANNING

We have argued in this chapter that effective health promotion is based on a systematic approach to planning. Indeed, planning is fundamental to the quality of health promotion. We have provided examples of a range of different planning models. While they differ to some extent in their orientation, there are several common features. They require the assessment and prioritization of needs and identification of objectives as a basis for appraising possible solutions and selecting the most appropriate courses of action. They also incorporate monitoring and evaluation elements. Perhaps the most important feature is that they provide a framework for integrating theory and empirical evidence into the various stages of the planning process. It is worth emphasizing that theory can be concerned with community participation and policy development as well as behaviour change.

Resistance to using planning models often derives from an association with reductionism and top-down styles of working. We would contend the reverse to be the case. When used appropriately, they can serve to open up the entire range of health promotion options and avoid any tendency towards being blinkered by custom and practice. Many health promotion programmes are destined to fail because they focus on too narrow a range of factors or are based on unsubstantiated assumptions. Rational planning processes will serve to expose such weaknesses and ensure that programmes address all relevant variables. Furthermore, the process of planning can be a vehicle for involving all stakeholders, ensuring wide ownership of plans.

The complex interplay of factors that influence health demands a coordinated response across a number of different sectors and at a number of different levels, from local to national and even supranational. The IFH approach is premised on the interrelationship between health and social and economic development, and seeks to strengthen the assets for health within communities by means of partnerships and policy.

Partnerships are seen to be the 'key mechanism for pulling together effective local planning and action' (Watson et al., 2000: 17). The involvement of communities and creating opportunities for participation on an equal footing are also instrumental to success. Building effective partnerships is undoubtedly challenging, but offers huge potential for developing whole systems approaches to promoting health, rather than reacting in a piecemeal fashion. However, this requires commitment from partners and new ways of working.

By way of conclusion, we would draw attention to the box which contains a proverb about the elephant. This has been used as an analogy for taking a whole systems approach to tackling health issues (Newcastle Healthy City Project, 1997). It draws attention to the fact that there are a number of different perspectives on complex systems – all of which may be true, but, equally, none represents a complete view. Understanding how the whole system operates depends on sharing knowledge. Members of the community concerned are more likely to interface with more components of the system and, hence, have a more complete picture than professionals, whose awareness may be confined to the remit of a particular agency.

Whole systems and elephants

There is an old Indian proverb about three blind people describing an elephant. One holds the trunk and says, 'This is a snake.' One holds the tail and says, 'No, it's a rope.' The third grabs a leg and says, 'You're both wrong. It is a tree trunk.'

Each person has offered their perception of the truth, but they have failed to describe the elephant. Even putting all three descriptions together would not make a recognizable elephant.

After Newcastle Healthy City Project, 1997

Furthermore, within complex systems, although all components could make a contribution to health and there are knock-on effects between the activities of different agencies, there is no single agency controlling and coordinating activity. Developing an intersectoral response to health issues and partnership working calls for a shift in emphasis away from the functioning of the 'parts' and towards their interrelationship and the functioning of the whole. The key to this is good communication, shared vision and clear strategic and operational objectives.

KEY POINTS

o The effectiveness and quality of health promotion programmes are dependent on good planning.

o The use of appropriate planning models ensures a systematic approach to planning.

o Consideration of equity at all stages of the planning process will prioritize action most likely to achieve narrowing of the gap in health status.

o The planning process can be a vehicle for involving all major stakeholders.

o Reference to theory and the development of clear objectives are essential, yet often neglected, components of the planning process.

o Partnerships between sectors and involving the community are essential for tackling the complex determinants of health and ill health.

o Successful partnerships require good leadership, a shared vision, clarity about roles and responsibilities, good communication, trust and respect.

o The development of partnerships is facilitated by having an appropriate infrastructure and the competencies required to work collaboratively.

o Investment for Health is an example of a partnership approach which recognizes the link between economic development and health.

5

INFORMATION NEEDS

Certitude is not the test of certainty. We have been cocksure of many things that were not so.

Oliver Wendell Holmes Jr (1841–1935) *Natural Law*

OVERVIEW

The purpose of this chapter is to consider the information required for programme planning. It will:

- consider the notion of need and different interpretations of health needs
- support the use of participatory approaches for identifying health needs
- note the importance of being aware of community profiles and wider contextual factors when responding to health needs
- emphasize the contribution of theory to understanding both the determinants of health and how to change them
- consider the nature of the evidence required to respond effectively to health needs.

INTRODUCTION

The first stage of systematic programme planning involves establishing what the problem is and determining what the causes are, along with any other contributory factors. Some understanding of the nature of the community, its members and the context in which they live is also needed before appropriate courses of action can be identified. Nutbeam (1998a) refers to this first stage as 'problem definition' and suggests that the research requirements include epidemiological and demographic analysis, along with a community needs analysis. The next phase of 'solution generation' on the other hand, draws on theory and models, evidence of effectiveness and practitioner experience. Nutbeam (1998a: 33) provides a useful summary of the key questions that should be addressed at each stage of programme planning and implementation.

- **Problem definition**: What is the problem?
- **Solution generation**: How might it be solved?
- **Innovation testing**: Did the solution work?
- **Intervention demonstration**: Can the programme be repeated/refined?
- **Intervention dissemination**: Can the programme be widely reproduced?
- **Programme management**: Can the programme be sustained?

In Chapter 2, we examined issues associated with the measurement of health status and the broad determinants of health and, in Chapter 3, the factors influencing behaviour and action. The purpose of this chapter is to apply these ideas more specifically to identifying the information needed for making decisions about possible interventions. We will begin by considering definitions of health needs before looking at different approaches to assessing needs and profiling the community. We will then focus on the development of possible solutions and, particularly, the application of theory and evidence to the rational selection of intervention strategies.

Advances in information technology in recent years, together with the development of new information systems and sources of data, have done much to improve access to health information. The establishment of Public Health Observatories in each of the NHS regions of the UK in 2000 is an example of an attempt to make information available to support efforts to improve health generally, but specifically the health of the worst off in society. The tasks of the Observatories are summarized in the box. However, it is still pertinent to note that, all too often, the information that is most readily available is not necessarily the most useful or revealing – a situation pithily summed up in Murphy's Law of Information (Williams and Wright, 1998: 182):

The information we have is not what we want.
The information we want is not the information we need.
The information we need is too expensive to collect.

The main tasks of public health observatories

Monitoring health and disease trends and highlighting areas for action
Identifying gaps in health information
Advising on methods for health and health inequality impact assessment
Drawing together information from different sources in new ways to improve health
Carrying out projects to highlight particular health issues
Evaluating progress by local agencies in improving health and cutting inequality
Looking ahead to give early warning of future public health problems

Association of Public Health Observatories, 2002

HEALTH NEEDS ASSESSMENT

Health needs assessment has been defined as 'a systematic method for reviewing the health issues facing a population, leading to agreed priorities and resource allocation that will improve health and reduce inequalities' (Cavanagh and Chadwick, 2005: 3).

The growing interest in health needs assessment has been attributed to the increasingly consumerist nature of society, economic concerns and the general squeeze on public funds, together with the current emphasis on effectiveness (Gillam and Murray, 1996). Within the UK, the restructuring of the NHS in the 1990s based on the notional 'internal market', focused attention on identifying needs as a basis for commissioning services. This was given further impetus – and a broader perspective – within the modernization agenda (Department of Health, 1997), which required health authorities and, more latterly, primary care trusts to work collaboratively with local authorities and the voluntary sector to identify needs and develop health improvement programmes. More recently, the Local Government and Public Involvement in Health Act (2007) placed a duty on local authorities and primary care trusts to undertake Joint Strategic Needs Assessment, defined as 'a process that will identify the current and future health and wellbeing needs of a local population' in order to inform local priorities and targets set out in Local Area Agreements and as a basis for 'commissioning priorities that will improve outcomes and reduce health inequalities' (Department of Health, 2007a: 3).

The nature of health needs

Given the debate about the nature of health and its determinants, the absence of a precise definition of health needs and the lack of a consensus about the means of assessing needs should come as no surprise. The interpretations of the term 'health needs' range from a narrow focus on heath service provision, through inclusion of a preventive element, to addressing social needs. There is an important distinction between health needs and healthcare needs. It will be clear from our earlier discussion that the broad remit of health promotion requires an analysis of needs that includes social and environmental concerns and also addresses wellbeing. However, in considering definitions of need, we will also draw briefly on interpretations of healthcare needs.

The traditional public health approach to assessing health needs has been to draw on epidemiological information to measure the disease burden or levels of ill health in communities. This stems from a conceptualization of health as the absence of disease. Robinson and Elkan (1996) are critical of this problem-focused approach, which they feel ignores needs that are unrelated to narrowly defined problems – the need to stay well, for example. They further challenge it on the grounds that it does not immediately suggest strategies to respond to any deficiencies identified. Liss (1990) raises the issue of how, on what basis, and by whom any deficiencies are identified and prioritized. Pickin and St Leger's (1993) lifecycle framework for assessing health needs is a development of this approach. It includes three main elements:

- measurement of health status, including both epidemiological and sociological analyses
- assessment of the resources available
- identification of ways of achieving maximum health gain.

Recognizing that needs will vary throughout a lifespan, the lifecycle framework also divides the population into a number of age groups with similar characteristics.

An alternative conceptualization of need – one that addresses the issue of what can be done – is based on the capacity to benefit. Culyer (1977) considers a need for healthcare to exist when there is potential to improve health status or avoid reduction in it, but only if an intervention exists that can achieve positive outcomes. This thinking is integral to Buchan et al.'s (1990) view that:

> people in need of a health service are defined as those for whom an intervention produces a benefit at reasonable risk and acceptable cost. The benefit may not necessarily be improved outcome. It may relate to information or reassurance or some other aspect of the care process.

A need is therefore determined not by the scale of the health problem, but the ability to benefit. These two approaches should not necessarily be seen as incompatible. The criteria used for identifying the key areas that should be addressed in the first health strategy document for England (Department of Health, 1991) included both the magnitude of the health problem (as assessed by its contribution to premature death and avoidable ill health) and availability of effective interventions.

Robinson and Elkan (1996) recognize the advantage of focusing on the capacity to benefit in that it encourages practitioners to specify what outcomes they are seeking to achieve. However, the ways in which these are framed will inevitably be influenced by value positions. Although in principle they could go beyond biomedical goals to include quality of life issues, in practice they are often defined rather narrowly as improved life expectancy. They are also critical of needs being defined by association with the effectiveness of an intervention – a view that overlooks the severity of a problem to the individual. However, they acknowledge Culyer's (1977) suggestion that, where no effective treatment exists, what is needed is research. We might also note the lack of precision about 'reasonable risk' and 'acceptable cost' and whether or not these should be defined in humanitarian or economic terms.

An emphasis on the capacity to benefit acknowledges that some interventions offer greater potential for gain than others. A key issue for health economists is the notion of 'allocative efficiency', which is concerned with achieving maximum benefits from available resources. Comparison of the respective gains from spending on different interventions is viewed as essential if resources are to be deployed to achieve the greatest good. Needs identified in this way will clearly be relative and heavily influenced by judgements, not least in relation to how benefits are defined and measured. The measures frequently used in this context include QALYs and DALYs, which, as we noted in Chapter 2, have been the subject of controversy.

Liss (1990) notes that the interpretations of 'needs' referred to above include matters of judgement in relation to what constitutes ill health, which health states *require* care and the services that *ought* to be provided. He suggests that there are two categories of assessors of need – the patient and the provider – that is, the doctor, but we might equally include the health economist or the planner. The identity of an assessor is clearly germane to any assessment of needs and Liss suggests that this should be included within the concept of need. Liss' (1990: 39) normative notion of a healthcare need is based on 'an "assessor" believ[ing] that healthcare ought to be provided'.

A further interpretation of healthcare needs derives from an instrumental perspective. Rather than focusing on deficiency states, needs are identified in terms of what needs to be done or what conditions need to be in place to maintain or improve health. Within the broader context of health promotion, a useful example is provided by the list of prerequisites for health identified in the Ottawa Charter (WHO, 1986) – peace, shelter, education, food, income, a stable eco-system, sustainable resources, social justice and equity – and updated in the Jakarta Declaration (WHO, 1997) to also include social security, social relations, the empowerment of women, respect for human rights and, above all, alleviation of poverty.

Liss' (1990) characterization of different views about healthcare needs provides a useful summary, one that could be applied more generally to health needs.

- **The ill-health notion** which equates a need for healthcare with a deficiency in health that requires healthcare.
- **The supply notion** which requires that acceptable treatment should also be available to respond to a deficiency.
- **The normative notion** which acknowledges that opinions about needs may vary and is based on an assessor believing that healthcare should be provided.
- **The instrumental notion** is based on the identification of care required to achieve certain states.

Bradshaw (1972) defined four types of social need, enshrined in his well-known taxonomy.

- **Normative need** is defined by experts or professionals often on the basis of a 'desirable standard' against which individuals or groups can be compared. However, normative needs may be defined differently by different professional groups and change over time. They cannot therefore be seen as absolute needs.
- **Felt need** is defined by lay people and equated with wants. It is limited as a measure of *real* need by people's perceptions, which may fail to recognize actual needs or else mis-represent wants as needs.
- **Expressed need** consists of felt need turned into action by seeking treatment or care.
- **Comparative need** is concerned with ensuring that people with similar characteristics receive equivalent levels of care and, if there is a shortfall, then individuals are in need.

Bradshaw (1994) acknowledges that there may be alternative views about normative needs and that comparative needs may themselves derive from normative judge-ments. Felt and expressed needs may differ widely, as illustrated in Figure 5.1.

The NICE guidance on health needs assessment (Cavanagh and Chadwick, 2005: 12) also recoginzes this diversity in its definition of health needs as:

Perceptions and expectations of the profiled population (felt and expressed needs)
Perceptions of professionals providing the services
Perceptions of managers of commissioner/provider organisations, based on available data about the size and severity of health issues for a population, and inequalities compared with other populations (normative needs)
Priorities of the organisations commissioning and managing services for the profiled population, linked to national, regional or local priorities (corporate needs).

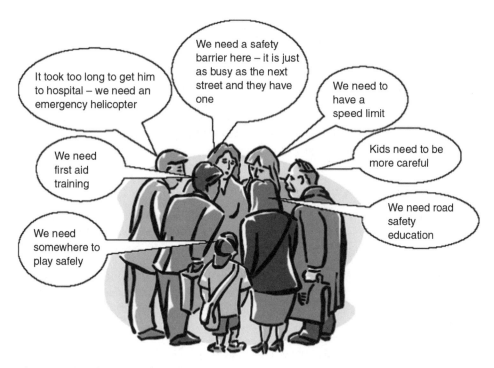

Figure 5.1   Alternative interpretations of need at the scene of an accident

It emphasizes the importance of balancing different needs when establishing priorities.

As we noted in Chapter 2, even what purport to be objective assessments of needs based on disease burden remain essentially ideologically driven. A number of tensions exist in identifying health needs and derive both from the ways in which health and its determinants are conceptualized and where the focus of attention lies. These are summarized in the box.

Tensions in health needs assessment

View of health:

- positive or negative view of health
- holistic or atomistic view of health
- biomedical or social interpretation of determinants
- professional or lay perspective.

Focus of attention:

- upstream (prevention) or downstream (treatment)
- individual or community.

Although Bradshaw's taxonomy provides a useful way to analyse different perspectives and, indeed, ensure that they are represented in any assessment of social needs, it offers little insight into the actual nature of need. Indeed, his assertion that 'real' need is likely to exist when all four types of need are present at the same time may be taken to imply that the individual 'types' are not sufficient in themselves as indicators of 'real' needs.

Two key issues remain unresolved – the distinction between needs and wants and whether needs are absolute or, ultimately, subjectively defined. Doyal and Gough's theory of human need sheds some light here.

Doyal and Gough's theory of human need

Doyal and Gough (1991: 9), in their meticulously constructed defence of the concept of objective and universal human need, recognize critics on both sides of the political spectrum:

> Many argue that it is morally safer and intellectually more coherent to equate needs with subjective preferences – that only individuals or selected groups of individuals can decide the goals to which they are going to attach enough priority to deem them needs.

Critics from the New Right are concerned about state collectivism and the intrusion of the 'nanny' state into matters of individual choice. In the absence of an agreed basis for identifying need, they advocate relying on individual preferences and market forces. Concerns on the Left and among minority and oppressed groups have their origins in the unequal power structure in society and the dominance of particular groups. The contention here is that needs are culturally determined and can only be fully understood by members of a group. They are therefore subjectively defined, but at the group collective level, rather than the individual. Doyal and Gough challenge both these positions, along with economic, sociological and postmodern interpretations of need as relative and contend that objective need does indeed exist. Furthermore, demonstrating that there are objective universal needs creates a moral imperative to meet those needs and effectively establishes them as fundamental rights.

The term 'need' has been used to refer to drives or motivational forces that arise from some disequilibrium – for example, the need for sleep when tired or food when hungry. Maslow (1954) identifies a number of such needs that can be ordered into a hierarchy premised on the requirement to satisfy basic needs, such as hunger and warmth, before higher-order needs can be addressed. The needs identified are felt to be common to different cultures. The levels of the hierarchy are set out in Figure 5.2.

Each level is assumed to be necessary for the achievement of the next, although there is no requirement for 100 per cent satisfaction before moving on to the next level. Maslow himself acknowledged that the hierarchy was not fixed. For example, for those who gain satisfaction from high-risk activities, such as mountaineering or hang-gliding, self-actualization needs may take precedence over safety needs.

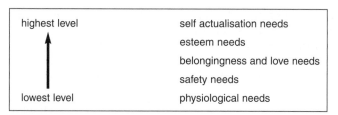

highest level	self actualisation needs
	esteem needs
	belongingness and love needs
	safety needs
lowest level	physiological needs

Figure 5.2   A representation of Maslow's hierarchy of needs

Doyal and Gough reject the interpretation of needs as drives on the basis that needs and drives can exist independently of each other. For example, individuals may have a drive to consume alcohol that cannot be construed as a need and, conversely, they may have a need to take more exercise, although they may not feel driven to do so. While recognizing that choices are constrained by biological factors, Doyal and Gough are wary of placing too great an emphasis on biological determinism.

An alternative way of looking at need is as a means of achieving a goal. Liss (1990) suggests that a goal therefore becomes a necessary precondition to there being a need. Hence, statements about need must conform to the pattern:

A needs X in order to G.

Wants would be distinguished from needs on the basis that wants can be expressed merely as preferences with no requirement to specify the relationship to goals. A further distinction between needs and wants can be made based on the nature of the goal. Doyal and Gough suggest that needs would only apply in relation to *universalizable* goals – that is, goals that are in everyone's interests to achieve. Wants, in contrast, would vary from person to person, reflecting personal preferences. Such wants would be guided by individual perceptions, whereas needs draw on a shared understanding about the avoidance of harm. For example, an individual may say that they *need* a cigarette, but, from a *universalizable* goal perspective, they *want* a cigarette and *need* to give up smoking.

Doyal and Gough's analysis of universalizable goals identifies two key elements: the avoidance of serious harm and the ability to participate in a social form of life. They propose that the universal prerequisites for achieving these goals and participating fully in society constitute basic human needs, which are identified as:

- physical health
- autonomy.

Autonomy is seen to include mental health, cognitive skills and opportunities to participate in society. In order to meet these basic needs, 11 categories of intermediate needs are identified, as seen in the outline of Doyal and Gough's theory of need in Figure 5.3. While basic and intermediate needs are universalizable, the ways in which these needs can be met may well vary.

Needs assessment will be concerned with assessing how well these basic and intermediate needs are being met. This raises the issue of what standard should be set concerning the satisfaction of needs. In relation to basic needs satisfaction, Doyal and Gough reject both absolute minimum standards and relative standards. Instead, they advocate an optimum standard for basic needs and propose a 'minimum optimorum' level for intermediate needs – that is, the minimum level of input of intermediate need satisfaction to achieve optimal basic needs satisfaction.

The remaining question concerns how needs will be assessed. Doyal and Gough support the notion of informed participation by those whose needs are being assessed, although they caution that this can favour those already in privileged positions who may be more influential than others without such advantages. They suggest that the development of indicators of intermediate needs will be fed, in an iterative way, by the development of new codified and experiential knowledge. They recognize that both qualitative and quantitative indicators will be needed, but place considerable emphasis on the latter:

> To chart both basic and intermediate indicators we ideally require social indicators which are valid, distributive, quantitative and aggregated, but which are open to revision. These indicators should be open to disaggregation between groups. In this way profiles of the need-satisfaction of nations, cultural groups and other collectives can be compiled. (Doyal and Gough, 1991: 169)

When differences arise between the views of needs established by expert-led approaches, which draw on codified knowledge, and community-based approaches, which are grounded in experience, dialogue is proposed as a mechanism for resolving the situation.

Needs, wants and demands

Equity is recognized as one of the fundamental tenets of health promotion. Principles of social justice would presuppose that health resources should be distributed in relation to needs. However, as is all too apparent, access to services and wider opportunities to promote health are not necessarily governed by needs. Some time ago, Hart (1971) used the notion of the 'inverse care law' to describe the generally poorer provision of services in those areas that are most deprived and have the greatest burden of ill health. An emphasis on needs rather than wants or demands is therefore integral to equity. Nutbeam (1998b: 7) captures this idea perfectly: 'Equity means fairness. Equity in health means that people's needs guide the distribution of opportunities for wellbeing.' The management of public services on market or quasi-market principles is necessarily demand-led. In contrast, a needs-led approach will be more consistent with a focus on social justice.

The defining characteristic of need in Doyal and Gough's theory of need is its instrumentality in achieving universal human goals. Wants, in contrast, are personal

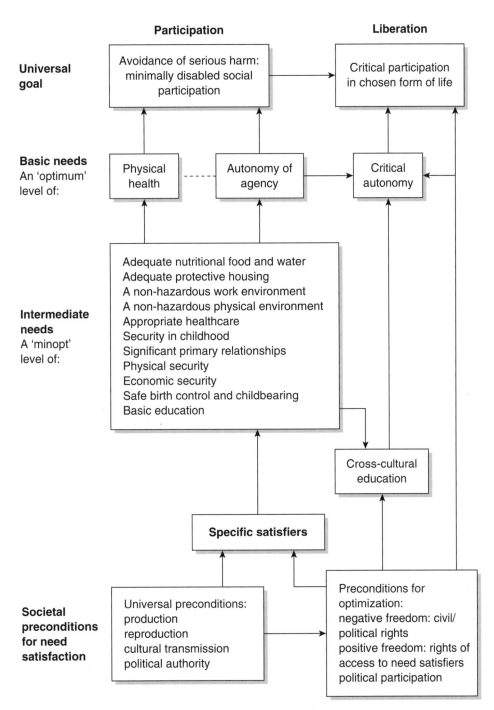

Figure 5.3   Doyal and Gough's theory of human need, in outline

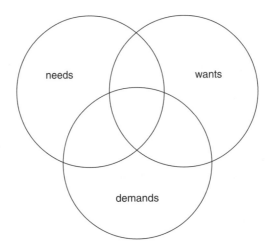

Figure 5.4   Needs, wants, demands

preferences and equate with what Bradshaw might term felt need. These subjective, personal preferences may overlap with an objective view of need or be completely different, as summarized in Figure 5.4.

In general economic terms, a demand is associated with the consumer's willingness to pay for desired goods or services (Bowling, 1997b). However, the complexity of the health and healthcare market calls for a broader interpretation. Mooney and Leeder (1997) describe demands as being based on wants, but also involving action directed at fulfilling the wants. There is a clear parallel here with Bradshaw's expressed need. Again, demands will overlap, to a greater or lesser extent, with wants and needs. Foreman (1996) suggests that health professionals effectively 'ratify' expressed needs or demands by providing services.

Clearly, those with most power will be better placed to articulate their wants and ensure that their demands are met – regardless of whether or not this is in the interests of the collective. Responding to demands may also ultimately conflict with the needs and longer-term interests of the individual. Robinson and Elkan (1996) offer the example of an individual demanding antibiotic treatment for a viral infection. Prescribing an antibiotic would serve no useful clinical purpose. Moreover, such unnecessary prescribing would contribute to the development of antibiotic-resistant strains of bacteria and, therefore, be against the longer-term interests of both the individual concerned and the wider population. There is an important distinction, therefore, between individual and collective interpretations of needs, wants and demands.

Whether or not we accept that there are objective needs, decisions about the best ways in which to achieve them will inevitably involve a degree of subjectivity. For some, the very nature of needs remains subjectively determined. Therefore, the issue of values – both personal and professional – cannot be ignored. At the most fundamental level, the distinction between needs, wants and demands is value-laden. There is also the related question of who should arbitrate when there are conflicting views (Bartholomew et al., 2001).

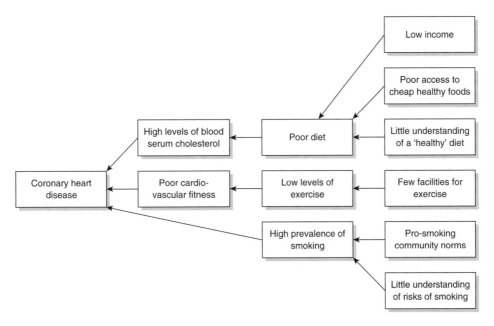

Figure 5.5   A reductionist assessment of need

A reductionist approach to needs assessment

The pursuit of the lowest-level causes of phenomena is referred to as 'reductionism'. Bringing a reductionist perspective to bear on the identification of needs would involve identifying the main health problems and constructing a causal chain that progressively homes in on factors that might be modified – that is, those factors that need to be changed to improve health status. Such a diagnostic approach would be very much in tune with the biomedical model of health promotion discussed in Chapter 1 and the public health approach to identifying needs referred to above. It could take either quality of life or disease as its starting point. This way of identifying needs would also equate with Bartholomew et al.'s view that a need is 'a difference between what currently exists and a more desirable state' (2001: 16). It typically draws heavily on epidemiological analyses and, by way of example, Figure 5.5 shows how it might apply to coronary heart disease.

The emphasis is on identifying modifiable risk factors. This approach has been criticized for attaching undue importance to behavioural risk factors. However, it could equally implicate social and environmental risk factors as the major determinants of problems. A further area of interest is the existence of any high-risk groups, defined as 'a group with a definable boundary and shared characteristics that have, or are at risk for, certain health and quality-of-life problems' (Bartholomew et al., 2001: 17).

As we will note below, reference can be made to major empirical studies and theoretical models to establish a framework for this type of enquiry. Such frameworks can be used to direct research at the local level towards identifying the key causative or contributory factors that should be considered when planning interventions. Analysis at the local level can then focus on identifying which of the generally recognized risk factors are the most pertinent in a specific context. Green and Kreuter (1991) suggest that one advantage of this approach is that it allows workers to direct their efforts at achieving maximum gains. However, it does not formally acknowledge the value of community insights or gaining the active involvement of members of the community.

Participation in needs assessment

The importance of community participation was recognized in the Ottawa Charter (WHO, 1986) and reaffirmed in the Jakarta Declaration (WHO, 1997): 'People have to be at the centre of health promotion action and decision-making processes for them to be effective.'

Arguments supporting public participation in needs assessment can be based on the rights of individuals to have a voice and also, more pragmatically, on the premise that participation fosters higher levels of motivation and enhances the effectiveness of interventions (Watson, 2002). Participation can be a means of bridging the gap between planners and the community. As we noted in Chapter 3, when a community recognizes the existence of a problem and identifies its own solution, then adoption of an innovation is likely to be much more rapid than when an external agency prescribes a solution for a problem the community was not aware of or does not consider to be a priority. Communities can also become a powerful voice for policy change when they are aware of unmet health needs.

Freire (1972) uses the term 'cultural invasion' for external agents bringing their own value systems to bear on the analysis of problems. The limitations of such top-down assessment of need are summed up by Gough (1992: 12):

> Experts and professionals can put their own interest before the wellbeing of their clients or research subjects. Often too they will be so ignorant of the reality of life for ordinary people that their proposals can be counterproductive or just plain stupid.

Mine risk education in Lao PDR: the importance of understanding behaviour

A survey and qualitative interviews revealed deliberate exposure to unexploded ordnance in contaminated areas in order to forage for scrap metal and clear farmland. Individuals were aware of the risk they were exposing themselves to, but such behaviour was driven by economic pressures. This insight called for a shift in emphasis from a zero risk strategy to include a range of risk reduction and risk avoidance approaches.

Durham and Ali, 2008

Knowledge held within the community must therefore become an integral part of any needs assessment (see box for example). It offers a complementary insight that should be considered alongside epidemiological and economic approaches. However, this raises the issue of the weight attached to the views of the public in contrast to those of so-called professionals (Foreman, 1996) and how to deal with any differences. Comparison of the professionals' views of priorities within an area with the actual priorities of the community that emerged from a rapid assessment of women's psycho–social health needs (Lazenbatt and McMurray, 2004) demonstrates only too clearly how professional assessments can differ markedly from those of the communities concerned, as shown in Table 5.1.

Table 5.1 Mean ranks of women's psycho–social health needs in Northern Ireland (lowest score = highest priority)

	GP team view n = 6	PRA team view n = 6	Community view n = 25
Physical environment			
Political boundaries	1.9	1.5	1.8
Transport	2.0	1.8	1.6
Lack of facilities	3.0	2.9	2.2
Disease			
Breast cancer	2.1	2.0	1.7
Cervical cancer	2.4	2.9	2.4
Heart disease	1.5	2.1	2.3
Psycho–social health issues			
Depression	2.1	3.1	3.2
Stress	2.7	2.9	2.9
Anxiety and fear	3.1	2.8	2.7
Lifestyle			
Smoking	2.1	3.1	3.2
Alcohol problems	3.0	3.1	4.4
Access to services			
Baby clinic	3.4	2.7	2.4
Well-woman clinic	2.8	3.2	2.3
Asthma clinic	1.9	1.9	3.2
Socio-economic			
Poverty	2.4	1.9	1.6
Unemployment	2.2	1.8	1.6
Low pay	3.0	2.8	2.7

Source: Derived from Lazenbatt and McMurray, 2004: 181

Stacey (1994) prefers the term 'people knowledge' to 'lay knowledge' as the term 'lay' often carries connotations of having less competence or worth. 'People knowledge' is often informal, experiential and mostly unwritten. It offers insights into the constellation of factors particular to specific situations from the perspective of those who are most familiar with them. The professional perspective, in contrast, draws on codified and systematized knowledge, often operating at a more general level.

Stacey is critical of the pressure to express lay understanding in official language and use acceptable research methods – that is, to operate within professionally defined parameters – and draws a number of lessons about participation:

- people's points of view should be understood in their own terms
- the distinction between people and professional is not rigid
- people knowledge is consistent and rational
- people are producers of health as well as consumers of healthcare
- lack of real influence in decisions alienates people from participation.

The Freirean notion of 'cultural synthesis' describes a situation in which professionals or external agents attempt to learn *with* the people about their experiences of the world.

Public participation in needs assessment can range from tokenistic consultation to having a controlling influence in arriving at what the needs are and how they should be prioritized. Arnstein's (1969) ladder of participation (see Figure 5.6) is a well-known device for distinguishing between genuine participation, mere tokenism and, indeed, attempts to manipulate. The degree of active participation increases progressively from none at the bottom to genuine control at the top.

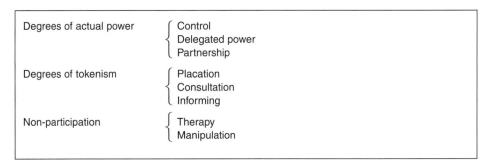

Figure 5.6 Arnstein's ladder of participation (after Arnstein, 1969)

Brager and Specht (1973) provide a similar analysis of the spectrum of participation (see Figure 5.7). Their depiction of the various levels is particularly pertinent to health promotion planning and needs assessment.

A further consideration – over and above the actual level of participation – is the motivation underpinning attempts to involve communities. Clearly, the chief beneficiary of participation in needs assessment and planning processes should be the

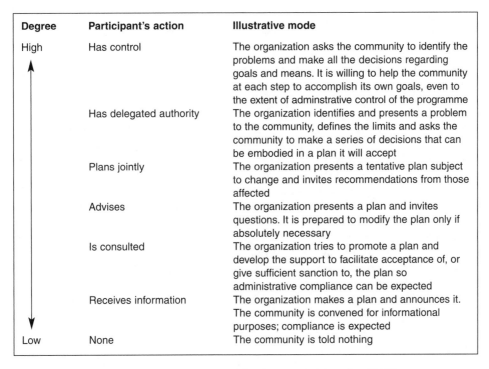

Degree	Participant's action	Illustrative mode
High	Has control	The organization asks the community to identify the problems and make all the decisions regarding goals and means. It is willing to help the community at each step to accomplish its own goals, even to the extent of adminstrative control of the programme
	Has delegated authority	The organization identifies and presents a problem to the community, defines the limits and asks the community to make a series of decisions that can be embodied in a plan it will accept
	Plans jointly	The organization presents a tentative plan subject to change and invites recommendations from those affected
	Advises	The organization presents a plan and invites questions. It is prepared to modify the plan only if absolutely necessary
	Is consulted	The organization tries to promote a plan and develop the support to facilitate acceptance of, or give sufficient sanction to, the plan so administrative compliance can be expected
	Receives information	The organization makes a plan and announces it. The community is convened for informational purposes; compliance is expected
Low	None	The community is told nothing

Figure 5.7   A spectrum of participation (after Brager and Specht, 1973)

community itself. Participation should not be a covert means of furthering professional or organizational interests – a situation graphically encapsulated in a French student poster from the 1960s (see box).

Community participation: declining the verb

Je participe
Tu participes
Il/elle participe
Nous participons
Vous participez
Ils profitent

A number of different vehicles have been used for consultation. These include citizens' juries, postal panels, face-to-face panels, local involvement networks (LINks), local user and carer groups and surveys and opinion polls. Jordan et al. (1998) suggest that consultation methods can be classified on the basis of whether or not:

- respondents are provided with any information
- respondents are involved in discussion or deliberation before recording their views.

Citizens' juries, for example, would be presented with information and involved in deliberation before reaching their decisions. In contrast, opinion polls would collect information from individuals on the spot.

A further issue relates to the representativeness of the various groups. Clearly, surveys can explicitly attempt to obtain representative samples. In contrast, the selection of jury members is usually more purposive and, despite membership generally rotating at intervals, cannot be regarded as being truly representative. There are similar concerns about the composition of user and carer consultation groups and citizen panels. Involving disadvantaged and vulnerable groups can be especially problematic and particular attention should be paid to overcoming any barriers to involvement.

Another pertinent issue is whether individuals are commenting on behalf of themselves or the group that they purport to represent – especially when there may be conflict between individual and community needs. Furthermore, within any community, the more articulate will inevitably be better placed to make their concerns known. Particular attention will therefore need to be paid to ensuring that the views of more marginalized groups are included. A variety of methods is likely to be needed to fully engage communities and the process itself can accordingly be resource intensive (Department of Health, 2007a).

The key aspects of the 'informed citizen process', which takes account of some of these concerns, are summarized by Blackwell and Kosky (2000):

- **information** – people must be presented with accurate, unbiased information
- **time** – sufficient time must be allowed to be informed and to be able to reflect
- **scrutiny** – opportunity must be provided to ask questions before making preferences
- **deliberation** – there must be a chance to reflect on information given
- **independence** – participants must have some control over how their findings are presented and to whom
- **authority** – participants must feel assured that their findings will be listened to.

In addition to improving understanding of health needs, participation can mobilize individuals and communities as agents for social change. The box provides an example of a project which has continued to inform sustainable change some ten years after its inception. It uses community-based participatory research, defined as:

A collaborative approach to research that equitably involves all partners in the research process and recognises the unique strength that each brings. [It] begins with a topic of importance to the community with the aim of combining knowledge and action for social change to improve community health and eliminate disparities. (Community Health Scholars Program, 2002 cited in Minkler et al., 2006: 294)

Case study: a community-based participatory research partnership for health promotion in Indiana

Initial partners:	University School of Nursing Healthy Cities Committee
Other key stakeholders:	included Members of City Council, newspaper editor, Fire Chief
Goal:	making the healthy choice the easy choice through changes in 'small p policies'
Methods used:	

- data from Census
- door to door survey of 1,000 households
- mobilising the community by raising awareness of health issues identified by the survey as compared with national health objectives (e.g. local smoking rate was double the national objective)
- five health priorities established (smoking, exercise, alcohol use and abuse, mental health, dietary choices)
- focus groups
- state-wide workshops including sessions on data interpretation, priority setting, policy change
- development of alliances between key stakeholders

Achievements:	increased concern about health among the community *early*: non-smoking areas in all City buildings *medium-term*: building a playground on city owned land by 1200 community volunteers *longer-term*: development of trails to encourage physical activity land use policy

Minkler et al., 2006

Rapid assessment and appraisal

Rapid assessment techniques have their origin in the broad move towards community participation and recognition of the need for local knowledge. They emerged in so-called developing countries as a response to inappropriate research by outside agencies – typified by overconfidence, lack of communication and consultation with the community or other professional groups, the use of theoretically rigorous, but time-consuming, methods and failure to translate research findings into action within a reasonable timescale (Vlassoff and Tanner, 1992).

Rapid assessment and appraisal attempts to overcome professional dominance and works towards developing a joint understanding of the needs of the community by bringing together the views of key stakeholders. It places emphasis on knowledge indigenous to a community and acknowledges the importance of qualitative research methods. However, it does not preclude the need for quantitative data, such as epidemiological information (Foreman, 1996).

A variety of terminology is used in relation to rapid assessment and appraisal, as summarized in the box below. In the literature, a clear distinction has not always been made – indeed, some authors have used the terms interchangeably. Rifkin (1992), however, identifies two broad strands, which helps to resolve the semantic confusion. One emerged from epidemiology and is concerned with collecting information on ill health and disease – usually referred to as 'rapid assessment' or 'rapid epidemiological assessment'. It draws on all forms of local data, including routinely collected data and the views of the community, but the role of the community members is generally as informants only.

Different terminology for rapid information collection approaches

REA   Rapid epidemiological assessment
RA   Rapid appraisal
RRA   Rapid rural appraisal
PRA   Participatory rural appraisal
PA   Participatory appraisal
PNA   Participatory needs assessment
RPA   Rapid participatory appraisal
REA   Rapid ethnographic assessment
PLA   Participatory learning and action

The second strand originated in the 'rapid rural appraisal' techniques developed for use in agriculture and rural development and the move from extractive to participative methods of research. It gives greater attention to the *process* of gathering data and involving communities in data collection and analysis. This latter approach is referred to as 'rapid appraisal'. The terms 'participatory rural appraisal' and 'participatory appraisal' are also used and, as these names imply, they place particular emphasis on community participation.

The distinction between the two broad strands revolves around the level and nature of participation and the emphasis on particular methodologies. Is the assessment merely community *based* or is it community *led*, taking its direction from issues raised by the community?

Notwithstanding this difference, there is some overlap between the two schools. Both take a holistic view of health and aim to collect information quickly and at low cost to inform planning at the local level.

The use of the term 'rapid' should not be taken to imply any sacrifice of rigour or attention to quality. Speed is achieved by using a battery of research methods and involving a range of professionals and lay people. Accuracy is also a major concern and triangulation is an important feature in relation to cross-checking the validity of findings (triangulation is considered more fully in Chapter 11). Rapid assessment and appraisal strategies usually incorporate opportunities, while still in the field, to reflect on findings and redefine data collection requirements in the light of any emergent conclusions or hunches. While there is considerable attention to validity, it should also be noted that rapid assessment and appraisal takes a realistic view of the level of precision required to meet the research objectives (Vlassoff and Tanner, 1992) and acknowledges that there are limits to what actually needs to be known (Heaver, 1992: 14):

> The principles apply here of optimal ignorance – not trying to find out more than is needed; and of appropriate imprecision – not trying to measure what does not need to be measured, or not measuring more accurately than is needed for practical purposes.

Ong et al. (1991) note that this approach goes beyond attempting to objectively assess the magnitude of a problem to address the strength of feeling in the community about the issue, which will inevitably be influenced by its wider ramifications. For example, although the actual number of people using hard drugs within a community may be small, drug use may have consequences for a much wider group and, therefore, be perceived to be a major problem.

Heaver (1992) identifies a number of advantages of these approaches over and above speed and economy:

- the information generated is accurate and context-specific as it draws on people's in-depth understanding of the local situation and provides opportunities for cross-checking
- plans drawn up by insiders are more likely to work than ones created by those outside the community because they take account of the local context
- the process is empowering – it enhances people's understanding of problems and enables them to have a voice in decisions made about the most appropriate course of action.

Annett and Rifkin (1990) represent the key information needs of a community as a pyramid (see Figure 5.8). Data can be collected from a number of different sources and using a range of different methods for each of the levels.

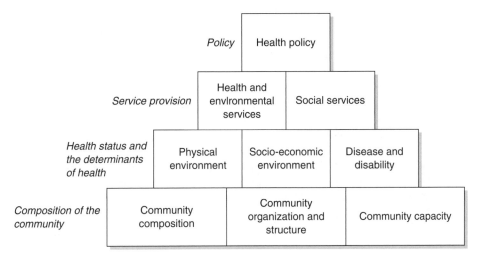

Figure 5.8   Information profile (derived from Annett and Rifkin, 1988)

The data collection methods used in rapid appraisal are many and varied. An example of the development of a food calendar by members of a coastal community in Guinea is provided in the box (below).

AN EXAMPLE OF USING A FOOD CALENDER

Extract from notes of a food and nutrition PRA:

Having heard about a 'hungry season' during the focused walk we decided to investigate the general diet and seasonal Variation...

... a team member drew out a six-season calendar framework in the sand as the women talked about their main staple food, rice, marked the top line with a grass frond to represent the rice, and allocated palm-nuts in each of the six sections according to the women's remarks on availability....discussion ensued ... and they insisted that one season be left empty, not because they have nothing to eat then, but because their own rice has been eaten or sold off to repay debts. They buy 'foreign' rice for that period ...

...the conversation about fish livened up 'Give me those nuts' said a lady in red, 'we can do this kind of writing'.

Calender of Main Elements of Household Budget

Season	Mist & fog			Hot & dry		Early rains		Rains		Late rain		Clear skies
	D	G	A	M	A	M	G	G	A	S	O	N
Own Rice	••• ••• ••• •••			••• ••• ••• •••		•• ••		•• ••				•• •• •• •••
Fish for Smoking	• ••• •••			• ••• •••		• ••• •••		••••• •••••		••• •••		••• ••• •••
Cash in	••• ••• •••			••• ••• •••		•••• ••••		••• ••• •••		••• •••		•• ••• •••
Cash out	• ••• •••			••• •••		•• ••		••••• ••••• •••••		••• •••		• ••• •••
Debt cycle	Repayments							Neglect debts				Repayments

Subsequent discussion of the calender with other members of the community resulted in a decision to explore the possibility of setting up a rice store.

Appleton, 1992: 79

The use of visual and oral methods is particularly appropriate where there are low levels of literacy. The methods used in participatory appraisal are limited only by the creativity of individuals involved in the process and include:

- Mapping
- Transects
- Social mapping
- Body mapping

- Timelines and trends, including seasonal trends
- Historical transects
- Photography
- Ranking and scoring exercises
- Sequence matrices
- Causal and flow diagramming
- Chapatti (Venn) diagramming
- Case histories
- Life histories
- Diaries
- Focus groups
- Observations.

Professionals may well require training in the use of these methods. Moreover, if they are to operate within a true spirit of participation, they will also need to abandon their expert role and go into a community prepared to learn from the people – communication and listening skills are therefore particularly important. Similarly, if members of the community are to be more than just informants, they will also need to develop skills in data collection methods and interpretation.

An important practical issue is the selection of key informants and ensuring that they are representative of the community. How this should best be tackled will require consideration of local contextual factors. Ong et al.'s (1991) rapid appraisal in the North West of England identified three groups of key informants:

- people with knowledge of the community because of their professional roles (such as health visitors, police, social workers)
- community 'leaders' (such as 'leaders' of voluntary associations, self-help groups, political groups)
- people centrally placed within the community (such as postal workers, local shopkeepers, school crossing patrols).

The data generated can be fed into any stage of the planning cycle (Vlassoff and Tanner, 1992) and, as we noted earlier, the approach is particularly useful in motivating communities. However, Rifkin's (1992) discussion generates some fundamental questions.

- Is participation viewed as a means or an end?
- Is participation active or passive?
- Does the community have control over the way in which the findings are used?
- Does the community have a say in planning processes?

The principles of participatory appraisal would require that the community should not merely be used as providers of information to slot into a conceptual framework already established by the researchers. True participation would involve the community members in developing the conceptual framework. It would also view them as equal partners in decision making – especially if the tokenism referred to by Arnstein (1969) is to be avoided.

It will be clear from our earlier discussion of empowerment in Chapter 3 that community involvement in rapid appraisal and participatory appraisal can be empowering. The value of community members' knowledge and experience can be formally acknowledged and they can exercise power and control in decision making and planning. However, there is always the risk of raising expectations that cannot be met, with consequent negative repercussions.

The key features of rapid and participatory appraisal can be summarized as:

- the community is involved in information collection and analysis – that is, they are done in/with/and by the community
- action-orientated nature
- attempts to include all perspectives
- use of multidisciplinary teams and interactive methods
- emphasis on communication and listening skills
- use of a range of data collection methods and triangulation
- analysis is carried out while still 'in the field'
- iterative nature
- incorporates critical reflection and self-criticism
- flexibility – the direction of research may be reorientated as new information becomes available
- an holistic view of health and its determinants
- optimal ignorance and appropriate imprecision.

While developing countries have paved the way in the use of these methods, there has also been increasing interest in the developed world. Indeed, Manderson and Aaby (1992) refer to an 'epidemic' in the use of rapid assessment procedures and Cornwall et al. (2001: iii) describe the spread of PRA through Kenya as being 'like a bushfire'. The approach has been particularly relevant when involving members of deprived and marginalized communities in identifying their needs and making them known. Often the technique has been used in geographically discrete areas, but it is equally applicable to more diffuse communities, such as refugees and asylum seekers (Vallely et al., 1999). It has also been used with young people as a means of giving them a voice. Morrow (2001), for example, adopted this approach with school pupils to build up a picture of how they see their social networks and communities.

Critical reflections on participatory appraisal

Participatory appraisal has grown rapidly in popularity. Cornwall et al. (2001) reflect on the consequences of the extensive use of PRA in Kenya and it having become almost a routine requirement of development organizations – many of which have done little to accommodate this participatory style of working within their own modes of operation. They feel that the range of meanings of participatory appraisal, different conceptualizations of what it involves, and the variety of practices carried out under its name threaten its quality and create difficulties in establishing quality standards. A concern is that people may subscribe to the rhetoric without fully embracing the principles.

While recognizing the potential offered by rapid appraisal and the rewarding nature of working in this way, Murray (1999) draws on the experience of five projects in the UK to identify a number of practical limitations. It tends to work best when there is a clearly defined, homogeneous community. Bias may occur if the informants selected have similar backgrounds and there is no conscious attempt to seek out any contradictory viewpoints. There may also be professional bias unless a multidisciplinary team is used and, in any event, there may be a degree of subjectivity in interpreting what people say. Any statistics generated may need to be interpreted with caution because of the rapid and highly focused nature of data collection.

The use of this approach requires training at the local level and the coordination of the various layers of activity can be demanding. Butcher and Kievelitz (1997) comment on the particular difficulty of developing analytical skills. Using the analogy of a jigsaw, Murray (1999: 444) suggests that rapid appraisal can provide 'key pieces of the jigsaw but not the complete picture' and that postal surveys and primary care data could help to complete the picture.

However, PRA appears to have a greater capacity to bring about change than the other methods. The changes documented after the technique was used in Edinburgh are listed in the box.

Changes recorded after use of a PRA in Edinburgh

- Local bus route altered to go into a council estate with 30 per cent increase in passengers
- Fenced-off play areas provided by the local council
- Use of community room for community education classes, residents' association and councillors' meetings
- Three companies tendering to build a local supermarket
- Improvements to medical facilities – additional telephone line, toys in the waiting area, ramp
- Patients spoken to with more respect

Murray and Graham, 1995

The London Health Economics Consortium (1996) carried out a review of practice in community needs assessments in four test-bed sites in the London area. It noted the lack of explicit attention to validity and practical problems with triangulation – particularly that of finding truly independent sources of information. There was concern about bias introduced by the selection of key informants. It also commented on a tendency to confuse causation with mere association and suggested that a more critical approach to causality was needed. The report noted that the findings of community needs assessments are often very similar, regardless of the areas in which they are carried out. The findings that commonly emerge are listed in the box.

> ### Common findings of needs assessment exercises
>
> - Pollution and the environment
> - Housing
> - Employment
> - Poor education and recreational facilities
> - Vandalism and crime
> - Transport
> - Loneliness, stress and mental health
> - Other diseases and disability
> - Information on, and availability of, general practitioner and social services
>
> London Health Economics Consortium, 1996

The chief concern that emerged from the study was the issue of priority setting. Particular problems concerned having too many options and the lack of criteria or appropriate mechanisms for choosing between them, the non-comparability of options, a reluctance to make decisions about rationing and a preference to view recommendations as *additional to* rather than *in place of* existing provisions – that is, incrementalism without loss.

Participatory appraisal techniques have both their critics and advocates. Some of the criticism centres on specific practical and methodological issues, in contrast to other more fundamental ideological concerns. The approach tends to work best when it conforms to a true spirit of participation and follows an agenda established by the community – a position that requires considerable skills in listening and facilitation on the part of those involved in the process. Problems tend to arise when the findings have to be slotted into a pre-existing agenda, which can lead to a mismatch between what the community is saying and what planners want to hear. As a method of working, it goes beyond merely providing a technical response to the issues of problem definition and solution generation to contributing to empowering communities by virtue of the value it places on individuals' contributions.

COMMUNITY PROFILES

Whichever way problems and needs are defined, additional information about the population or community is needed before decisions can be made about health promotion interventions and how they will be implemented. Bartholomew et al. (2001) emphasize the importance of getting to know the community as well as analysing its problems. A community profile will include information relevant to the assessment of needs, together with this wider contextual information.

Haglund et al. (1990: 91) define a community profile as:

blending quantitative health and illness statistics and demographic indicators with qualitative information on political and socio-cultural factors. The profile includes a community's image of itself and its goals, its past history and recent civic changes, and its current resources, readiness and capacity for health promotion activities.

It provides a basis for setting priorities and planning. 'It should define community strengths as well as potential problem areas' (Rissel and Bracht, 1999: 59) and help to ensure that there is a good match between the characteristics of a community and any proposed intervention (see the box). The profile is the product of a process of community analysis. The term 'community diagnosis' has also been used, particularly in the North American context. Comparing community diagnosis with needs assessment, Stuart (in Quinn, 1999: 685) stated that:

> Diagnosis is much broader and aims to understand many facets of the community including culture, values and norms, leadership and power structure, means of communication, helping patterns, important community institutions and history. A good diagnosis suggests what it is like to live in a community, what the important health problems are, what interventions are likely to be most efficacious, and how the program would be best evaluated.

Although the two terms are synonymous, our preference here is to use 'community analysis', which we feel gives a better sense of the broad remit of the process and an emphasis on the positive aspects of a community. It reduces the risk of misinterpretation arising from associating the word 'diagnosis' with a narrow focus on the identification of problems.

Different communities, different interventions

Community A:

- traditional
- homogeneous
- family ties and hierarchies within families important
- religious
- church leaders respected
- school curriculum controlled at national level – no provision for sex education
- general reluctance to talk about sex
- media are tightly controlled
- strong censorship laws
- strong sense of community.

Community B:

- progressive
- heterogeneous
- variety of different family structures and ties
- few members of the community belong to any religion
- schools are required to provide sex education, although the quality varies between schools

(Continued)

(Continued)

- young people laugh and joke among themselves about sex, but feel uncomfortable talking to their parents or teachers about it
- little control over the media
- censorship is very liberal and there is a considerable amount of sexually explicit material in the media
- no real sense of community.

Responding to the problem of HIV/AIDS would demand completely different intervention strategies in these two communities.

As with the assessment of needs, a community analysis may be undertaken from a biomedical perspective or adopt community development principles and a more participative approach. It will include both quantitative and qualitative information derived from a variety of different sources, both primary and secondary.

Haglund et al. (1990) identify four main features of a community that would require consideration:

- specification of geographical boundaries
- assessment of social institutions – health, education and so on
- identification of social interaction patterns
- examination of social control mechanisms and norms, both formal, via institutions such as the police, school and church, and informal, via values, norms and customs in the community.

While establishing geographical boundaries is important in delimiting the area of enquiry, it should be noted that communities are not necessarily defined in geographical terms – they can be based on shared characteristics, such as ethnicity, gender, sexual orientation and disability. The concept of 'community' will be discussed further in Chapter 9.

Bartholomew et al. (2001) comment on the importance of assessing community competence, capacity and social capital because of their relevance as:

- **inputs** – factors that contribute directly to health promotion intervention
- **throughputs** – factors that will affect successful programme implementation
- **outputs** – the products of programmes.

'Community competence' focuses on how a community is currently functioning. The concept of 'community capacity' is closely related. It includes the notion of current competence, but also the potential within the community to respond to issues of common concern. Smith et al. (2001) note that, although there has been increasing emphasis on the concept of community capacity, there has been relatively little attempt to define it. The box provides an overview of some of the definitions used.

> ### Some definitions of 'community capacity'
>
> … a wholistic representation of capabilities (those with which the community is endowed and those to which the community has access) plus the facilitators and barriers to realization of those capabilities in the broader social environment.
>
> Jackson et al., 1997, in Smith et al., 2001: 33
>
> … the characteristics of communities that affect their ability to identify, mobilize and address social and public health problems.
>
> McLeroy, 1996, in Bartholomew et al., 2001: 26
>
> … the degree to which a community can develop, implement and sustain actions for strengthening community health.
>
> Smith et al., 2001: 33

The National Civic League (2002) in the United States has developed a Civic Index to assist communities in assessing their capacity to deal with issues of concern. It covers ten broad areas:

- citizen participation
- community leadership
- government performance
- volunteerism and philanthropy
- inter-group and intra-group relationships
- civic education
- community information sharing
- capacity for cooperation and consensus building
- community vision and pride
- regional cooperation.

Reference to our earlier discussion of social capital in Chapter 2 will confirm the considerable overlap with community capacity. However, social capital tends to focus on the networks, relationships and structural conditions rather than the resources that can be tapped into, material or otherwise (Smith et al., 2001). Eight verifiable domains of social capital have been identified and are listed in the box. The notion of social cohesion is also closely related and refers to the bonds within communities based on shared social and cultural commitments. The Home Office's Community Cohesion Review Team (2001) draws on the work of Ferlander and Timms to identify the principal characteristics of community cohesion:

- commitment to common norms and values
- interdependence as a result of shared interests
- identification with the community.

The domains of community cohesion are listed in the box, along with the domains of social capital.

The domains of social capital and community cohesion

Domain	Description
Social capital	
Empowerment	People feel that they have a voice that is listened to, are involved in processes that affect them, can themselves take action to initiate changes
Participation	People take part in social and community activities. Local events occur and are well attended
Associational activity and common purpose	People cooperate with one another by forming formal and informal groups to further their interests
Supporting networks and reciprocity	Individuals cooperate to support one another for either mutual or one-sided gain. An expectation that help would be given to, or received from, others when needed
Collective norms and values	People share common values and norms of behaviour
Trust	People feel that they can trust their co-residents and local organizations responsible for governing or serving their area
Safety	People feel safe in their neighbourhood and are not restricted in their use of public space by fear
Belonging	People feel connected to their co-residents, their home area, have a sense of belonging to the place and its people
Community cohesion	
Common values and a civic culture	Common aims and objectives, common moral principles and codes of behaviour, support for political institutions and participation in politics
Social order and social control	Absence of general conflict and threats to the existing order, absence of incivility, effective informal social control, tolerance, respect for differences, intergroup cooperation
Social solidarity and reductions in wealth disparities	Harmonious economic and social development and common standards, redistribution of public finances and opportunities, equal access to services and welfare benefits, ready acknowledgement of social obligations and willingness to assist others
Social networks and social capital	High degree of social interaction within communities and families, civic engagement and associational activity, easy resolution of collective action problems
Place attachment and Identity	Strong attachment to place, intertwining of personal and place identity

Forrest and Kearns, 2000, in Community Cohesion Review Team, 2001

It would be invidious even to attempt to draw up a generic checklist of all the issues that need to be considered before the detailed planning of interventions to improve the health status of a population can begin. However, they fall into five broad categories that are applicable regardless of whether there is a professional or community-led approach to data collection and whichever ideological position underpins the endeavour:

- the health status of the population – identification of problems and any groups particularly 'at risk'
- the key determinants of health status and disease – behavioural and environmental at micro, meso and macro levels
- motivation and capacity to respond – individually and collectively
- channels of communication and patterns of influence
- characteristics of the community and power structures within it and wider society.

Prioritization of health needs

Regardless of the approach taken, it is likely that a number of different health needs will emerge in view of the wide range of factors – both upstream and downstream – which impact on health status. Some prioritization will be necessary. Cavanagh and Chadwick (2005) propose two initial selection criteria:

- impact – in terms of the severity or magnitude of the problem
- changeability – the feasibility of change.

Decisions can be based on the perceptions of the community, service providers and managers, health data, and local, national and organizational priorities. The acceptability of change and the availability of resources are also important considerations. Clearly, the respective emphasis on these different criteria and the value attached to the views of different groups of stakeholders will be influenced by the approach taken to health needs assessment and its underpinning ideology.

SOLUTION GENERATION

Following on from establishing what the priority health needs are and analysing the characteristics of a community, the challenge is 'translating the findings into effective action' (Cavanagh and Chadwick, 2005: 9). The white paper *Choosing Health* (Department of Health, 2004: 14) raises concerns that:

> Too often in the past we have devoted too much time and energy to analyzing the problems and not enough to developing and delivering practical solutions that connect with real lives. (cited by Cavanagh and Chadwick, 2005: 9)

The principal dilemma for those involved in health promotion planning is the selection of an appropriate intervention or combination of interventions. To an extent, the options considered will be constrained by ideological commitments. As we have noted in Chapter 1, those who subscribe to the ideology of empowerment will opt to work in participative ways. In contrast, more authoritarian, top-down approaches would be consistent with a preventive model. The range of options can be represented using models – either iconic or analogic (see the box). Beattie (1991) provides a useful analogic taxonomy of the range of different health promotion approaches.

Iconic and analogic models

- **Iconic models** are descriptors or characterizations that offer a simplified view of a recognized aspect of reality.
- **Analogic models** provide a framework to assist understanding of reality and use analogies or metaphors that need not necessarily currently exist (Rawson, 1992).

Beattie's model, as represented in Figure 5.9, incorporates two fundamental dimensions – the mode of intervention, which ranges from authoritative to negotiated, and the focus of intervention, which is either on the individual or the collective. An individual's personal and professional values will have a bearing on the preferred mode of operation. Furthermore, imperatives within the workplace may direct the activities of practitioners – regardless of whether or not the implicit values are consistent with their own.

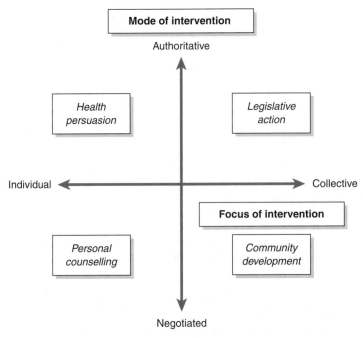

Figure 5.9   Beattie's model of health promotion (Beattie, 1991)

Rawson notes that the advantage of analogic models over iconic models is that they have a theoretical structure, which can assimilate new forms of practice. However, the disadvantage is that 'they may seem remote from the detail of reality' (1992: 211). Clearly, the demarcation between authoritative and negotiated approaches is not absolute. Rather, they represent polar extremes, with some possible gradation between the two. For example, we have already observed that community participation can range from a minimum, tokenistic consultation to the community having genuine control and a recognized decision-making role. Similarly, there is the possibility of differing levels of authoritarian control. Indeed, we might postulate that this could even include the instrumental use of participative methods – not because of any commitment to negotiated styles of working, but because it is the best way to achieve predefined goals. The focus of intervention will also be subject to parallel variation. A collective approach could involve change at the group, setting, community or population level.

Notwithstanding an ideological commitment to broad styles of working, the rational selection of specific methods will be based on a combination of:

- theory
- evidence about effective practice
- context
- professional judgement based on experience.

The role of theory

Recourse to theory will be useful both in pursuing the cause of health problems and in identifying what should be done to tackle them – referred to respectively by the National Cancer Institute (2005) in the USA as 'explanatory theory' and 'change theory'.

In short, theory supports the identification of key relevant variables. Explanatory theory will guide the search for modifiable risk factors. For example, if the proportion of young people taking up smoking has been implicated as the problem, a health action model (HAM) analysis would direct attention towards exploring the principal determinants of young people's behavioural intention concerning smoking – that is, their belief, motivation and normative systems and self concept. Furthermore, investigation of any factors that facilitate or act as a barrier to their translating intentions into practice would also be required.

In contrast, change theory will inform decisions about the most appropriate strategy. It will make clear any assumptions underpinning the chosen strategy and also check that all the necessary elements of the intervention are in place (see the box).

A view of theory and professional practice

Like an expert chef, a theoretically grounded health education professional does not blindly follow a cookbook recipe, but constantly creates it anew, depending on the circumstances. Without a theory, she or he has only the skills of a cafeteria line worker.

National Cancer Institute, 1997

Unless a full, rational appraisal of the problem and possible solutions is undertaken, interventions might easily:

- address wrong or inappropriate variables – that is, miss the target completely
- tackle only a proportion of the variables required to have the desired effect – that is, hit only a few of the total possible targets and not enough to achieve any meaningful change (Green, 2000).

Theory, then, can make an important contribution to solution generation by virtue of its explanatory and predictive capabilities. Indeed, Eiser and Eiser's (1996: 43) review of the effectiveness of video for health education is adamant on this point:

> Interventions without a clear theoretical rationale almost always fail or achieve only a semblance of success that disappears when submitted to critical examination.

However, this type of theoretical analysis of problems and possible solutions is not without its critics. It has been aligned with authoritarian, individualistic approaches and the preventive model discussed in Chapter 1. A particular concern is that it objectifies human experience and is therefore inconsistent with the central tenets of health promotion – holism and empowerment. Buchanan (1994) attributes scepticism about the relevance of theory to health promotion practice to a narrow view of theory equated with the natural sciences and positivism. This interpretation of theory would see it as establishing the relationships between factors (independent variables) and some outcome (dependent variable). It should also be possible to predict the changes in outcome that would be caused by manipulation of the independent variable/s and, indeed, verify this by testing. The role of the health promoter would therefore simply be to identify and change the relevant independent variables to achieve the desired outcome. Failure to achieve success would demand a more thorough and detailed analysis of the variables and evermore precise targeting and tailoring of interventions. 'Targeting' involves designing interventions to suit the characteristics of particular subgroups (such as age, gender, ethnicity, social class, occupational group) whereas 'tailoring' adapts interventions to meet the specific requirements of individuals. Kreuter and Skinner (2000: 1) offer the following definition of tailoring:

> Any combination of information or change strategies intended to reach one specific *person*, based on characteristics that are unique to that person, related to the outcome of interest, and have been *derived from an individual assessment*.

Noar and Zimmerman (2005) argue that although there are numerous health behaviour theories, there is no consensus about which offers most precision in explaining health behaviour. Further, despite the similarity between the constructs of different theories, the use of different terminology gives the illusion that they are different. They call for more empirical testing and comparison of theories in order to refine them as a means of understanding health behaviour.

Buchanan, in contrast, contends that human action is not governed in the same law-like way as natural processes and, hence, the methods used to study natural phenomena cannot be applied to human behaviour. The role of human agency in constructing reality is well recognized in this regard (see the box).

Human agency and reality

Human beings are not 'things' to be studied in the way one studies ants, plants or rocks, but are valuing, meaning attributing beings to be understood as subjects and known as subjects ... To impose positivistic meanings upon the realm of social phenomena is to distort the fundamental nature of human existence.

Hughes, 1976: 25

Buchanan (1994: 274) does not reject the need for theory per se, but calls for a broader conceptualization of theory that recognizes that 'knowledge is contingent and contextual rather than universal, determinate and invariable'. The purpose of theory, then, is not to offer universal explanations or predictions, but to clarify understanding of complex situations. It therefore needs to interplay with a range of contextual factors. Buchanan proposes Aristotle's notion of 'phronesis' or 'practical reason' as a means of understanding the unique features of each situation. This contrasts with *episteme* or 'theoretical knowledge' based on universal laws that Aristotle himself recognized could not capture the complexity of the social world. Practical reason (Buchanan, 1994: 279) is the:

ability to recognize, acknowledge, pick out and respond to the singular salient features of a complex and unique situation. It is not deduction from abstract generalizations ... Practical reason is the thinking process involved in deciding what to say or how to do that which best suits the particular situation at hand. Practical reason is involved in weighing which of the available courses of action is more appropriate given the specific circumstances.

Theory, then, can provide important insights into the nature of problems and the strategies that could be adopted. As Kurt Lewin is famously noted to have said, 'there is nothing so practical as a good theory' (Marrow, 1969). However, as we have noted above, an abstract analysis alone is insufficient. A complementary understanding of specific contextual factors is also required before a decision can be made about the most appropriate course of action.

Case study: the use of the health belief model to understand factors associated with the acceptability of solar disinfection of drinking water in Nepal

Uptake of solar disinfection (SODIS) 9%

Beliefs

Beliefs about susceptibility and seriousness:
Don't know what causes diarrhoea
Diarrhoea is a normal situation

(Continued)

(Continued)

Headache, not diarrhoea, was the main reported health problem
Barriers:
Heavy workload
No bottles available
No place to expose bottles all day
Temperature/taste of water different
Solar Disinfected water was seen as a 'leftover' and not culturally acceptable
Effectiveness of preventive measures:
Don't know if SODIS works or not
Self-efficacy:
Solar disinfection is easy to understand

Cues to action

Ill family members
Turbidity of water
Presence of researcher during data collection

Efforts to increase uptake would need to address the beliefs of the community.

Derived from Rainey and Harding, 2005

Health promotion has a plethora of theories to draw on. A key issue concerns the selection of appropriate theory for the task in hand – see box for an example of the use of the health belief model. The factors that influence health status range from micro-level individual factors to macro-level policy and environmental issues. The various levels of an ecological approach identified by the National Cancer Institute (2005) are:

- intrapersonal level
- interpersonal level
- community level

  - institutional or organizational factors
  - community factors
  - public policy.

Clearly, each level will have its own repertoire of theory to draw on. Relevant theory at the intrapersonal level might, for example, include the health belief model (HBM), and theory of planned behaviour (TPB); at the interpersonal level, social cognitive theory; and, at the community level, diffusion of innovations. Some theories will bridge different levels – for example, the health action model (HAM). Comprehensive multi-level approaches will therefore need to combine different theories from the different levels of analysis. McLeroy et al. (1993: 305) contend that *'no single theory*, certainly no psychological theory, is adequate for developing truly effective and comprehensive health education programmes'. They also note that there are no guidelines for selecting individual theories, let alone combinations of theories. The National Cancer Institute (1997) cautions against attempting to fit a square peg into a round hole! The 'Which theory?' box lists some key questions to consider when assessing how well a theory is suited to the task.

Which theory?

- Does it include all relevant variables?
- Is it parsimonious (does not include any redundant variables)?
- Does its use make logical sense in the particular situation?
- Has it been used by others for similar purposes?
- Are there any published studies that use the theory for similar purposes?
- Is it consistent with the values integral to the work?

The application of theory

The choice of theory will clearly be influenced by ideological perspectives. By way of illustration, let us pursue the example of high levels of heart disease in a socially dis-advantaged community, where it is recognized to be a problem by both professionals and the community itself.

A major risk factor is the diet of many members of the community, which is known to be high in saturated fats and refined carbohydrates. An authoritarian or preventive approach would search for the key variables to address by means of the application of cognitive behavioural or psycho-social theory – for example, the HAM would identify the main factors associated with dietary practice and the stages of change model would assess the readiness of the community to change. A two-pronged strategy might be adopted. One strand would focus on attempting to change behavioural intention concerning a healthy diet and develop skills in preparing healthy meals at low cost. The selection of actual methods should also be informed by a range of relevant theories – learning theory, diffusion of innovations theory and communication theory. The other strand would be concerned with making healthy foods available at lower cost – for example, by working with local shops to gain their cooperation. The selection of methods to achieve this would be enhanced by reference to diffusion of innovations theory and organizational change theories. Should the remit of the programme be more ambitious and attempt to influence food policy more generally, then recourse to policy theory would be needed.

In contrast, a negotiated approach would draw on community development theory to identify ways of working with the community to enable it to identify the main causes of the problems it is experiencing and the most feasible solutions. These might include the need to empower people to achieve a healthy diet on a low income, either individually or by working collectively to reduce food costs by setting up food cooperatives. Both may require some form of learning and, again, communication and learning theory will be important as will community organization theory. Should any environmental change and political action be needed – for example, getting the council to set aside land for allotments so that people can grow their own food, then additional lobbying and advocacy skills will be needed, together with an understanding of how to influence political processes derived from policy theory.

An overview of both these approaches is presented in Figure 5.10.

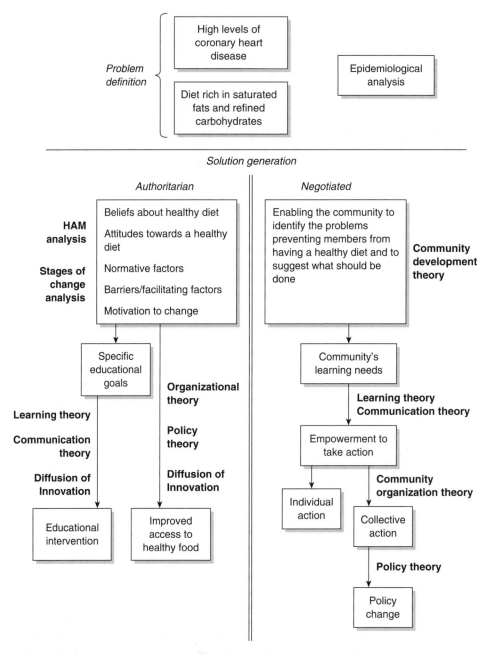

Figure 5.10   Choice of intervention – the contribution of theories

Evidence-based practice

The latter part of the twentieth century witnessed a move towards evidence-based practice in health and social care generally, but also in health promotion. Indeed, the 51st World Health Assembly (WHO, 1998c) urged all member states to 'adopt an evidence-based approach to health promotion policy and practice, using the full range of quantitative and qualitative methodologies'.

While evaluation has been recognized as being integral to good practice in health promotion, there is now even greater emphasis on the *utilization* of evaluation evidence in practice. The need for such evidence of effectiveness has been a major driver for the production of systematic reviews, and groups such as the Cochrane Collaboration have played a leading role. Some of the major sources of systematic reviews and other evidence to be found online are listed in the box.

Selected online sources of evidence and systematic reviews

	Website
Health Information Resources	www.library.nhs.uk/evidence/
NICE evidence base	www.nice.org.uk/aboutnice/whoweare/ aboutthehda/evidencebase/
NHS Quality Improvement Scotland	www.nhshealthquality.org/nhsqis/92.html
Health Evidence Bulletins Wales	http://hebw.cf.ac.uk/
NHS Centre for Reviews and Dissemination, including access to: DARE: Database of Abstracts of Reviews of Effects, NHS EED: NHS Economic Evaluation Database and HTA: Health Technology Assessment Database	www.york.ac.uk/inst/crd
Evidence from systematic reviews of research relevant to implementing the 'wider public health' agenda	www.york.ac.uk/inst/crd/wph.htm
The Evidence for Policy and Practice Information and Coordinating Centre (EPPI-Centre)	www.eppi.ioe.ac.uk/cms/
The Cochrane Collaboration	www.cochrane.org

(Continued)

(Continued)

Cochrane Public Health Group	www.vichealth.vic.gov.au/cochrane
Campbell Collaboration	www.campbellcollaboration.org
International Union for Health Promotion and Education (IUHPE)	www.iuhpe.org
Reviews of health promotion and education online (RHP&EO)	www.rhpeo.org
WHO Reproductive Health Library	www.who.int/rhl/en/

Much of the discussion about evidence-based practice in the past has focused on ways of measuring effectiveness. A particular concern has been the emphasis on positivist methodology and the use of randomized controlled trials (RCTs). We will focus on the issue of evaluation and the generation of evidence in Chapter 11. However, we should note, in passing, that there is a developing consensus – endorsed by WHO (1998a) – on the value of methodological pluralism for health promotion evaluation.

Notwithstanding these concerns and the ongoing debate, it is still the case that greater weight is attached to evidence from experimental or quasi-experimental studies – see, for example, the hierarchy of evidence for assessing interventions given in the box.

Levels of evidence for studies on the efficacy of public health interventions

Level of evidence	Type of evidence
1++	High-quality meta-analyses, systematic reviews of RCTs, or RCTs (including cluster RCTs) with a very low risk of bias
1+	Well-conducted meta-analyses, systematic reviews of RCTs, or RCTs (including cluster RCTs) with a low risk of bias
1–	Meta-analyses, systematic reviews of RCTs, or RCTs (including cluster RCTs) with a high risk of bias*
2++	High-quality systematic reviews of, or individual, non-randomized controlled trials, case–control studies, cohort studies, controlled before-and-after (CBA), interrupted time series (ITS), correlation studies with a very low risk of confounding, bias or chance and a high probability that the relationship is causal

(Continued)

(*Continued*)

2+	Well-conducted, non-randomized controlled trials, case–control studies, cohort studies, controlled before-and-after (CBA), interrupted time series (ITS), correlation studies with a low risk of confounding, bias or chance and a moderate probability that the relationship is causal
2–	Non-randomized controlled trials, case–control studies, cohort studies, controlled before-and-after (CBA), interrupted time series (ITS), correlation studies with a high risk of confounding bias or chance and a significant risk that the relationship is not causal*
3	Non-analytic studies (for example, case reports, case series)
4	Expert opinion, formal consensus

* Studies with a level of evidence '–' should not be used as a basis for making a recommendation (NICE, 2005: 31)

Furthermore, some of the central concerns of health promotion – participation, empowerment, policy development and environmental change – present a greater challenge for robust evaluation than individually orientated behaviour change. It is perhaps not surprising, therefore, that there is less evidence to draw on in relation to these areas than is the case for others. Tilford (2000) notes that, as health promotion has evolved from health education, there has been a time-lag in evaluations focusing on the social rather than the individual determinants of health. However, there is considerable interest in developing appropriate indicators for complex concepts, such as social capital (Campbell et al., 1999; Cooper et al., 1999; Community Cohesion Review Team, 2001; Coulthard et al., 2001) and the application of theoretical frameworks to evaluation of comprehensive multi-level interventions (see, for example, Pawson and Tilley, 1997).

Comparatively little attention has been given to the ways in which practitioners use evidence in planning health promotion interventions. Ideological commitments will, again, influence views about the credibility and utility of different types of evidence and its appeal to practitioners. However, over and above the issues associated with evaluation methodology, systematic reviews (and, indeed, published evaluations more generally) are recognized as having a number of limitations for the end-users. These are summarized by Tilford (2000) as being:

- insufficient attention to the quality of interventions
- the theoretical basis of interventions is not always made clear
- insufficient information on the process of implementation of interventions
- the tendency for reviews to focus on health education rather than the broader sphere of health promotion
- the short-term follow-up time of many studies
- the dominance of studies from the USA.

She notes that the mismatch between the types of interventions that have been rigorously evaluated and those commonly used in practice further limits the relevance of the evidence base for practitioners. It is self-evident that innovative approaches will have little, if any, evidence to draw on.

South and Tilford's (2000) study of the use of research by health promotion specialists in England found two different interpretations of evidence-based practice among practitioners. On the one hand, it was associated with using sound empirical research and, on the other, it was conceptualized more broadly as additionally drawing on theory, principles of good practice, the academic literature and national policy. Some practitioners used a systematic approach to retrieve and appraise evidence, whereas, for others, this was done on a rather more ad hoc basis or, alternatively, seen as falling within the general context of keeping up to date. Practitioners also used their professional judgement to make decisions about the appropriate level of evidence required. The valuable contribution of research to planning interventions was recognized, but only as one element alongside theory and professional expertise.

Nutbeam (1996) identifies three levels of practice that differ in the extent to which they are based on research evidence – planned, responsive and reactive. *Planned* health promotion is based on a rational and systematic review of evidence concerning health needs, effectiveness of interventions and contextual factors. *Responsive* health promotion involves addressing the expressed needs of the community in ways it sees as most appropriate – the use of research evidence is only one factor in the decision-making process. Although this style of working is consistent with the rhetoric of the Ottawa Charter, Nutbeam (1996: 321) cautions that:

> the interventions chosen may not be effective or efficient, and not tackle fundamental problems even though they are strongly supported by the community.

Reactive health promotion takes the form of a rapid and often high-profile response to a problem or crisis. Political imperatives may drive both the pace and type of response – for example, the early public awareness campaigns about HIV. The short timescale of this knee-jerk type of response does not allow sufficient time for rigorous evidence-based planning.

Although evidence-based practice had been narrowly equated with evaluation research, a broader interpretation will provide a more secure base for practice. This view, as we have noted, is reflected in the field, where there is some concern that other forms of evidence may be omitted from decisions about interventions (South and Tilford, 2000). Green (2000) has argued for a greater emphasis on the contribution of theory to evidence-based practice. Furthermore, empirical evidence and theory are not alternatives, but should be inextricably linked. In short, research evidence about the effectiveness of interventions should contribute to the development of intervention theory, which will itself shape subsequent interventions and the ways in which they are evaluated. Sackett et al. (1996: 71) also draw attention to the importance of professional expertise in their definition of evidence-based medical practice as 'integrating individual clinical expertise with the best available external clinical evidence from systematic research'.

A combination of these elements should allow state-of-the-art solutions or interventions to be identified and an appropriate selection made. McLeroy et al. (1993) refer to this as the 'theory of intervention' – statements or summaries of what we know about the relative effectiveness of different intervention strategies with particular populations.

Professional judgement and context

We have already noted the importance of the professional perspective in our discussion of the contribution of both theory and evidence-based practice to solution generation. At grass-roots level, this derives from experience and is grounded in familiarity with particular contexts and specific groups, which enables the most appropriate course of action to be identified. Adherence to the professional values of health promotion will also make some approaches more acceptable and preclude others. These values have been discussed at length in Chapter 1.

Realist approaches to evaluation are attracting considerable attention and will be discussed more fully in Chapter 11. Unlike other approaches, they focus particularly on attempting to understand the contexts and mechanisms underpinning observed outcomes (Pawson and Tilley, 1997). However, much of the research evidence about effectiveness and theoretical analyses remains largely context-free. Health promotion, though, does not operate within a vacuum. Effective health promotion interventions must be designed to have a good fit with contextual factors and local circumstances. For example, any attempt to bring about organizational change will need to give due regard to the culture and norms within the organization. Similar attention should be given to the range of relevant contextual factors, regardless of the level of the proposed intervention – be it individual, group, community, organization, environmental or policy change.

We noted above the broad range of factors included within a community profile that are relevant both to understanding needs and the contextual factors that will influence the response. McLeroy et al. (1993) emphasize that this understanding should include the capacity of families, social networks, communities and organizations to address the needs of their members and that health promotion interventions should take a form that strengthens this. Otherwise, health promotion interventions risk becoming a substitute for these local mechanisms, reducing the community's capacity to cope independently – effectively becoming a de-powering, rather than an empowering, influence.

Over and above contributing to strategic decisions, contextual information also informs operational planning. It identifies who the most appropriate target groups are and what channels are most appropriate for reaching them. It also identifies any gatekeepers. Indeed, it may be more appropriate to target gatekeepers than those it is hoped will ultimately benefit. For example, attempts to improve the nutrition of young children will need to target families, particularly mothers. In patriarchal societies, improving women's access to contraception may require working with men to gain their support. Similarly, if access to interventions is controlled by gatekeepers, their cooperation will be needed. For example, schoolteachers have an important gatekeeper function in relation to young people's access to health education materials. If there are important opinion leaders or referent groups, then it is also wise to work with them.

Understanding what channels of communication exist will increase the potential for success. This might be something as obvious as access to radio or television and details of listening audiences at particular times of day, if a mass media campaign is being

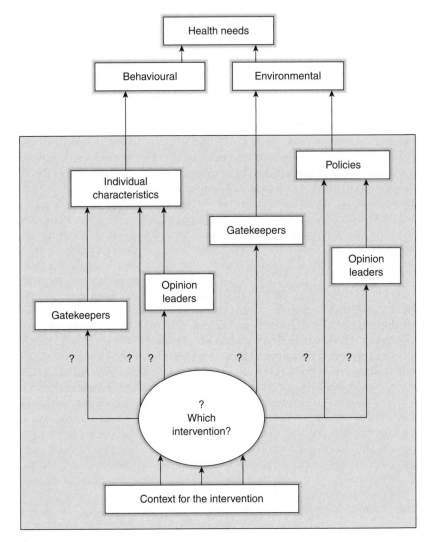

Figure 5.11   Contextual factors and choice of intervention

planned, or details of social interaction networks, if a peer education programme is being developed. Larkey et al. (1999), for example, used systematic network measurement techniques to identify individuals who were most centrally and socially connected before offering them the opportunity to train as peer health educators for their worksite dietary change intervention. Similarly, effective lobbying and advocacy is dependent on being able to identify and target those with most political power and influence. An overview of how these various strands fit together is provided in Figure 5.11.

INFORMATION AND HEALTH PROMOTION PLANNING

This chapter has focused on identifying the information needed to plan interventions. A theme running through the chapter has been the tension between different approaches to defining needs and proposing solutions – particularly between:

- participative, bottom-up and professionally led top-down approaches
- subjective and objective interpretations
- reductionist and interpretive perspectives.

This will inevitably influence the ways in which health needs are defined and prioritized and the types of solution proposed.

Health promotion, by its very nature, is action-orientated towards improving health status – whether this is viewed as addressing specific problems or creating conditions that are supportive of health. Health promotion interventions are more likely to be successful if they respond to the needs recognized by individuals or a community and are based on an analysis of environmental, social and behavioural determinants. Identifying appropriate solutions requires recourse to theory, research evidence of effectiveness, analysis of contextual factors and professional judgement. Furthermore, the use of participative approaches at all stages will draw on the practical knowledge and experience of the community.

Whichever approach is adopted, information is needed to answer the following key questions.

- What is the nature of the problem?
- Who is affected?
- What are the causes?
- What are the contextual factors?
- What do we need to do to tackle it?
- How should we do it?

KEY POINTS

- ○ Assessing health needs is the first stage of systematic programme planning.

- ○ Understanding of contextual factors and community profiles should also inform the planning process.

- ○ The approach to health needs assessment will be influenced by ideology.

- ○ Participatory approaches place people at the centre of the process and are consistent with the principles of health promotion.

- ○ Developing effective responses to health needs requires reference to relevant theory, existing empirical evidence, and the insight of practitioners and the community.

6

HEALTHY PUBLIC POLICY

He has sat on the fence so long that the iron has entered his soul.

David Lloyd George (1863–1945)

OVERVIEW

This chapter will look at the role of policy in influencing health and establishing supportive environments for health. It will:

- define healthy public policy
- consider the process of policy making and implementation
- identify the contribution of health education to policy development through awareness raising and development of political skills
- outline the contribution of advocacy to policy making and consider advocacy strategies
- consider the role of power in the policy process and how to bring pressure to bear
- examine the contribution of Health Impact Assessment to building healthy public policy.

INTRODUCTION

The defining feature of health promotion has been its emphasis on the environmental determinants of health rather than individual behaviour. Healthy public policy has been seen as the vehicle for 'creating supportive environments to enable people to lead healthy lives' (WHO, 1988: 1). The use of public policy measures to protect health is not new. Many of the health improvements in the UK in the nineteenth century were achieved by public policy, such as the Public Health Acts of 1848 and 1875, which attempted to control aspects of the environment – water supply, sewage disposal, slaughtering of animals, parks and open spaces, isolation hospitals and the beginnings of housing control (McKeown and Lowe, 1974; Jones and Sidell, 1997).

The rediscovery of the importance of environmental influences on health underpinned the emergence of health promotion and the 'New Public Health' movements in the latter part of the twentieth century. However, contemporary conceptualizations of the environment have broadened to include social and economic as well as physical aspects. Furthermore, simple causal sequences linking environment and disease have been replaced by complex causal webs of factors affecting health status. The policy response required is similarly more complex and wide-ranging. Jones and Sidell (1997) trace three main strands that have influenced the development of healthy public policy:

- public health, the 'New Public Health' and, alongside these, health education and health promotion
- social welfare reforms and the welfare state
- new social movements, such as women's and civil rights movements and the environmental movement.

This chapter considers the role of policy in two broad ways. First, the development of policy explicitly to tackle health issues – policy as the solution to health concerns. There are clear links with the sections on media advocacy and persuasive communication in Chapters 7 and 8 and community activism in Chapter 9. Second, the effects on health of policy designed for other purposes and the use of Health Impact Assessment to identify these potential effects. However, we will begin by examining the WHO position on healthy public policy.

HEALTHY PUBLIC POLICY – THE WHO POSITION

The central role of healthy public policy has been a consistent theme running through major WHO documents on health promotion as discussed in Chapter 1. The Ottawa Charter (WHO, 1986) – which has been a constant source of reference in the development of health promotion and the 'New Public Health' – identified building healthy public policy and the creation of supportive environments as two of its five priority action areas. This commitment has been reaffirmed in subsequent statements.

The Jakarta Declaration (WHO, 1997) noted the importance of multisectoral and partnership working along with a commitment to healthy public policy. The pursuit of social responsibility for health involves decision makers in the public and private sectors adopting polices and practices that:

- avoid harming the health of individuals
- protect the environment and ensure the use of sustainable resources
- restrict the production of, and trade in, inherently harmful goods and substances, such as tobacco and armaments, as well as discourage unhealthy marketing practices
- safeguard both the citizen in the marketplace and the individual in the workplace
- include equity-focused health impact assessments as an integral part of policy development (WHO, 1997: 3).

Healthy public policy was the specific focus of the second International Conference on Health Promotion held in Adelaide, which defined it as 'characterized by an explicit concern for health and equity in all areas of policy and accountability for health impact' (WHO, 1988: 1).

The recommendations of the Adelaide Conference formally recognized that the activities of a number of different government sectors influence health status and that there should be accountability for health impacts. This would include effects on the social and physical environments, which may influence the possibility and ease of making healthy choices or, alternatively, effects that are directly health-enhancing or damaging. Health was also seen as a fundamental right and sound social investment.

A central concern was equity and narrowing the health gap in society by means of policies that attach high priority to disadvantaged and vulnerable groups. Furthermore, developed countries were considered to have an obligation to ensure that their own health policies impacted positively on developing nations.

Healthy public policy was seen to be important at all levels of government, from national to local, and 'public accountability for health … an essential nutrient for the growth of healthy public policy' (WHO, 1988: 2). Community action can therefore provide the motive force for policy development. The other side of the coin is that governments should assess and report the impact of policies in a way that can be understood by all groups in society.

Although government was seen to have a key role, other groups – such as the private and business sectors, non-governmental and community organizations – were also identified as important influences that could be harnessed for health promotion.

The Fifth Global Conference on Health Promotion held in Mexico identified the central responsibility of governments for health and social development. It acknowledged that in order to achieve equity and health for all, '… health promotion must be a fundamental component of public policies and programmes in all countries …' (WHO, 2000a). A strong theme to emerge from the Mexico conference was the need to 'work with and through existing political systems and structures to ensure healthy public policy, adequate investment in health and facilitation of an infrastructure for health promotion' (WHO, 2000b: 21). This was held to require:

- democratic processes
- social and political activism
- a system of equity-orientated health impact assessment
- reorientation of health services
- improved interaction between politicians, policy makers, researchers and practitioners
- strengthening existing capacity for implementing health promotion strategies and supporting synergy between different levels – local, national and international.

The responsibility of governments in relation to health promotion was reiterated in the Bangkok Charter (WHO, 2005), along with the need to 'make the health consequences of policies and legislation explicit, using tools such as equity-focused health impact assessment'. Further, the Charter also emphasized the importance of establishing mechanisms for global governance to address the harmful effects on health of trade, products, services and marketing strategies.

Recognition of the importance of policy also emerges in the 'Health for All' literature. *Health for All in the 21st Century* 'guides action and policy for health at all levels (international, regional, national and local), and identifies global priorities and targets for the first two decades of the twenty-first century' (WHO, 1998e: 2). International and national policies and actions are seen as the means of securing the right to health (WHO, 1998e: 20):

through adoption of international and national human rights instruments Member States assume specific responsibilities and duties to promote and protect the health of their populations by:

- ensuring that sustainable health systems are accessible to all people
- promoting intersectoral action to address the determinants and prerequisites of health.

It could be argued that all of the regional targets identified by 'Health for All 2000' ('HFA 2000'), (WHO, 1985) and latterly *Health for All in the 21st Century* ('Health21') (WHO, Regional Committee for Europe, 1998) demand a policy response. For example, achieving Target 10 below will be dependent on environmental policy.

European Health21 Target 10 — A Healthy And Safe Physical Environment: By the year 2015, people in the Region should live in a safer physical environment, with exposure to contaminants hazardous to health at levels not exceeding internationally agreed standards.

Similarly, let us briefly consider:

European Health21 Target 12 — Reducing Harm From Alcohol, Drugs And Tobacco: By the year 2015, the adverse health effects from the consumption of addictive substances such as tobacco, alcohol and psychoactive drugs should have been significantly reduced in all Member States.

Achieving this target, to an extent, involves behavioural choices. However, it will also be influenced by tobacco, alcohol and drug policies. At a more general level, poverty and social inequality are known to be associated with substance misuse and so addressing this requires consideration of broader areas of policy, such as employment, economic and social policy.

More specifically, European Health21 Target 21 states:

By the year 2010, all Member States should have and be implementing policies for health at country, regional and local levels, supported by appropriate institutional infrastructures, managerial processes and innovative leadership.

One of the keys to successful implementation of 'Health21' has been identified as strengthening the capacity for policy making. Governments are expected to take a lead in developing policy based on sound research and evidence and have an obligation 'to ensure that health is explicitly considered in the development of public policy'

(WHO, 1998e: 42). Policy analysis is also required to ensure that the policies and activities across different sectors are aligned in relation to achieving health goals. International and foreign policy should also consider health impact.

The key issues to emerge are:

- the centrality of healthy public policy to health promotion at all levels, from international to local
- the link between healthy public policy and supportive environments
- the multisectoral scope
- the need for public participation
- governmental responsibility and accountability for considering health in the development of public policy – national and international.

HEALTHY PUBLIC POLICY – MEANINGS AND SCOPE

Health, as we noted in Chapter 1, is both a relative and contested concept. The notion of policy is equally nebulous, as encapsulated in the metaphor, 'Policy is rather like the elephant – you recognize it when you see it, but cannot easily define it' (Cunningham, 1963: 229).

The term 'policy' is subject to variation in meaning and usage in different contexts. Hogwood and Gunn (1984), for example, suggest that policy can be characterized as:

- a label for a field of activity
- a statement of aspiration or purpose
- specific proposals
- (government) decisions
- formal authorization
- a programme
- output(s)
- outcome(s)
- a theory or model
- a process.

Another grassroots view of policy that emerged from a qualitative study (Green, 1995: 108) of the development of sex education policy by schools is that it is a written document, which may or may not guide practice: 'We don't actually look at [the policy] in school … Basically we've got a piece of paper if anybody asks and I think that is the bottom line.'

This illustrates the point that, while policy is often associated with government activity, it also exists outside of government circles and is developed at the local as well as regional and national levels.

Colebatch (1998) identifies three key elements of policy:

- **authority**: the implication that there is official endorsement
- **expertise**: applied to a problem area and identifying what should be done about it
- **order**: decisions are not arbitrary but consistent and structured.

Jenkins (1978: 15) provides a useful definition that focuses on the instrumentality of policy and emphasizes that it should not merely be aspirational, but also within the control of those responsible for making policy:

> A set of interrelated decisions taken by a political actor or group of actors concerning the selection of goals and the means of achieving them within a specified situation where these decisions should, in principle, be within the power of these actors to achieve.

While the implication of this definition is that policy is concerned with action, it can equally involve inaction – deciding what *not* to do. Ignatieff (1992, in Walt, 1994: 40) draws attention to the longer-term view of policy in his acerbic commentary on short-term economic policy:

> A policy ought to be something more than a galvanic twitch. It ought to have legs for distances longer than those implied in a 'dash for growth'. It ought to have some end in view larger than seeing an addled government through the next month ... policy is not about surviving till Friday. Nor is policy to be confused with strategy, which is about getting through to Christmas. Policy is the selection of non-contradictory means to achieve non-contradictory ends over the medium to long term.

What, then, is healthy public policy? There is a clear distinction between 'public health policy', which focuses narrowly on healthcare and, frequently, illness management, and 'healthy public policy', which has a much broader remit (Hancock, 1982). Healthy public policy is concerned with the role of government and the public sector in creating the conditions that support health. Milio (1988: 264), who has played an influential role in shifting the emphasis from health policy to healthy public policy and raising its profile within WHO, offers the following definition of public policy:

> Simply put, public policy – the guide to government action – sets the range of possibilities for choices made by public and private organizations, commercial and voluntary enterprises, and individuals. In virtually every facet of living, the creation and use of goods, services, information and environments are affected by government policies – fiscal, regulatory, service provision, research and education, and procedural.

Further, she contends that healthy public policy should be:

- ecological in perspective
- multisectoral in scope
- collaborative in strategy.

Draper (1988: 217) has defined the goal of healthy public policy as being:

> to make government activity across the board contribute as much as possible to health development, while recognizing the tradeoffs that are an inevitable and necessary part of the policy process.

The key characteristics of healthy public policy are listed in the box.

Characteristics of healthy public policy

- Commitment to social equity
- Recognition of the important influence of economic, social and physical environments on health
- Facilitation of public participation
- Cooperation between health and other sectors of government

After Draper, 1988

Given the plethora of factors that influence health status (discussed in Chapter 2), the scope of healthy public policy is necessarily wide-ranging. Some indication of that breadth is provided by Terris (in Tesh et al., 1988) in an editorial submitted to the Yale Symposium on Healthy Public Policy.

> The logic of our discipline makes it necessary to support a healthful standard of living through full employment and adequate family income; improved working conditions; decent housing ... ; effective protection from environmental discomforts ... ; good nutrition that will foster optimal physical and mental development; increased financial support to public education and elimination of financial barriers to higher education; improved opportunities for rest, recreation, and cultural development; greater participation in community activities and decision making; an end to discrimination against minority groups based on race, gender, age, social class, religious belief, national background or sexual preference; and freedom from the pervasive fear of violence, war and nuclear annihilation.

Policy can support health in a number of different ways (Milio, 1986, in Abel-Smith, 1994):

- fiscal/monetary – incomes and incentives
- regulation – economic and environmental
- provision of goods and services
- supporting participation
- research, development, information, education.

In the UK, the Independent Inquiry into Inequalities in Health chaired by Sir Donald Acheson (1998) made 39 detailed recommendations about future policy development to tackle inequalities in health linked to socioeconomic status, gender and ethnicity, and variations throughout the life cycle. These are summarized in the box.

Policy and health inequality: recommendations of the independent inquiry into inequalities in health (*The Acheson Report*)

General recommendations

1   We recommend that, as part of health impact assessment, all policies likely to have a direct or indirect effect on health should be evaluated in terms of their impact on health inequalities, and should be formulated in such a way that by favouring the less well off they will, wherever possible, reduce such inequalities.

2   We recommend a high priority is given to policies aimed at improving health and reducing health inequalities in women of childbearing age, expectant mothers and young children.

Specific recommendations are also made about:

- poverty, income, tax and benefits
- education
- employment
- housing and environment
- mobility, transport and pollution
- nutrition and the Common Agricultural Policy
- mothers, children and families
- young people and adults of working age
- older people
- ethnicity
- gender
- equity within the National Health Service.

Acheson, 1998

The specific areas identified include both upstream and downstream policies. The former would include, for example, the development of preschool education to meet the needs of disadvantaged families or reducing the fear of crime and violence and creating a safe environment. In contrast, the latter would focus on policies intended to prevent disease, such as fluoridation of drinking water or ensuring equitable access to healthcare. Furthermore, because of the synergistic effect between many of the recommendations, the report advises policy development across a broad front rather than 'cherry picking' those areas that are most amenable to change.

Tesh et al. (1988) welcome the growing acceptance within the policy field that health has little to do with medical care, together with the move away from monocausal models and reductionist analyses and towards recognition of the complex interplay of factors that impact on health. However, they have a number of concerns about the adoption of multifactorial models of causality. First, they offer little insight into exactly how to prevent disease. Because everything is interlinked, any one action may appear insignificant, yet it is unlikely that sufficient resources will be available to tackle everything. The enormity of the task can become a reason (excuse) for not taking action and thus lead to inertia.

Second, because all elements of a multicausal web appear equally weighted, policy makers are provided with an opportunity to appear to be responding to a problem while at the same time opting for interventions that are less socially disruptive or costly and may well be less effective than some other course of action – for example, providing smoking cessation clinics rather than tackling poverty or encouraging people to improve their diet rather than addressing the issue of whether or not those on low incomes or receiving state benefits can afford a healthy diet.

This also provides the opportunity to effectively opt out of responsibility for a health issue by attributing major responsibility elsewhere. For example, there would be no need to address the activities of the food industry if the major influences on a healthy diet were perceived to be acceptable minimum levels of income and awareness of what constitutes a healthy diet.

The third point is that an emphasis on cause overlooks those who are more likely to experience ill health – notably those of lower socio-economic status. Recognition of the 'primacy of poverty' (Tesh et al., 1988: 258) presupposes that all elements of the web are not equal, but that some have more fundamental significance. Therefore, constructing a hierarchy of causes may be necessary to target those that are likely to have the greatest impact on health.

Clearly, when considering policy options, there will be a need to make tradeoffs in choosing one course of action rather than another and between those groups that benefit and those that bear the costs – a distinction that is frequently not clear-cut (Draper, 1988; Tesh et al., 1988). Tuohy (in Tesh et al., 1988) contends that the criteria and processes used to make these tradeoffs should be made explicit and proposes the common themes emerging at the Yale Symposium on Healthy Public Policy as a starting point:

- the importance of ensuring healthy minimum standards of living – internationally as well as intra-nationally
- the establishment of participatory decision-making structures – but these need the support of a balanced structure of interests and power.

Christoffel (in Tesh et al., 1988: 259) asserts that 'Knowing how to solve a public health problem is not enough when powerful interests are threatened by the solution, which seems to be the case most of the time'. He sees the major problem for health as not being an overall shortage of resources, but an uneven distribution of them. The redistribution of resources would require that some (albeit a minority) lose and these are, in general, those who hold 'critical political power' (in Tesh et al., 1988: 260). Christoffel concludes that the main barrier to healthy public policy is the concentration of wealth and power among those who stand to lose.

While the role of the state has been at the forefront of thinking about healthy public policy, it is important to also recognize the importance of non-governmental policy on health, at all levels. Bunton (1992: 130) writes:

> The concept anticipates a new culture of public policy that is pluralistic and looks beyond state administrative planning structures to develop and implement policy, calling for multisectoral, multilevel, and participatory initiatives.

Delaney (1994c) makes the distinction between policy as *problematic* for health promotion and policy as the *solution*. The former focuses on identifying the negative impacts of policies on health status. The growing field of health impact assessment is concerned with analysing the potential health impact of policies (we will return to this below). The latter is concerned with the use of policy to tackle the problems and create conditions that are supportive of health.

Choice and control

Recognition of the duty of governments to create conditions that support health and enable community participation is a core principle of health promotion. Individuals are also seen as having a responsibility – individually and collectively – to contribute to health. A fundamental question is, what should be the respective roles and responsibilities of the individual and the state for controlling the determinants of health?

As we observed in Chapter 1, one of the core ethical principles of health education has been a commitment to voluntarism, or, free choice. This was aptly summarized in the North American Society of Public Health Educators Code of Ethics: 'change by choice not coercion' (Society of Health Education and Health Promotion Specialists, 1997). Milio (1981: 277) contends that: 'There is no "free choice" but only "choice" within a limited number of options … '. The key issue is what options will be made available and how health promoting or damaging those options are. For example, Swinburn (2008) argues that commercial interests are driving the obesity epidemic and that policies, laws and regulations – so-called hard paternalism – may be needed to bring about 'the environmental and social changes that eventually, will have a sustainable impact on reducing obesity' (see box).

Roles of government in obesity prevention

Leadership

Providing a visible lead
Reinforcing the seriousness of the problem
Demonstrating a readiness to take serious action
Examples:
Being visible in the media
Role modelling healthy behaviours (at an individual level)
Role modelling healthy environments (at a government agency level)
Creating mechanisms for a whole-of-government response to obesity
Lifting the priority for health (versus commercial) outcomes

Advocacy

Advocating for a multi-sector response across all societal sectors (governments, the private sector, civil society, and the public)

(Continued)

(Continued)

Examples:
Advocating to the private sector for corporate responsibility around marketing to children
Creating a high-level taskforce to oversee and monitor multi-sector actions
Encouraging healthy lifestyles for individuals and families

Funding

Securing increased and continuing funding to create healthy environments and encourage healthy eating and physical activity
Examples:
Establishing a health promotion foundation (e.g. using an hypothecated tobacco tax) to fund programs and research
Moving from project funding to program and service funding for obesity prevention
Creating centres of excellence for research, evaluation and monitoring

Policy

Developing, implementing and monitoring a set of policies, regulations, taxes and subsidies that make environments less obesogenic and more health promoting
Examples:
Banning the marketing of unhealthy foods to children
Subsidising public transport and active transport more than car transport
Requiring 'traffic light' front-of-pack labelling of food nutrient profiles
Restricting the sale of unhealthy foods in schools

Derived from Swinburn, 2008

The concern of healthy public policy should be to ensure that the environment does not damage health and that there is an equitable distribution of 'health-important resources'. Furthermore, it should make 'health-damaging choices the more costly ones, and health-improving choices less costly, to both organizations and individuals' (Milio, 1981: 303).

Healthy public policy is generally seen, therefore, as a vehicle for tackling structural and environmental threats to health – as both protective and opening up healthy choices by removing constraints to action. However, we should also note that, over and above making the healthy choice the easy choice, policies can make it the *only* choice (Tones and Tilford, 1994). Beattie (1991) sees legislation and policy as an authoritarian approach directed at the collective (see Figure 6.1).

Curtailing individual choice can clearly be defended when exercising that choice may put others at risk. For example, it would be difficult to uphold the rights of individuals to choose to drive through residential areas at excessive speed or while intoxicated or subject others to inhaling tobacco smoke.

However, control takes on a more coercive complexion when applied to behaviour that only places the individual concerned at risk. Such an approach equates with a

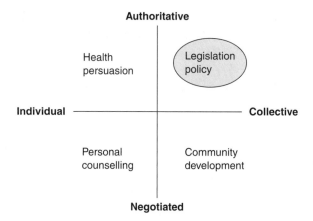

Figure 6.1   Health promotion – alternative approaches (after Beattie, 1991)

narrow, preventive model of health education and leaves health promoters open to accusations of health fascism. The anti-health lobby has been quick to pick up on this element of coercion and frequently uses arguments about liberty and civil rights in its activities. For example, FOREST (The Freedom Organisation for the Right to Enjoy Smoking Tobacco, 2008) describes its purpose as 'to protect the interests of adults who choose to smoke or consume tobacco in its many forms'. The pro-gun lobby in the United States and the opponents of pool fencing in Australia take a similar stance.

To what extent should government intervene in people's lives? Jochelson (2005) characterizes alternative perspectives in the debate about this as, on the one side, interventionists who see government's role as enhancing individual freedom by creating opportunities and reducing inequities in society and, on the other, libertarians who see government intervention as undermining individual freedom and therefore advocate minimal interference. She points out that 'Almost every government intervention in the public health arena has been criticized … as a sign of tyranny, nanny statism, or the end of individual freedom' (2005: 29) despite the capacity to bring about changes which individuals are unable to do on their own. She proposes the use of the term stewardship rather than nanny state to describe 'public health measures that set new social standards and bring about changes that individuals on their own cannot make'. Further, 'stewardship also implies that a government protects its citizens against harm from others' (2005: 31).

In relation to the views of the public, the survey by the Kings Fund, referred to in Chapter 1 (see box on page 22), revealed strong support 'across the social spectrum for government action to prevent illness and improve health' (2004: 4). Three types of measures government can take were identified:

- Encouraging measures that inform and advise, warn about health risks and encourage employers to promote health.
- Enabling measures that help to create favourable social, economic and environmental conditions.
- Restrictive measures prevent actions that put others' health at risk or actively discourage people from putting their own health at risk. (2004: 4)

Public support was greatest for encouraging and enabling measures and for those interventions which require others to make changes to their lives rather than individuals to their own.

Health education and health promotion – lifestyle and structure

Healthy public policy is generally associated with attempts to influence the structural determinants of health. Health education, in contrast, is seen as a means of influencing lifestyle. However, this representation is overly simplistic and ignores the complexity of the interplay between these various elements.

As we have noted earlier, structural factors can have a major influence on lifestyle and behaviour – and vice versa. Similarly, a major goal of policy may be to widen access to education, as evidenced by, for example, efforts to secure universal primary education. Education policy will influence the content of education generally and, more specifically, the opportunities afforded for health education.

Within England and Wales, educational policy on sex education has been instrumental in shaping schools' response (Green, 1997 and 1998). Furthermore, the introduction of health-promoting schools initiatives has policy implications from the national level down to individual schools (see Chapter 10). Conversely (as we will discuss in more detail in Chapters 7, 8 and 9), health education is the means of raising awareness of issues that need to be addressed and getting them onto the political agenda.

Critical consciousness raising, as we note in Chapter 7, is at the heart of Freirian approaches to education. Furthermore, health education can develop the skills required for political activism, including lobbying and advocacy skills.

Thus, it can be seen that representing health education and healthy public policy as competing options for promoting health is to create a false dichotomy. As Figure 6.2 illustrates, health education is a major driver in the process of policy development.

DEVELOPING POLICY – FROM RHETORIC TO REALITY

The potential for organizations and communities to influence public policy will inevitably be dependent on the structure of the state. Walt (1994) notes that, in contrast to more authoritarian regimes, liberal democracies will, at least in theory, encourage participation and that participation can be both direct and indirect.

Direct participation involves explicit attempts to shape the development of policy by means of involvement in the policy-making process or lobbying and advocacy. Alternatively, indirect participation consists of exercising influence via electoral processes. Walt also notes that opportunities for participation may be limited in relation to 'high politics' where consideration of major issues may be dominated by small 'élites'. High politics has been defined as 'the maintenance of core values – including national self-preservation – and the long-term objectives of the state' (Evans and Newnham, 1992, in Walt, 1994: 42).

In contrast, there may be greater opportunity for participation in more run-of-the-mill issues of policy – that is, 'low politics'. Generally, individuals have little direct influence on the role of policy making and their voice is more likely to be heard as part of a collective

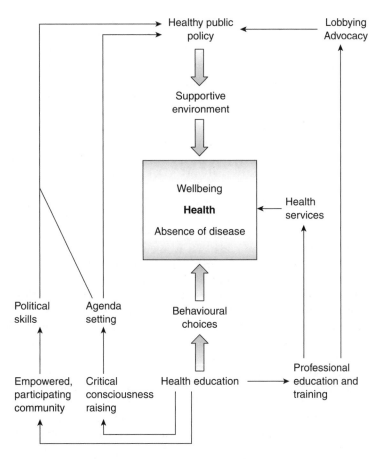

Figure 6.2   Health education and health promotion (after Tones and Tilford, 1994)

or via organizations. However, public opinion can be an important contextual factor (Milio, 1988) and, in particular, in terms of the political risk of alienating public opinion.

Walt (1994) identifies a number of other contextual factors that influence policy development and, following Leichter (1979), categorizes these as being:

- **situational factors**: temporary conditions or situations
- **structural factors**: relatively stable elements of society polity
- **cultural factors**: the values within communities and society
- **environmental factors**: factors external to the political system or international factors, such as international trade agreements, international aid and the activities of transnational corporations.

Understanding the machinery of government and the relative roles of local, national and supranational organizations is clearly a necessary precondition for those seeking to influence policy. However, Delaney (1994c) contends that this is insufficient in itself. Healthy public policy is essentially a political undertaking (Draper, 1988; Tesh et al., 1988; Signal, 1998) and analysis of the location of political power and influence is of critical importance to the process of policy development. Yet Signal (1998) comments that the politics of health promotion receive comparatively little attention.

There are several different perspectives on the politics of policy making. Walt (1994) distinguishes between pluralist and elitist views. 'Pluralist interest group theory' presupposes that power is distributed among a number of different interest groups within the policy arena and that no single group dominates. The alternative position is that 'the political arena is dominated by "ruling élites"' and that the state acts 'in the interests of capital accumulation or that major interests are incorporated into a "corporate" non-competitive network' (Delaney, 1994c: 7). The former is consistent with neo-Marxist interpretations and the latter with the new institutionalism.

Hogwood and Gunn (1984: 71) note that the concentration of power in elite groups is seen as deriving from 'office-holding, political power, or the way the state is structured to favour the interests of the dominant class'. Norsigian (Tesh et al., 1988), writing from a feminist perspective, contends that women have a major role in supporting health by their childrearing, caregiving, homemaking and food production and preparation roles, yet have a very limited role in policy making.

Signal (1998) applies these three perspectives to the politics of health promotion. 'Pluralist interest group theory' is seen as offering a micro-level analysis of the interest groups within the policy arena and their influences on public policy. Identifying the key players and the location of support and opposition is necessary for building alliances to achieve desired policy changes and tackling any opposition.

Signal uses 'the new institutionalism' as a meso-level theory to explore the effects of institutional characteristics in shaping the process of policy making – focusing on the effects of organizational structure, together with the ways in which organizations operate, the rules that guide their operation and the ideas integral to their functioning. Clearly, there will be a stronger impetus to address issues of healthy public policy among those organizations that have a 'health promotion mandate' or those that perceive health issues as falling within their legitimate sphere of activity. Furthermore, wider recognition of health being part of an organization's accepted remit will lend authority to its voice within the policy arena. Key issues to consider in assessing the potential of different interest groups are summarized in the box.

Assessing the potential of different interest groups

- How well organized is the group?
- What resources are available – financial, time, skills, experience?
- What strategies are used to influence the political process?

After Signal, 1998

We noted in Chapter 4 that institutions vary considerably in their degree of openness and the extent to which they interlink with other institutions and involve communities.

This will inevitably impact on alliance building and responsiveness to the community's needs.

Finally, Signal draws on neo-Marxist theory to analyse macro-level political and economic factors that set the broad context for policy. She refers to two traditions within neo-Marxist analysis – the functional perspective and the political class perspective. The former is concerned with the organization of the state in relation to capital accumulation and emphasizes the importance of locating health promotion policy development within the broader economic and social policy context.

The political class perspective focuses on power and the capacity to take collective action among the three main political class groupings – organized capital, organized labour and political parties. In particular, it draws attention to the need to harness the forces of business, labour (and the trades unions) and political parties in the interests of healthy public policy.

We might summarize the key points as follows:

- know your potential allies and adversaries
- know the structures with which you are working
- know the context within which you are working.

Rational and incremental approaches

There are two broad schools of thought about the process of policy making – the 'rational' and the 'incremental'. The former conforms with the principles of rational decision making discussed in Chapter 7 and assumes:

- clear explication of goals
- identification of all the alternatives for addressing the issue
- rational and objective appraisal of each alternative
- selection of the most appropriate alternative.

The view that policy is the product of such rational processes is considered to be overly idealized. A more realistic interpretation is offered by incrementalism, which describes policy as evolving gradually 'on the basis of previous decisions and pragmatic considerations' (Delaney, 1994b: 219).

Lindblom (1987) – one of the main proponents of incrementalism – suggests that the complexity of many problems is such that analysis is beyond the capacity of our small minds. As Lindblom and Woodhouse (1993: 66) state:

It is impossible to unambiguously calculate even how a single complex policy will interact with another, much less how it will interact with all others. Nor does anyone really ever attempt such a task.

The choice is therefore between inaction in the face of the enormity of the task of ensuring that the right course of action is being taken or at least making some headway. The notion of 'bounded rationality' accepts that rational decision making will inevitably be constrained by factors such as cost and practicability. A further factor limiting the practical feasibility of purely rational approaches is that policy makers are not value-free (Walt, 1994). Indeed, we have identified the core values of health promotion in Chapter 1 and, clearly, health promotion policy should be consistent with these core values.

Incrementalism is characterized by:

- lack of a clear distinction between goals and the means of achieving them
- consideration of a restricted number of alternatives
- identification of the major consequences rather than all consequences
- no ideal policy option – the best option is the one that policy makers agree is the most appropriate
- achieving small changes to existing policy rather than major change (after Walt, 1994).

Incrementalism is also typical of pluralist, democratic approaches. Decisions about policy are arrived at by means of bargaining and compromise between different interest groups – referred to as 'partisan interaction' and 'mutual adjustment' (Lindblom, 1979; Lindblom and Woodhouse, 1993). Each attempts to pursue its own interests, but, to accommodate the interests of other groups, may be prepared to fall back to a compromise position (Janis and Mann, 1977: 34):

> Whenever power is distributed among a variety of influential executive leaders, political parties, legislative factions, and other interest groups, one centre of power can rarely impose its preferences on another and policies are likely to be the outcome of give and take among numerous partisans. The constraints of bureaucratic politics, with their shifting compromises and coalitions, constitute a major reason for the disjointed and incremental nature of the policies that gradually evolve.

Small changes are held to be more feasible than radical ones. Incrementalism, therefore, tends to maintain the status quo (Delaney, 1994c) or support gradual change and so has been challenged on account of its inherent conservatism. The incrementalist view is that small changes can be made quickly and a series of small changes can, when judged as a whole, achieve major change. It is, therefore, associated with serial policy making – that is, revisiting and readjusting policy (Walt, 1994). It is also consistent with the environmental maxim attributed to Dubos: 'think globally, act locally'.

The notion of mixed scanning (Etzioni, 1967) adopts a middle-ground position and attempts to capitalize on the strengths of both rational and incremental approaches. It involves developing a broad overview of the policy field as a basis for distinguishing between those areas that can be approached incrementally and those requiring a more thorough analysis of options before making major strategic decisions.

Conflict and consensus models

'Conflict models' see groups as having their own interests and competing to ensure that they achieve their own goals. The issue of tobacco control offers a clear illustration in which the interests of the transnational tobacco conglomerates cannot be reconciled with those of public health or, indeed, the consumer when, as Action on Smoking and Health (ASH, undated) reminds us, 'Tobacco is unique: the only product that kills when used normally'. British American Tobacco (BAT), as part of its strategy to be seen as a responsible company, initiated a process of social reporting in 2001–2 (see BAT, 2008) based on the company's audit of its social and ethical performance. The stakeholder dialogue that was set up to contribute to this was met with the following response from ASH (2002a):

[There is] no public health benefit to justify the time and cost. We see little benefit coming from it in public health terms, and that is our objective. There are virtually no areas where BAT and ASH can find common cause - we characterize BAT's relationship with public health as a zero sum game. Our efforts and limited resources are best spent in pressing for meaningful public policy measures at national, European and international level that control the activities of tobacco companies and reduce smoking. An invitation to a stakeholder dialogue, is an invitation to spend our funds on BAT's initiative, when we believe we can spend our money and time better in other ways. Where we do believe there is potential common ground we retain the option to meet with tobacco companies on a case-by-case basis.

While ASH was prepared to provide information, it defended its reluctance to engage in a fuller dialogue on the grounds of the unethical activity of the tobacco industry, summarized in its own report on the social impacts of the activities of the tobacco industry (ASH, 2002a).

Bunton (1992) sees the state as having an important role when major corporations bring power to bear to thwart public health interests. Equally, the state must balance economic and other interests with public health concerns. For example, the Chief Medical Officer's Report (2003) addressed concerns about possible negative economic effects to support the introduction of a ban on smoking in public places in England as well as emphasizing the health benefits. It noted:

- A policy of creating smoke-free workplaces and public places would yield an overall net benefit to society of £2.3 billion to £2.7 billion annually, equivalent to treating 1.3-1.5 million hospital waiting list patients.
- Smoke-free laws help rather than hinder the hospitality industry. For example, New York has seen an increase in both taxable sales from eating, drinking and hotel establishments and restaurant employment (up 18% compared to 5% in the area round about) since going smoke-free; and New York City, Los Angeles and San Francisco have seen tourism revenues and employment continue to grow.
- The vast majority of good quality, published research confirms this positive result for business. Studies that claim to show that going smoke-free is bad for business tend to be poor in quality and sometimes funded by the tobacco industry. (Chief Medical Office, 2003)

International agreements may also be necessary to meet the challenge to health posed by multinational companies or, indeed, when the activity of one country has negative effects on the health of others. Pursuing tobacco control as an example, the Framework Convention on Tobacco Control – the first treaty negotiated by WHO – came into force in 2005 to address the global problem of tobacco consumption. It includes measures to reduce both the demand for and supply of tobacco products (see box).

WHO Framework Convention on Tobacco Control

Core demand reduction provisions – articles 6–14:

- Price and tax measures to reduce the demand for tobacco, and
- Non-price measures to reduce the demand for tobacco, namely:
    - Protection from exposure to tobacco smoke;
    - Regulation of the contents of tobacco products;
    - Regulation of tobacco product disclosures;
    - Packaging and labelling of tobacco products;
    - Education, communication, training and public awareness;
    - Tobacco advertising, promotion and sponsorship; and,
    - Demand reduction measures concerning tobacco dependence and cessation.

Core supply reduction provisions – articles 15–17:

- Illicit trade in tobacco products;
- Sales to and by minors; and,
- Provision of support for economically viable alternative activities.

WHO, 2008b

As well as conflict arising from different sectional interests vis-à-vis an issue or problem, Bunton (1992) also suggests that it can arise from the reactions to change and forces for innovation competing with forces of inertia. Furthermore, conflict theorists contend that power may be exercised in framing the political agenda. Powerful insider groups may effect closure to confine debate to their own areas of concern, excluding other issues and, indeed, interest groups (Jones and Sidell, 1997).

Clearly, conflict models are marked by a power struggle that results in some groups 'winning' or an impasse. The power strategies that are used in groups and organizations to exert control are summarized in the box. Variations between different groups in their access to resources will influence the pressure that they can bring to bear. The structure of the policy environment may be such that some groups are excluded and, where there are steep social gradients, the most disadvantaged will have greatest difficulty in making their voices heard (Bunton, 1992).

Power strategies

Physical power: coercive power, either real or threatened.
Resource power: (also referred to as reward power) deriving from possession of valued resources that may or may not be material.
Position power: (also referred to as legitimate power) associated with position or status.
Expert power: attributed to individuals on account of acknowledged expertise.
Personal power: emanates from the personality and is associated with charisma.

(Continued)

(Continued)

Negative power: the inappropriate use of power outside the recognized domain of interaction. Its intention is subversive, for example not passing on information.

After Handy, 1993

Lindblom and Woodhouse (1993: 128) identify three methods for conflict resolution:

- non-rational and irrational persuasion, as via propaganda campaigns or symbolic rhetoric
- logrolling — that is, steam rollering — vetoes, bribery or other interpersonal means for inducing acquiescence without actually persuading on the merits
- informed and reasoned persuasion.

Profound differences in ideological commitments between different groups make it unlikely that reasoned persuasion will be effective and it may therefore be necessary to resort to less rational and more persuasive – or, indeed, coercive – strategies. A 'consensus model' is premised on the view that it is possible to reach agreement and is consistent with pluralism and the 'muddling through' notion of incrementalism.

Bunton (1992) contends that the development of healthy public policy can be built on cooperation and collaboration. Agreements are reached by means of negotiation and bargaining – partisan mutual adjustment. The role of health promotion is to influence the process to maximize health gain via persuasion techniques, such as 'information dissemination, incentives and sanctions' (Bunton, 1992: 146). Hogwood and Gunn (1984) note Dror's criticism that, while approaches emphasizing consensus may be acceptable during periods of relative stability, they are unlikely to achieve major innovation or offer solutions to complex problems.

Lindblom and Woodhouse (1993: 120) contend that, overall, the level of fundamental disagreement in society is surprisingly small:

> Instead, politics normally proceed on the basis of what some call the 'underlying consensus' in a society. Is this agreement brought about by reasoned persuasion, or does much of it evolve through social indoctrination processes … ? Who has the capacity and incentive to use schooling and other socializing institutions to bring about widespread agreements?

Their views draw attention to the narrowness of contemporary debates and raise the question: why has there not been a greater challenge to issues such as inequality? Furthermore, any attempts to do so have, to date, been relatively modest and have avoided tackling root causes.

The players – terminology

'Policy actors' are those individuals, groups or organizations involved in policy making. Their level of involvement may well vary at different stages of the policy development process. For example, groups that are at the forefront of lobbying activity may have a less prominent role in the formulation and implementation of policy. However, an important consideration at each stage is not only who is included, but, equally, who is left out. 'Stakeholders' are all those who stand to be affected, in whatever way, by the introduction of a policy and who may be, but are not necessarily, involved in policy making.

The 'policy keeper' is the agency that, either by mandate or its own initiative, holds a policy and moves the policy forwards during any phase of policy making (Milio, 1988). The identity of the policy keeper may change during these different phases. Milio provides the example of the non-governmental National Nutrition Council in Norway acting as policy keeper in advocating a national food and nutrition policy, but, once this became part of the government agenda, a ministerial office assumed the role of policy keeper.

There are various different groups that seek to influence policy. The term 'interest or pressure group' is generally used for groups that exist outside government. Walt (1994) identifies the common feature of interest groups to be aiming to achieve goals without becoming part of the formal mechanism of government – that is, attempting to influence from outside rather than inside government. If they do gain formal political power, then they cease to be an interest group and become part of the institutional process of government.

Lindblom and Woodhouse (1993) note the lack of precision in the term 'interest group'. They suggest that business interest, for example, cannot be seen as a 'group' in the conventional sense, but that businesses are organized bureaucracies dominated by a small number of executives. Some of the so-called interest groups may, in fact, be highly influential individuals who take on interest group activity to influence the direction of policy. Somewhat unusually, Lindblom and Woodhouse also suggest that government departments and officials may seek to shape the development of policy by lobbying on behalf of their own interests – operating in substantially the same way as private interest groups – for example, the ministry of health trying to influence fiscal policy on tobacco or transport policy. They (1993: 75) therefore define 'interest group activity' rather more broadly to include the activity of government officials that falls outside the usual channels of authority and spheres of activity:

> interactions through which individuals and private groups not holding government authority seek to influence policy, together with those policy-influencing interactions of government officials that go well beyond the direct use of their authority.

Milio (1988: 266) subscribes to this broader view and refers to the major players as interest groups:

> any organized groups or parts of groups whose resources, authority, status, influence or survival is affected by a policy. Such groups include political parties; parliamentary committees, ministerial offices and bureaucratic units; commercial enterprises; and voluntary, professional, religious, communications or minority organizations.

Interest groups fall into two broad divisions – those concerned with protecting the interests of their members, such as Trades Unions, Disability Rights groups and Gay Rights groups, and those coming together around a specific issue, such as abortion, pollution or opposition groups to local planning developments. It follows that membership of the former will be restricted to particular groups, whereas in the latter it will be open to anyone with an interest in the issue.

The terminology for these groups varies – Walt (1994) suggests 'sectional' and 'cause' groups. She also notes a further distinction between 'insider' and 'outsider' groups. Insider groups are respected by policy makers, there are often close working relationships, and, because of their recognized legitimacy, these groups tend to be consulted on policy issues and invited to participate in policy making. Outsider groups, in contrast, have greater difficulty in gaining access to the policy process and may resort to direct action to make their voices heard. Walt cites the activities of Greenpeace, drawing attention to the pollution generated by industry, or anti-abortion groups demonstrating outside clinics. Less extreme activity would involve advocacy and lobbying on behalf of a cause.

An alternative strategy would be to move from outsider to insider status. Walt notes that groups such as the Family Planning Association in the UK and HIV activist groups in a number of countries have achieved insider status by providing services and building up acknowledged expertise in particular areas. Walt also draws attention to the important role of non-governmental organizations (NGOs) in developing countries and Constantino-David's witty categorization (see the box). While not formally recognized as interest groups, NGOs may consciously seek to influence policy or ensure the public accountability of the state.

Non-governmental organizations

BINGOS	big NGOs
GRINGOS	government run or inspired NGOs
BONGOS	business-orientated NGOS
COME'NGOs	NGOs set up opportunistically and which do not last long

Constantino-David, 1992, in Walt, 1994: 116

Generally, members of the public do not, as individuals, engage directly with policy-making processes. Their influence is more usually via action groups or contributing to creating a collective opinion, such that adoption of a particular policy becomes the most prudent course of action for politicians seeking to maintain their popularity with the electorate. There are notable exceptions and committed individuals have managed to secure policy change. A well-known example is the case of Victoria Gillick, who challenged a Department of Health circular stating that young people under the legal age of consent could receive confidential contraceptive advice and treatment. She succeeded in 1984 in winning an appeal court ruling that girls under 16 should not be given contraceptives without their parents' consent, although this was subsequently overturned by a House of Lords decision in *Gillick* v *West Norfolk and Wisbech Area Health Authority and another* [1986] 1 AC 112. More recently, Laura Ahearn is known for her work in attempting to change policy on the prevention of child sexual abuse and the introduction of 'Megan's Law' in the United States.

A 'policy network' is the 'collection of actors and organizations which influences decision making in a policy sector' (John, 1998: 205). A network is made up of a number of 'policy communities'. John (1998: 83) suggests that this term implies that 'the participants know each other well and ... share the same values and policy goals' and defines it (1998: 204) as 'a restricted set of actors and organizations which influence decisions on a policy sector'. Walt (1994) contends that policy communities are characterized by an ongoing interchange of information and ideas.

Smith (1997) distinguishes between 'policy communities' and 'issues networks'. The former have limited membership (possibly with the conscious exclusion of some groups), regular and frequent contact, common values and a relationship based on exchanges of resources. Issues networks tend to be larger and more variable in their composition and the interests of members and arrangements for contact may be more ad hoc. Access to, and sharing of, resources will also vary, along with the power that different members command. Several government departments may be included within an issues network. For example, some 14 government departments were identified by the White Paper on Tobacco (Department of Health, 1998b) as contributing to tackling smoking, plus all those reviewing their internal smoking policies.

Coalitions

In that networks include different public, private and commercial organizations, it is likely that a range of different viewpoints will be represented. 'Coalitions' may, therefore, develop between groupings sharing similar values. They can become a major force within the policy arena. Coalitions have been defined (Feighery and Rogers, 1989, in Butterfoss et al., 1993: 316) as:

> an organization of individuals representing diverse organizations, factions or constituencies who agree to work together to achieve a common goal.

and (Brown, 1984, in Butterfoss et al., 1993: 316):

> an organization of diverse interest groups that combine human and material resources to effect a specific change the members are unable to bring about independently.

The key elements can be summarized as:

- unity in working towards a common goal
- pooling of resources
- increased capacity to achieve the goal.

Butterfoss et al.'s (1993) review of the literature on coalitions identifies three types of coalition, based on Feighery and Rogers (1989):

- **grassroots coalitions**: generally set up by volunteers to respond to a crisis, such as closure of a local hospital
- **professional coalitions**: formed by professional organizations
- **community-based coalitions**: usually initiated by an agency, but involving professionals and grass-roots leaders.

The review also identifies a number of factors associated with the importance of coalitions and these are summarized in the box.

The importance of coalitions

- Coalitions spread responsibility across a number of organizations and enable them to become involved in a broader range of issues.
- Coalitions both demonstrate and mobilize public support for an issue.
- Coalitions can maximize the power brought to bear on an issue and achieve a 'critical mass'.
- Coalitions can minimize duplication of effort.
- Coalitions provide access to a wider range of talent and resources – human and material – and can 'enhance the leverage' of groups.
- Coalitions are a vehicle for recruiting additional groups – across a range of constituencies – to a cause.
- The flexibility of coalitions enables them to draw on new resources as situations change.

After Butterfoss et al., 1993

Herman et al. (1993) draw attention to the issue of recruitment. Their study of the development of a coalition among a number of organizations to address inadequate state-subsidized family planning found that recruitment relied heavily on existing interpersonal and inter-organizational networks. While, on the one hand, this supported the rapid mobilization of an effective coalition, it also resulted in gaps in representation and the exclusion of some groups. Rogers et al. (1993) also note the lack of representation from key community constituencies in local tobacco control coalitions.

We have already considered the issue of inter-sectoral working and healthy alliances in Chapter 4. However, we should note here some of the factors associated with the success of coalitions. Granner and Sharpe's (2004) review of the literature identified a number of factors associated with the effectiveness of coalitions (see box).

Factors associated with coalition functioning

Member characteristics and perceptions

Member benefits
Member participation
Member satisfaction and commitment
Members skills and training
Representativeness of members
Member recruitment
Member expectations
Ownership

(Continued)

(Continued)

Organizational or group processes

Conflict resolution
Decision making
Clear mission
Quality of action plan
Formalized roles and procedures
Technical assistance
Resources available

Organizational or group characteristics and climate

Community context and readiness
Group relationships/collaboration
Communication
Strong leadership

Impacts and outcomes

Linkages to other groups/community
Policy advocacy/change
Empowerment/social capital
Community capacity
Institutionalization

Butterfoss et al.'s (1993) analysis indicates that one of the key elements in coalition formation is the development of a clear goal to which all members can subscribe. Individual interests then become subsumed within a collective purpose. Indeed, development of a spirit of cooperation is fundamental to cohesive, effective coalitions. While a whole range of factors related to structure, leadership and interpersonal factors will affect the maintenance of the coalition, member satisfaction is important – members need to perceive the coalition as beneficial. Achieving some short-term success will increase motivation and the credibility of the coalition. However, this should not detract from a focus on the overall goal. Clearly, evaluation of outcomes is essential in demonstrating progress and sustaining momentum. Feighery and Rogers (1989) found that the following influenced members' satisfaction with the coalition:

- it is managed effectively
- it has good communication among membership
- it has low costs of, and barriers to, participation.

Gottlieb et al. (1993) recommend:

- formalization of agreements, mission statements, and goals and objectives
- attention to the process of group formation
- clarification of expectations.

POLICY MAKING

The main stages in policy making are problem identification, policy formulation, implementation and evaluation. While this may be taken to imply a chronological sequence, in reality, the process may be more iterative and complex. Milio (1988: 266) suggests that it is a 'continuous, but not necessarily linear, social and political process'. Springett (1998) also notes that, in practice, there is often no clear distinction between policy development and implementation and the two strands frequently develop in parallel.

Delaney (1994c: 7) cites the questions posed by Anderson (1975) as a means of identifying key issues at each stage and proposes adding 'Why?' and 'Why not?' to expose more fundamental concerns – particularly the location and operation of political power:

1 Problem formation. What is a policy problem? How does it get on the agenda of government?
2 Formulation. How are the alternatives for dealing with the problem developed? Who participates?
3 Adoption. How is a policy alternative adopted or enacted? Who adopts?
4 Implementation. What is done, if anything, to carry a policy into effect? What impact does this have on policy content?
5 Evaluation. How is effectiveness measured? Who evaluates? What are the consequences?

Milio (1988) also offers a series of generic issues to consider in relation to policy making and these are set out in the box.

Policy making – issues to consider

- Agenda setting – whether or not a given public issue is an appropriate problem for public policy
- Problem framing – determining the definition and scope of the problem
- Priority setting
- Option setting – finding possible optional solutions, including goals and strategies
- Criteria selection – by what criteria options should be chosen
- Policy selection – who bears the responsibility to decide
- Means choice – how, and by whom, the policy should be implemented
- Success indicators – determining the criteria and sources of evaluation
- Changing goals or means – how the policy should be reformulated.

After Milio, 1988: 266

Milio (1988: 265) contends that those seeking to influence policy making need to identify 'points of entry into policy-making processes, sources of support, and strategies to enhance the feasibility of specific health promotion policy options in any given policy sector'. In the same way that healthy public policy should make the healthy choice the easy choice, efforts to influence policy should make the healthy policy option the most attractive option. Clearly, both insiders and outsiders will need political skills and acumen to effectively exert influence within the policy arena.

Ideally, policy should be based on sound evidence and there is clearly a need to produce relevant information to inform the policy-making process. De Leeuw (1993) notes that epidemiological research findings are often not translated into effective policies. Discussion tends to centre on:

- what information is needed by policy makers
- how information can be used to influence the development of policy.

However, she contends that it is naïve to suppose that information will automatically be assimilated into policy making and achieve change by means of rational processes. The reality is that policy making is heavily influenced by assumptions, vested interests and power positions. Bearing in mind our various earlier discussions, it will be apparent that the relative power of the key groups of players is of paramount importance. At a government level, conflict between ministers is a well-known phenomenon. Powles' (1988) analysis of the development of a food and nutrition policy in Victoria, Australia, provides an example of attempts to reconcile the conflicting interests of different groups and, in particular, to address the concerns of the Victorian Employers Federation, which represented the interests of food-processing companies. Crucial elements in achieving a resolution (albeit at the expense of protracting the process and considerably lengthening the document) were the tenacity of individuals and clarity about where it might be possible to make concessions to alternative positions and where not – for example, refusal to negotiate on the concept of dietary guidelines.

Key assumptions in the policy-making process concern 'cause and effect' and 'intervention effect' – that is, if we do X then Y will follow. While data can be collected to establish the nature of a problem and predictions can be made about the effects of policy change (see the box for an example), the challenge is to convert research findings into a form that conveys a powerful message that appeals to dominant values. It is also important to understand the power structures within the policy arena and how to manipulate them. As Milio (1988: 265) suggests, the development of 'policy relevant' information requires consideration of the following issues:

- how to extrapolate the policy implications of data
- how to propose feasible policy options
- how to judge the social and political responses to issues and proposals
- who to contact, when and how.

The anticipated effect of smoking legislation

Prior to the introduction of a ban on smoking in enclosed public places in Scotland, a study by the Health Economic Research Unit on likely impact (Ludbrook et al., 2005) provided evidence that:

(Continued)

(Continued)

- A complete ban would bring about greater reduction in exposure to environmental tobacco smoke than partial restriction.
- This would reduce mortality and morbidity from lung cancer and coronary heart disease with a saving of 219 deaths per year.
- Banning smoking in public places would also reduce the prevalence of smoking (conservatively estimated by 2%) leading to a further saving of 260 lives per year.

The notion of 'creative epidemiology' is concerned with making research findings and epidemiological data more accessible: 'It is particularly concerned with placing unfamiliar or complicated data in perspective against data that are more familiar to people' (Chapman and Lupton, 1994: 160). For example, expressing death rates from smoking-related diseases in conventional epidemiological terms as rates per 100,000 or as relative risk – while undoubtedly essential in establishing evidence of the effects of smoking on health – has little impact outside professional circles. The statement that, in the UK, 120,000 smokers will die each year as a result of their smoking habit (ASH, 2002a) is easier to visualize and more attention-grabbing. The information becomes even more dramatic when converted to a toll of 328 lives *per day* – equivalent to a major air crash. This instantly raises the profile of smoking-related deaths from hidden daily occurrences to a major national tragedy.

Other strategies for gaining attention include comparison with issues that already stimulate public concern, such as smoking kills around six times more people in the UK than road traffic accidents (3391), other accidents (8933), poisoning and overdose (3157), murder and manslaughter (495), suicide (4485) and HIV infection (180) *all put together* (20,641 in total – 1999 figures) (ASH, 2002a).

Similarly, information can be manipulated to emphasize the potential risk for individuals – for example, half of all teenagers smoking today will die of tobacco-related causes if they continue to do so (ASH, 2001).

Chapman and Lupton (1994) provide a detailed account of the various strategies that might be used and cite an example of the use of creative epidemiology that convinced politicians of the effects of tobacco sponsorship on children and led to the Federal Government in Australia supporting a ban on tobacco sponsorship. Data were collected on cigarette brand preferences in four states in Australia and were found to correspond with the major football sponsors in each state. Steve Woodward, the then Australian Director of ASH, converted the data into visually appealing graphs that were distributed to all politicians and the media.

Agenda setting

The 'policy agenda' has been defined (Kingdon, 1984, in Walt, 1994: 53) as:

> the list of subjects or problems to which government officials and people outside of government closely associated with those officials are paying serious attention at any given time.

A key question concerns how issues get on to – or fail to get on to – the policy agenda. Jones and Sidell (1997) refer to the well-known UK example of the effective 'burying' of Sir Douglas Black's report, *Inequalities in Health* (Department of Health and Social Security, 1980) by tactics such as producing a limited number of copies and its publication on an August bank holiday, which ensured minimum publicity. Whitehead's update on inequality, *The Health Divide* (1987), suffered a similar fate and there was only tacit reference to inequality in the first national health strategy 'Health of the Nation' (Department of Health, 1992).

Notwithstanding the lack of national political attention, sound research evidence demonstrating inequality to be a major public health issue generated a groundswell of opinion at local and national levels, including public health professionals, academics, pressure groups and the public. Against this backdrop, inequality has received progressively increasing government attention – initially with the 'variations' agenda (Department of Health, 1995) and more latterly with the response to the publication of the *Independent Inquiry into Inequalities in Health* (Acheson, 1998). Tackling inequality and social exclusion now forms a central plank of the national health strategy.

Hogwood and Gunn (1984) suggest that an issue is most likely to get on the policy agenda if any of the following apply:

- it has reached crisis proportions
- it has achieved particularity – that is, it exemplifies a larger issue
- it has an emotive aspect
- it is likely to have wide impact
- it raises questions about power and legitimacy in society
- it is currently 'fashionable'.

However, the influence of 'agenda setters' (see the box) can also be pivotal. As we have already noted, the elitist viewpoint (Hogwood and Gunn would also include anything other than the most naïve pluralist interpretation) acknowledges that there may be unequal access to the policy agenda. John (1998: 147) suggests that:

> the distribution of power is the underlying factor, but it is more normal in radical accounts to stress the salience of ideas and political language which marginalizes certain interests and ideas. Power is expressed through the hegemony of certain ideas. Created by the middle or upper classes and by economic interests, ruling ideologies ensure that certain issues are off the agenda and others are on it.

Agenda setters

- Organized interests
- Protest groups
- Political party leaders
- Senior government officials and advisers
- Informed opinion
- Mass media

After Hogwood and Gunn, 1984

The notion of 'bounded pluralism' has been applied to gaining access to the policy agenda. Elite groups may have dominant influence over major issues, of high politics, whereas there may be much more open debate on more minor and less politically sensitive issues. In addition to what gets on to the policy agenda, an important consideration is what is kept off. Elite groups may take on a gatekeeper function in relation to major – potentially politically damaging – issues (Walt, 1994; Jones and Sidell, 1997). Efforts to confine the agenda to safe issues can simply involve filtering out more contentious ones, but also, and perhaps rather more sinisterly, implicitly or explicitly shaping people's perceptions of what they want and need (Lukes, 1974). Reich (2002) maintains that policy change is dependent on the political will of leaders. The role of policy advocates, therefore, is to create that political will. This requires political analysis to identify the key stakeholders and their intentions, potential losers and winners, and where support and opposition will lie. It also requires the adoption of appropriate political strategies.

ADVOCACY

Healthy public policy depends on political vision and leadership and Draper (1988: 218) contends that leadership 'must begin with the people who have a strong professional responsibility for public health'. It also requires an effective advocacy function yet advocacy tends to be an underdeveloped element of health promotion and public health practice. Radius et al. (2008) propose improving the professional preparation of health educators to take on an advocacy role and the capacity of institutions to provide training and appropriate developmental experience. Furthermore, the evidence base is not well developed, largely due to the reactive and iterative nature of even the most well-planned advocacy initiatives (Chapman and Wakefield, 2001).

Defining advocacy

Advocacy was identified as a key strategy by the Ottawa Charter (WHO, 1986). The term 'advocacy' has traditionally been used to describe activity on behalf of those in a less powerful position. The International Union for Health Education (1992) identified three main areas in which advocates can operate:

- influencing government to develop healthy policies and legislation
- influencing commercial and other organizations to consider the health impact of their activities and exert pressure on governments and citizens
- influencing individuals and groups to make healthy choices and support initiatives to promote health.

Advocacy for health has been defined as:

A combination of individual and social actions designed to gain political commitment, policy support, social acceptance and systems support for a particular health goal or programme. (WHO, 1998f: 5)

Wallack et al. (1993: 27) suggest that:

Advocacy is a catch-all word for the set of skills used to create a shift in public opinion and mobilize the necessary resources and forces to support an issue, policy, or constituency. Advocacy involves much more than lobbying in support of a certain piece of legislation. Health professionals routinely engage in a wide array of advocacy activities, including patient advocacy, client advocacy, and policy advocacy, all designed to make the system function better to meet health and safety goals...

They draw on Amidei (1991, in Wallack et al., 1993: 28) to identify several characteristics of advocacy:

- Advocacy assumes that people have rights, and those rights are enforceable.
- Advocacy works best when focused on something specific.
- Advocacy is primarily concerned with rights and benefits to which someone or some community is already entitled.

Policy advocacy is concerned with ensuring that institutions work the way they should. Patient and client advocacy are concerned with ensuring that individuals obtain their rights. Our concern here is with the broader area of policy advocacy – specifically, healthy public policy advocacy and issues affecting collective rights. The related activity of lobbying is taken to apply narrowly to attempts to persuade members of government to take up a cause.

Walt (1994) distinguishes between 'commercial lobbyists', who will take on any cause, and 'cause lobbyists', who are seeking to further the specific cause to which they subscribe. Both may adopt similar tactics and seek close relationships with civil servants as well as elected representatives.

In contrast, the target of advocacy may range wider than government circles to generate support among interest groups, the media and the general public. Based on the premise that democratic governments tend to act in line with major public opinion – or at least not risk alienating it – the overall intention of public health advocacy is to create a climate of support for healthy policy options.

As Milio (1981: 304) argues:

The development of organized advocacy for the public's health may well be necessary to demand that government use its resources for health-making purposes. If so, advocacy must go far beyond the usual voicing of discontent, or of admonitions to individuals to change their ways. The message must be conveyed in ways that create widespread and informed public debate. Usable translations of the message are necessary. Explanations are needed of the complexities of the health problem, of alternate health strategies, and of their costs and gains. The true costs of not preventing illness must be addressed, as well as the protections that are possible for those whose livelihoods might be harmed during transitions. Workable formats for presenting the message and convenient forums for discussion are needed for the general public and for its subgroups, for the mass media and specialized professional media, for policymakers, and for scientists and methodologists. Such groundwork seems essential to effective policy-influencing action. Its ultimate strategic purpose is to make health-promoting policy decisions easier for policymakers to choose.

Chapman and Lupton's (1994: 6) influential text defines public health advocacy as:

> the process of overcoming major structural (as opposed to individual or behavioural) barriers to public health goals. Numbered among such barriers are some of the most formidable political, economic and cultural forces imaginable. These forces include political philosophies that devalue health and quality of life at the expense of economic outcomes; political and bureaucratic opposition or inertia to health-promoting legislative or regulatory provisions and policies, and to the participation of consumers in healthcare planning; the marketing of unsafe and unhealthy products, often by transnational corporations of immense influence and wealth; and the pervasiveness of major cultural values such as racism and sexism, which find expression in institutional values and personal attitudes and behaviours relevant to public health issues.

Wise (2001) contends that, although the overall aim may be to change the legislative, fiscal, physical and social environment, advocacy is fundamentally a political process that aims to influence political decisions. She draws on Wallack (1998) to distinguish between advocacy and public education or social marketing. Although they may use the same media to communicate their messages, the latter are predicated on the assumption that problems are due to lack of information and focus on filling the information gap. Advocacy, on the other hand, focuses on the *power* gap and problems are seen to be due to lack of sufficient power to achieve social change. Advocacy, therefore, attempts to mobilize support and political involvement. McCubbin et al. (2001) note two interrelated facets of advocacy as a health promotion strategy:

- prescriptive or campaign-style advocacy
- empowering or community development-style advocacy.

Strategies

Effective advocacy involves identifying and assessing the power of opposition groups and supporters as a basis for targeting action to build support and develop coalitions, along with undermining the opposition.

Advocacy relies on the tactical use of persuasive communication. Presenting the evidence is not enough. Effective advocacy must, in Klein's words, be 'logically persuasive, morally authoritative, and capable of evoking passion. A campaign message must speak at one and the same time to the brain and to the heart' (American Cancer Society/International Union Against Cancer, 2003: 17). Further, effective advocacy campaigns often use a 'simplifying concept' – catchy phrases which communicate more complex ideas such as 'global warming' and 'second-hand tobacco smoke'. Symbolic representations can also be useful, for example the red ribbon for HIV awareness (see box) or white wrist band as the symbol of the Make Poverty History campaign.

Symbolic representation of a cause

The red ribbon – a powerful symbol of HIV awareness.

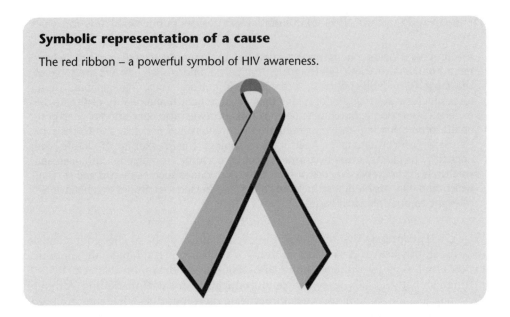

Advocacy involves framing issues to convey their fundamental essence and constructing arguments to appeal to potential supporters. The various players present what is in the best interests of their group by filtering information from factual reality. Their stated reason for their stance on policy is the 'publicly acceptable justification of their material or political interests' (Milio, 1988: 267). Dorfman et al. (2005) refer to two main frames which shape dialogue about the health consequences of corporate action – market justice and social justice and argue that public health advocates must articulate the latter.

Given that there is no objective reality, public health policy initiatives are open to a range of interpretations (Chapman and Lupton, 1994). These will inevitably be influenced by values and ideological commitments. Milio suggests that we need to understand how a policy will affect major stakeholders and how they frame their support or opposition. For example, the Acheson inquiry (1998) noted strong evidence that fluoridation of water improves the dental health of children and significantly reduces inequality in dental health. However, notwithstanding the sound supportive evidence, attempts in the UK to add fluoride to drinking water have been variously interpreted as:

- offering all children the benefits of protection from dental caries
- offering particular benefits for disadvantaged children who are more vulnerable to caries
- compensating for a deficiency in the drinking water in some geographic areas and restoring it to normal levels
- contaminating drinking water
- mass medication
- an infringement of liberty
- state interference
- placing children at risk of toxic effects.

Effective advocacy requires careful framing of arguments and, conversely, understanding of the way the opposition is framing its own arguments so that an appropriate response can be mounted (see the box for an example).

Responding to the opposition

Advocates of smoke-free restaurants in the United States had difficulty countering the tobacco industry's arguments that this would be unfair to smokers. They responded by shifting the message to 'smoke-free workplaces' (which clearly include restaurants) and upholding the rights of ALL workers to a healthy, smoke-free environment – a message which was simple, logically strong, carried moral authority and aroused public passion.

American Cancer Society/International Union Against Cancer, 2003

Efforts to sway public and political opinion will need to draw on a whole repertoire of proactive and reactive, creative, dramatic and news-grabbing tactics (Chapman and Lupton, 1994). An example is provided in the box.

Advocacy in action

Surfers against Sewage (SAS) launched the Return to Offender campaign in April 2006 at the opening of the O'Neill Highland Open international surf contest in Thurso, Scotland. Companies identified from litter collected on local beaches were contacted by competitors to persuade them to:

- improve 'the anti-littering' message on their products
- look at using less harmful packaging to ensure products can break down naturally without putting wildlife at risk
- promote recycling and/or reuse wherever appropriate, including more involvement with community 'anti-litter' initiatives.

SAS, 2008

The media can be particularly effective in bringing issues to public attention and influencing opinion. Chapman and Lupton (1994: 19) note that relatively few key decision makers need to be convinced before action is taken and that highly placed individuals – politicians, senior bureaucrats and heads of non-governmental organizations – are 'often highly sensitive to the ways in which the media are framing issues and setting public expectations about the roles they should perform'. Furthermore, where there is dispute, the media can become the 'battlegrounds on which each side seeks to secure the most powerful connotations for its cause, and to attribute to its adversaries the most negative associations' (Chapman and Lupton, 1994: 99). They contend that the success of an advocacy campaign can hinge on the way in which issues are framed in

Table 6.1   Framing the debate – arguments of supporters and opponents of pool fencing

Supporters	Opponents
Expert opinion favours pool fencing	Expert opinion discredits pool fencing arguments
Community supports for pool fencing revealed by survey	Community supports discredited
Personalizing the issue by presenting the human face of infant drowning	State intrusion into the home
Parents as fallible	Supervisory negligence responsible for drowning
	Drowning as a consequence of trespass
	Fencing swimming pools is arbitrary when there are many unfenced water sources
Aesthetics versus saving a child's life	Hysteria and emotional claptrap
Need to ensure consistency with other safety standards	Overkill to fence all pools even in households where there are no children
Vocal selfish minority are opposed to pool fencing	Opponents portrayed as ordinary citizens and proponents as paid civil servants
Votes versus children's lives	
Defenders of the innocent and helpless	

Source: After Chapman and Lupton, 1994

the media and how they are reframed to respond strategically to the efforts of the opposition. Chapman and Lupton's analysis of the themes emerging in press reports of the debate about fencing domestic swimming pools in New South Wales is summarized in Table 6.1 (see also the box).

Alternative frames for charitable action

Archbishop Helder Camara of Brazil said, 'When I feed the hungry, they call me a saint. When I ask why they have no food, they call me a Communist.'

Cited by Wallack et al., 1993

Given that many – if not most – public health pressure groups have insufficient funds to buy advertising space in the media to publicize their causes, maximizing free media coverage becomes essential. Like the well-known acronym for giving information to politicians – KISS (keep it short and simple) – gaining access to the media demands brevity rather than protracted rational argument. Presenting the human side of an issue is both powerful and emotive. Witness, for example, the moving address to the 13th International AIDS Conference in 2000 by Nkosi Johnson given in the box on the facing page. At the age of 11, he was South Africa's longest-surviving child with HIV. His words were televised worldwide and were influential in changing the attitudes of individuals, companies and governments to people with AIDS.

Nkosi Johnson's speech to the 13th International Aids Conference

Care for us and accept us – we are all human beings.
We are normal.
We have hands.
We have feet.
We can walk, we can talk, we have needs just like everyone else.
Don't be afraid of us – we are the same.

Nkosi Johnson AIDS Foundation, undated

The association of a celebrity with an issue or cause can attract considerable publicity. Well-known individuals, such as Arthur Ashe, Rock Hudson, Ervin (Magic) Johnson and Freddie Mercury, brought the issue of HIV and AIDS to the forefront of public attention by generating substantial media coverage. Similarly, the association of Diana, Princess of Wales with the landmine issue, gave it considerable international prominence.

Chapman and Lupton (1994: 99) note that:

> newsworthiness requires that issues be framed through the transformation of facts and arguments into metaphors, labels and symbols, to allow them to be told as news 'stories'.

We will consider the issue of media advocacy more fully in Chapter 8. The box provides a set of tips for gaining media coverage (see also Chapman, 1994).

Tips for getting items into the media

- Get to know the media – know what types of stories they publish.
- Develop good relationships with local journalists and local radio and television.
- Build up a list of contacts of people who handle your sort of story.
- Be realistic about the amount of interest your story will attract.
- Find a local angle.
- Use concrete examples rather than abstract ideas.
- Find a human interest angle.
- Think visual and use a good picture.
- Involve celebrities.

Teenage Pregnancy Unit, 2000

While the media may be very effective in raising awareness of issues, Walt (1994) notes that policy makers are unlikely to be influenced by a single account and poses the question of how long media coverage has to be sustained before an issue is put on to the policy agenda. Finnegan and Viswanath (1999: 123) also refer to the need for sustained action on the part of community groups:

> The mass media can be highly effective in building the community agenda for public policy change on behalf of public health, but media attention alone is seldom sufficient without sustained efforts by empowered community groups and coalitions.

Campaign groups will therefore need to consider strategies for maintaining the visibility of issues over a protracted period. Furthermore, Walt raises the issue of what controls the media agenda. In some parts of the world, state control of the media casts doubt on its impartial reporting. Similarly, economic interests may dictate what gains coverage. Newspaper editors and radio and television producers occupy a key gatekeeping role. Over and above dominant ideological frameworks shaping the content of the media, there may also be more conscious filtering of information. Walt refers to the 'propaganda model' of Herman and Chomsky, which is based on the view that the media are controlled to further the interests of the state and powerful groups. Factors that may affect the filtering of news coverage include ownership, profit orientation, advertising and sources of information.

Returning to the more general issues of advocacy, Baum (2001: 107) suggests that successful advocacy strategies should:

- set an agenda
- frame the issue for public consumption
- advocate specific solutions.

The 'A' Frame for Advocacy developed by the Johns Hopkins Center for Communication Programs (undated) identifies six stages in the advocacy process.

1 **Analysis** of the problem, the need for policy change, stakeholders and, specifically, supporters, opponents, decision makers and vote swingers, policy-making structures and processes and means of influencing decision makers.
2 **Strategy** based on clear objectives suited to the context.
3 **Mobilization** of potential partners and coalition building to maximize collective resources and power.
4 **Action** achieving maximum visibility for the cause using credible messages and appropriate channels, including the media.
5 **Evaluation** to identify what has been achieved and what still needs to be done.
6 **Continuity** planning for the longer term, keeping coalitions together, keeping arguments fresh and adapting them to current circumstances.

Having clear objectives is a key factor in coordinating activity during the various stages. Furthermore, advocacy efforts are more likely to be successful if decisions about the most appropriate courses of action are based on an analysis of contextual factors and the location of power and influence. Chapman and Lupton (1994: 130) also caution that those involved in advocacy should be clear about their goals and not lose sight of 'the big picture'. Moreover, advocacy should not become an end in itself, but a means of achieving public health goals.

Key questions to guide an advocacy strategy are therefore:

- What are the public health objectives?
- Who are the main stakeholder groups?
- What alliances/coalitions can usefully be formed?
- Who is the target? Who has the power to bring about change?
- What is the message?
- How can the message be framed to appeal to the target group/s?
- Which channel/s will be most effective for reaching the target?
- What other action will achieve visibility for the cause and a supportive climate of public opinion?
- What opposition is there?
- How can opposition be countered?
- How will you know you have been successful and what milestones are there en route to success?

ADOPTION AND IMPLEMENTATION

Whether polices are adopted or not will depend on a range of factors. Bunton (1992: 137) suggests that these would include:

> how the policies are conceived, how they are introduced, the group's commitment to them, the local resources available to assist their introduction, and a range of other socio-economic factors.

Furthermore, he notes that policies may be modified and considerably watered down during the process of development and implementation. This may be the product of powerful interests bringing their weight to bear or, alternatively, the decisions and routines established by what Lipsky (1997) terms 'street-level bureaucrats' – workers in public services, such as welfare departments, schools, health services and so on.

Walt (1994: 165) also sees that the implementation of policy requires the cooperation of many different groups and that 'policy formulation, even in the form of a legal statute, is not a sufficient condition for implementation'. Hogwood and Gunn (1997) contend that the perfect implementation of policy is extremely unlikely and specify the conditions that would need to exist for this to happen:

- circumstances external to the implementing agency not imposing crippling constraints
- adequate time and sufficient resources being made available
- the required combination of resources being available
- the policy being based on a valid theory of cause and effect
- the relationship between cause and effect being direct and few, if any, intervening links
- dependency relationships being minimal
- understanding of, and agreement on, objectives
- tasks being fully specified, in the right sequence
- perfect communication and coordination
- those in authority being able to demand and obtain perfect compliance.

Springett (1998) notes that inter-sectoral policy is notorious for failure during implementation. Clearly, ensuring that the conditions specified are met is particularly problematic when a number of different agencies and sectors are involved. Colebatch (1998: 56) states that there is held to be a problem in implementation when 'the outcome was likely to be quite different to the originally stated intentions'. By way of illustration, he quotes the title of the seminal work by Pressman and Wildavsky (1973) – *Implementation: How Great Expectations in Washington are Dashed in Oakland: or, Why It's Amazing that Federal Programmes Work at All, This Being a Saga of the Economic Development Administration as Told by Two Sympathetic Observers Who Seek to Build Morals on a Foundation of Ruined Hopes*. The problems identified by Pressman and Wildavsky include having a large number of participants and diversity of goals, such that approval needed to be obtained at a number of different points.

Colebatch provides a useful overview of the ways in which implementation problems are perceived. The vertical perspective assumes a top-down approach and sees implementation as requiring compliance with the directives of those in authority. In contrast, a horizontal perspective recognizes that participants have their own agendas and interpretations of policy. It also acknowledges that the flow of influence is not only vertically within organizations, but that there is negotiation with people external to them.

The horizontal perspective views the implementation of policy rather more flexibly than the vertical. It would see implementation as a collective action that evolves to be compatible with the policy goals and the perspectives of participants rather than a strict adherence to top-down directives.

A further distinction is between normative frameworks, which are concerned with what 'ought to be', and empirical frameworks, which are concerned with 'what is'.

Colebatch equates the vertical perspective on implementation with normative frameworks and the horizontal with empirical frameworks. He notes, too, that there can be two coexisting accounts of the implementation process – the *sacred*, which presents the ideal, and the *profane*, which is a more realistic account of what actually happened.

The means of securing policy implementation will inevitably vary according to the perspective. The vertical perspective will focus on policy goals and compliance, whereas the horizontal will pay greater attention to processes and the people involved.

HEALTH IMPACT ASSESSMENT

We turn our attention now to the wider issue of health impact assessment (HIA). As we noted earlier, the notion of healthy public policy is not just concerned with the development of policies to tackle health issues, but also requires an appraisal of the health impact of all policies. Health impact assessment is 'a combination of procedures, methods and tools by which a policy, programme, product, or service may be judged concerning its effects on the health of the population' (Smith et al., 2006). Furthermore, its capacity to assess differential impact on various groups within the population makes it an important tool in efforts to achieve equity in health. HIA can apply to policy, programmes, projects and industrial and commercial activity but our concern here is principally with policy.

Kemm (2001) suggests that healthy public policy is dependent on predicting the health consequences of different policy options and ensuring that the policy process gives consideration to these potential consequences at all stages. The Gothenburg consensus paper on HIA (European Centre for Health Policy, 1999: 1) sees the purpose of HIA as being to:

improve knowledge about the potential impact of a policy or a programme, inform decisionmakers and affected people, and facilitate adjustment of the proposed policy in order to mitigate the negative and maximize the positive effects.

HIA therefore leads to informed policy making and provides the opportunity to adapt decisions to avoid potential harm. It is considered to add value to policy and decision-making processes (National Assembly for Wales, 1999). The various benefits of HIA are listed in the box.

The benefits of health impact assessment

Health impact assessment can:

- promote equity, sustainability and healthy public policy in an unequal and frequently unhealthy world;
- improve the quality of decision making in health and partner organizations by incorporating the need to address health issues into planning and policy-making;
- emphasize social and environmental justice (it is usually those who are already disadvantaged who suffer most from negative health impacts);
- encourage public participation in debates about public policy issues;
- give equal status to both qualitative and quantitative assessment methods;
- make values and politics explicit, and open issues to public scrutiny;
- demonstrate that health-relevant policy is far broader than health-care issues.

Scott-Samuel and O'Keefe, 2007: 212

Within the UK, the importance of assessing the impact of government policy on health and inequality was recognized in the health strategy document, *Saving Lives: Our Healthier Nation* (Department of Health, 1999) and the recommendations of the Acheson report, referred to in the box on page 255. The National Assembly for Wales (2002) demonstrated its commitment to developing the use of HIA by setting up a series of pilot projects and the publication of *Developing Health Impact Assessment in Wales* (National Assembly for Wales, 1999).

The move towards a more integrated approach to health and development has focused the attention of governments and international organizations, such as WHO and the World Bank, on HIA. Within the European Community, Article 152 of the Amsterdam Treaty states that 'A high level of human health protection shall be ensured in the definition and implementation of all Community policies and activities' and an EU Council resolution of June 1999 calls for the establishment of procedures to monitor the impact of Community policies and activities on public health and healthcare (UK Health for All Network, 2001).

Furthermore, Scott-Samuel and O'Keefe (2007) note the effect that public policy decisions and the activity of multilateral organizations and transnational companies can have on global health. They argue that HIA should be applied to foreign policy-making, global public policy and the operation of transnational companies and bodies.

Identifying the potential health impact of policy is necessarily complex – given the plethora of factors that interact to influence health status, both directly and indirectly. Moreover, policy development in one sector may have a knock-on effect in another – for example, education policy on sex education may well have repercussions for the Department of Health meeting its targets for reducing teenage pregnancy and the rate of sexually transmitted infection (Green, 1998). The Social Exclusion Unit (1999) identifies 28 government programmes that impact on teenage parenthood. Lee et al. (2006) note the difficulty of elevating the priority attached to health concerns in traditionally non-health policy agendas such as foreign policy and security.

Morgan defines HIA as:

> a methodology which enables the identification, prediction and evaluation of the likely changes in health risks, both positive and negative (single or collective) of a policy programme, plan or development action on a defined population. These changes may be direct and immediate or indirect and delayed. (1998, in Kemm, 2001: 80)

The key questions to consider in planning to undertake a HIA are summarized in the box.

Key questions concerning HIA

What   ... policies will be screened and what are the criteria for deciding?
              ... impacts will be assessed? Will these include health outcomes, determinants, risks and equity?
How   ... will HIA happen? Will it be integrated or conducted separately? Will it be a voluntary or legal requirement?
              ... can we infer causality between policy and outcome?
When   ... will HIA be introduced into the policy process?
Who   ... does the assessment? Will this be the policy proponent or an external agency?
              ... pays?
Where ... at international, national or local levels?

After European Centre for Health Policy, 1999: 8

To have maximum influence, HIA will need to be integrated into the various stages of policy making. There is general agreement that HIA should be carried out early enough for there to be sufficient fluidity in the decision-making process to respond to the findings. Although, optimally, HIA will be predictive in order to enable remedial action to be taken, the National Assembly for Wales (1999) identifies three types of assessment:

prospective   predicts the effects of policy before it is implemented

retrospective identifies the consequences of a policy already implemented (such evidence may inform future prospective assessments)

concurrent aims to identify consequences as policies are implemented, particularly when negative impacts are anticipated and there is some uncertainty about them, and allows prompt action to be taken should any negative consequences arise.

Banken (2001) identifies two conceptual streams that have informed the development of HIA – namely, environmental impact assessment, which focused on the environmental consequences of projects, and the public health emphasis on the social and environmental determinants of health. Lerer (1999) notes that the current focus tends to be on identifying health hazards and health-risk management, but there is clearly scope to broaden this. Although HIA is usually concerned with policies in the non-health sector, Kemm (2001) suggests that it also has a role in identifying the indirect and unanticipated consequences of health-sector policy. Latterly, there have been links with the inequality and human rights agendas.

The potential remit, then, is enormous and this raises questions about the feasibility of assessing the health impact of all policies. There are two responses to this. The first is to filter out for scrutiny only those policy areas that are likely to have health consequences. The second, more radical approach, is to make HIA an integral part of all public policy development and part of the mindset of those involved (Barnes and Scott-Samuel, 2000: 2):

> In the longer term it [HIA] has the potential to make concern for improving public health the norm and a routine part of all public policy development.

This latter approach undoubtedly has the advantage of institutionalizing concern for health. Kemm (2001) sees ownership of HIA by the policy proponent as the ideal state – one that supports shared understanding of values and, at a more practical level, allows HIA to be embedded in all stages of policy development. This is in marked contrast to the situation in environmental impact assessment, where there is usually an external regulatory authority.

Banken (2001) is also supportive of institutionalization of HIA, but cautions that raising health to superordinate status may be perceived by other players in the policy arena as health imperialism, resulting in some resistance. She (2001: 30) emphasizes that the aim should not be to increase the power of public health actors, but to 'add health awareness to policy making' by enabling those in non-health sectors to 'produce public health knowledge for use by decisionmakers'. Clearly, this may require the development of skill and awareness among those involved. She also suggests that enabling non-health actors to produce this kind of information needs to be followed through with quality control to ensure rigour and avoid tokenism. As Bartlett (1989, in Banken, 2001: 31) notes:

> the politics of bureaucracy provide an environment in which the effectiveness of impact assessment can be tempered, subverted, and broken in the absence of adequate provisions for external accountability.

It has been suggested that the use of an alternative term to HIA might advance the cause more effectively. Kemm (2001) suggests 'overall policy appraisal' and Banken (2001) 'human impact assessment'.

The main stages in the process of HIA identified by the technical briefing for the World Health Organization Regional Committee for Europe (2002) are:

1   **Screening** to quickly establish whether a particular policy, programme or project is relevant to health. This assessment may involve the use of checklists or other tools (see, for example, Department of Health, 2007b). It will flag up if there is a need for a more detailed assessment.
2   **Scoping** to identify the relevant health issues and public concerns that need to be addressed during appraisal. It generates questions, maps out possible connections, and sets the boundaries and terms of reference for the appraisal.
3   **Appraisal** to identify, and when possible quantify, the potential impacts on health and wellbeing in the context of available evidence and the knowledge, experience and opinions of stakeholders. It can be a *rapid* or an *in-depth appraisal*, depending on the level of detail and quantification needed to inform the policy decision, and may include mitigation and health-promoting measures.
4   **Reporting,** that is, communicating with stakeholders about the expected impacts on health and about how the policy, programme or other development could be modified to minimize negative and maximize positive impacts.
5   **Monitoring** of compliance with recommendations and of expected health impacts following the implementation of the policy or programme. This allows the existing evidence base to be expanded.

The final stage often includes evaluation of the quality of the HIA process to inform future assessments (AHPO, 2007). Although the stages are presented sequentially, the process is essentially iterative and should conform with the key principles of HIA (see box).

Key principles of HIA

- A social model of health and wellbeing
- An explicit focus on equity and social justice
- A multidisciplinary, participatory approach
- The use of qualitative as well as quantitative evidence
- Explicit values and openness to public scrutiny

Barnes and Scott-Samuel, 2000: 2

During the appraisal stage all significant health impacts should be identified and the implications of each should be considered in relation to quantity and quality of life. Resource costs in the healthcare and other sectors can also be considered. However, it is unlikely that sufficient information will be available to allow this to be done in monetary terms (National Assembly for Wales, 1999). The various impacts identified may well have contradictory effects on health or, indeed, on different groups and, in principle, this could be reduced to an overall net effect. However, it is more useful to maintain an overview of the various pathways that might improve or harm health. See the example in the box.

Health impact assessment

Extract from the assessment of the impact of the operational phase of the Merseytram Scheme on lifestyle

Lifestyle	Direction/scale	Likelihood
Travel behaviour		
Increase in sustainable, healthier transport modes	+	probable
Modal shift from bus to tram	−	probable
Modal shift from car to tram	+	possible
Physical activity		
Some increase in cycling, walking reduced risk of developing heart disease, diabetes (2), obesity, fall in hypertension, etc.	++	probable
Reduction in health inequalities between Merseytram zone and elsewhere	+	possible
Mobility		
Increase in mobility, increased access to job, education opportunities, social networks	++	probable
Reduction in health inequalities between Merseytram zone and elsewhere	+	probable
Safety		
Low, but increased risk of accidental injury involving the tram and pedestrians, cyclists	−	possible
Reductions in fear of crime associated with public transport increased use of tram	+	probable
Electromagnetic effects – the National Radiological Protection Board has concluded that there is no clear evidence that electromagnetic fields emanating from alternative or direct currents to which people are exposed to everyday activities can give rise to adverse health effects	negligible	probable

Derived from Prashar et al., 2004: 13

Kemm (2001) also emphazises the importance of differentiating between winners and losers by including consideration of which groups are affected as well as the nature and magnitude of health impacts. For example, in the development context, the construction of a dam may secure a supply of potable water, support irrigation schemes to increase agricultural yields and increase health and prosperity for some, but may require others to relocate, losing homes and farmland, and shift the distribution of diseases such as schistosomiasis. Douglas et al.'s (2001) case study of three possible scenarios for developing transport policy in Edinburgh differentiated the effects on various subgroups of the population, as shown in Table 6.2.

Table 6.2 Health impacts on different population groups under transport scenario 1 (low spend) and scenario 3 (high spend)

	Accidents		Pollution		Physical activity		Access to goods and services		Community network	
	1	3	1	3	1	3	1	3	1	3
Young children										
Affluent	+	+	+	+	+	−	−	+	−	++
Deprived	+	+	−	+	+	+	+	+	−	++
Adolescents										
Affluent	−	++	+	+	−	+	+	++	+	++
Deprived	+	+	−	+	−	++	+	++	+	++
Elderly										
Affluent	−	++	−	+	−	++	−	+	−	++
Deprived	−	+	−	+	−	++	−	++	−	++
Working people										
Affluent	0	+	+	+	−	+	−	++	−	+
Deprived	−	+	−	+	−	++	+	++	−	++
Unemployed										
Deprived	−	+	−	+	−	+	+	++	+	++

Key:
++ very positive impact   0 no impact   − very negative impact
+ positive impact   − negative impact

Source: After Douglas et al., 2001

It is axiomatic that HIA should be based on sound evidence. Kemm (2001) distinguishes two main approaches to assessment. One is characterized by a 'tight focus', based on an epidemiological model of exposure and dose–response relationships. Outcomes are usually defined in terms of death and disability, but could potentially be extended to include additional dimensions. The other 'broad focus' adopts a more wide-ranging approach and draws on informed opinion and local knowledge. A combination of the two is held to be most likely to generate a complete picture. HIA, therefore, relies on both qualitative and quantitative information and a multidisciplinary input. Kemm (2001: 82) suggests that this multidisciplinary input is particularly relevant to:

- **situational validation** — will the policy objectives be relevant to the problem?
- **societal vindication** — will the policy have instrumental value for the health of society as a whole?
- **social choice** — will the fundamental ideology of the policy be compatible with health?

While acknowledging the persuasiveness of quantitative data and providing guidance on the production of robust quantitative HIA, Mindell et al. (2001) express a number of reservations:

- not everything that can be quantified is important
- not everything that is being quantified at the moment should be
- not everything that is important can be quantified.

Communities may well have different perceptions of risks and benefits than professionals. The National Assembly for Wales (1999: 6) considers community participation to be essential:

> The involvement of the public is particularly important as many judgements within Health Impact Assessment are value judgements rather than scientific judgements.

Lerer (1999) also advises including communities and an ongoing iterative consultation with major stakeholders. The Gothenburg statement (European Centre for Health Policy, 1999: 5) proposes that HIA should include:

- consideration of *evidence* about the anticipated relationships between a policy, programme or project and the health of the population
- consideration of the *opinions*, experience and expectations of those who may be *affected* by the proposed policy, programme or project.

Careful consideration will need to be given to ways in which to involve the public. Mittelmark (2001) notes that the trend towards more technical and complex methods of assessment, along with the use of inaccessible jargon, makes it difficult for the average citizen to participate. He calls for an approach to HIA that is user-friendly and inclusive and cites the example of the People Assessing Their Health (PATH) project in Eastern Nova Scotia. This involved members of the community in developing local HIA tools suited to the needs of the community. As we have noted, commitment to participation is a central concern of health promotion and is supported by the Gothenburg statement's list of values governing HIA (see the box). Furthermore, there are clear links with health advocacy and ensuring that there are opportunities for individuals who stand to be affected by policy to have a say in shaping its development.

The Gothenburg statement's values governing HIA

- Democracy
- Equity
- Sustainable development
- Ethical use of evidence.

European Centre for Health Policy, 1999

Notwithstanding the rhetoric about the importance of participation, Mathers et al. note some tension between the participatory and knowledge-gathering dimensions of HIA. They note the tendency to give 'pre-eminence to expert and research generated evidence' (2005: 58).

While decision makers need to be confident that the conclusions of HIA are robust (Mindell et al., 2001), predicting the consequences of policy will inevitably be associated with some uncertainty. In some instances, there will be evidence on which to draw, whereas in others, predictions may need to be based on informed opinion, experience of similar situations and theory. Examples of evidence and data collection methods (from Taylor and Blair-Stevens, 2002) include:

- Depth/key informant interviews
- Focus group discussions
- Equity audits
- Surveys/questionnaires
- Secondary analysis of existing data
- Community profiling
- Health needs assessment
- Expert opinion
- Documentary sources.

Identifying indirect effects may be particularly problematic, especially if they operate via complex systems. It may be possible to extrapolate precise figures and attach confidence intervals to these, but, equally, predictions are often expressed as crude ordinal scales from very certain to very uncertain (Kemm, 2001) or very positive impact to very negative impact, as shown in Table 6.2. The National Assembly for Wales (1999: 6) recognizes this and suggests that those involved:

> should make the best assessment they can using the information and skills available to them and by accepting that some degree of uncertainty may be unavoidable.

The Gothenburg Consensus (European Centre for Health Policy, 1999) emphasizes the importance of taking into account the values and goals within a given society and suggests that the process of HIA should be informed by the core values identified in its Statement, given in the box on page 293. Furthermore, it identifies three categories of HIA that can be instigated following the scoping exercise:

- **rapid health impact appraisal**: based on existing knowledge and the exchange of information between experts, decision makers and representatives of those affected by the proposed policy
- **health impact analysis**: involving a more in-depth analysis based on existing evidence and, if necessary, the generation of new data
- **health impact review**: used when policies are very broad, it aims to produce a convincing estimation of the major impacts of a policy on health without disentangling the detailed impacts of the various policy components and is more concerned with broad relationships than precise cause-and-effect ones.

While it is not possible here to pursue in detail the actual process of conducting risk assessment, numerous guides and checklists are available – see, for example, European Centre for Health Policy (1999), Barnes and Scott-Samuel (2000), Kemm (2007), Department of Health (2007b), The Welsh Health Impact Assessment Support

Unit (2004) and a collection of guides at the HIA Gateway (http://www.apho.org.uk/default.aspx?QN=P_HIA). However, we will conclude with the list of recommendations developed by Douglas et al. (2001: 152):

> screen to select policies for HIA
> negotiate
> share ownership
> be timely
> define and analyse the policy
> define and profile the population
> use an explicit model of health
> be aware of underlying values
> be systematic
> think broadly
> use appropriate evidence
> involve the community
> take into account local factors
> recognize differences within communities
> monitor impacts continuously following an initial prospective HIA
> make practical recommendations.

HEALTHY PUBLIC POLICY, HEALTH PROMOTION AND HEALTH EDUCATION

We have established that healthy public policy is a central concern of health promotion. It is a means of upholding the rights of individuals to health by creating a supportive environment – one that:

- does not threaten health
- provides the conditions to:
  - make the healthy choice the easy choice
  - encourage the participation of citizens.

While policy can be explicitly developed to further health goals, the contention is that all policy should consider potential impacts on health – direct and indirect.

A key theme running through this discussion has been the location and exercise of power. Advocacy and participation in HIA have been identified as ways of influencing policy development.

Health education and healthy public policy have been seen by some as competing options – the former associated with individual behaviour change and victim blaming, and the latter with an emphasis on structural factors and enabling. However, making healthy public policy a reality is dependent on the skills and awareness of those involved. Health education, viewed more broadly, can therefore be a major driver in developing healthy public policy by virtue of its contribution at a number of different levels – from consciousness raising and the development of the skills needed for advocacy and community activism through to professional training and lobbying.

KEY POINTS

o   The development of healthy public policy is central to health promotion practice.

o   Public health professionals can be important advocates for policy to improve public health and need to understand policy processes.

o   Health education has a key role in the development of healthy public policy by raising awareness of health issues among 'policy actors' and also by developing political skills among those seeking to influence policy.

o   Health Impact Assessment is a means of assessing the potential effect on health and health equity of any policy in order to recommend ways of minimizing negative and maximizing positive effects.

7

EDUCATION FOR HEALTH

Those that know, do. Those that understand, teach.

Aristotle (384–322 BC)

OVERVIEW

The purpose of this chapter is to consider the contribution of education to health promotion. It will:

- establish the central importance of health education as the major driver within health promotion
- consider the ethical implications of alternative approaches to health education
- understand the factors involved in communication and their relevance to health education
- distinguish different types of learning
- identify key source, message and audience factors of relevance to communication, health education and efforts to persuade
- consider the appropriateness of different learning methods for achieving particular learning outcomes
- explore the potential of health education as a strategy for social and political change.

INTRODUCTION

In Chapter 1, we provided a technical definition of 'health education' as a planned process designed to achieve health- and illness-related learning. Discussion focused on its philosophical and ideological dimensions – attempting to answer the question of what education ought to be about. Its role was seen to involve more than traditional attempts to persuade individuals to comply with received wisdom about health behaviour and include empowerment and social and political change. The term 'new health education' is used to distinguish this broader conceptualization. We now turn attention to the technical aspects of what is involved in achieving educational goals, together with the nature and dynamics of the learning process.

In Chapter 1, a number of different kinds of influences on learning were identified. These were arranged on a spectrum of coercion. At one end of this spectrum was empowerment, which fulfils the requirement of voluntarism that characterizes true education and the model of health promotion that is espoused in this book. Other activities, indicative of a much wider range of potential interventions, were also represented on the spectrum. Some may be ideologically neutral; others, such as brainwashing, are unacceptable in the context of our empowerment imperative.

Procedures to promote learning

Education	Indoctrination	Advising
Teaching	Propaganda	Social marketing
Instruction	Conditioning	Lobbying
Training	Facilitating	Brainwashing
Persuasion	Counselling	Advocating

The negative connotations of at least some of the activities listed in the box will doubtless be obvious through their association with coercion. For others, there may be more debate. It is interesting, for instance, to consider the use of 'propaganda', which currently has negative associations, but this was not always so. For instance, in the early days of health education, 'health propaganda' was considered perfectly acceptable. The use of propaganda by politicians and dictators – particularly in wartime – has resulted in a more tarnished image.

Notwithstanding ethical and ideological considerations, all the various activities listed in the box have in common a capacity to influence learning to a greater or lesser extent and potentially contribute in some way to health education. However, in line with the emphasis we are placing on empowerment, we will give particular attention to health education's radical imperative and its concern to create social change. We will, however, start by examining a process that is a prerequisite for *all* kinds of learning. That process is communication.

THE COMMUNICATION PROCESS

The word 'communication' is sometimes used to refer to the whole educational process. For instance, Fletcher (1973: 2) viewed communication as synonymous with learning, as the first of his principles of communication demonstrates:

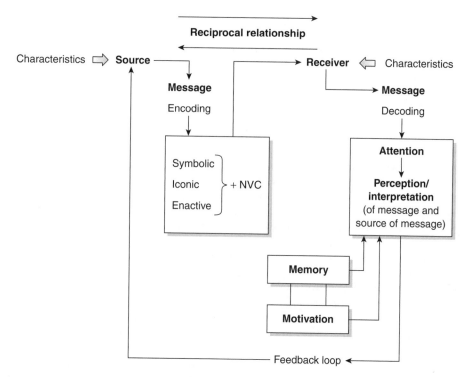

Figure 7.1   A communication model

> The purpose of communication is not just to deliver a message but to effect a change in the recipient in respect of his knowledge, his attitude or, eventually, in his behaviour.

However, there is an important distinction. Whereas communication is a necessary prerequisite for learning, it is learning per se that is responsible for change. The communication process itself is essentially concerned with the transmission and reception of messages. While in many instances some learning will also take place, it is also possible to envisage situations in which it does not, for example telling someone it is raining when they already know this to be the case. Further, mere transmission of information is not the same as the relatively permanent change in knowledge, disposition or capability which is central to our earlier definition of learning. Nonetheless, the form and effectiveness of communication will have some bearing on the achievement of learning goals.

The model shown in Figure 7.1 developed out of work in telecommunications. An information source sends a message via a transmitter and this, hopefully, reaches its destination and is decoded by a receiver. Inevitably, the process is afflicted to a greater or lesser extent by noise. This is not just technical interference, but may refer to psychological as well as physical 'noise'. It would thus include any distortions resulting from individuals' beliefs and attitudes, as well as defects or limitations of their sensory systems.

Key features of the communication process

The communication process involves three components:

- a sender
- a message
- a receiver.

Terminology may differ. For instance, the sender may merely be described as the 'communicator'. More commonly, the originator of the message may be called the 'source' – in which case, the receiver is likely to be defined as the 'audience' (even if it is an audience of one). The source may be personal or 'mediated' – that is, it may be in the form of a poster or leaflet or any other variety of mass media. Whenever the source is present in person, non-verbal communication (NVC) will accompany the message. The source constructs or, more accurately, *encodes* the message and it is the task of the receiver to decode it.

The coded message may be 'symbolic', using spoken or written language (or, of course, mathematical and scientific symbols). Alternatively, it may be 'iconic', using pictorial or diagrammatic presentations or 'enactive'.

As stated, it is the task of the receiver to decode the message. First of all, the message must reach the receiver's senses (if this does not happen, communication and learning fails at this initial stage). It is obviously the responsibility of the communicator to avoid such failure. Secondly, the receiver must pay attention to the message for as long as it takes to achieve the goals of the communication. Thirdly, the processes of perception are brought into play – the message must be correctly interpreted. Attention and accurate perception will be determined by past experience (stored in the memory) and current motivation (also partly determined by past experience).

The nature and success of the communication process will be influenced by the characteristics of both the source and the receiver. The source (and his or her non-verbal communication – NVC) is an integral component of coding and transmitting messages. For instance, the receiver's perception of the source may influence whether or not he or she pays attention or interprets the message appropriately. As we will note later, the credibility of the source will also have a major effect – not only on communication, but on learning. Indeed, identification and manipulation of source characteristics are two of the main concerns in devising 'persuasive communication'. Clearly, receiver characteristics are all-important in the decoding process – cultural beliefs, language skills, intellectual capabilities and personality traits will influence attention and, in particular, perception and interpretation of messages.

Figure 7.1 includes an 'immediate feedback loop', which shows the reciprocal relationship between communicator and receiver, between source and audience. (Note also the 'long-term' feedback system in Figure 7.2.) As has frequently been remarked, communication is (or should be) a two-way process. A critically important part of this reciprocity is the (immediate) feedback loop, which forms an integral part of the interaction. The only way in which communication can be maximized is when the source of the message constantly checks the reactions of the receiver (often by accurately perceiving his or her NVC). Successful communication occurs when the receiver's interpretation of the message exactly matches the communicator's intended message.

Readability

Written communications constitute one of the most common forms of symbolic coding used by health educators. The use of such materials assumes that the target audience is literate. Clearly, it is incumbent on communicators to ensure that their written materials match the audience's level of competence. Key issues influencing the ease of reading appear to be sentence length, the number of words, word length, the inclusion of 'difficult' words and writing in the passive voice. A plethora of tests of readability – or 'reading ease' – have been developed to assess the degree of difficulty of written communications, for example Flesch, FOG (frequency of gobbledygook) and SMOG (subjective measures of gobbledegook). Some express the results as a score associated with the level of difficulty, whereas others use a school grade equivalent (see box). The Infomatics Review (undated) recommends writing at the 6th–8th grade level (11 to 14 years) to communicate effectively with a general audience in the USA. A study in the UK of the coverage of diabetes on 15 internet sites found that they required the reading ability of an educated 11- to 16.9-year-old and yet the average ability in the UK is equivalent to a 9-year-old (Boulos, 2005).

Grade level* of current periodicals

Periodical	Grade Level	School Age
Times of India	15	–
London Times	12	17–18
Los Angeles Times	12	17–18
Sydney Sun-Herald	12	17–18
China Daily	12	17–18
New York Times	10	15–16
Washington Post	10	15–16
The Sun (UK tabloid)	9	14–15
Daily Mirror (UK tabloid)	9	14–15
Reader's Digest	9	14–15

*Assessed using Dale-Chall formula

Derived from Impact Information, 2005

While readability tests offer some insight into the intelligibility of written material, none of these tests measures the *actual* level of understanding of the target audience. Only a direct test of people's ability both to read and to understand a particular communication will do that. Moreover, communicators need to be aware of the cultural interpretations and emotional reactions of their audience to written communications. It is essential, therefore, to undertake a comprehensive pretest of communications.

The US National Cancer Institute (undated) provides guidance on developing print materials for audiences with low literacy levels (see box). It cautions that it involves more than using short words and sentences, and needs the same attention to research, planning and applying the principles of communication as with any other audience – but with particular attention to the key aspects identified in the box.

Designing print materials for low literacy audiences – and improving the quality for everyone!

- Include only the information needed to convey the behavioral objective and support the intended audience in attaining it.
- Organize topics in the order the reader will use them.
- Present the most important points first and last.
- Group information into chunks, with a clear, ordered format.
- Respect the intended audience – don't talk down.
- Follow these guidelines:

  - Use short sentences and paragraphs.
  - Write in the active voice.
  - Clarify concepts with examples.
  - Avoid jargon, technical terms, abbreviations, and acronyms.
  - Include a glossary if necessary (but define key words within the sentence).
  - Give the reader an action step he or she can take right away (e.g., call your clinic, send in a request).
  - Use graphics and design to make the reader's job easier and to increase comprehension and recall; make sure they support, rather than compete with, the text.
  - Don't assume that pictorial signs, symbols, and charts are more effective than words for low-literacy intended audiences.
  - Avoid using all capital letters; they are more difficult for everyone to read, particularly so for less skilled readers.
  - Use captioned illustrations that are relevant to the subject matter and model the desired behavior.
  - Use headings and subheadings to convey a message and help reinforce the flow and content.
  - Use bullets and other graphic devices to highlight key messages and to avoid large blocks of print.
  - Avoid right-justified margins.

- Pretest all materials with the intended audience.

National Cancer Institute, undated

Reflections on empowerment

People have a right to information and communication can serve to meet that need. Communication may therefore be seen as essentially empowering – provided due consideration is given to accessibility to the target audience. However, the source–audience relationship frequently involves an imbalance of power. The selection and manipulation of symbols may reflect cultural assumptions or more conscious efforts on the part of the communicator to persuade.

A goal of an empowerment model of health promotion, and indeed health literacy, would be to enhance the ability of the audience to obtain information and, moreover, to question the content and challenge the sources of messages directed at them. More generally, empowerment seeks to shift the power balance between communicators and audiences.

Daghio et al. (2006) advocate involving lay people in the production of written materials to redress any imbalance, through the following process:

1 priority setting to identify the topic
2 critical appraisal of evidence
3 collective writing of the key messages
4 calculation of readability scores
5 assessment of readability by an independent reading panel
6 assessment of comprehensibility by an independent panel.

HEALTH EDUCATION AND LEARNING

Clearly, learning is linked to communication as shown in Figure 7.2, which also indicates the centrality of selection of methods and development of the message.

In Chapter 1, we distinguished between two often conflicting approaches to health promotion – the preventive medical model and the empowerment model. The contribution of health education to each was characterized as:

- **Health education as persuasion** – associated with 'coercing' people into adopting 'approved' behaviours to prevent disease and improve health.
- **Health education as empowerment** – concerned to strengthen individuals' capacity to control their own health (*self*-empowerment) and work collectively to achieve support-ive environments for health (*community* empowerment).

It is also useful to note a radical variation on the empowerment model of health education that is primarily concerned with developing the capacity to achieve social and political change in the interests of promoting public health. While this is integral to the empowerment model described in this book, efforts which focus on developing this capacity may be distinguished as 'critical health education'.

Patient education can also be legitimately located under the health education umbrella. However, perhaps because of its association with the medical model, it has become marginalized by mainstream health promotion. This is unfortunate. Not only is the education of patients a task of major importance, it can be comfortably accommodated within the general empowerment model of health promotion. Indeed, empowering strategies typically result in more effective preventive outcomes than so-called victim-blaming approaches. In fact, the only real logical distinction between patient education and other varieties of health education is the fact that it is, by definition, concerned to promote the health of people who have been defined as patients!

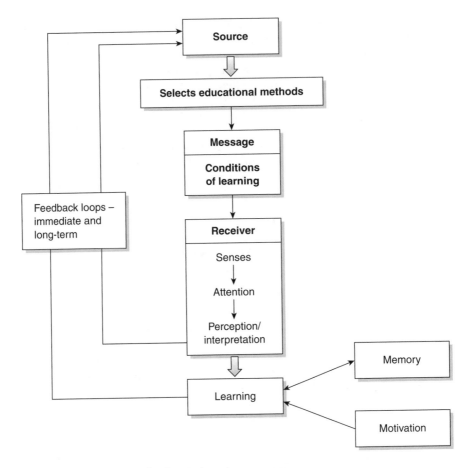

Figure 7.2   The communication to learning process

The role of health education is to create the conditions necessary for achieving the required learning. The key questions which will inform the selection of methods are:

- What learning is required?
- Who is the target (group)?
- How large is the group?
- What are the contextual factors?

A theme running through this book is that, regardless of whether the focus is on policy, behaviour or empowerment, achieving change is ultimately dependent on learning. Clearly, the actors will differ and the type of learning required will vary. The adoption of a systematic approach to planning and the application of theory should produce a clear specification of what type of learning is required and by whom. For

Table 7.1   Targets of change and strategies for different ecological levels

Ecological level	Targets of change	Strategies and skills
Intra-personal	Developmental processes Knowledge Attitudes Values Skills Behaviour Self-concept, self-efficacy, self-esteem	Tests and measurements Educational approaches Mass media Social marketing Skills development Resistance to peer pressure
Interpersonal	Social networks Social support Families Workgroups Peers Neighbours	Enhancing social networks Changing group norms Enhancing families Social support groups Increasing access to normative groups Peer influence
Organizational	Norms Incentives Organizational culture Management styles Organizational structure Communication networks	Organizational development Incentive programmes Process consultation Coalition development Linking agents
Community	Area economics Community resources Neighbourhood organizations Community competences Social and health services Organizational relationships Folk practices Governmental structures Formal leadership Informal leadership	Change agents Community development Community coalitions Empowerment Conflict strategies Mass media
Public policy	Legislation Policy Taxes Regulatory agencies	Mass media Policy analysis Political change Lobbying Political organizing Conflict strategies

Source: Derived from McLeroy, 1992

example, this could involve attempts to shift the attitudes of those holding the balance of power in policy development or consciousness raising and the development of community activist skills with a community group or assertiveness skills with young women. The framework developed by McLeroy (1992) (see Table 7.1) provides a useful overview. Green (2000) contends that, without a full theoretical analysis, interventions risk addressing inappropriate variables or failing to tackle the whole combination of variables required to bring about the desired effect.

A taxonomy of health learning

It is worth reiterating here our earlier definition of learning as a 'relatively permanent change in capability or disposition'. This might involve change in:

- knowledge and understanding
- ways of thinking
- beliefs
- values
- attitudes

and

- the acquisition or development of skills.

In terms of designing effective interventions for influencing learning, four key principles emerge from the seminal work of Gagne (1985):

- there are various different and separately identified types of learning and learning outcome
- learning is hierarchical – typically 'lower-order' learning outcomes must be fulfilled before higher levels of learning can be attained
- successful learning requires that learning-specific *internal* and *external* conditions be supplied – where internal conditions relate to previously acquired capabilities and dispositions and external conditions are provided by the deliberate organization of external events to facilitate learning
- those who seek to influence learning – via persuasion, training, education and so on – must check that the necessary internal conditions have been met and then provide the appropriate external conditions by using the right educational methods for the situation.

The simplest classification of learning has been mentioned in Chapter 3, which categorizes it as cognitive (concerned with knowledge and beliefs), affective (concerned with values and feelings), and conative (concerned with purposeful action and change).

Learning also includes the development of skills. The term 'skill' is often used in a general sense merely to indicate a high level of competence. Three kinds of skill are of particular relevance to health promotion. These are: psycho-motor, social interaction and problem-solving or decision-making skills.

The cognitive domain

A detailed technical analysis of cognitive learning is beyond the scope of this chapter. At a common-sense level, it is clear that a distinction may be made between the rote learning of facts and acquiring deeper levels of understanding. While factual data may be useful, understanding is necessary for the transfer of learning and its application to problem solving. As we noted in Chapter 3, beliefs are best conceptualized as cognitive constructs and, as indicated in our discussion of the HAM, perhaps the most important goal of health education is to create or modify health-related beliefs.

Cognitive skills – problem solving and decision making

Problem solving is usually categorized as a cognitive skill. For instance, Gagne (1985) defines it primarily as a 'cognitive strategy' that 'enables the learner to select appropriate information and skills and to decide when and how to apply them in attempting to solve the problem'.

Problem-solving ability can be enhanced through two main types of learning – first, the acquisition of new principles and associated concepts and, second, the development of generalizable problem-solving skills. For instance, consider the case of diabetic labourers working on building sites. Two problems they face are finding ways to inject themselves at work and eat regularly and appropriately. Forward planning might allow them to come up with a workable solution. Furthermore, a thorough understanding of the need to balance dietary intake, exercise and insulin will enable them to have greater control over their lifestyle. This learning can be generalized so that they can successfully apply problem-solving skills in a variety of different situations. However, such transfer of learning is only likely to occur where there is a good deal of similarity and common ground between the different types of problem to be solved.

As mentioned above, it is difficult in practice to distinguish between problem-solving skills, social interaction skills and decision-making skills. They all tend to be viewed as part and parcel of 'life skills' (or 'action competences') that form an integral part of education for empowerment. They will be discussed more fully in the context of critical health education later in this chapter.

Decision making is closely related to problem solving and the terms are often used synonymously. Decision making is frequently conceptualized as rational, but as we noted in the discussion of the HAM, may also be influenced by emotional and social pressures. Janis and Mann (1977) distinguish between 'cold' decisions taken in a calm detached state and 'hot' decisions which involve issues that matter more to the individual and are hence more emotionally charged. These include issues of immediate safety as well as longer-term issues such as the choice of a lifetime partner. The Conflict Model of Decision Making (Janis and Mann, 1977; see also Horan, 1977; Newman and Brown, 1996) focuses on these decisions that matter. The model is based on the tension between maintaining and changing current behaviour. Three main groups of influence have a bearing on the quality of decision making – awareness of the risk associated with current activity (and indeed change); recognition that there may be a better alternative; the amount of time to assess alternatives. Depending on the mix between these variables, five different patterns emerge which influence the way information is processed and decisions taken, as outlined below:

- **Unconflicted inertia** – no serious risk is recognized with current behaviour, therefore there is little stress associated with continuing.
- **Unconflicted change** – serious risk is recognized with continuing current behaviour and none with change, therefore little stress is associated with change.
- **Defensive avoidance** – serious risk is associated both with current activity and change, with no hope of a better solution, therefore stress is high. Decision making may be cut short or postponed.

- **Hypervigilance** – the risks of changing and not changing are both recognized, but there is insufficient time to pursue all options. Stress is high (akin to panic) and decisions may be taken on partial information, or responsibility delegated to others.
- **Vigilance** – the ideal when there is recognition of the risk of continuing current behaviour and ample time to appraise the alternatives.

High quality, vigilant decision making involves:

- seeking out a wide range of alternatives
- carefully assessing the known risks and costs associated with each, as well as any benefits
- searching for additional information
- reassessing the alternatives in the light of new information
- planning implementation including contingency plans to deal with anticipated risks.

Before moving on to affective learning, we will briefly consider other types of skill development.

Psycho-motor skills

The relevance of psycho-motor (or motor) skills to health education is doubtless self-evident. They range from simple to complex and the following examples will serve to illustrate this particular kind of learning:

- competence in cardio-pulmonary resuscitation
- use of a toothbrush for the efficient removal of plaque
- using a condom.

Social interaction skills

The skills involved in interacting with other people are fundamental to social health. Furthermore, capabilities such as assertiveness are of importance in empowering individuals and groups and increasing the likelihood of their gaining control over their lives and the political systems that govern them. Health literacy, as we noted in Chapter 3, involves the acquisition of cognitive and social skills to obtain, understand and use health information along with the motivation to do so.

There is an important parallel with psycho-motor skills learning – as the late Michael Argyle, one of the key authorities in researching social interaction, has amply demonstrated. Indeed, in the 1960s, he made particular reference to a 'motor skills model' of social interaction (Argyle, 1978), shown in Figure 7.3. Social interaction skills, like psycho-motor skills, involve accurate perception of and response to both external environmental cues and internal proprioceptive cues. In learning to drive a car, the learner must respond appropriately to visual information about the road situation and to those muscular sensations involved in controlling the steering wheel. Similarly, socially skilled communicators will accurately interpret the non-verbal cues provided by other people – such as facial expressions – and, at the same time, will be in control of their own non-verbal responses, such as gesture and tone of voice. A socially skilled person makes an appropriate choice from a wide repertoire of

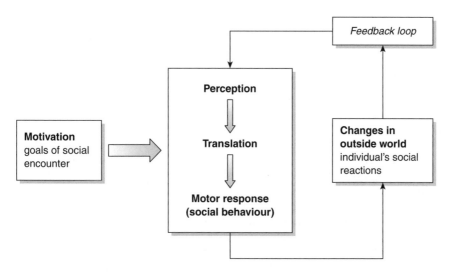

Figure 7.3   Motor skills model of social interaction (after Argyle and Kendon, 1967)

Table 7.2   Key features of non-verbal communication (NVC)

Channel	Examples
Proxemics	Personal space, territory, body orientation, seating arrangement, body angle
Haptics (touch)	Playful, ritualistic, aggressive, affection
Chronemics (time)	Waiting time, punctuality, duration, urgency
Kinesics	Direction of gaze, facial expression, smiling, gestures, head movements, posture, gait
Physical appearance	Body shape, weight, height, hair and skin colour, clothing, cosmetics, adornments
Vocalics	Tempo, pitch, loudness, dialect, fluency, pauses, articulation, breathiness
Artefacts	Volume of space, size, ventilation, furniture arrangement, decor, lighting, temperature

potential responses on the basis of incoming interpersonal information, then he or she reacts in the most appropriate way.

It will be apparent that the ability to interpret and use non-verbal communication (NVC) is also of central importance to the acquisition of social interaction skills. For instance, respect, empathy and genuineness have been described as the 'holy trinity' of counselling. It is relatively easy to *say* the right things, but a lack of genuineness or empathy is readily revealed by what has been called 'non-verbal leakage'. NVC is of paramount importance in communicating feeling and attitudes. Numerous studies have demonstrated, for example, that when there is a contradiction between verbal and non-verbal messages, the non-verbal is more powerful. A verbal expression of interest can so easily be undermined by tone of voice and facial expression. Table 7.2

sets out some of the key features of NVC. For a review of social skills training, readers are advised to consult Trower et al. (1978) and, particularly, Dickson et al. (1989).

The affective domain

We now turn our attention to affective learning. The different aspects of affective learning are encapsulated in the motivation system of the health action model (HAM), discussed in Chapter 3. These include values and attitudes along with emotional states and associated drives such as fear. The model identifies two sets of influences on motivation. The first operates via the mediation of the belief system, while the second provides a direct input into the motivation system itself – for instance, by using emotive imagery to generate anxiety or other feelings directly.

We have consistently challenged the use of coercive methods to achieve the goals of health promotion on the grounds that it conflicts with empowerment. Yet the use of 'persuasion' and 'attitude change' techniques has traditionally been associated with coercion. Clearly, any attempt to change attitudes should be subject to ethical scrutiny.

It is important to distinguish between *deliberate* attempts to persuade and coerce by generating emotional responses and, on the other, those situations in which emotional responses occur as an almost *incidental* effect of learning. For instance, to the extent that people come to understand and accept the reality of personal risk or realize the ways in which social injustice is associated with ill health, it is quite probable that emotions will be roused. In the first instance, it may involve anxiety or concern over personal vulnerability. In the second instance, it may result in feelings of indignation and commitment to take political action. Moreover, while the deliberate use of attitude-change techniques are most closely associated with attempts to manipulate rather than empower – and, thus, are ethically dubious – there is, paradoxically perhaps, a situation where persuasion rather than empowerment is justified. As we noted in Chapter 6, the use of persuasion is standard practice for lobbyists and other political activists seeking to bring about changes in health-related policy. It is presumably acceptable, therefore, for health promotion activists to become skilled in the use of attitude-change techniques. There is, of course, a difference in degree between, say, a community health worker utilizing persuasive techniques with a local politician and advertisers' use of persuasive messages to persuade young children to pester their parents to buy them unhealthy products.

The conative domain

Conative learning is associated with proactive behaviour and is central to self-direction and autonomy. Conation influences whether cognition (knowing) and affect (feeling) result in behaviour. It is an essential, yet often overlooked, aspect of learning in general and health-related learning. It clearly has particular relevance to empowerment. Huitt (1999) attributes this lack of attention to the fact that it is so closely enmeshed with the cognitive and affective domains. However, some key aspects derived from Huitt's review are summarized in Table 7.3 and the implications for health education are identified.

Huitt draws on Bandura's social cognitive theory to identify past experience of achieving mastery as an important influence on self-efficacy and a predictor of future

Table 7.3   Aspects of conative ability

Aspects of conation	Sub-components	Implications for health education
Direction	Awareness of human needs	Exercises to enable individuals to identify their own needs
	Visions and dreams – awareness of what is possible	Raise awareness of possibilities
	Making choices	Develop decision-making capability
	Setting goals:	Encourage setting difficult but attainable goals
	• Mastery goals – concerned with developing competence	Develop self-efficacy beliefs
	• Performance goals – concerned with achieving outcomes	
	• Social goals – concerned with the individual fitting into a group or group performance	
	Develop plans	Enable individuals to develop a clear view of their desired specific outcome and to identify the steps to take to achieve this
		Encourage commitment – ideally writing plans down or at least telling others of intentions
Energizing	Potential for positive returns from the effort must outweigh any negative aspects of change and fear of failure	Attention to early gains
		Attention to self-efficacy beliefs
Persistence	Linked to the level of motivation, expectation of success, high self-esteem, previous experience of success or failure, praise for effort and public display of achievement of outcomes	Praise
		Reinforcement
		Public acknowledgement of success

Source: Based on Huitt (1999)

success. Enabling learners to be successful and experience success can therefore help individuals to be successful in other areas of their lives.

FACILITATING LEARNING

The purpose of health education is to achieve health- or illness-related learning and the task of the health educator is to marshal those methods that provide the conditions needed to ensure efficient learning. There is a considerable repertoire of methods on which to draw, backed up by numerous manuals on their detailed application. Educational methods range from formal, top-down, didactic ones to participatory methods and the target from a single individual (as in the one-to-one encounter) to whole populations. Figure 7.4 attempts to order selected educational methods with respect to the size of the target group and the level of participation. Our purpose here is not to review the utility of specific methods, but, rather, to draw out key principles

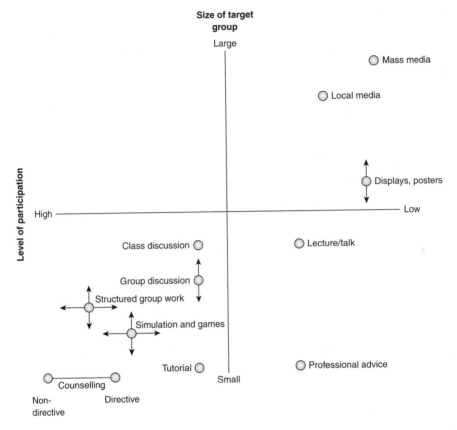

Figure 7.4   Health education methods

that will inform approaches to promoting learning. Clearly, ideology will have some influence but, over and above such concerns, the selection of an appropriate mix of activities will be governed by:

- the type of learning required
- the characteristics of the learner
- the characteristics of the teacher
- other factors – context, availability of resources, time, feasibility.

The need for participation

A fundamental principle of Carl Rogers' approach to education is that we cannot teach, but can only facilitate learning (Barrett-Lennard, 1998). Work undertaken some time ago at the Industrial Training Research Unit at the University of Wales Institute of Science and Technology (Belbin et al., 1981) found that poor learners were characterized by a passive attitude towards learning, used a narrow range of learning methods and frequently inappropriate methods. The active involvement of the learner is therefore essential – encapsulated in the maxim:

> I hear and I forget
> I see and I remember
> I do and I understand.

Not only does active involvement maximize learning, it also contributes to empowerment. It underpins life and health skills teaching and the development of action competences and, as we will see, is central to Freirean approaches. A digest on National Standards for School Health Education in the USA (Summerfield, 1995: 3) affirmed that:

> the most effective methods of instruction in health are student-centred approaches: hands-on activities, cooperative learning techniques, and activities that include problem solving and peer instruction to help students develop skills in decision making, communication, setting goals, resistance to peer pressure, and stress management.

Similarly, in England and Wales, curriculum guidance on health education (National Curriculum Council, 1990: 7) stated:

> While there is a place for direct teaching, the use of audio-visual aids, visits and contributions from visitors, much of the teaching of health education will be based on the active involvement of pupils.

The guidance goes on to list methods suited to this active learning approach (see the box).

Teaching methods suited to active learning

- Games
- Simulations
- Case studies
- Role plays
- Problem-solving exercises
- Questionnaires
- Surveys
- Open-ended questions and sentences
- Groupwork of various kinds

National Curriculum Council, 1990

Tones (1993) attributes the shift from formal to more participatory methods of health education over the last 50 years to ideological considerations – notably a commitment to participation and empowerment. A further influence has been the development of theory that has supported their use and evidence of greater effectiveness of these

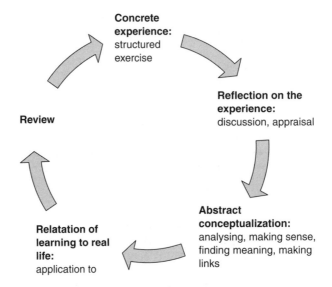

Figure 7.5   The experiential learning cycle (after Kolb et al., 1971)

approaches. This shift has been accompanied by an increasing awareness of the importance of process as well as content. Furthermore, there has been a gradual move away from seeing learners as empty vessels to be filled with knowledge towards acknowledging and building on their prior learning and experience. The role of the health educator has correspondingly changed from expert to facilitator and the role of the learner from passive acceptance to active involvement.

A number of different terms refer to methods for achieving active learning – 'experiential learning', 'participatory learning', 'active methods', 'student-centred learning', 'confluent education'.

The notion of the 'experiential learning cycle' derives from the work of Kolb et al. (1971), shown in Figure 7.5. The cycle begins with a new experience or some device for drawing on the learner's past experience, followed by reflection and sharing of learning. This is followed by processing, which involves an analysis of the learning in cognitive, affective and conative domains and its relevance. The learner may appreciate the need for additional skills or knowledge. Anderson (undated) suggests that the role of the 'teacher' or the trainer at this point, can be to provide input that is outside the experience of the group. Provided the input is linked to the learner's needs and experiences, this is not seen as compromising commitment to active learning. Finally, if it is to be meaningful, learning should be applied to the real world, with opportunities for subsequent reflection and review.

Ryder and Campbell (1988) draw on the work of Settle and Wise (1986) and Brandes and Ginnis (1986) to contrast experiential methods with more traditional approaches, as shown in Table 7.4.

The mainstay of experiential learning is structured groupwork. The effective functioning of groups as a means of promoting learning is dependent on good

Table 7.4 Contrasting teaching styles

Experiential	Traditional
Role of learner active: • negotiating content • negotiating ground rules • communicating with other learners • displaying work • management of resources • maintaining behaviour as agreed	Role of learner passive: • teacher determines content • teacher sets rules • talk between learners discouraged • teacher controls display of work • teacher manages resources • teacher maintains standards of discipline
Teacher as facilitator or guide	Teacher as expert – transmits knowledge
Uses active methods: • collaboration • groupwork • starts from what the learner knows or is concerned about • not confined to the classroom • regular review and evaluation (of self and group performance)	Focuses on memory, practice and rote learning: • individual and competitive • concerned with academic standards • confined to the classroom • emphasis on tests and grades
Subject matter integrated	Traditional boundaries between subjects
Uses the intrinsic motivation of students	Motivation external and based on rewards and punishments
Focuses equally on cognitive and affective domains	The affective domain is neglected
Students encouraged to reflect on, and talk about, their learning	Little attention to learning behaviour
Process is valued as well as content	Little attention is paid to process

Source: After Ryder and Campbell (1988)

facilitation and attention to two broad areas of functioning, although there may be some overlap – namely:

- task-orientated functions – designed to achieve specific leaning
- group-orientated functions – designed to build and maintain the cohesiveness of the group.

The selection of appropriate methods is made easier if learning objectives are formulated precisely – and optimally if framed as behavioural objectives (that is, they specify what the learner will be expected to be able to *do*, under what conditions and over what timescale – see Hubley, 1993) – for example:

Following the groupwork session, participants will:

- when asked, list the main routes of transmission of HIV (knowledge)
- demonstrate to the group, using a condom and banana as visual aids, the correct way to put on a condom (skills)
- in a role-play situation, use three different strategies to refuse pressure to have unprotected sex (skills).

M Memorizing	U Understanding	D Doing
Facts	Concepts	Skills
Methods of learning		
Association: • visual • verbal Repetition: • written • verbal • aura • visual Self-testing	Listening Questioning: • ourselves • others Discussing Comparing Solving problems Acting out Experiencing Imagining	Practice Demonstration Teaching others Trial and error Doing and reviewing

Figure 7.6 Appropriate learning strategies (after Belbin et al., 1981, in Anderson, undated)

Clearly, the development of knowledge will require different methods from those used in the development of skills. Belbin et al. (1981) produced a simple taxonomy using the acronym MUD to distinguish between appropriate methods for memorizing, understanding and doing (see Figure 7.6). The development of skills requires the opportunity to learn from the practical experience of trying out the skill. Complex skills may need to be broken down into components and, once each of these has been mastered, grouped together to achieve competence in relation to the whole.

Ryder and Campbell observe that, in experiential learning, the affective and cognitive domains tend to flow together to achieve confluent learning. They cite Rogers' (1983) view that the personal involvement in learning central to experiential approaches necessarily touches feelings, even when it has a cognitive orientation or the impetus comes from outside.

In some instances, it will be possible to identify detailed and specific learning objectives, leading to sharply focused interventions. Furthermore, as we will note below, messages can be tailored with increasing sophistication to match the characteristics and precise learning needs of individuals. This effectively demands greater precision – and potentially control – on the part of those responsible for designing interventions. This approach may be more relevant in the context of vertical rather than horizontal programmes and is certainly less applicable when the objectives are couched in broader terms, such as the development of empowerment or social capital. While it would, in principle, be possible to conduct a detailed analysis of the constructs of empowerment and put together an appropriate collection of methods to address each of these, an alternative approach would be to use methods that are more wide-ranging and have a multidimensional impact. These allow the learner to take from the learning experience whatever meets his or her own learning needs and achieve confluence between the different learning domains rather than compartmentalization of knowledge. The potential of the creative arts for contributing to community health has begun to receive attention and we will conclude this section with a brief consideration of their role in health promotion.

The creative arts and health promotion

The capacity of the arts in general to enhance wellbeing is well recognized, as is their capacity to improve communication by increasing aesthetic appeal and arousing emotions and, indeed, to raise awareness of oppression and social inequality. However, in contrast to the visual and performing arts, the explicit use of the arts to promote health is characterized by participation and active involvement in the creative process – hence, the term creative arts projects (see the box for a couple of examples).

Examples of Walsall's community arts team projects

Truck Stop Rock

A singer/songwriter interviewed 42 truck drivers and turned the findings into a song entitled '10, 20, 30, 40, 50 a day', about a chain-smoking truck driver. It was felt that the music provided a way into talking to the truck drivers and that they were much more open than they would have been talking to health professionals.

Issues raised included the problems of healthy eating and exercising when on the road and the problem of loneliness. As well as the song raising the awareness of drivers, haulage companies are beginning to talk about work-based clinics.

Comedy

Theatre workers went into 'spit and sawdust' working men's clubs where they helped members and health workers to devise a comedy routine on men's health – including men's reluctance to admit that they are ill and see a doctor. When the routine was performed, nurses were available to carry out health checks and 200 of the 300 men who saw the routine had a check-up.

The follow-on project is developing a cabaret along similar lines.

Carlisle, 2002

The materials produced may take a number of forms – from posters and leaflets to banners, artworks, music and drama performances – and may or may not have an additional educational purpose. For example, a giant mobile developed by pupils on the importance of clean air and the polluting effects of smoking displayed in a school entrance hall communicated the message to the whole school community without a word being said. However, it is important to distinguish the effects it had on two major constituencies. Those who developed the mobile benefited from having participated in the creative process. On the other hand, for those who had not taken part, it was simply a means of communicating a message – comparable to professionally developed materials, albeit benefiting from local relevance and a certain homophily between the designers and the audience (Green and Tones, 2000).

Participating in creative arts projects will contribute to the learning of those taking part in a number of ways. Learning may be concerned with substantive content and developing knowledge, raising awareness and changing attitudes. Additionally, the process itself may be empowering as a result of its developing skills, which, together with the concrete evidence provided by the successful production of materials, will contribute to self-efficacy beliefs, confidence and a sense of control. Clearly, if others recognize the value of the 'products' or artefacts, then there will be further enhancement of self-esteem. In short, it will influence the basic constructs of empowerment (and indeed health literacy). The development of these attributes will apply outside the boundaries of the arts projects to more general areas of people's lives. If those involved feel that they are achieving worthwhile goals, then the meaningfulness of their involvement will lead to an enhanced sense of coherence (Antonovsky, 1984) and the achievement of salutogenic goals. Furthermore, contact with other individuals may generate a sense of social connectedness, contributing to a sense of community and the development of social capital. An illustration of these effects deriving from a community arts project is provided in the box.

Case study: lantern festival

A lantern festival was one of a number of creative arts activities set up to tackle social isolation in a new and rapidly growing housing development. The area was characterized by an influx of newcomers, the absence of an infrastructure to support social cohesion and a consequent lack of a sense of community, little social connection and the absence of lay support networks.

Lantern-making workshops to prepare for the 'festival' were led by a professional artist in the local doctor's surgery and schools.

The event itself was highly symbolic and involved a procession around the houses, lighting the streets and drawing people out of the isolation of their own homes, and culminated in a party. From small beginnings with only 15 families taking part in 1990, it went on to become an annual event and, by 1996, 400 families were involved.

Preparation for the festival brought people together in a mutually dependent way. Over and above the social contact, people developed skills – not just in making lanterns, but also all the other activities needed to make the event a success – and frequently passed these skills on to others. Involvement contributed to self-efficacy beliefs, self-confidence, self-esteem and a sense of community. There are clear links between this and the main elements of a sense of community identified by McMillan and Chavis (1986: 6):

(Continued)

(Continued)

- membership – a feeling of belonging
- influence – making a difference
- integration and fulfillment of needs
- shared emotional connection – 'the commitment and belief that members have shared and will share history, common places, time together, and similar experiences'.

Rigler, 1996; Tones and Green, 1999

A review of good practice in community-based 'arts for health' projects commissioned (HEA, 1999a) noted that the quality of the artefacts was of central importance in generating a sense of pride and influencing the extent to which the participants took the activity seriously. It also saw no conflict between an emphasis on the rigorous teaching of basic skills (and, if necessary, correcting them) and commitment to participation. Rather, it found that this contributed to the quality of the artefacts. The participatory models that were found to work best were 'well-structured, well-organized and specifically related to the acquisition of skills or of resources for self-expression' (HEA, 1999b: 5).

Creative arts projects have also been used to explore health needs. Their capacity to put people in touch with their feelings and engage their imagination to envisage how things *might* be is particularly valuable in this regard. The materials produced can themselves have a powerful advocacy function. For example, one community arts project involved different generations in depicting their views about the health of their community through the medium of art. A display of their work was described by one observer as 'chilling' (Tones and Green, 1999). It communicated to policy makers the fear of crime and going out at night, the problem of traffic and the issue of loneliness more powerfully than perhaps any other medium could.

The creative arts can also have a role in developing awareness of issues and the motivation to take action about them. This critical consciousness raising is a central concern of Freirian approaches and liberatory education which will be discussed more fully later. In particular, creative arts can contribute to critical reflection on reality and the belief that change is possible. The use of theatre has been popular in this regard and notably forum theatre, which is attributed to Freire's fellow Brazilian, Augusto Boal.

In forum theatre, members of the audience with ideas for change go on stage and act out their ideas, becoming transformed from spectators in to 'spectactors'. This enables the audience to envisage change, act it out and reflect collectively on outcomes and potentially empowers the audience to take social action. The use of theatre to achieve social change has been referred to as 'theatre of the oppressed' (Paterson, 1999).

Theatre is becoming more widely used in health education – for example, in HIV, AIDS and drugs education. However, theatre can only be included under the umbrella of 'creative arts' if the audience actually participates. There is a well recognized repertoire of theatre in education (TIE) activities to encourage such participation – role play, simulation and problem solving. The use of theatre can be particularly relevant to developing empathy, clarifying values and exploring moral dilemmas.

Day (2002) provides an example of the use of forum theatre in schools to enable young people to put themselves in other people's shoes and try out moral behaviour with regard to the homeless and refugees. Ball (1994) identifies a number of commonalities between health education and theatre to provide a philosophical basis for theatre in health education. These are:

- the need for affective as well as cognitive involvement
- utilization of active learning
- concern to explore attitudes and values
- role-taking
- self-empowerment
- concern with what it is to be human
- a community dimension.

In summary, creative arts offer the potential for enhancing learning in relation to both cognitive and affective issues and have a particular capacity for developing individual empowerment, a sense of community and social capital.

The HEA (1999b: 2) review of arts for health projects proposes a broad range of possible outcomes, which would include:

- enhanced motivation – within the project and in the participants' lives generally
- greater social connectedness
- people perceiving that they have a more positive outlook on life
- reduced sense of fear, isolation and anxiety
- increased confidence, sociability and self-esteem.

Participation was identified as a key element linking the arts activity with health outcomes and the principal contributions of projects (HEA, 1999b) were seen as:

- development of interpersonal skills
- opportunities to make new friends
- increased involvement.

The study by Comedia (Matarasso, 2001) identified some 50 social impacts deriving from participation in arts projects. While they might all influence empowerment and health in a general way – for example, in terms of enhanced educational opportunity and increased employability – a selection of immediate relevance to health is provided in the box.

Selected social impacts of arts projects

- Increase people's confidence and sense of self-worth
- Provide a forum to explore personal rights and responsibilities
- Reduce isolation by helping people to make friends
- Develop community networks and sociability
- Build community organizational capacity

(Continued)

(Continued)

- Encourage local self-reliance and project management
- Help people extend control over their own lives
- Be a means of gaining insight into political and social ideas
- Facilitate effective public consultation and participation
- Strengthen community cooperation and networking
- Help feel a sense of belonging and involvement
- Create community tradition in new towns or neighbourhoods
- Help community groups to raise their vision beyond the immediate

After Matarasso, 2001: 159–60

Characteristics of the learner

Using educational approaches and content suited to the age and stage of development of the learner is fundamental to good educational practice. The notion of 'cognitive matching' (Bruner, 1971) underpins the concept of the spiral curriculum, which introduces ideas in a simple form and revisits them with increasing sophistication and levels of abstraction as the learner matures.

The work of Piaget has been influential in relation to understanding the cognitive development of young people. While a full discussion of developmental psychology is beyond the scope of this chapter, a summary of Piaget's developmental stages is provided in the box. Ryder and Campbell (1988: 101) characterize the development in reasoning through these stages as:

- taking things at face value
- exploring relationships between tangible entities
- recognizing relationships involving unseen events
- abstract conceptualization.

Approximately 20 per cent of adults do not reach the stage of having developed full formal operational thought and the capacity for hypothetico-deductive reasoning.

Piaget's developmental stages

Sensory-motor	0 – 1½/2 years
Pre-operational	1½/2 – 7/8 years
Concrete operations	7/8 – 11/12 years
Formal operations	11/12 – 15 years/adolescence

Piaget and Inhelder, 1969

As well as consideration of the stage of development, the need to 'start where children are' has informed the development of school-based health education projects. For example, 'Health for Life' (HEA, 1989) was based on extensive research into children's conceptualization of health and health-related issues. It used the 'draw and write' technique which, despite some recent criticism (Backett-Milburn and McKie, 1999), has proved valuable in enabling children to express their views (Williams et al., 1989a; Williams et al., 1989b; and Pridmore, 1996).

While the relevance of didactic methods for teaching young people is questionable, the use of these methods is particularly inappropriate to the needs of adult learners. The idea that adult learners have different learning needs to those of children and the use of the term 'andragogy' to refer to adult learning has been associated particularly with the work of Knowles, who built on the earlier work of Lindeman dating back to the 1920s. Knowles' seminal text, *The Adult Learner: A Neglected Species*, was published in 1973 and is now in its fifth edition (Knowles et al., 1998).

The core principles of adult learning that can usefully inform the development of health education interventions for adults are:

- adulthood is associated with a self concept of being self-directed and in control – adults therefore need to feel responsible for their own learning
- adults have large reserves of experience on which to draw, so learning should utilize this experience
- the willingness to learn is associated with its contribution to carrying out roles and coping with life situations
- the relevance of the learning needs to be clear and immediate rather than deferred
- the motivation to learn is internal and linked to coping with real-life situations.

Over and above the stage of development, within any group there will be differences in preferred learning style, linked to personality.

There are several different instruments for assessing learning styles. Perhaps the best-known of these is the Myers-Briggs Type Indicator (MBTI), developed from Jungian theory and first published in 1962 (see the box). The 'Health Skills Project' used a simpler version, based on two dimensions – 'doer-intuiter' and 'feeler-thinker' – to identify four basic personality types as shown in Figure 7.7.

The Myers-Briggs Type Indicator

On the basis of the four dimensions below, there are 16 possible combinations:

- extraversion (E) v introversion (I)
- seeing (S) v intuition (N)
- thinking (T) v feeling (F)
- judging (J) v perceptive (P).

Teaching methods will vary in their appeal according to an individual's learning style. For example, extraverts (spelt as in Myers-Briggs) often learn by explaining to others, whereas this may not appeal to introverts who prefer to have a logical framework to order their learning. The tendency is also to teach in one's own preferred

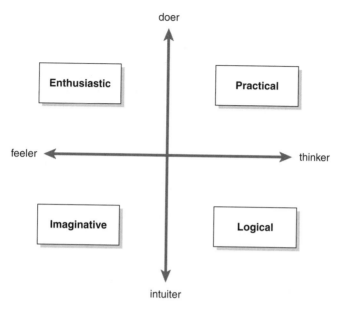

Figure 7.7   Personality types (based on Anderson, undated)

learning style, but, given that in any group there is likely to be a mix of styles, variety is essential to ensure that the needs of all learners are met at some point.

In addition to developmental and personality factors, the effective facilitation of learning also requires sensitivity to issues such as gender, ethnicity and culture. Such sensitivity is central to the core values of health promotion, as well as being instrumental to success. Clearly, educational interventions are more likely to be effective if they are perceived to be personally relevant. A key consideration is the extent to which interventions are designed to suit the specific requirements of individuals – that is, the extent to which they are targeted or individually tailored.

Targeting and tailoring

Reference to social marketing theory would indicate that health education is more likely to be effective if there is a good fit between the message and the characteristics of the target group.

The notion of 'targeting' applies the principle of market segmentation to the design of materials for specific subgroups in relation to particular characteristics, such as age, gender, ethnicity, social class, occupation. In contrast, 'tailoring' refers to adapting the educational approach to meet the needs of the individual (Kreuter and Skinner, 2000):

> any combination of information or change strategies intended to reach one specific person, based on characteristics that are unique to that person, related to the outcome of interest, and have been derived from an individual assessment.

Kreuter and Skinner provide a useful analogy, comparing off-the-peg clothing (targeted) and bespoke tailored clothing (tailored).

Holt et al. (2000) identify a number of empirical studies that have demonstrated the superior effectiveness of tailored materials, but also note that factors such as personality and locus of control play a part. They suggest that developments in information technology offer considerable potential for tailoring health education materials to suit individual psycho-social and behavioural profiles. However, their effectiveness will ultimately be dependent upon being able to identify, with some precision, all relevant variables.

Kreuter et al. (2000) contend that tailoring is currently relatively crude and its comparative advantage over targeted or mass-produced material has not been fully revealed. The most commonly used approach is 'behavioural construct' tailoring, which draws on theories of behaviour. Constructs such as stages of readiness to change, identification of barriers to change and self-efficacy for changing behaviour are frequently used. As yet, however, there is little advantage over well-designed non-tailor-made materials that address these constructs. This could, perhaps, be expected, given that little attention is paid to cultural and personality factors. Kreuter et al. suggest that the inclusion of a wider range of variables, including non-behavioural factors such as preferred learning styles, would increase the relative advantage over non-tailored material.

The stages of change model (Prochaska and DiClemente, 1983) offers the possibility of designing interventions that are appropriate to the various stages, and can be applied to both targeting and tailoring. Miilunpalo et al. (2000) describe the basic elements of the model as being:

- **motivational** – concerned with attitudinal readiness, intention building and decision making
- **behavioural** – tentative performance up to regular practice.

Progression through the stages of change from pre-contemplation to contemplation, preparation, action and maintenance is marked by a shift in emphasis from motivation to behaviour. Figure 7.8, developed from Cabanero-Verzosa (1996), indicates how learning needs will vary depending on the stage an individual or group is at.

A key concern is whether or not the individuals at a particular stage are, in fact, a homogeneous group. Miilunpalo et al. (2000), for example, suggest that, in relation to physical activity, the precontemplation stage may be subdivided into two groups – 'negative precontemplation' in which individuals may be consciously resistant to change, and 'neutral precontemplation', in which little consideration, if any, has been given to the possibility of change. The findings of Dijkstra and de Vries (2000) also confirm that the precise tailoring of smoking interventions would need to recognize that there are subgroups within the precontemplation stage.

The principles of targeting and tailoring support the development of interventions to suit particular needs. Clearly, tailoring is more challenging in that messages are designed for individuals and depend on an analysis of pertinent individual-level factors. However, we should also note that the process of checking out individual characteristics is integral to the interchange that takes place in one-to-one counselling.

Stages of change

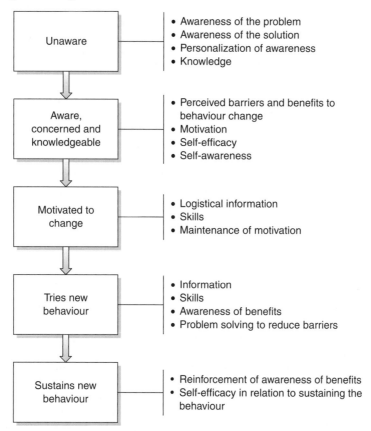

Figure 7.8 Learning needs and stages of change

For example, 'motivational interviewing' (Rollnick et al., 1992) was developed as a means of helping people to work through ambivalence about behaviour change and is structured to respond to different needs at the various stages of change. Furthermore, well-designed experiential groupwork has the capacity to achieve highly individualized learning outcomes. However, one-to-one counselling or small groupwork may only be feasible in relatively small-scale projects. Targeting and tailoring offer the potential for improving the effectiveness of larger-scale programmes by means of individualization of messages.

Characteristics of the teacher

Social learning theory – which has been a major influence on the development of health education interventions – recognizes the contribution of the characteristics of the teacher to the learning process through 'modelling'. Ryder and Campbell (1988) cite McPhail et al.'s (1972) research for the 'Lifeline Project' on moral education, which found that young people were critical of being told how to behave when this was not reflected in the behaviour of their teachers. This applies to a whole range of 'teacher' behaviour, but is particularly pertinent to fundamental principles such as integrity and respect.

These principles are also integral to Rogerian and Freirian approaches. Rogers refers to 'realness' or 'genuineness' as a key attribute of a facilitator, along with acceptance, trust and valuing of the learner. He also notes the importance of being able to empathize with the learner (Rogers, 1967). The 'Health Skills Project' (Anderson, undated) used the acronym REG to summarize these requirements – respect, empathy and genuineness. To avoid any gender bias, it also offered RUBY – respect, understanding and be yourself. Reference to Freire's message to the coordinator of a 'cultural circle' in the box reveals similar views about what makes a good coordinator. More information about cultural (or culture) circles is provided later in this chapter (page 344) and in Chapter 9 (page 427).

To the coordinator of a cultural circle

In order to be able to be a good coordinator for a 'cultural circle', you need, above all, to have faith in man [*sic*], to believe in his possibility to create, to change things. You need to love. You must be convinced that the fundamental effort of education is the liberation of man, and never his 'domestication'. You must be convinced that this liberation takes place to the extent that man reflects upon himself in relationship to the world in which, and with which, he lives ... A cultural circle is a live and creative dialogue, in which everyone knows some things and does not know others, in which all seek, together, to know more. This is why you, as the coordinator of a cultural circle, must be humble, so that you can grow with the group, instead of losing your humility and claiming to direct the group, once it is animated.

Freire, 1972: 61

Over and above the content of any message, the style of interaction adopted by the health educator can contribute to empowerment to a greater or lesser extent as shown in Figure 7.9.

Our discussion of communication of innovations theory in Chapter 3 also highlighted the importance of the change agent's characteristics, particularly the principle of homophily (Rogers and Shoemaker, 1971). The growth in popularity of peer education in recent years is premised on the notion that peer educators will automatically have more credibility than other teachers and that people learn best from those who share similar characteristics. Given the growth in popularity of peer education in recent years and the development of what Frankham (1998) refers to as the 'dogma' of peer education, we will briefly consider its relevance for enhancing learning.

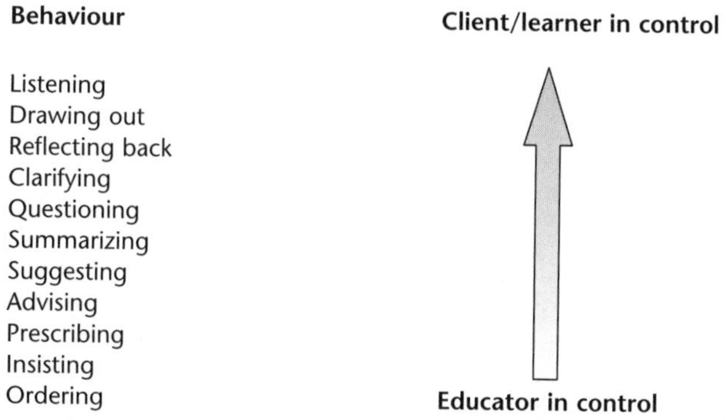

Behaviour   **Client/learner in control**

Listening
Drawing out
Reflecting back
Clarifying
Questioning
Summarizing
Suggesting
Advising
Prescribing
Insisting
Ordering   **Educator in control**

Figure 7.9   Empowering or de-powering educator behaviour

Peer education

Peer education has been defined (Sciacca, 1987, in Milburn, 1995: 407) as 'the teaching or sharing of health information, values and behaviours by members of similar age or status groups'.

There is some variation in the terminology associated with peer education (see the box), which Milburn (1995) suggests signals subtle difference in roles and styles of working – particularly regarding the level of control and authority.

Peer education – the terminology

- Peer education
- Peer training
- Peer tutoring
- Peer counselling
- Peer facilitation
- Peer leader
- Peer helper.

A number of claims have been put forward to support the use of peer education. Turner and Shepherd (1999) identify the following. Peers are:

- a credible source of information
- acceptable sources
- more successful than professionals
- able to reinforce learning through ongoing contact
- positive role models.

Peer education:

- is empowering for those involved
- is beneficial to those involved

- utilizes established channels of communication
- provides access to those who are hard to reach through conventional methods
- is more cost-effective.

Furthermore, the use of peers as educators may enable groups to be reached who would ordinarily be difficult to access. The 'Child-to-Child' movement (Aarons and Hawes, 1979; and Hawes and Scotchmer, 1993), for example, which was set up in 1979 to mark the International Year of the Child and has subsequently expanded to involve more than 70 countries, recognized the potential of children to reach younger brothers and sisters, families, out-of-school youth and the wider community. A key principle of the programme is that action should be based on children's own observations and conclusions and that there is the opportunity for reflection on action. The assumptions underpinning the programme are summarized in the box and they are particularly concerned with the benefits for those taking part.

The 'child-to-child' programme

Basic assumptions:

- Primary education becomes more effective if it is linked closely to things that matter most to children and their families and communities.
- That education in and out of school should be linked as closely as possible so that learning becomes part of life.
- That children have the will, skill and motivation to help educate each other – and can be trusted to do so.

Hawes, in Hubley, 1993: 181

Clearly, peer education is more than a device for educating 'others'. Those who take on the role of peer educator stand to benefit from improved knowledge, skills, self-confidence, self-esteem and standing within their social group. This may derive from the training they receive, but may also stem from their role as 'educators', as summed up in the aphorism *qui docet discit* – he who teaches learns!

Fundamental questions in the development of peer education projects concern who is a peer and who defines this, together with the related issue of how peer leaders/educators are selected. Age has often been seen as a key determining factor – many projects have focused on young people and there has been interest in peer education programmes for senior citizens. However, other commonalities may also be relevant, such as common status (being a pupil in a school, for example, or a member of the workforce of a company) or experience that is relevant to the programme (such as breastfeeding or quitting smoking).

Turner and Shepherd (1999) note that the principles of social learning theory (Bandura, 1986) would suggest that the effectiveness of peers as educators will be influenced by their standing within the group. Michell's (1997) study, for example, revealed that 13-year-olds have a very clear grasp of their social map and the pecking order within it. In many instances, peer education projects have paid little regard to this and peer leaders have been volunteers or, alternatively, selected as 'suitable' by project coordinators. In contrast, others have included provision for groups to select their own peer leaders – such as the 'Smoking and Me' project – (HEA, 1991) – or have even used systematic network measurement techniques for identifying those individuals who are most centrally and socially connected (Larkey et al., 1999).

Peer education projects fall into two broad groups: those that tap into existing social and friendship groups and those in which groups are more artificially constructed for the purpose of 'receiving' peer education (Milburn, 1995). Furthermore, the method of delivery can be through 'formal', planned sessions or informal social contacts. There is no rigid boundary between the two approaches and, whichever is used, the involvement of peer leaders in the selection and development of methods helps to ensure relevance. Backett-Milburn and Wilson (2000) noted that young peer leaders were aware of the advantages of informal approaches in that they could choose the right moment and adapt what they said to suit the needs and experience of the person they were speaking to.

Turner and Shepherd (1999) assert that many peer education projects lack a sound theoretical base and that, given its diversity, peer education will need to draw on a number of theories. The box provides a list of the theories that they identify as being relevant to peer education.

Theories relevant to peer education

- Social learning theory (Bandura, 1986)
- Social inoculation theory (Duryea, 1991)
- Role theory (Sarbin and Allen, 1968)
- Communication of innovations theory (Rogers and Shoemaker, 1971)
- Differential association theory (Sutherland and Cressy, 1960)
- Subculture theories (for example, Cohen, 1955).

A review of the effectiveness of peer education interventions with young people (EPPI-Centre, 1999) found some evidence of their producing positive changes in behaviour. However, it noted that the lack of methodologically sound evaluations meant that the intuitive appeal of the approach was not backed up by much hard evidence. Similarly, Frankham (1998) expresses concern about the way that claims made for the relevance of peer education for young people are repeated as dogma without being substantiated by research evidence. She takes the 'key tenets of the faith' and subjects them to critical scrutiny in relation to peer sex education.

- The claim that young people talk openly to each other about sensitive issues, such as sex and drugs:
    - little factual learning takes place between friends and the content of conversations in groups is limited by the need for girls to protect their reputation and boys to be seen as 'one of the lads'

- young people are more likely to turn to friends for advice than parents, but friends are not necessarily seen as credible sources
- giving advice to friends can be seen as 'breaking the unwritten rules of friendship'.

- The claim that peer pressure is a powerful influence on young people's behaviour:

  - young people appear to choose peer groups that suit their preferences, rather than their preferences being dictated by the group (a view endorsed by Michell, 1997) and allegiance to such groups is concerned more with identity formation than being pressured to fit in
  - the portrayal of young people as a homogeneous group or, alternatively, as members of stable subgroups, appears to be erroneous – there are several subgroups and the boundaries between them are relatively fluid.

- The claim that peer education is participatory and empowering:

  - peer educators facilitating sessions with groups may feel the need to set themselves up as experts and model the behaviour of those who trained them
  - peer educators often see maintaining control of the group as part of their purpose – it may, therefore, be difficult for young people to use participatory forms of education
  - peer leaders may not be representative of young people generally and the agenda that they set may reflect their own needs rather than responding to others' needs.

Frankham (1998: 190) concludes that peer education 'seems to sit (often uneasily) at the intersection of two cultural domains – the professional cultures of health education and the peer cultures of young people who are the intended recipients'. Young peer educators are confronted with the challenge of bridging both worlds. She also sees an inherent contradiction in submitting to peer influence in the context of peer education, but resisting it in other areas of life. Milburn (1995) also notes the ethical dilemma of placing peer educators in a position in which they feel responsible for influencing behaviour when the principal determinants of that behaviour are social and environmental factors beyond their control.

The EPPI-Centre review (1999) called for a clearer understanding of the processes involved in peer education and the ways in which they impact on outcomes. Backett-Milburn and Wilson (2000) concur with this view. Their process evaluation of a young people's peer education project noted the reluctance of adults to relinquish control to young people and that this was attributed to concerns about passing on inaccurate information. They emphasize the importance of distinguishing between concerns that can be addressed by means of the quality of the training given to peer educators and the more general concerns about handing over power to young people, such as fear that they might talk about sensitive subjects, such as sex, in ways that adults might not approve of.

The insight into the peer education process provided by Backett-Milburn and Wilson (2000) allows us to identify a number of key factors that impinge on it:

- **the recruitment process** – the extent to which peer educators are recognized as natural leaders within the group
- **setting** – the formality of the setting and consistency with the informality of peer education, the opportunity to maintain protected time for peer education, enthusiasm and commitment of staff, good liaison and evidence of success as a motivational factor

- **organizational context** – role of various stakeholders in decision making and the extent to which power rests with the peer educators themselves
- **personal development of participants** – the development of the skills and acquisition of information needed to be peer educators
- **ongoing support for peer educators** – whether or not this is in place as they carry out their role.

Peer education offers the opportunity to capitalize on the shared characteristics of 'the teacher' and the 'learner' to enhance learning. However, it needs to be based on a full understanding of the social context in which it takes place (Milburn, 1995; Frankham, 1998). Furthermore, to maximize its potential, the peer educators need to be fully involved in developing the agenda and making decisions about process and content rather than merely acting as agents delivering a professionally defined programme.

Other factors

Educational interventions will necessarily be influenced by contextual factors. These can be thought of as falling into two broad groups. First, there is a set of factors that will determine the practical feasibility and acceptability of different methods and this is largely outside the control of those responsible for implementing interventions. This would include the availability of resources (financial and other), size of the target group, experience of the staff and so on. Cultural and professional norms will also influence the acceptability of programmes – to both recipients and key gatekeepers.

Second, there are several contextual factors that health educators might consciously seek to control to enhance the quality of the learning environment. Ryder and Campbell (1988) see part of the educator's role as that of providing an appropriate learning climate. This can include psycho-social as well as physical factors. Some of the key factors identified by the 'Health Skills Projects' are listed in the box.

Selected key factors that influence the learning climate

Physical factors

- Space – appropriate for comfort and closeness
- Seating – to allow eye contact with all participants
- Bright, stimulating environment
- Protected from outside distractions
- Convenient timing for participants – and sufficient for the task

Psycho-social factors

- Appropriate style of leadership
- Negotiated ground rules

(Continued)

(Continued)

- Appropriate size of group
- Unfinished business' or members' mental baggage cleared away
- Any conflict is brought into the open and dealt with
- Clear expectations and purpose
- Reactions of the group are checked out regularly
- High levels of trust and cooperation
- Constructive feedback
- Appropriate use of humour
- Interactions between all members of the group – and leader's attention shared evenly
- Good group management skills.

Adapted from Anderson, undated

We have considered the various elements which impact on learning. We now turn our attention to consider attitude change in more detail and then go on to conclude the chapter by considering critical health education and strategies for social and political change.

PERSUASION AND ATTITUDE CHANGE

Attitude change has occupied a prominent part in traditional health education as health educators have searched for ways to persuade individuals to adopt healthy practices. We have already noted the potential conflict with empowerment.

We identified earlier four interrelated motivational constructs featured in the HAM – drives, emotional states, values and attitudes. Attitudes were conceptualized as specific rather than general and deriving from 'higher-order' motives. Emotional states can result from basic drives, such as fear, while attitudes emerge from values. Both values and emotional states may influence attitudes – that is, determine the importance attached to certain objects, people or courses of action. Rokeach (1965: 80) emphasizes the importance of hierarchy:

A grown person probably has tens of thousands of beliefs, hundreds of attitudes, but only dozens of values. A value system is an hierarchical organization — a rank ordering — of ideals or values in terms of importance. To one person truth, beauty and freedom may be at the top of the list, and thrift, order and cleanliness at the bottom: to another person, the order may be reversed.

The significance of the hierarchical dimension for health education is doubtless obvious. Given the enduring power of values, attempts to change attitudes may be ineffectual or counterproductive *unless* these underlying values are acknowledged. The enduring nature of values established during primary socialization is illustrated in the box.

Enduring values – the law of primacy

Give me a child for the first seven years, and you may do what you like with him afterwards.

Jesuit maxim, cited by the UK National
Child Development Survey (Davie et al., 1972)

Apparently, the Communist regime in the USSR required an additional year.

Give us the child for eight years, and it will be a Bolshevist forever.

Lenin, speech to the Commissars of
Education, Moscow, 1923 (Lenin, 1969)

From the plethora of theories, we will use the Yale-Hovland model as a framework for this relatively brief analysis of attitude change. It was explicitly designed to develop efficient ways to influence public attitudes. An early concern, for example, was with finding the best way to convince American servicemen – in the middle of a general euphoria over victory in Europe in the Second World War – about the (erroneously) anticipated long and difficult struggle with Japan.

The general framework of the approach derived from Lasswell's (1948) recommendation to examine: 'who says what to whom via what medium and with what effect?'. Hovland et al., therefore, researched the relative contributions of the message, the source of the message, the characteristics of the audience for whom the message was intended and the nature of the action resulting from the process of attitude change (for a more complete review of the early work, see Hovland et al., 1953).

Figure 7.10 has been adapted from McGuire and colleagues (McGuire, 1989) who have made a major contribution to the development of the Yale-Hovland model and its evaluation. Our adaptation aims to accommodate the model to the analysis of communication and learning presented at the beginning of this chapter and to our subsequent discussions of mass media and methods in Chapter 8. The figure provides a matrix relating source, message and audience factors to the various key stages in the communication and learning processes. The idea of a 'channel' has also been included and allows us to consider and contrast the relative roles of mass media and inter-personal methods.

Figure 7.10 not only shows the various stages in the communication to learning process, but gives an indication of the relative ease or difficulty in achieving the necessary change. Certain stages are of greater relevance to typical attitude-change initiatives. For instance, although it would be essential to understand and remember information associated with attitude change and the actions ensuing from that, the learning of principles and concepts would not normally be of concern – indeed, genuine understanding might militate against persuasive pressure! The cells in the matrix (following McGuire's formulation) can be used as a convenient evaluation device in the form of a checklist to assess to what extent various intermediate, process and outcome objectives have been achieved.

Level of difficulty in achieving each stage **LOW** ↑	Communication characteristics				
	Communication and learning outcomes	Source	Message	Channel	Audience
	Exposure to message				
	Attention: • attract • sustain				
	Perception/interpretation				
	Recall of essential information				
	Understanding of message*				
	Beliefs: Accept truth of message				
	Positive attitude to recommended action				
	Acquisition of skills**				
	Adopt approved action				
↓ **HIGH**	Sustain approved action				

Key: * In-depth understanding is rarely needed – it may even be a disadvantage!
       ** The acquisition of skills would be incidental to an attitude-change programme.

Figure 7.10   Relationship of major communication variables to the communication to learning process (adapted from McGuire, 1989)

Before proceeding further, a cautionary note should be introduced. Psychology is replete with studies that have demonstrated statistically significant effects of particular approaches to attitude change. These are most commonly achieved in the laboratory. The effect is real, but their applicability to real life may be limited, insignificant or completely irrelevant. This is typically due to the fact that minor effects revealed in the laboratory are completely submerged by much more powerful real-life influences – often in combination with other equally powerful influences. As a full discussion of the complicated field of attitude theory is beyond the scope of this book, a selection of factors that do seem to be relevant to real concerns for health promoters will be outlined below.

Source factors

Reference was made earlier in this chapter to the role of the communicator or 'source' in both the communication and learning process. The real and perceived characteristics of the source are considered to be pivotal in the attitude-change endeavour and have been extensively researched. We must content ourselves here with merely listing the most important features identified by research:

- power and leadership
- source credibility:
  - legitimate and expert authority
  - perceived trustworthiness
  - source attractiveness
- homophily and referent authority
- group pressure.

Message factors

Considerable research effort has also been devoted to the relative effectiveness of different ways of presenting persuasive messages in producing changes in attitudes and behaviour. Five key aspects emerge:

- repetition, primacy and recency
- sidedness
- the use of positive affect
- fear appeal
- arousal.

Repetition, primacy and recency

One of the most common assumptions is that, generally speaking, the more frequently a message is repeated, the more effective it will be. By contrast, a good deal of laboratory evidence has been accumulated to demonstrate that a message delivered first or last in a sequence of different persuasive attempts is more likely to be influential.

Sidedness

An important consideration in the construction of the message is whether greater attitude change would be produced by a one-sided persuasive argument or if both sides were presented. This is referred to as 'sidedness'. The outcome would seem to depend on the audience. If it is well educated, intelligent or both, a two-sided approach should be adopted. If the audience is uneducated/unintelligent or it could be guaranteed that it would never be exposed to the counter-arguments, the one-sided approach might be used.

One of the findings to emerge from the work on sidedness was that people exposed to two-sided messages who already favoured the advocated measure (such as fluoridation), maintained their support, even when exposed to attempts to change their commitment. This phenomenon provoked not only further research, but also, ultimately, resulted in deliberate measures designed to 'inoculate' individuals against attempts to persuade them to adopt unhealthy practices, such as smoking. McGuire (1970: 37, cited by Pfau, 1995: 100) played a substantial role in this research and his position is clear:

> We can develop belief resistance in people as we develop disease resistance in bio-logically overprotected man or animal, by exposing the person to a weak dose of the attacking material strong enough to stimulate his defences but not strong enough to overwhelm him.

Pfau distinguishes inoculation 'proper' from *'social inoculation'*. He defines this latter as an approach that uses a combination of strategies designed to anticipate future anti-health arguments and pressures. The essence of the technique involves 'threat and *refutational preemption'*. The threat might be an anticipated challenge to existing attitudes, such as a threat to existing negative feelings about smoking. Pfau (1995: 103–4) summarizes the situation as follows:

> adolescents commence the transition from the primary to middle grades with strong attitudes opposing smoking. 'They have *already been persuaded* that smoking is bad' (Pfau and Van Bockern, 1994: 420) ... these attitudes often do not persist during the two years following the transition from elementary school to junior high school. The large majority of adolescents began this transition with negative attitudes toward smoking, but those attitudes deteriorated during the next two years. Adolescents grew more positive towards smoking, more positive towards peer smoking, and less likely to overtly resist smoking (Pfau and Van Bockern, 1994) ... at the point of tran-sition from the primary to middle school grades, adolescents possess reasonably established attitudes opposing smoking. What is needed at this point is a strategy to protect these antismoking attitudes from deterioration during the turbulent middle school years.

'Refutational preemption' is the proposed strategy. Individuals are made aware that there may at some future point be an 'attack' on their attitude which is vulnerable to change, i.e. there is a threat. They are exposed to weak negative messages. The process of countering these messages prepares them to deal with any subsequent exposure 'in real life' to potentially stronger messages. Typically, the approach has involved peer-leadership as discussed earlier in this chapter, peer modelling and videos.

Interestingly, the analogy of immunization can be further extended to include the use of 'booster' doses of education to maintain immunity. Botvin (1984) added these to his successful 'life skills training model', which demonstrated a reduction of 50 per cent or more in school students' recruitment to smoking.

A further consideration is whether or not greater attitude change would result when conclusions are explicitly drawn for the audience or when the audience is allowed to reach its own conclusions on the basis of the information included in the message. Again, it seems to depend on the audience. A more informed or intelligent audience would demonstrate a greater shift in opinion and attitude by drawing its own conclusions, whereas less experienced or less intelligent people might need to be told much more directly what they should believe!

Positive affect

The majority of communications will produce an affective reaction of some kind in the audience, whether revulsion, humour or just interest. However, we are concerned here with *deliberate* attempts to design a message to produce affective responses that will lead to attitude and behaviour change.

Two important situations merit discussion. These relate to generating *positive* affect – that is, creating positive emotional responses in the audience – and, by contrast, the use of negative affect – an approach more usually described as 'fear appeal'. Although there is some evidence for the success of approaches seeking to generate positive affect (see, for instance, Monahan, 1995; Zajonc, 1980; and Murphy and Zajonc, 1993), most research has concentrated on the creation of negative affect in the form of fear appeal. Monahan (1995) observes that there is little evidence to suggest that positive affect can change strongly held negative attitudes. A qualitative study by Lewis et al. (2007) into the views of drivers about road safety messages found that emotional messages were judged to be more effective than rational, information-giving messages in attracting attention, maintaining interest and being remembered. Further, they found that positive emotional appeals accompanied by the provision of strategies can contribute to the perceived persuasiveness of messages and would have a role in road safety education – an area traditionally dominated by the use of fear appeal.

In all events, there can be no real objection to using positive messages as, at the very least, they attract attention and are likely to be more memorable than dry, factual data. Provided, of course, that messages fulfil the ethical requirement of not being economical with the truth. In contrast, there may be fundamental objections to the use of negative affect in changing attitudes and behaviour, irrespective of the question of effectiveness.

Fear appeal – creating negative affect

The use of fear appeal in general – and for health promotion in particular – is still highly controversial, both regarding the ethics of its use and its relative effectiveness. Research into the use of fear to bring about an attitude change was famously triggered by the work of Janis and Feshbach (1953). Their influential study into the use of different levels of fear appeal in persuading individuals to brush their teeth regularly seemed to demonstrate that there was actually an inverse relationship between level of fear and (reported) tooth-brushing behaviour. Those experiencing a very high level of fear were least likely of all to change their dental practices, while those experiencing a relatively neutral presentation were most likely to report an increase in dental hygiene. The results of those receiving the mid-level of arousal were, naturally, located somewhere in the middle!

Innumerable studies into the use of fear followed this counter-intuitive result, but none replicated Janis and Feshbach's results, though they did demonstrate the complexity of the situation. Indeed, Hale and Dillard (1995: 70, 78), in a review, appear to be convinced about the effectiveness of using negative affect.

> Three quantitative reviews (Boster and Mongeau, 1984; Mongeau, in press; Sutton, 1982) all show reliable and compelling evidence that fear is persuasive. [These] and several newer studies, perhaps the best of the lot, concluded that perceived fear and the attitude of the target were positively correlated, as were perceived fear and behavior ... abandoning the use of fear would be to abandon an effective persuasive strategy ... Fear appeals have enormous persuasive potential and can promote better health.

A more recent meta analysis (Witte and Allen, 2000) indicates that strong fear appeals are more persuasive than weak. The results also indicate that fear appeals appear to 'motivate adaptive danger control actions such as message acceptance and maladaptive fear control actions such as defensive avoidance or reactance' (Witte and Allen, 2000: 591). To avoid such defensive responses, strong fear appeals need to be accompanied by equally strong efficacy messages, including both response efficacy and self-efficacy. Witte and Allen conclude that 'Fear appears to be a great motivator as long as individuals believe they are able to protect themselves' (2000: 607). This conclusion is echoed in the National Cancer Institute's (undated) guidance on developing health communications (see box). Nonetheless, it acknowledges that the effectiveness of such approaches is widely debated. Furthermore, from an ethical standpoint, fear appeal should only be used when it is possible for individuals to take action to reduce the threat and associated fear. It is, therefore, incumbent on those using fear appeal to ensure that the audience is aware of and able to undertake required action.

Threat and fear appeal

To be effective, a threat appeal should include:

- A compelling threat of physical or social harm
- Evidence that the intended audience is personally vulnerable to the threat
- Solutions that are both easy to perform (i.e., intended audience members believe they have the ability to take the action) and effective (i.e., taking the action will eliminate the threat)

National Cancer Institute, undated: 61

Key questions concerning the use of fear appeal are:

- What exactly do we mean by fear?
- What level of arousal justifies using the word 'fear'?
- What is the effect of given levels of fear?
- How do audience factors influence perceptions of fear-arousing stimuli and reactions to these?

Witte and Allen (2000: 591) define fear as a 'negatively valenced emotion, accompanied by a high level of arousal'. It is distinct from, but closely influenced by, the related cognitive variable 'perceived threat', itself made up of two dimensions – perceived severity and perceived susceptibility.

Arousal

Some insight into the effect of arousal on learning is provided by the so-called 'Yerkes–Dodson law' (Yerkes and Dodson, 1908). It has also been applied in the attitude change field, although some workers have questioned the generalizability of this phenomenon (Winton, 1987, for example). In short, the Yerkes–Dodson law demonstrated that both a very low level of arousal and a very high level of arousal resulted in poor learning. This is entirely consistent with common sense – an individual who is totally disinterested will neither be motivated to learn nor to perform. An individual whose state of arousal has resulted in an attack of panic and is paralysed with terror will also not be in a position to learn or act. Moreover, complicated and intricate learning tasks are disrupted at lower levels of arousal (i.e. more easily) than simple tasks.

The Yerkes–Dodson Law is often described in terms of an inverted 'U' curve where some optimal level of arousal figures at the top of the 'U'. While the effect of extreme levels of arousal is unchallengeable, it is more problematic finding evidence of a smooth curve – although a nicely constructed piece of research by Krisher et al. (1973) into the uptake of mumps vaccination did produce results consistent with the curvilinear predictions of Yerkes–Dodson.

It also seems clear that the shape of the curve or the level of 'threshold arousal' will depend on the nature of the proposed actions. For example, presenting immediate action opportunities that are perceived to be attainable would increase the likelihood that a relatively high level of arousal might lead to action. Without such opportunities, high levels of arousal can backfire and be associated with denial and avoidance.

Again, as noted above by Leventhal (1980), audience characteristics would also be important. High self-esteem and self-efficacy certainly tend to result in vigilance and people having such characteristics would be able to cope with relatively high levels of arousal without resorting to defensive behaviour or succumbing to paralysis! However, Witte and Allen (2000) note that personality factors and demographic characteristics such as gender appear to have little influence on the way fear appeal messages are processed.

Audience factors

The final aspect of attitude change under consideration here is the contribution of the audience itself. As emphasized in Chapter 4, detailed information about the target group of a health promotion intervention should be an essential part of effective planning. Attitude change theory, too, urges persuaders to know their audience. It is, self-evidently, important to know people's existing attitudes and the values from which they are derived.

At a macro level, there is evidence that there may be social class differences in reactions to persuasive messages (see our discussion of social marketing in Chapter 8).

At the micro level, there also seems to be some variation in individuals' suggestibility, which can render them more amenable to persuasive influences. Moreover, reference has already been made to the importance of self-esteem in several contexts. It is generally accepted that individuals having high self-esteem (and belief in their capacity to control their lives) are better able to make vigilant decisions following exposure to health education messages – whether or not they use fear appeal. Yet high self-esteem may confer some protection against persuasive attempts to change attitudes. To pursue this further, we will consider the notions of cognitive dissonance and reactance.

Dissonance and reactance

Cognitive dissonance theory (Festinger, 1957) is one of a group of so-called 'balance theories' that contend that a state of imbalance between psychological components, such as belief, attitude and behaviour, results in an uncomfortable state of dissonance and creates pressure for change. Accordingly, an imbalance between one's beliefs and attitudes and behaviour should result in a change of one or more of these in order to restore 'consistency' or 'congruence'. In Chapter 3, we located 'dissonance' in the motivation system of the HAM, equating it with such emotional states as guilt and anxiety in terms of its capacity to influence intentions to act. For instance, a smoker who is health-conscious and concerned about his family's welfare is likely to experience a high degree of dissonance about exposing his family to passive smoking. Clearly, this dissonance could readily be resolved by quitting or only smoking outdoors. However, smokers who feel unable to do this often resort instead to denying the risk.

Festinger and colleagues performed an ingenious series of experiments demonstrating the effects of dissonance and attempts to reduce it (for a comprehensive account, see Aronson, 1976). One example will suffice to indicate the lengths to which people will go to achieve dissonance reduction. Aronson was concerned with the way dissonance reduction was related to the justification of cruelty in the context of significant US policy decisions. He described a notorious situation at Kent State University when four students were shot and killed by the Ohio National Guard during a demonstration against the Vietnam War. According to Aronson (1976: 121, citing Michener, 1971), the guilt and dissonance experienced by the community in relation to respectable students could only be assuaged by modifying beliefs and attitudes so that the killing could be justified:

> several rumors quickly spread to the effect that: (1) both of the slain women were pregnant (and therefore, by implication, were oversexed and wanton); (2) the bodies of all four students were crawling with lice; and (3) the victims were so ridden with syphilis that they would have been dead in two weeks anyway.

Two of the more important generalizations from research are, first of all, that dissonance is proportional to the seriousness of the issue that creates the dissonance. Second, it seems clear that the level of dissonance is also proportional to the level of self-esteem. Someone having high self-esteem who 'acts out of character' or in contradiction to moral values that he or she has espoused is likely to experience such discomfort that the mere contemplation of the act is likely to result in its rejection.

The second audience characteristic of relevance to attitude change is 'reactance'. One of the important facts of life is that most people do not like to be bludgeoned into taking action, even if they believe it is for their own good. Brehm (1966: 9), who studied this characteristic extensively, provides a key definition.

> Reactance is the motivational state experienced whenever any behaviour that the audience might have freely engaged in is either eliminated or threatened; its aim is to re-establish freedom of choice. Freedom will be re-established by changing attitude in a direction away from the advocated position.

Sutherland's commentary on the negative reaction to the historic establishment of the (English) General Board of Health in 1850 provides a common-sense example of reactance in the field of public health. In his words:

> Many local 'interests', however, resented the central power of the Board, and particularly Chadwick's thrustful, tactless methods, and these probably led *The Times* to comment: 'We prefer to take the chance of cholera and the rest than to be bullied into health'. (Sutherland, 1979: 7)

The objections to healthy public policy illustrated above clearly involved a clash of political and economic interests. This, though, is not the same as the psychological phenomenon of reactance. The 'law of reactance' developed by Brehm and colleagues (Brehm, 1966; and Brehm and Brehm, 1981) makes the simple, but highly relevant, point that, whenever individuals feel that their freedom of action will be curtailed, they tend to react against the message and its source. Dowd (2002) distinguishes reactance and resistance. Resistance always involves some sort of obstructive or oppositional behaviour. In contrast, reactance is characterized as a motivational psychological attribute which may be expressed through developing a negative attitude to the message (even if the individual was initially favourably disposed towards it) or through behaviour. Crossley (2002) cites as an example the tendency among gay men to reject safer sex messages despite being made aware – through years of intensive health education – of the risks they might incur.

Resistance to health promotion messages is held to involve:

1 a challenge to the idea that 'unhealthy' or ' risky behaviours' are 'irrational';
2 a recharacterisation of 'unhealthy' or 'risky' behaviours as an intelligible response and assessment of 'risks' in a risk laden society;
3 an argument for the need to understand such activities rather than simply explain them away;
4 a characterisation of the 'dominant' health promotion perspective as dominant or 'hegemonic' – a perspective which imposes and/or prioritises a medical/scientific 'world view' over the 'lay' perspective. (Crossley, 2002: 108)

Some individuals appear to have a greater tendency to be oppositional than others. For instance, Dowd (2002) indentifies an association between reactance and Type A behaviour linked to the individual's need to have a sense of control. This is somewhat paradoxical given the emphasis of health promotion on enabling individuals to have control over their health.

Even the best intentioned health education can therefore backfire, resulting in reactance and oppositional behaviour – either at an individual or a group level. What, then, is the best strategy to adopt? Crossley argues that greater exposure to 'accurate' information fails to engage with alternative 'world views' about risk. Rather than repeating simple messages, she advocates critical discussion and debate which allow concerns to be brought out into the open.

Channels and methods for attitude change

Reference was made earlier to the importance of taking into account both the channel used to deliver persuasive messages and the particular methods used. Mass media are often deliberately employed to change attitudes by utilizing influential sources and messages that are deliberately tailored to specific audiences and take account of their characteristics. We will consider the role of mass media more fully in Chapter 8. However, we should note the limited capacity of mass media to bring about attitude change. Participatory and interpersonal methods, as discussed earlier, offer much more potential in this regard.

In contrast to the persuasive role of health education, we will now turn our attention to its more radical and emancipatory role – arguably, its most important function for health promotion. We use 'critical health education' as a generic term to describe this function.

CRITICAL HEALTH EDUCATION – STRATEGIES FOR SOCIAL AND POLITICAL CHANGE

Although critical education incorporates all of the categories of learning described in this chapter, its major concerns are essentially affective. It aims to motivate people to take action to achieve the various goals that characterize health promotion's ideological commitments. The key difference between critical education and the kinds of attitude change that we have discussed above is that the attitudes to be changed relate to achieving social and political outcomes that, in turn, address issues of equity and social justice. It is therefore closely linked to empowerment and informed by critical theory. It is essentially political (see box).

Health promotion as a political enterprise

Health promotion is an inherently political enterprise. Not only is it largely funded by government, but the very nature of its activity suggests shifts in power. Its recognition that peace, shelter, food, income, a stable ecosystem, sustainable resources, social justice and equity are basic prerequisites for health implies major redistribution in power and wealth.

(Signal, 1998: 257)

In discussing the application of critical theory to research, Tones and Tilford (2001: 164) cite Harvey (1990: 2), as follows:

> At the heart of critical social research is the idea that knowledge is structured by existing sets of social relations. The aim of a critical methodology is to provide knowledge which engages the prevailing social structures. These social structures are seen by critical social researchers as *oppressive* structures. [Our emphasis]

Again, discussing implications of critical theory for health promotion research, Connelly (2001: 118) leaves no doubt about the social activist goals of health promotion.

> Reality is produced and reproduced by the causal powers of generative mechanisms whether these are our activities and attitudes or our encounters with social structures. Why we should want to strengthen some or undermine other generative mechanisms emerges from the inescapable reality of making ethical and political decisions in the light of our human interest in emancipation and enlightenment.

We have emphasized the relationship between health education and healthy public policy. We have also asserted the primacy of education in achieving health promotion outcomes. Accordingly, critical health education is viewed here as potentially the most powerful means of achieving the supportive environments needed to empower choice. Although, as noted earlier in this chapter, health education can achieve individual empowerment, at this point, our focus is primarily on those empowering strategies that influence the physical, socio-economic and cultural environment. In other words, to build environments that facilitate healthy choices and remove the barriers that militate against these. There are five separately identifiable (but frequently overlapping) approaches to achieving this end:

- activism and social action
- critical consciousness raising
- providing 'life skills' and 'action competences'
- community organization
- media advocacy.

We will consider activism, social action and community organization more fully in Chapter 9 and media advocacy in Chapter 8. For the purpose of this chapter, we will focus more specifically on the contribution of education and learning.

As we explained earlier, health education is concerned with health- (or illness-) related learning. Moreover, we argued that education and policy development and implementation were mutually interdependent; it is rare to find examples where healthy public policy does not in fact involve – and, indeed, depend on – health-related learning. On the other hand, social action has not infrequently been contrasted with 'traditional' health education and its focus on individuals. Our view is that *critical* health education is the major means for achieving social action.

Persuasion and other forms of education are central to achieving change through 'non-violent disruption' exemplified by Ross and Mico (1980) as Gandhi's civil disobedience and Martin Luther King's civil rights movement. Ross and Mico also included the work of Saul Alinsky, whose radical approach is relevant to current conceptions of the social determinants of health. Alinsky's (1969, 1972) main concerns were with alienation and social disadvantage. His approach included the recruitment and training of a cadre of leaders and, in the words of Minkler and Wallerstein (1997: 243):

> This *social action organizing* emphasized redressing power imbalances by creating dissatisfaction with the status quo among the disenfranchised, building community-wide identification, and helping community members devise winnable goals and non-violent conflict strategies as means to bring about change.

For further discussion of Alinksy's approach, see Pruger and Specht (1972).

Freudenberg (1978, 1981, 1984) has been consistently associated with a radical approach. He (1984: 40) reminded us that radical action for health is not a recent phenomenon and described how, between 1910 and 1920, Dr Alice Hamilton investigated health conditions in the lead and mercury industries:

> When employers refused to allow her on their premises, she set up clinics in the back rooms of bars and social clubs. ... she also instructed them on how to protect themselves against toxic exposure and she lobbied forcefully for stricter regulations of these metals.

A flavour of activism in the field of health and safety is provided by a case study of the work of the Delaware Valley Toxics Coalition (DVTC). As Freudenberg (1984: 41) reports:

> Among their educational methods were demonstrations at polluting companies, testimony of victims of poisoning at public hearings, and written reports by scientists, physicians and epidemiologists. They developed a flair for using the media creatively. [See Chapters 6 and 8 on media advocacy.] At one city council hearing, a union member who was appearing in support of the bill sprayed an unmarked canister into the chamber. 'Stop that,' the legislators shouted, 'you're poisoning us.' The unionist replied, 'This can has only air, but everyday we have to work with chemicals we know nothing about.' His testimony made headlines in the local paper.

Critical consciousness raising – the Freirean perspective

Paulo Freire, who died in 1997, is probably the best-known advocate of a radical, libertarian approach to education for social change. His work originated with literacy programmes for impoverished cane-cutters in plantations near Recife in Brazil in 1958. He rapidly realized that de-powered individuals viewed reading and writing as alien to them. The way to achieve literacy was therefore by developing a radical challenge to poverty and the social systems that created it. Only in this way could illiterate workers be empowered. Freire's emancipatory approach has inspired not only those concerned to promote social justice, but also those who seek to promote the health of the disadvantaged. His approach mirrors the empowerment model we propose in this book in that it not only seeks to liberate people from environmental barriers derived from oppressive power structures, but also to free them from their perceptions of an 'external locus of control' revealed in 'magical thinking'.

Following our earlier discussions of the meaning of education, we can say that Freire is committed to 'true education' – that is, to voluntarism and depth of understanding rather than persuasion and propaganda. Indeed, he (1972: 43) criticizes the 'activism' of revolutionary leaders who fail to genuinely educate the populace:

> [Unless] one intends to carry out the transformation *for* the oppressed rather than *with* them ... the oppressed ... must intervene critically in the situation which surrounds them and marks them: propaganda cannot achieve this ... It is my belief that only this latter type of transformation is valid. The object in presenting these considerations is to defend the eminently pedagogical character of the revolution.

In justifying his educational approach, Freire (1972: 67) cites Mao Tse-tung:

> We should not make the change until, through our work, most of the masses have become conscious of the need and are willing and determined to carry it out ... There are two principles here: one is the actual needs of the masses rather than what we fancy they need, and the other is the wishes of the masses, who must make up their own minds instead of our making up their minds for them. (From the selected works of Mao Tse-tung, 1967)

Over and above any radical concerns, Freire's humanistic approach to education frequently includes references to the intrinsic value of people. These are essentially similar to Rogerian notions of 'unconditional positive regard' – a mainstay of non-directive counselling, which affirms that, although individuals' behaviour may be a cause for condemnation, their essential humanity must be respected. Freirean observations are also often reminiscent of the transactional analysis notion of healthy 'life positions' (Berne, 1964; Harris and Harris, 1986). It is argued that, as a result of early socialization and life experiences, individuals adopt basic attitudes to the self. There are four such positions, deriving from the extent to which people accept that they and other people are 'OK'. Turner (1978) adopted the term 'OK Corral' to describe the matrix shown in Figure 7.11.

As will probably be apparent, the 'healthy' state is depicted in the top right cell, indicating an individual belief that the people in question feel content with themselves and have good self-esteem, but also trust others and feel concern for them. In other words, we have a remarkably concise definition of mental and social health, having links to such concepts as a 'sense of coherence'.

The pedagogy – educational methods

An emancipatory curriculum such as Freire's includes both cognitive and affective factors and the pedagogical methods employed take this into account. They are concerned with creating a level of critical awareness and translating that awareness into action.

A core feature is *'conscientizacao'*, or 'conscientization' which, in the words of the translator of *Pedagogy of the Oppressed* (Freire, 1972: 16, footnote), 'refers to learning to perceive social, political, and economic contradictions, and to take action against the

| I'm OK
You're not OK | A | I'm OK
You're OK | B |
| I'm not OK
You're not OK | C | I'm not OK
You're OK | D |

Key:
A Distrustful, B Optimistic, C Despairing, D Depressed

Figure 7.11   The OK Corral (Turner, 1978: 72)

oppressive elements of reality' and is most readily translated as 'critical consciousness raising'.

The link between consciousness raising and action is defined in terms of 'praxis'. Praxis is the interactive process of reflection and action. Action without reflection is mere 'activism'; reflection without action can involve mere detached intellectualism. The method is primarily 'dialogical' and involves problem-solving approaches.

Freire compared traditional educational approaches that treat learners as empty vessels to be filled by a teacher, referred to as 'banking', with a problem-posing approach that seeks to engage learners and put them in control of their learning. The distinction between 'banking' and 'problem-posing' is not new, as we noted earlier in our analysis of rote learning, problem solving and decision making. The novelty here lies in the purpose of education – that is, it is radical, political and essentially affective.

The banking approach is not viewed merely as a technical method of teaching, but has deep ideological connotations – namely, in respect of the emphasis on the inequality of the teacher–learner relationship and the consonance between 'banking' and political domination. It is characterized as follows:

- The teacher teaches and the students are taught.
- The teacher knows everything and the students know nothing.
- The teacher thinks and the students are thought about.
- The teacher talks and the students listen – meekly.
- The teacher disciplines and the students are disciplined.
- The teacher acts and the students have the illusion of acting through the action of the teacher.
- The teacher chooses the programme content and the students (who were not consulted) adapt to it.
- The teacher confuses the authority of knowledge with his own professional authority, which he sets in opposition to the freedom of the students.
- The teacher is the subject of the learning process, while the pupils are mere objects.

The specific techniques employed by Freire in problem posing include the use of 'culture circles' – that is, informal group work. The culture circles explore their thematic universe, which is composed of a complex of generative themes that refer to key social and cultural issues. The culture circle (or 'thematic investigation circle') is presented with 'codifications of reality' – in other words, pictures or other triggers to discussion that incorporate major social issues, of which the participants are not yet conscious. The 'decoding' process works through dialogue and group members typically:

- reflect on aspects of their reality, such as poor housing
- search for a root cause of the problem
- consider implications and consequences
- devise a plan of action.

Because of its relevance to community development, we will revisit Freirean methodology in Chapter 9. It has also been adapted for a variety of health promotion purposes. For instance, Macdonald and Warren (1991) amalgamated the Freirean approach with Frankena's (1970) model for analysing the philosophical basis of educational programmes and applied this to primary healthcare (as prescribed by WHO). Figure 7.12 outlines this amalgamation.

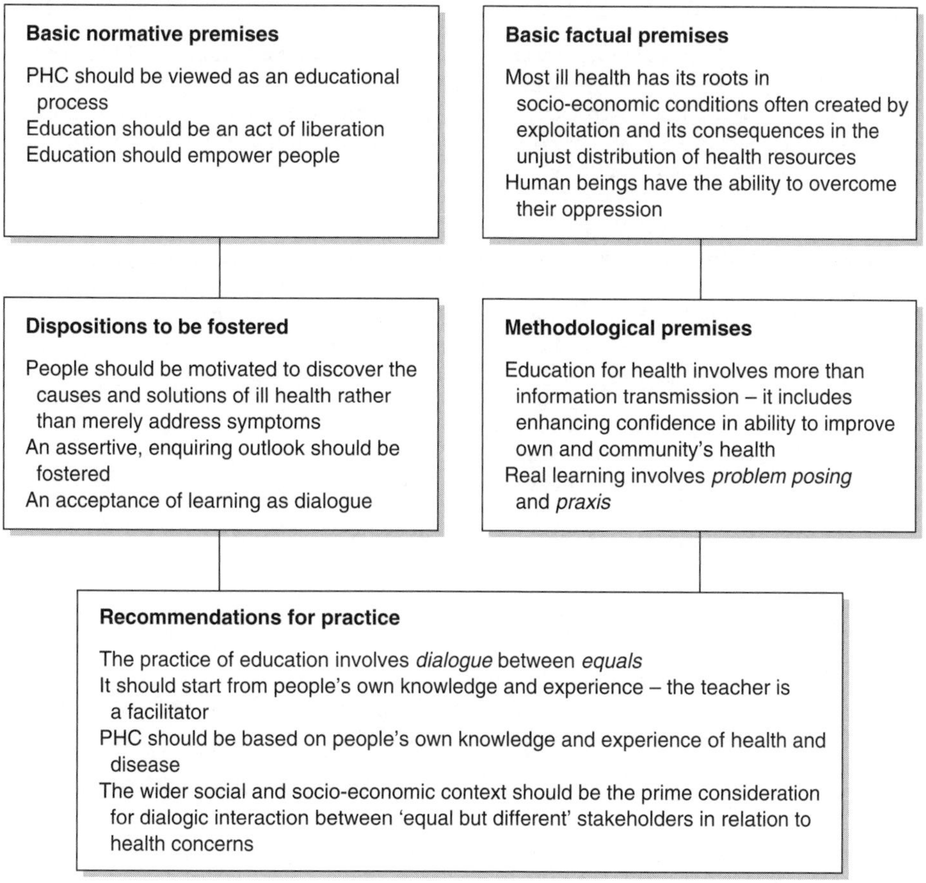

Basic normative premises

PHC should be viewed as an educational
  process
Education should be an act of liberation
Education should empower people

Basic factual premises

Most ill health has its roots in
  socio-economic conditions often created by
  exploitation and its consequences in the
  unjust distribution of health resources
Human beings have the ability to overcome
  their oppression

Dispositions to be fostered

People should be motivated to discover the
  causes and solutions of ill health rather
  than merely address symptoms
An assertive, enquiring outlook should be
  fostered
An acceptance of learning as dialogue

Methodological premises

Education for health involves more than
  information transmission – it includes
  enhancing confidence in ability to improve
  own and community's health
Real learning involves *problem posing*
  and *praxis*

Recommendations for practice

The practice of education involves *dialogue* between *equals*
It should start from people's own knowledge and experience – the teacher is
  a facilitator
PHC should be based on people's own knowledge and experience of health and
  disease
The wider social and socio-economic context should be the prime consideration
  for dialogic interaction between 'equal but different' stakeholders in relation to
  health concerns

Figure 7.12   An analysis of the application of Freirean principles to primary healthcare (PHC) using Frankena's model

One of the most substantial and detailed analyses of the application of Freirean notions to health promotion has been provided by Wallerstein and Bernstein (1988) in relation to a substance misuse prevention programme (ASAP). It is particularly interesting because it could, at first glance, be seen as 'mainstream', preventive health promotion. It is also of interest as it links Freirean theory with protection motivation theory (Rogers, 1975), a theoretical model that has frequently been applied to health education. Its emphasis throughout is on empowerment, which is linked with principles of community organization and the use of peer leaders. See the box for selected aspects of the ASAP programme.

Case study: the ASAP alcohol and substance misuse prevention programme

This involved a collaboration between an emergency centre and local schools in New Mexico.

Goal: 'to reduce excess morbidity and mortality among multi-ethnic middle and high school students' by empowering youth 'from high-risk populations to make healthier choices in their own lives, to play active political and social roles in their communities and society, and, as community participants, to effect positive changes'. (Wallerstein and Bernstein, 1988)

Groupwork: peer facilitators used a five-step questioning strategy that moved from the personal to the social and action levels. Using 'coding' devices of trigger videos (for example, depicting the life of an Indian woman who came to the emergency centre drunk and who had been raped), participants were asked to:

- describe what they could see and feel
- as a group, define the many levels of the problem
- share similar experiences from their lives
- question why this problem exists
- develop action plans to address the problem.

This discussion was guided by the acronym 'SHOWED':

S   What do we See here?
H   What is really Happening?
O   How does her story relate to Our lives?
W   Why has she become an alcoholic?
E   How can we become Empowered by our new social understanding?
D   What can we Do about these problems in our own lives?

Wallerstein and Bernstein, 1988: 386

An update on the progress of the ASAP programme (Wallerstein and Sanchez-Merki, 1994) provides an interesting theoretical model that combines the Freirean principles of 'listening, dialogue and action' with the protection motivation theory emphasis on the interaction of threat appraisal (severity and susceptibility), coping appraisal (self and response efficacy) and protective behaviour.

The programme evaluation focused on three 'self-identity changes'. Stage one was labelled 'action orientation of care' and there was evidence of changes in such measures as 'recognition (emotionally and cognitively) of one's personal connection and susceptibility to the problem'. Stage two – 'individual responsibility to act' – revealed, for example, 'evidence of increased self-efficacy to talk and help others and their own self-articulated behaviour changes reinforced their self-confidence and their own recognition of their personal changes in self perception and in perception of others'. Stage three – 'social responsibility to act' – indicated changes such as student involvement in peer education and 'tribal council presentations'.

The use of photo novella

Prior to offering a few final thoughts on Freire's radical approach, Wang and Burris' (1994) discussion of their use of the photo novella provides an illustration of how Freirean 'coding' can be part of radical empowering education. In fact, the use of photography (rather than just photographs) might be seen as an empowering operation in its own right that fits remarkably well with the general dialogical process. The photo novella ('picture stories') gives just such a function for photographs, which are used not only to document people's lives and as a basis for consciousness raising, but also as a deliberate device to influence policy.

Wang and Burris' project was located in China's Yunnan province. The use of documentary photography has a long tradition in consciousness raising, and Wang and Burris added an extra empowering dimension by providing intensive training in the use of the photo novella for 62 rural Chinese women (many of whom were illiterate) to use cameras to document their lives and circumstances. This technique proved to be especially effective in stimulating consciousness and praxis – doubtless helped by the fact that, as the authors observe, many of their older women subjects were familiar with the 'culture circles' and 'study sessions' from the days of Mao Tse-tung.

In the authors' (1994: 185) words:

> The photographs taken by the village women are an exquisite history of a place, a community, and a way of life that is unseen by most outsiders and that is undocumented by insiders and outsiders alike ... the rural Chinese women we worked with had little money, power, or status. For these ... women to photograph their lives evokes a double power: it records for future generations what is happening now, and it enables the village women to define for themselves and others, including policymakers, what is worthy to remember and where change must occur.

The Freirean perspective – problems and prospects

The ideological approach intrinsic to Freire's pedagogy is entirely consistent with the commitments and concerns of empowering health promotion. However, there are problems to be addressed by those health promoters seeking to utilize Freirean enlightenment.

For example, it has been argued that Freire's focus on overtly oppressive state control and class is not relevant to all societies and cultures. However, Freire himself argued that his approach could be adapted to fit all those situations in which there was oppression and a lack of empowerment. The techniques can, and have, been applied to different contexts – for example, as a feminist challenge to male hegemony.

However, in accordance with the ever-present threat of false consciousness, a greater challenge to Freirean ideology and practice is the suggestion that Freire's ideas have been co-opted and thus emasculated (Kidd and Kumar, 1981; Zacharakis-Jutz, 1988). Kidd and Kumar refer to the co-option threat in terms of the emergence of a 'pseudo-Freirean' perspective that appears, superficially, to have radical credentials, but, in fact, does not significantly challenge the status quo and its power structure. Referring to adult education (in all its many aspects), Kidd and Kumar (1981: 28) identify the following features of pseudoradical education:

- naming the central problem as 'poverty' rather than as 'oppression' (that is, ignoring the primacy of power)
- identifying the cause of poverty as the self-inflicted deficiency of the poor rather than oppression (that is, the problems of the poor are acknowledged but considered to be due to a 'culture of poverty' created by the shortcomings of the poor themselves)
- proposing, as treatment, to change the behaviour of the poor by means of a transmission of information and skills
- converting Freire's method into a 'neutral', apolitical classroom technique (for example, the use of group discussion – *any* kind of group discussion – rather than true dialogue leading to praxis, and the conversion of 'problem posing' into 'discovery learning' where the learner is helped to 'discover' the correct, predetermined answer to the problem)
- defining 'action' as coping activity (that is, the acquisition of personal competences other than those associated with political challenges to authority).

Freirean practice – difficult and dangerous

It should be stated that the emancipatory practices associated with critical consciousness raising and praxis are difficult to achieve and there is clearly a temptation to follow 'pseudo practices'. In certain circumstances (as Freire himself acknowledged), the pedagogy of the oppressed can be physically dangerous to both educator and learner. We are reminded of a cartoon embodying advice to would-be radical educators, that showed an ostrich with its head in the sand. The novice educators are counselled not to ignore reality in that way, but an accompanying picture showing the ostrich on the receiving end of a fusillade of rifle fire also advises them not to stick their heads above the parapet!

The effectiveness of the approach may be increased and the risks reduced if the oppressed and powerless could enlist the support of an alliance of those who possess both goodwill and power – see the empowerment model in Chapter 1. Moreover, the process of praxis may be facilitated and, again, the element of risk reduced if consciousness can be supplemented by the acquisition of key 'protective' skills and those that facilitate the attainment of power. We will now, therefore, examine this latter suggestion and consider the role of life skills and action competences as part of critical health education.

Life skills, action competences and health

Life skills teaching enjoyed a good deal of popularity in the UK, originally for personal and social education in schools and, subsequently, for health education generally (see Hopson and Scally, 1981, 1980–2). At this point, we will concern ourselves with the application of life skills teaching and action competences to critical education – inside or outside the school sector. We will further consider the relevance of life skills and action competences to the health promoting school in Chapter 10.

Hopson and Scally (1981) summarized the key elements of life skills teaching in terms of providing a 'survival and growth kit for an age of future shock':

> a school should provide a basic survival kit for young people ... they need to be taught skills like values clarification, decision making, how to cope with crises, intellectual and emotional problem solving, helping, assertiveness, relationship building, how to find appropriate information and use personal and physical resources which are available in the community. They need to be made aware of themselves, others and the world around them, in order to become more self-empowered people.

The reference to *self*-empowerment is perhaps revealing. Critics of a radical persuasion saw the reference to self as evidence that the life skills approach was effectively blind to socio-economic circumstances. While it is true that many life skills do indeed refer to individual empowerment and sometimes to an acceptance of the social status quo (for example, skills such as how to present yourself at interview in order to get a job), the following points should be noted.

- Many skills are indeed concerned with invidual growth and development and include, for example, preventive health skills, such as stress management.
- The armamentarium of life skills includes large numbers of transferable skills that may be applied to a wide variety of situations – both conformist and revolutionary! Indeed, we noted earlier that lack of literacy skills is essentially de-powering and intimately associated with Freire's adult education approaches. Again, skills involved in working with groups could be used in taking action to achieve changes in health policy.
- A number of what might be called 'skills for radicals' are incorporated in Hopson and Scally's life skills menu.

Hopson and Scally identified the skills needed in different contexts, as shown in Figure 7.13.

There is a good deal of overlap and congruence of purpose between life skills and action competences. Although Hopson and Scally's work is firmly committed to Freirean principles, the action competence approach is, on the face of it, somewhat more radical. This is doubtless due to its overt commitment to critical theory and,

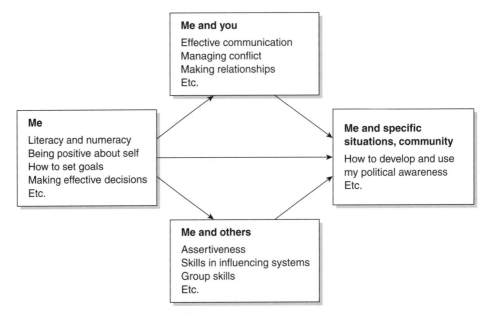

Figure 7.13   Life skills and community action (after Hopson and Scally, 1980–2)

thus, critical education. The work on action competences is very much associated with The Danish School of Education (see, for example, Jensen, 1991, 2000) and its emphasis on education for democracy in school and community. Jensen and Schnack (1997) also argue that it is central to environmental education. They see environmental problems as having their origin in society and ways of living, and that the solution requires developing the capacity to envisage alternatives and to act at a societal as well as an individual level. Fien refers to the notion of political literacy which has parallels with Freire's formulation of critical thinking and praxis, as can be seen in the following definition:

> The ultimate test of political literacy lies in creating a proclivity to action, not in achieving more theoretical analysis. The politically literate person would be capable of active participation (or positive refusal to participate) ... The highly politically literate person should be able to do more than merely imagine alternatives ... The politically literate person must be able to devise strategies for influence and for achieving change. (Crick and Lister's (1978: 41) use of the term, as cited by Fien, 1994: 43)

Wals and Jickling (2000) also support this view in their comprehensive discussion of the role of environmental education, which they consider should be essentially emancipatory with reference to social, political and economic matters and concerned with 'recognizing, evaluating and potentially transcending social norms' (see also Fien and

Table 7.5 Philosophical implications of a critical theory approach in environmental education

Type of science	Human interest served	Related ideologies	Environmental education
Seeks to explain the empirical world in terms of underlying structures and mechanisms and the events that set them in motion. This requires not only empirical analysis and hermeneutic understanding, but also theoretical accounts of the mechanisms. It is the development of valid theories of the 'abstract real' and their use in explaining concrete events and experiences that are the fundamental tasks of critical science.	The goal is *emancipation* – freeing people from the ideological (and material) constraints to their understanding. Self-determination or the full development of human potential requires knowledge, not only of the empirical and hermeneutic kind – valuable though it is – but also of the critical sciences. These aim to expose people to exactly how and why their society operates, thereby allowing them to become fully involved in its transformation to the sort of society they want. Radical, ecocentric environmentalism draws on critical science.	The critical sciences are fundamentally radical. They oppose the domination of the empirical sciences in a capitalist society, for example, because these do not tackle, and so implicitly promote, the basic inequalities on which such societies are built. They fault the hermeneutic sciences because they present a false ideology of human self-determination. The critical sciences are potentially dangerous as they would unmask society's ideology and expose its role in the promotion of vested interests that continue to exploit both people and nature.	Environmental education aims to empower people so that they can become agents of social change and sustainable development. It enables them to reflect, and act, on the structures and mechanisms that shape the social use of nature in ways prefiguring future democratic and sustainable society. Such education draws heavily on critical knowledge of the environment and education and can be termed 'education for sustainability'.

Source: Huckle, 1993: 62, cited in Fien, 1994: 24

Trainer, 1993). The philosophical implications of critical theory when applied to environmental education are listed in Table 7.5.

Mogensen (1997) describes praxis and critical thinking in environmental education as a holistic combination of feeling and reason – a dialectical process of examining situations from multiple perspectives and 'constantly challenging, querying, criticizing, breaking down parts of existing practice with the aim of reconstructing a new and alternative practice'.

According to Schnack (2000), critical thinking and praxis are essential in the context of what he calls 'the dissolution of tradition'. He also makes the point that action competence for health and environmental education should include the traits associated with C. Wright Mills' (1959) concept of 'sociological imagination' – that is, 'the capability of shifting perspective backwards and forwards between the individual, personal level, which is often seen as the purely private sphere, and the social, structural level'.

THE PRIMACY OF EDUCATION

In this chapter, we have reiterated and emphasized the point that, following the 'formula' health promotion = healthy public policy × health education, education is a sine qua non for contemporary health promotion. Indeed, it is challenging to find a situation in which education cannot be identified as being a major component in health promotion.

The importance of education for achieving sustainable development is recognized in the following quotation.

> Ethical values are the principal factor in social cohesion and, at the same time, the most effective agent of change and transformation. Achieving sustainability ... will need to be motivated by a shift in values. Without change of this kind, even the most enlightened legislation, the cleanest technology, the most sophisticated research will not succeed in steering society towards the long-term goal of sustainability. *Education in the broadest sense will by necessity play a pivotal role in bringing about the deep change required in both tangible and non-tangible ways.* [Our emphasis] (UNESCO-EPD report, 1997: 32, cited in Fien, 2000: 47)

This is equally applicable to the contribution of health education to health promotion and public health, not only in relation to their need to engage with environmental concerns, but also in relation to achieving other health goals – notably empowerment.

KEY POINTS

o Effective communication is central to health education and requires consideration of source, message and audience factors.

o The development of health education interventions requires clear specification of intended learning outcomes – cognitive, affective, conative and skills.

o The selection of methods also requires consideration of the characteristics of the teacher and learner.

o The use of participatory methods is consistent with the principles of empowerment. It is also more effective and less likely to induce reactance among learners.

o Methods such as creative arts, which have a multidimensional impact, can achieve confluence between different learning dimensions.

o The use of targeting and tailoring can increase the effectiveness of large-scale programmes by making messages more relevant to individuals.

o A power imbalance between teacher and learner can be a barrier to learning. Peer education can enhance learning by capitalizing on the shared characteristics of teacher and learner.

(Continued)

(Continued)

○ Factors to consider in the design of messages to influence attitudes include sidedness, implicit versus explicit conclusions, inoculation and refutational pre-emption, and the use of affect – either positive or negative.

○ The use of fear appeal is controversial from an ethical standpoint and can backfire. However, fear can be a useful motivator provided individuals both believe they can and are able to do something to protect themselves.

○ Health education can raise awareness of the factors influencing health and can empower individuals and groups to take action to tackle these factors.

○ Within the critical theory tradition and in line with Freirean approaches, health education can be involved with critical consciousness raising in relation to oppressive social structures and enabling learners to seek solutions.

8

MASS COMMUNICATION

Nothing is easier than leading the people on a leash. I just hold up a dazzling campaign poster and they jump through it.

Joseph Goebbels, cited in Rhodes, 1976

OVERVIEW

This chapter focuses on the use of mass media in health promotion. It will:

- consider the potential and limitations of mass media interventions for health promotion
- note the incidental effects of mass media as part of the wider environmental influences on health
- identify pathways though which mass media exert an effect on the individual
- consider theoretical and technical issues involved in planning mass media interventions
- identify the key elements of social marketing
- explore the use of media for advocacy purposes.

INTRODUCTION

This chapter begins by considering the more conventional role of mass media in persuading individuals to adopt healthy behaviours. Notwithstanding their potential to reach large numbers of people, mass media are not without their limitations in achieving behaviour change. Social marketing attempts to address these by applying marketing principles to the design of programmes and we will examine its contribution to health promotion.

Finally, we will turn our attention to a less widely acknowledged role of mass media, but one which is central to our view of health promotion – that is, its contribution to the development of healthy public policy.

MASS COMMUNICATION AND HEALTH PROMOTION

The term 'mass communication' is often used interchangeably with 'mass media'. In the interest of clarity, it is worth giving brief consideration to the use of the terms 'communication' and 'media'. Applying our earlier definition of 'communication' as the business of transmitting messages from a source to a receiver would limit the scope of 'mass communication' in a way that is certainly not intended by those who use it. The intended meaning is more in line with 'education' – as we have used it in Chapter 7, but with an emphasis on its persuasive dimension. The educational messages are, however, mediated by the use of a range of electronic and print media which have the advantage of being able to contact very large numbers of people at any one time. Their limitations derive from the fact that, as the messages are mediated, interpersonal contact is not possible. It is therefore very difficult precisely to tailor communications to the audience and impossible to react immediately to people's reactions to the mediated messages.

What exactly is a mass audience? It is meaningless to refer to precise numbers as it is not so much the actual numbers that are important but the one-way, top-down nature of communication. For instance, a typical 'block' lecture to the public or a student group has more in common with mass media than with interpersonal education, despite relatively small numbers.

Schramm and Roberts (1972: 392, cited by Reardon, 1981: 195) refer to the 'latitude of interpretation and response' that characterizes mass media:

> Characteristics of the mass communication situation, such as the receiver's freedom from many of the social constraints which operate in interpersonal communication, greatly attenuated feedback, and lack of opportunity to tailor messages for specific people allow any individual receiver a good deal more latitude of interpretation and response than he has when speaking face-to-face with friend, colleague or acquaintance.

Issues for health promotion

There are four main areas of interest and debate for health promotion in respect of mass media.

- The unhealthy influence of mass media generally, for example, encouraging health-damaging behaviours such as excessive alcohol consumption, or copycat violence, or even reducing the stock of social capital – see Putnam's (1995) suggestion that the decline in social capital is substantially due to the increase in television viewing.
- The specific marketing of unhealthy products using mass media.
- The acceptability of using mass media to achieve health promotion goals and associated debate about the relative effectiveness of mass media compared with alternative interpersonal approaches.
- Debate about the use of persuasive messages to 'sell health' rather than empower choice.

Mass media

The variety of available media is substantial including television and radio; print media such as newspapers, magazines, billboards and mass mailshots; and the plethora of communication channels opened up by modern information and communication technology. However, despite the shared characteristics mentioned above, it is unwise to treat mass media as completely homogeneous. It is obvious that there are differences between, for example, advertisements which deliver a health promotion message, coverage of health issues in documentary and news programmes, and the inclusion of health issues in drama or soap operas – so-called 'edutainment'. Equally, paying for media time (or space) for advertising one's message is different from using public service announcements (PSAs) which are delivered by mass media channels without charging.

It is also important to make a clear distinction between mass media and superficially similar devices, such as videos that are used to trigger discussion and involve interpersonal interaction with a teacher. A video endlessly repeated in a shopping mall is an example of mass media; the same video used as an aid to discussion and learning is a 'learning resource' or visual aid.

We should also be aware of rapidly evolving possibilities offered by interactive digital media including websites, chat rooms, email lists, newsgroups, mobile phones, CD-ROMS and so on. While some usage may exhibit the characteristics of mass communication, these media also have the potential to tailor messages to suit the user's needs and include opportunities for feedback (Bernhard, 2001).

The advantages and disadvantages of various channels are summarized from a practical perspective by the National Cancer Institute (undated) – see Table 8.1.

Table 8.1   Advantages and disadvantages of selected mass media channels

Mass Media Channels	Activities	PROS	CONS
Newspaper	Ads Inserted sections on a health topic (paid) News Feature stories Letters to the editor Op/ed pieces	Can reach broad intended audiences rapidly Can convey health news/breakthroughs more thoroughly than TV or radio and faster than magazines Intended audience has chance to clip, reread, contemplate and pass along material Small circulation papers may take PSAs	Can be costly, time-consuming to establish May not provide personalized attention Organizational constraints may require message approval May lose control of message if adapted to fit organizational needs
Radio	Ads (paid or public service placement) News Public affairs/	Range of formats available to intended audiences with known listening preferences Opportunity for direct intended audience	Reaches smaller intended audiences than TV Public service ads run infrequently and at

(Continued)

Table 8.1 *(Continued)*

Mass Media Channels	Activities	PROS	CONS
	talk shows Dramatic programming (entertainment education)	involvement (through call-in shows) Can distribute ad scripts (termed 'live-copy ads'), which are flexible and inexpensive Paid ads or specific programming can reach intended audience when they are most receptive Paid ads can be relatively inexpensive Ad production costs are low relative to TV Ads allow message and its execution to be controlled	low listening times Many stations have limited formats that may not be conducive to health messages Difficult for intended audiences to retain or pass on material
Television	Ads (paid or public service placement) News Public affairs/ talk shows Dramatic programming (entertainment education)	Reaches potentially the largest and widest range of intended audiences Visual combined with audio good for emotional appeals and demonstrating behaviors Can reach low income intended audiences Paid ads or specific programming can reach intended audience when most receptive Ads allow message and its execution to be controlled Opportunity for direct intended audience involvement (through call-in shows)	Ads are expensive to produce Paid advertising is expensive PSAs run infrequently and at low viewing times Message may be obscured by commercial clutter Some stations reach very small intended audiences Promotion can result in huge demand Can be difficult for intended audiences to retain or pass on material
Internet	Web sites E-mail mailing lists Chat rooms Newsgroups Ads (paid or public service placement)	Can reach large numbers of people rapidly Can instantaneously update and disseminate information Can control information provided Can tailor information specifically for intended audiences Can be interactive Can provide health information in a	Can be expensive Many intended audiences do not have access to Internet Intended audience must be proactive – must search or sign up for information Newsgroups and chat rooms may require monitoring

(Continued)

Table 8.1   *(Continued)*

Mass Media Channels	Activities	PROS	CONS
		graphically appealing way	Can require maintenance over time
		Can combine the audio/ visual benefits of TV or radio with the self-paced benefits of print media	
		Can use banner ads to direct intended audience to your program's web site	

Source: National Cancer Institute (undated)

MASS MEDIA – CAPABILITIES AND FUNCTIONS

What, then, can we expect from mass media? Implicit in such a question is frequently an expectation of mass behaviour change – especially when posed by politicians and practitioners. However, such expectations – either in pursuit of profit or social welfare and health goals – will typically fail to materialize. Mass media are not a 'magic bullet' that will generate dramatic and widespread success, despite the hopeful expectations of some decision makers. These unrealistic expectations reflect a model of mass media which is now rather disparagingly referred to as the 'direct effects' model or 'hypodermic model'. It derives from the assumptions that:

- mass media have a direct effect on the audience
- mass media act like a hypodermic syringe – advertisers fill it with a powerful message and inject it into the population at large
- if it does not achieve the desired result, a bigger syringe is needed (more intensive media blitz) with a more powerful content (new, more persuasive message)!

Mendelsohn (1968) challenged the direct effects model, preferring to use the metaphor of an aerosol spray, arguing that, as the mass media message was sprayed on to the target population, most of it 'drifted away', only a small amount actually hit the target, and only a very small proportion 'penetrated'. Klapper (1960, cited in Wallack, 1980: 15) made a similar point in relation to its effect:

> Within a given audience exposed to particular communications, reinforcement, or at least constancy of opinion, is typically found to be the dominant effect, minor change as in intensity of opinion is found to be the next most common, and conversion is typically found to be the most rare.

Nonetheless, mass media can have dramatic repercussions, sometimes unintended! For instance, Orson Welles' dramatic radio broadcast of H.G. Wells' *War of the Worlds*, which included news flashes about a Martian invasion, famously created widespread panic in America (Cantril, 1958).

There is some evidence that mass communication can be effective in increasing awareness of health risk. Indeed, WHO (2002b: 42) notes that:

> Although newspapers, magazines, radio and television are often criticized for inaccurate and biased reporting, in industrialized countries they remain the most influential sources for everyday information on risks to health. The rapid spread of these media in developing countries, together with improvements in literacy, mean that this is increasingly true in low and middle income countries.

However, relatively few studies have demonstrated effectiveness in achieving behaviour change. For example, Hawks et al.'s (2002: xiii) review of what works in preventing psychoactive substance use found that:

> The use of the mass media on its own, particularly in the presence of other countervailing influences, has not been found to be an effective way of reducing different types of psychoactive substance use. It has however been found to raise information levels and to lend support to policy initiatives. Combined with reciprocal and complementary community action, particularly environmental changes, media campaigns have proved more successful in influencing attitudes towards psychoactive substance use and use itself. Health warnings associated with illicit psychoactive substance use have been an effective way of communicating the hazards of such use particularly to heavy users if combined with other economic and environmental initiatives.

Notwithstanding the view that mass media are more effective when combined with other methods than when used alone, Zimmerman et al. (2007) demonstrated that an intensive television campaign could be effective in improving safer sexual behaviour among high risk youth, provided it was well planned. Key elements included audience segmentation and targeting, along with formative research with the target group to develop the persuasive appeal of the message.

Yanovitzky and Stryker (2001) suggest that the direct model fails to account for alternative pathways of influence which might lead to behaviour change. They argue that paying ever more attention to improving the persuasive appeal of messages ignores the well recognized knowledge–behaviour gap, i.e. the fact that knowledge alone is rarely sufficient to motivate behaviour change. Drawing on an analysis of media coverage of youth binge drinking, they propose two additional pathways of influence:

1 the influence of mass media on social norms and the acceptability (or otherwise) of behaviours mediated through social influence;
2 the effect of policy changes in response to the issue.

Wellings and Macdowall (2000) distinguishs these approaches as the 'risk factor model', which is concerned with changing individual behaviour, and the 'social diffusion model', which sees mass media as activating the forces for social change.

Furthermore, Katz and Lazarsfeld (1955) described the influence of mass communications on the audience as a two-step process. Communications instigated by national leaders and transmitted via mass media (in those days, chiefly radio and the press) were 'intercepted' by opinion leaders (see the diffusion of innovations theory, Chapter 3). Opinion leaders were, almost by definition, more open to, and receptive of, mass media information. They also tended to be sought out for advice by what Katz and Lazarsfeld rather archaically called the 'rank and file'.

It is interesting to note that, some 30 years ago, Lazarsfeld and Merton (1955), in challenging simplistic views of mass communication effects, identified three conditions for mass media effectiveness:

1 **Monopolization** – the success of any given influence attempt was most likely where there was no opposition or counter-messages (and, arguably, where there was a limited overall volume of media activity).
2 **Canalization** – success was most likely to occur where persuasive messages were consistent with the audience's existing motivation and could be 'plugged in' to these existing prejudices, desires and wishes.
3 **Supplementation** – mass communication would be more likely to succeed when this supplemented, and was supported by, interpersonal influences.

The potential for health communication, as identified by The US National Cancer Institute, is shown in the box and could equally apply to mass media communication.

The role of health communication

Communication alone can:

- Increase the intended audience's knowledge and awareness of a health issue, problem, or solution
- Influence perceptions, beliefs, and attitudes that may change social norms
- Prompt action
- Demonstrate or illustrate healthy skills
- Reinforce knowledge, attitudes, or behavior
- Show the benefit of behavior change
- Advocate a position on a health issue or policy
- Increase demand or support for health services
- Refute myths and misconceptions
- Strengthen organizational relationships.

National Cancer Institute, undated: 3

The strengths of mass media lie in their ability to reach large audiences and groups who would be difficult to reach through more interpersonal methods. They have limited capacity to develop skills and achieve sustained attitude and behaviour change unless they form part of a more comprehensive programme. However, well planned and executed mass media interventions of sufficient intensity can raise awareness of health issues and risks and lend credibility to local programmes. Furthermore, mass media can raise the profile of health issues on the public agenda and take on an advocacy function in relation to social and political change – as we discuss in more detail later in this chapter. Over and above more 'traditional' usage, mass media can therefore contribute to empowerment and social change and the model of critical health education set out in the previous chapter. Overall, the health promotion role of the media can be summarized as:

- general information dissemination
- specific focused campaigns, either through direct influence on individuals or indirectly through influencing social and cultural norms
- countering the advertising and marketing of 'unhealthy' products
- advocating for policy change.

The National Social Marketing Centre (2006: 99) identifies 10 situations when mass media use is most appropriate:

1 When wide exposure is desired.
2 When the time frame is urgent.
3 When public discussion is likely to facilitate the educational process.
4 When awareness is a main goal.
5 When media authorities are 'on-side'. Where journalists, editors and programmers are 'on-side' with a particular health issue, this often guarantees greater support in terms of space and editorial content.
6 When accompanying on-the-ground back-up can be provided.
7 When long-term follow up is possible.
8 When a generous budget exists.
9 When the behavioural goal is simple.
10 When the agenda includes public relations.

Theoretical considerations

Murphy and Bennett (2004) note that many mass media campaigns have been criticized for being atheoretical or relying on inappropriate theories and models. The Communication Evaluation Expert Panel (2007: 233) endorsed:

> the use of explicit program logic models that incorporate theoretical constructs into descriptions of the causal pathways through which program effects are expected to come about. They found that theory-based logic models help to keep message strategies linked to psychosocial predictors and performance measures on mark.

Klapper (1995) emphasizes that in order to understand and use media effectively, it is important to view mass communication in the context of broader theories of the individual and society. The problem, then, becomes, not a shortage of theory, but rather which theories to select from the plethora of theories available.

Clearly, no single model or theory will suffice. The design of mass media interventions should conform with the principles of health promotion planning and include:

- definition of goals and specific objectives for the mass media programme
- specification of the audience and identification of audience characteristics including any sub-groups

- development of the message and pretesting with the target group
- selection of channels that will maximize reach
- selection of a 'source' to maximize appeal and credibility with the target audience
- implementation
- evaluation – both formative and summative.

The development of mass media campaigns will also need to consider theory at a number of different levels. By way of example, these might include the following.

- At the individual level:
  - behavioural theories such as health action model, health belief model, theory of reasoned action, protection motivation theory
  - communication theory
  - theories concerning persuasion and attitude change (including the use of fear appeal)
  - stage models of change.

- At the interpersonal level:
  - social cognitive theory.

- At the organizational/community/societal level:
  - organizational change theory
  - diffusion of innovations theory.

These various theories have been discussed at some length earlier in this text and, notwithstanding their undoubted relevance to the development of mass media campaigns, we do not propose to reiterate them here. We will, however, consider at this point some additional theoretical insights.

Berger (1991) identifies four separate analyses that can be applied to mass communication:

- a Marxist analysis
- a semiological analysis
- psychoanalytic criticism
- sociological analysis.

A Marxist perspective

Marxist media theory demonstrates the ways in which capitalism exercises control over the proletariat by, among other means, use of mass media. Many of the key concepts of Marxism can be applied to the analysis of mass media. McQuail (1994) provides a very succinct summary:

- mass media are owned by the bourgeois class
- media are operated in the interest of the bourgeoisie
- media promote working-class false consciousness
- media access is denied to political opposition.

The notion of 'hegemony' is one of a number of key Marxist notions that Berger thought relevant to the role of mass media in society. Berger (1991: 49) defines hegemony as:

> a complicated intermeshing of forces of a political, social, and cultural nature [that] transcends but also includes two other concepts – culture, which is how we shape our lives, and ideology, which, from a Marxist perspective, expresses and is a projection of specific class interest ... Ideology may be masked and camouflaged in films and television programmes and other works carried by mass media but the discerning Marxist can elicit these ideologies and point them out.

Unsurprisingly, mass media would provide an invaluable tool for creating false consciousness and reducing potential threats to the status quo. Similarly, and in relation to the key notion of alienation, Berger (1991: 43–4) argues that:

> the media play a crucial role. They provide momentary gratifications for the alienated spirit, they distract the alienated individual from his or her misery (and from consciousness of the objective facts of his or her situation) and, with the institution of advertising, they stimulate desire, leading people to work harder and harder. (Advertising has replaced the Puritan ethic in America as the chief means of motivating people to work hard.)

and, in respect of the consumer society:

> people must be driven to consume, must be made crazy to consume, for it is consumption that maintains the economic system. Thus the alienation generated by a capitalist system is functional, for the anxieties and miseries generated by this system tend to be assuaged by impulsive consumption ... Advertising generates anxieties, creates dissatisfactions, and, in general, feeds on the alienation present in capitalist societies to maintain the consumer culture. There is nothing that advertising will not do, use, or co-opt in trying to achieve its goals, and if it has to debase sexuality, co-opt the women's rights movement, merchandise cancer (via cigarettes), seduce children, or terrorize the masses, all of these tactics and anything else will be attempted. One thing that advertising does is divert people's attention from social and political concerns into narcissistic and private concerns. Individual self-gratification becomes an obsession and, with this, alienation is strengthened and the sense of community weakened.

Bearing in mind our early comments on policy and WHO's imperative to deal with inequity in particular and social issues in general, the implication of the above analysis for fostering healthy public policy needs no further comment!

Insights from semiology

'Semiology' is the science of signs (from the Greek, *semeion*, which means sign) and derives originally from linguistics. Its founding father was Saussure (1915). Semiology is used virtually interchangeably with 'Semiotics' – a term devised by the American Pierce (1839–1914). Although language was the original sign system subjected to semiotic scrutiny and 'discourse analysis', the methods of study were increasingly applied to signs of all kinds.

One especially relevant application of discourse analysis to mass media is embodied in the concept of 'myth'. Despite the sense in which it is used in everyday parlance, 'myth' does not necessarily mean false beliefs. Chapman and Egger (1983: 167) define it as:

> any real or fictional story, recurring theme or character type that appeals to the consciousness of a group by embodying its cultural ideals or by giving expression to deep, commonly felt emotions.

They provide a revealing demonstration of the ways in which myth frequently figures in cigarette advertising in its embodiment of major interests and concerns in a given society. An example of an Australian advertisement for Winfield cigarettes is provided in the box.

Case study: creating the myth of the Winfield smoker

Some key features of the advertising campaign:

- It used Paul Hogan – a comedian who later enjoyed international fame for his movie portrayal of *Crocodile Dundee*. Hogan was originally a painter on the Sydney Harbour Bridge and was discovered in a talent show prior to becoming 'Winfield Man'. He personified the anti-hero 'rags-to-riches' myth of the working-class male who had made it to the top from humble beginnings without losing the common touch – and thus appealed to the market segment targeted by this particular brand of cigarettes.
- The word 'anyhow' was used in all Winfield advertising – 'Anyhow, Have a Winfield!'. This word is allegedly associated in Australian minds with another expression, 'she'll be right', which connotes a fatalistic outlook on life (and death), but with a touch of optimism in the face of adversity. As Chapman and Egger indicate, 'the word "anyhow" is probably intended to act as a pat on the back to people on low incomes, with high mortgages, with bad marriages, with bleak prospects, etc. It is saying "yes, we know your life is dull/bleak/wearying/unrewarding, but ... anyhow ... "'.

Chapman and Egger, 1983

Sociological and psychoanalytic insights

We have already noted that social and cultural factors will influence the acceptability of messages, their wider dissemination through social channels and the extent to which they might ultimately influence behaviour.

At a practical level, it is possible to 'prescribe' key elements of effective, persuasive messages. Nicholson (2007) summarizes these as including grabbing attention, being easy to understand, personally relevant, provoking the audience to think about or discuss the message/campaign and ultimately motivating action. However, she goes on to raise the question of what actually contributes to the appeal of campaigns such as the highly successful 'truth' anti-smoking campaign. Notwithstanding criticism and legal action, the 'truth' campaign (see box) has produced a substantial decline in youth smoking (Farrelly et al., 2005). In contrast, exposure to the Philip Morris' 'Think. Don't Smoke' campaign, aired around the same time, was not only ineffective in reducing youth smoking, but was associated with more positive beliefs and attitudes about the tobacco industry (Farrelly et al., 2008). She quotes Salovey's comments:

> If the principles of psychology were a series of main effects — meaning that x works better than y — rather than more qualified statements that reflect interactions between variables, then we wouldn't need a science of human behavior to deduce them. They'd be obvious.

She speculates that the unprecedented success of the 'truth' ads was because they 'simply tapped into what motivates teenagers'. In particular, their 'anarchistic vibe', taking on big corporations and fast-paced 'gritty' style, was thought to appeal to free-spirited rebellious teens. In contrast, the Philip Morris ad spoke down to teenagers, telling them what to do. Over and above message factors, it should also be evident that there are differences in source factors too. Notably, the 'truth' campaign capitalized on peer influence, homophily and source credibility.

> We're a dependable source of real facts and information. The minute we lose that quality and start bending and manipulating facts to our gain, then we're no better than the tobacco industry. (Truth, undated)

Case study: the truth campaign

The truth campaign started in 2000 and was run by the American Legacy Foundation, funded under the terms of the 1998 Tobacco Master Settlement Agreement against the four largest US tobacco companies.

'Truth' is a hard-hitting media campaign that uses edgy television, radio and print ads featuring youth-led activism against tobacco companies and exposing the industry's deceptive marketing techniques. Some examples of the campaign's advertisements include a commercial that features 'a youth piling body bags outside a tobacco company's headquarters and another that exposes how the industry purposefully markets towards young people' (Krisberg, 2005).

The emphasis is NOT on telling young people what to do but on 'exposing how the tobacco industry has been manipulating our generation and others before it' (see www.thetruth.com/aboutUs.cfm).

The latest campaign 'The Sunny Side of Truth' uses heavy irony to present positive messages about tobacco.

> Sure, truth has been tough on Big Tobacco. And for good reason: they make a product that kills over 1,200 people a day, so someone has to say something.

(Continued)

(Continued)

> But after all these years, we thought we'd give Big T a break and look at the sunnier side for once. Like if every 1 of every 3 youths who smoke will eventually die from it, that means 2 live! See how easy that is (see www.thetruth.com.)

The website also provides access to popular elements of contemporary youth culture – blogs, videos, games and free music remixes.

Uses and gratification theory

Uses and gratification theory provides some insight into the appeal of messages and also into the limitations of the 'hypodermic model' of media operation and the reason why so little of the contents of the 'aerosol' manage to penetrate. Rather than seeing the audience as homogenous passive recipients, uses and gratification theory asserts that individuals interact selectively with messages.

Those watching a television programme may or may not focus on the message. Even if they do concentrate, there is absolutely no guarantee that they will interpret the message in the ways intended by the programme's producers, indeed quite the opposite may occur in practice. Moreover, they will not only actively select what they watch, they will interpret it in accordance with the principles of wish fulfilment.

According to uses and gratification theory, people *use* the media to *gratify* their desires and satisfy their prejudices. A journalist (Sarler, 1996), commenting on criticisms of a deceased 'agony aunt' colleague (Marjorie Proops) for encouraging sexual irresponsibility, made the point rather nicely:

> People knew Miss Proops' views, as surely as they know the views of all journalists who write on a regular basis ... When they wrote to her, they knew in advance what she would say ... An estimated 3 per cent of the population did write to her, comfortable in the certainty that she thought what they thought. Not that she could form their thoughts for them ... And as one reader said, 'You put that so well; it's just what I have been thinking for ages.'

Berger (1991: 86–91) provides the following comprehensive list of a wide range of typical gratifications offered by the media which clearly illustrates this particular theory of mass media use:

- to be amused
- to see authority figures exalted or deflated
- to experience the beautiful
- to have shared experiences with others/sense of community
- to satisfy curiosity and be informed
- to identify with the deity and the divine plan
- to find distractions and diversion
- to experience empathy
- to experience, in a guilt-free and controlled situation, extreme emotions, such as love and hate, the horrible and the terrible, and similar phenomena

- to find models to imitate
- to gain an identity
- to gain information about the world
- to reinforce our belief in justice
- to believe in romantic love
- to believe in magic, the marvellous and the miraculous
- to see others make mistakes
- to see order imposed on the world
- to participate in history (vicariously)
- to be purged of unpleasant emotions
- to obtain outlets for our sexual drives in a guilt-free context
- to explore taboo subjects with impunity
- to experience the ugly
- to affirm moral, spiritual and cultural values
- to see villains in action.

Elaboration Likelihood Model

The Elaboration Likelihood Model (Petty and Cacioppo, 1986) suggests that there are two routes through which messages might change attitudes. The first is the central route which involves messages being subjected to considerable thought and scrutiny, i.e. high levels of elaboration. The second peripheral route does not involve the same level of critical thinking and relies more on the general appeal of the message and the way it is conveyed, including the credibility and attractiveness of the source. The way campaigns are branded would also exert an influence.

The route taken is influenced by both motivational and ability factors. The former includes the relevance of the message and compatibility with previously held beliefs and attitudes. The latter includes the ability to process information logically and have the time to do so. While both routes can influence attitudes and, indeed, behaviour, the high elaboration central route is more likely to achieve enduring attitude change.

Prospect theory – framing the message

Prospect theory (Kahneman and Tversky, 1979) indicates that the choices people make are influenced by whether messages are conveyed in terms of benefits (gain framed) or negative consequences (loss framed) and the level of uncertainty about each. People appear to be less likely to accept risks and uncertainty when choosing between options when they have something to gain and more likely when they have something to lose. Rothman and Salovey (1997) have applied this thinking to health education. They propose that preventive messages should be framed positively to focus on gains. In contrast, there is a high level of uncertainty associated with going for a screening procedure such as a mammogram. In this situation, messages which focus on potential losses are held to be more effective.

Mass media and supportive environments for health

As we observed above, in addition to the specific use of mass media to influence individual attitudes and health behaviour, they can also have more general health enhancing or damaging effects. The mass media, therefore, are part of the wider environmental influences on health. From a health promotion perspective, the action implication is to control and minimize harmful effects and to maximize any beneficial effects.

The general health-damaging consequences of mass media have been well documented and range from Putnam's view that it undermines 'social capital' (as noted above) to specific effects, such as glorifying the use of firearms. However, there is considerable debate about the alleged *direct* effects of, say, the portrayal of violence on film or television and, for example, copycat killings. Indeed, uses and gratification theory would suggest that negative inclinations are already present, that mass media events are merely used as an adjunct to trigger negative behaviour and perhaps shape the form it takes. Nonetheless, mass media clearly exert a 'normative effect', as we noted in Chapter 3. Even if they do not exactly exert pressure on individuals to adopt behaviour that they would not otherwise have adopted, they often signal that such behaviour is normal and acceptable. Before commenting further, it is important to point out that at this point we are not discussing deliberate persuasive advertising. Rather, we are concerned here with 'incidental' effects exerted via a variety of media. For example, the review by Gunasekera et al. (2005) of popular movies noted the normative depictions of negative health behaviours (see box).

> ### The top 200 movies of all time and health-related behaviour
>
> Excluded from the study: films released or set prior to the HIV era (1983), animated films, films not about humans; general release or parental guidance films.
>   In the 87 remaining, there were:
>
> - 53 sex episodes in total appearing in 28 movies (32%)
> - one suggestion of condom use – the only reference to birth control
> - no depictions of the consequences of unprotected sex such as unwanted pregnancy or STDs
> - 8 per cent showing cannabis use, 7 per cent other illicit drugs – which were also portrayed positively and without negative consequences
> - 32 per cent showing alcohol use, 68 per cent smoking

The portrayal of alcohol and alcohol consumption by the media has been subjected to substantial research. Hansen (2003) analysed British primetime television over a five-day sample period which covered 28 soap operas (13.6 hours), 14 dramas (13.4 hours) and 47 news programmes (22.3 hours). The study found that:

- 85.4 per cent of the programmes contained some reference to alcohol or alcohol-consumption
    - all of the drama programmes
    - 92.9 per cent of soap operas
    - 76.6 per cent of news programmes
- the total number of visual and verbal references to alcohol (381) was more than double the total number of references to non-alcoholic drinks (170)
- the hourly rate of visual references to alcohol was 10.6 in soaps, 4.3 in drama and 1.9 in news
- the hourly rate of drinking scenes in soaps was 7, drama 3.1 and news programmes 1.3.

Hansen noted that:

> The most noticeable aspect of alcohol consumption and alcohol images on television was the way that they featured prominently in terms of frequency of occurrence, yet were rarely in the foreground narratively or thematically. In this respect, alcohol and alcohol consumption are 'naturalised' by the programmes, as a normal, frequent, and common aspect of social interaction.
>
> ... Television offers a very selective — and, in Soaps and Drama, remarkably uniform — image of alcohol consumption as a routine, pleasant and unproblematic component of social interaction, a marker of celebrations, achievements, romance and sexual relations, and an integral component of 'having a good time'. Conversely, television Soaps and Drama offer little portrayal of the wide range of potentially serious personal and social consequences of alcohol consumption generally, and excessive drinking more particularly. (2003: 7-8)

Finn (1980) reminded us of the wide range of media which might contribute to perceptions and norms about alcohol in a study of the way in which greetings cards perpetuate stereotyped images, such as jolly drunks supporting lamp posts.

Researchers and those working in health promotion and public health have typically recommended that television companies should adopt a healthier and more responsible approach to alcohol use specifically and health issues more generally.

As we have noted, over and above deliberate attempts to use the media to convey health messages or advertise products which can affect health, the media have more subtle effects. Not only do they exert an influence through the foreground narrative or theme, the background content is also important. Furthermore, in addition to such incidental coverage, some companies have deliberately attempted to exploit the potential of these background influences through product placement. For example, the tobacco industry has paid for specific brands of cigarettes or for smoking more generally to appear in movies (Smoke Free Movies, undated; Victorian Smoking and Health Program, 1995) – see box. Such expenditure provides testimony in itself to the faith of the tobacco industry in the effectiveness of this type of exposure.

Product placement

Definition:

> Product placement (also known as 'embedded advertising') occurs when a product or brand gains exposure, apparently incidentally, for example in a film, or a photograph, or even an advertisement for something else. While brand exposure obviously provides a distinct benefit to a particular company, it is not essential. The simple activity of smoking can also be enhanced by its association with a broad variety of desirable personalities or characteristics.

Victorian Tobacco and Health Program, 1995

(Continued)

(Continued)

Example:

> Not only did Philip Morris arrange for Lois Lane (Margot Kidder) to smoke Marlboros, but *Superman II* also included a classic fight scene in which Superman and the bad guys throw a Marlboro truck back and forth across Lexington Avenue. The truck was produced solely for the movie and exists nowhere else.

Smoke Free Movies, undated

What can be done to minimize this negative influence? On the one hand, the capacity of the public to engage with the media more critically can be developed by improving *media literacy*. Media literacy includes the skills needed to deconstruct media messages and, where relevant, 'identify the sponsor's motives' (National Cancer Institute, undated: 248). Such awareness, it might be assumed, would offer some protection against clandestine attempts to persuade.

On the other hand, these media influences are pervasive and it would be unrealistic to expect people constantly to engage in critically appraising them – notwithstanding peripheral effects which bypass critical scrutiny (see the elaboration likelihood model) and indirect effects through influences on social norms. In the interests of developing supportive environments for health, it is important that their potentially negative influence on health is recognized and steps taken to ameliorate it.

There is some reluctance to take action to control the media – often linked to support for the freedom of the press. Defoe and Breed (1989) have argued for a compromise approach involving 'collaborative consultation', in which health promoters work with media and persuade them to adopt a responsible approach to their programming.

A number of Codes of Practice have been developed, for example in relation to junk food and alcohol. However, they tend to focus on explicit advertising rather than more incidental coverage. Nevertheless, the Television Advertising Standards Code, developed by the British Broadcast Committee of Advertising Practice (2004), refers to any coverage of alcohol in all advertisements (see box). There are further requirements for specific advertisements about alcohol, especially in relation to limiting their appeal to young people.

Alcohol: Television Advertising Standards Code

Rules which apply to all advertising

11.8.1(a)
(1) Advertisements must not suggest that alcohol can contribute to an individual's popularity or confidence, or that refusal is a sign of weakness. Nor may they suggest that alcohol can enhance personal qualities.

(Continued)

(Continued)

(2) Advertisements must not suggest that the success of a social occasion depends on the presence or consumption of alcohol.

11.8.1(b)
Advertisements must not link alcohol with daring, toughness, aggression or anti-social behaviour.

11.8.1(c)
Advertisements must not link alcohol with sexual activity or success or imply that alcohol can enhance attractiveness.

11.8.1(d)
Advertisements must not suggest that regular solitary drinking is acceptable or that drinking can overcome problems.

11.8.1(e)
Advertisements must neither suggest that alcohol has therapeutic qualities nor offer it as a stimulant, sedative, mood-changer or source of nourishment, or to boost confidence. Although they may refer to refreshment, advertisements must not imply that alcohol can improve any type of performance.

Advertisements must not suggest that alcohol might be indispensable or link it to illicit drugs.

11.8.1(f)
Advertisements must not suggest that a drink is to be preferred because of its alcohol content nor place undue emphasis on alcoholic strength. (This does not apply to low alcohol drinks. See 11.8.3).

11.8.1(g)
(1) Advertisements must not show, imply or encourage immoderate drinking. This applies both to the amount of drink and to the way drinking is portrayed.
(2) References to, or suggestions of, buying repeat rounds of drinks are not acceptable. (Note: This does not prevent, for example, someone buying a drink for each of a group of friends. It does, however, prevent any suggestion that other members of the group will buy any further rounds.)
(3) Alcoholic drinks must be handled and served responsibly.

11.8.1(h)
Advertisements must not link drinking with the use of potentially dangerous machinery, with behaviour which would be dangerous after consuming alcohol (such as swimming) or with driving.

British Broadcast Committee of Advertising Practice, 2004

Soap operas and edutainment

There is considerable evidence for the impacts of soap operas. They illustrate, par excellence, the uses and gratification theory in practice. Viewers identify with the characters, the characters reappear in other media, such as popular magazines, and so fiction and reality appear to blend seamlessly. Clearly, soap operas are not real – indeed, analysis demonstrates that they caricature reality (for example, in the amount of alcohol apparently consumed and the high incidence of unnatural deaths and criminality!). They do, however, mirror viewers' constructions of reality and focus on common concerns, interests and prejudices. Verma et al. (2007) explored the coverage of selected behaviours which impact on health in the four leading British soap operas. Alcohol-related behaviour occurred in total 19.3 times per programme hour and unhealthy food behaviour 6.1 times in contrast to healthy food behaviour 2.9 times. They argue that, while the depiction of unhealthy behaviour may reflect what the programme producers feel is normal behaviour, there is an opportunity to convey healthier norms.

> Engaging the makers of these programmes in a health promotion agenda may be a fruitful method of promoting healthy behaviours among a wide cross-section of the population – perhaps by the establishment of voluntary liaison with public health policymakers. (Verma et al. 2007: 576)

Soap operas can also be used more directly to convey health messages. For example, the makers of the UK soap drama *Hollyoaks* were congratulated in a parliamentary debate on their storyline covering sexually transmitted infection and the consequence of unprotected sex (HC Deb, 2001–2). The use of entertainment media for educational purposes has become referred to as 'edutainment' – defined in the *American Heritage Dictionary of the English Language* (2000) as 'The act of learning through a medium, particularly media-based, that both educates and entertains' (see also Zeedyk and Wallace, 2003).

An example of a highly successful edutainment initiative is provided by Soul City (see box).

Case study: Soul City

A multimedia project which reaches 16 million South Africans through:

- Soul City targeted at adults, and
- Soul Buddyz targeted at 8- to 12-year-olds.

It tackles a range of health and development issues and aims to 'impart information and impact on social norms, attitudes and practice' (Soul City Institute, 2008).

It recognizes that health does not rely solely on individual choice, but requires an enabling environment. It therefore includes a multimedia advocacy strategy. A national lifeskills programme for use in schools has also been developed with the Departments of Education and Health (Peltzer and Promtussananon, 2003).

The success of the Soul City approach is based on its two guiding principles:

- *Research* – including consultation with experts, formative research and pretesting with audiences.
- *Partnerships* – with organizations active in the issues being dealt with, which allows integration with local initiatives.

Advertising and counter-advertising

Freudenberg (2005) identifies advertising as one of the corporate behaviours that promote disease if the product is harmful in itself or can be used in ways that damage health. Advertising therefore makes up part of the wider environmental influences on health. Controls on advertising and voluntary agreements have been used to limit the effect, for example banning tobacco advertising in many countries. However, there are concerns about the effectiveness of voluntary agreements (see, for example, Munro, 2006).

Efforts to counter the negative influence of advertising include using the media to deliver alternative messages. These frequently rely on humour to undermine the original message or the use of shock tactics to expose the reality of negative health consequences of products being marketed. They also adopt similar styles to the original advertisements – indeed, campaigns such as the BUGA UP campaign, which we will discuss in more detail later, use graffiti to modify billboard advertising and change tobacco marketing messages into anti-tobacco messages.

Warning labels on products have also been used. These have generally taken the form of written warnings about the health hazards associated with using the product. Canada was one of the first countries to introduce picture warnings. In the UK, from 1 August 2008, tobacco manufacturers were required to include picture warnings covering 40 per cent of the back of packs of cigarettes or tobacco products (see Figure 8.1) as well as having an approved written warning on the front. These warnings are selected in rotation from a set of 14. A study by Hammond et al. (2007) found that the effectiveness of warnings on cigarette packs was influenced by the design and 'freshness' of the warning. Prominent warnings were more likely to be effective and this was further enhanced by the inclusion of pictorial images.

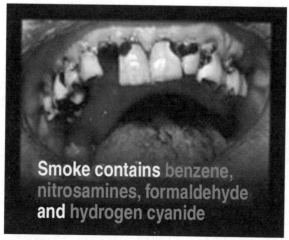

Figure 8.1   Picture warning to appear on tobacco products

MASS MEDIA IN PRACTICE

The two case studies which follow illustrate how mass media campaigns have been used with some degree of success to influence behaviour.

Case study 1: Truly Clean Hands campaign – 'Hohoro Wonsa'

Location: Ghana, December 2003–May 2004.

Target audience: mothers with children under 5.

Aim: to reduce diarrhoeal diseases by improving hygiene behaviours, specifically washing hands with soap.

Message: single clear message – 'without soap your hands are not truly clean'.

Development: based on in-depth qualitative research that revealed hygiene behaviours were driven by fear of contamination, desire to care for children and conforming with social norms. Not washing hands regularly with soap appeared to be due to habit, belief that water alone is sufficient and failure to perceive contamination without the sensory cue of dirt on hands.

The target audience was involved in creative development and pilot testing of the materials.

Campaign:

- mass media

  - TV aired prime time, six times per day in English and Twi across three major TV networks
  - radio aired prime time six times per day in ten local languages across 18 stations
  - 32 billboards placed nationally

- community events

  - 132 direct contact consumer events in five of the twelve regions
  - launch activities across the 12 regions in 120 of 138 districts

- posters and stickers were distributed at the events and via schools.

The different communication channels were linked by a common slogan and a song was developed for the campaign. The common message across all channels was: 'after visiting the toilet or cleaning a child's bottom there remained things on your hands that could not be removed unless the hands are washed with soap' (Scott et al., 2008: 394).

Effect (assessed by pre-post survey):

There was a high level of awareness of the campaign:

- 82 per cent of the target population were reached by the campaign (44 per cent through one channel only, 36 per cent by at least two)
- 56 per cent were reached by the TV campaign, 48 per cent by radio, and less than 3 per cent by print materials
- 69 per cent knew the campaign song.

TV and radio had greater reach and impact on self-reported hand washing than community events. However, exposure to TV and radio campaigns was associated with higher socio-economic status – unlike the community events which may be better able to reach lower socio-economic mothers.

The greatest impact was achieved by exposure to a community event, plus at least one mass media channel producing a 30 per cent increase in self-reported 'washing hands with soap' after visiting the toilet or cleaning a child's bottom.

The authors concluded that despite the cost of production and broadcasting of mass media campaigns, the cost per head reached can be less than for direct contact community events. Difficulty in reaching all the target audience, especially lower socio-economic groups, coupled with the additive effect of exposure to one or more channels, supported the use of a number of complementary channels.

(See Scott et al. (2008) for a full account of the campaign and its effects and conclusions.)

Case study 2: 1% or Less campaign

Location: Hawaii six-week intervention, June–July 2004.

Target group: statewide multiethnic community.

Aim: to reduce saturated fat intake by encouraging individuals to switch to low-fat milk (1 per cent fat or less).

Message: 1% or less is best.

Development: existing commercials developed for use in West Virginia were adapted to suit the local context. At a 'surface level', this involved using local actors, accents and humour. At a 'deep level', the campaign tapped into traditional Hawaiian values of interdependence and family and used children to deliver the message.

The campaign drew explicitly on the theory of reasoned action.

To advise on the development of the campaign and establish local ownership, a '1% or Less Commission' was set up involving local physicians, health educators, nutritionists and representatives from the Departments of Health and Education. Partnerships were also developed with the local university, supermarkets and dairy, which was involved in providing free milk for the tasting sessions.

Campaign:

- mass media:

  - radio (budget $40, 000) commercials were aired 1936 times across 12 radio stations
  - television (budget $100, 000) advertisements were aired 505 times across four TV channels

- 585 'shelf talkers' (shelf edge displays) were displayed in the dairy section of supermarkets
- posters were displayed on all Oahu buses during the campaign
- 150 posters were distributed to the Department of Motor Vehicles, worksites, hospitals and physicians' offices
- PR activities, including a press conference launch by the State of Hawaii's Governor's Office, which generated free TV and newspaper coverage
- taste tests in supermarkets and at community events – participants received an information brochure plus promotional material and a money-off coupon for low-fat milk.

Effect (assessed by cross-sectional telephone surveys at baseline, immediately after the campaign and three months later. Milk sales were also assessed.):

- 37.8 per cent recalled the campaign initially and 27.6 per cent after three months
- of those aware of the campaign:
    - 82.2 per cent got it from TV, 4.1 per cent from radio, 5 per cent from newspapers, 4 per cent from magazines
    - the primary message was recalled correctly by 33.8 per cent
- consumption of low-fat milk by milk drinkers increased from 30.2 per cent to 40.8 per cent immediately after the campaign, falling to 35.9 per cent three months later
- it is estimated that some 65,000 people changed to low-fat milk immediately after the campaign, with a sustained effect on 32,000
- in the largest county, low-fat milk sales increased from 32.1 per cent before the campaign to 41 per cent in September 2004 and 38.8 per cent in October 2004.

Other effects: from September 2004, schools stopped offering 2 per cent milk and replaced it with 1 per cent.

(For a full account of the 1% or less campaign, see Maddock et al., 2007.)

The case studies in context

The two examples share common features including having clear objectives, a simple message, adaptation of the message to suit the audience and the intensity of the campaign involving a number of channels. Further, one of them has an explicitly stated theoretical framework.

It is interesting to note commonalities with the principles set out by Aldoory and Bonzo (2005) for the development of injury prevention campaigns. These were identified following a review of the research literature and theoretical perspectives. In their view, campaigns should:

- be multi-component multichannel – incorporating interpersonal, mass media and printed sources
- use a mix of voices to spread campaign messages – both authority figures and peers
- focus on simple steps to injury prevention – i.e. on changes which are easy to make
- encourage the confidence to change
- emphasize benefits over risks
- address and reduce constraints/barriers to action – perceived and real
- work with opinion leaders
- consider mediating factors in message design such as age, sex, ethnicity, level of education.

In addition:

- the success of fear appeals depends on the amount of efficacy information.

Overall, it appears that what you get out depends on what you put in, in terms of planning, understanding the audience, involving the audience and having adequate resources to implement a campaign of sufficient intensity. Even so, the achievements are relatively modest. Probably the most systematic and comprehensive approach to achieving behaviour change has been provided by 'social marketing'.

SOCIAL MARKETING AND HEALTH PROMOTION

According to Solomon (1989), 'The field of social marketing was probably born in 1952, when Wiebe (1952) raised the question, "Why can't you sell brotherhood like you sell soap?"' He reviewed four examples of what would now be called health promotion campaigns and concluded that their effectiveness was proportional to the extent that they were similar to commercial product marketing. Kotler et al. (2002) identified further seminal events and landmarks in the rise of social marketing. These included an article by himself and Zaltman (1971) and, most recently, the formation of the Social Marketing Institute in 1999.

Kotler et al. (2002: 19–20) define social marketing as follows:

> Social marketing is the use of marketing principles and techniques to influence a target audience to voluntarily accept, reject, modify, or abandon a behaviour for the benefit of individuals, groups, or society as a whole ... [it] is largely a mix of economic, communication, and educational strategies ... As a last resort, the social marketer may turn to the law or courts to require a certain behaviour.

Rather more succinctly, the Social Marketing Institute (undated) define it as 'the use of commercial marketing concepts and tools in programs designed to influence individuals' behavior, to improve their wellbeing and that of society'.

While it would be generally accepted that mass media campaigns utilize communication and educational strategies, reference to economics and legal measures moves beyond the preserve of traditional mass communications. Social marketing, therefore, is more than mass communication and can also involve interpersonal and policy development. Katz and Lazarsfeld's principle of 'supplementation' mentioned earlier is relevant here. Mass media are more effective when supplemented by additional interpersonal strategies.

Much of the early development of social marketing was in the USA. In England, social marketing began to receive more attention following the publication of the *Choosing Health* white paper (Department of Health, 2004). This noted that while a range of lifestyle choices (many unhealthy!) were marketed to people, there was no attempt to market health. The consultation therefore:

> took evidence from people who help make the less healthy choices the sexy ones — marketers and advertisers. They told us that the power of 'social marketing', marketing tools applied to social good, could be used to build public awareness and change behaviour, making behaviour that harms health less attractive and encouraging behaviour that builds health. (2004: 21)

Nonetheless, Kotler et al. (2002: 20) identify a number of differences between commercial and social marketing:

> Social marketers focus on selling behaviours, whereas commercial marketers position their products against those of other companies, the social marketer competes with

the audience's current behaviour and associated benefits. The primary benefit of a 'sale' in social marketing is the welfare of an individual, a group, or society, whereas in commercial marketing the primary benefit is shareholder wealth.

Kotler et al. (2002: 21–2) also:

> resent the notion that social marketing has the same motivations and therefore the same processes as those found in organizations for profit. Commercial ventures are 'in it' for the shareholders. We're in it for the public good. We don't like the association.

The National Social Marketing Centre (2005) makes the point that social marketing does not merely 'import' commercial marketing techniques, but also draws on non-governmental and community sector expertise.

Key features of social marketing

Lefebvre and Flora (1988: 301) identify eight essential characteristics of social marketing:

1 a consumer orientation
2 an emphasis on voluntary exchanges of goods and services between providers and consumers
3 research in audience analysis and segmentation strategies
4 the use of formative research in product or message design and the pre-testing of these materials
5 an analysis of distribution (or communication) channels
6 use of the marketing mix
7 a process tracking system with both integrative and control functions
8 a management process that involves problem analysis, planning, implementation and feedback functions.

There are clearly commonalities with Solomon's ten key concepts (see box) and the model developed by the National Social Marketing Centre (see Figure 8.2). We will briefly consider the most significant elements.

Ten key concepts of social marketing

- marketing philosophy
- the marketing mix
- a hierarchy of communication effects
- audience segmentation
- understanding relevant markets
- information and rapid feedback systems
- interpersonal and mass media interactions
- utilization of commercial resources
- understanding the competition
- expectations of success

Solomon, 1989

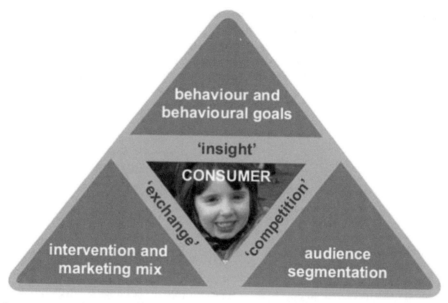

'customer triangle' nsmc © 2006

Figure 8.2   Elements of social marketing (French and Blair-Stevens, 2007: 35)

Consumer orientation

The core feature and underlying philosophy of social marketing is its consumer or customer orientation. Figure 8.2 graphically places the consumer at the heart of the enterprise. The consumer can be the public, professionals or policy makers. The key issue is understanding them within their social context – what is important to them, what motivates them and what factors influence their behaviour (National Social Marketing Centre, 2007). Lefebvre and Flora (1988) emphasize that social marketing should address clients' needs and interests. They argue that instead of being product or expert driven, social marketing should be responsive to consumer needs.

Exchange

The 'primary operational mechanism is based on exchange theory' (Lefebvre and Flora, 1988: 302). This involves an exchange of something valued by two or more parties. In commercial marketing, it is typically a consumable product that is exchanged for money. In social marketing, it more typically involves ideas or behaviour. Similarly, costs can include time and effort rather than money. Lefebvre and Flora (1988) stress that the approach should encourage voluntary exchange and reject the use of high pressure persuasion. While the notion of profit tends to be alien to social programmes, the concept can equally embrace social benefits such as health and wellbeing.

Audience segmentation

Meeting the needs of the 'audience' in relation to the development of either a product or a message will clearly be enhanced if the audience can be segmented into homogenous subgroups which share key characteristics. Segmentation can be based on a range of variables including traditional geographical and demographic factors. However, greater precision can be introduced by considering so-called psychographic factors such as lifestyle, personality, stage of readiness for change, and perceptions of costs and benefits. Although not strictly the intended audience, the views of any gatekeepers may also be important.

Channel analysis

This involves identifying which channels or combination of channels will be most effective in conveying the message to the target audience. Consideration will need to be given to the reach and credibility or persuasive appeal of different channels. These would include opinion leaders as well as mass media and the identification of what Lefebvre and Flora (1988) refer to as 'life path points' such as grocers, restaurants, bus stops, hairdressers. Maximizing interaction between media and interpersonal interventions is likely to increase effectiveness in line with Lazarsfeld and Merton's key principle of 'supplementation'.

Financial constraints may encourage social marketers to use commercial resources by working with commercial agencies. For instance, Solomon suggests that advertising agents might be persuaded to lend their support to enhance their own agency's brand image of social responsibility. Such tactics should be approached with caution as association with certain commercial ventures might well undermine the integrity and credibility of health promotion. For instance, to accept support from manufacturers of powdered baby milk for antenatal education would be unwise.

The marketing mix

The so-called 'marketing mix' refers to the classic four 'Ps' – Product, Price, Place, Promotion.

The main principle for marketing health is that health **products** should be tangible, attractive and accessible. Certainly, a major problem with many health promotion 'products' is that they can be intangible and their accessibility is limited – for instance, a lack of exercise facilities or, more importantly, access to a decent job, money and respect. As for attractiveness, a number of traditional health promotion goals may look distinctly unappealing to the potential customer! Kotler et al. (2002) describe three levels of product. These are core products (benefits), actual products (behaviour) and augmented products (tangible objects or services).

Price is clearly important for all marketing. This may involve actual financial expense but, typically, includes social, psychological and environmental 'costs'. Reference to the health belief model indicates that preventive behaviour will only occur if the perceived benefits outweigh the costs. The implication for social marketing is, in Kotler et al.'s words, 'managing the costs of behaviour change'. Kotler et al. provide examples of the costs of tangible objects (bike helmets, condoms, sunscreen, earthquake preparedness kits) and services (swimming classes and family planning services). Non-monetary costs include time, effort and energy – for instance, parking one's car before using a mobile phone or using public transport. A third category of non-monetary cost is labelled 'psychological risks and losses', such as embarrassment or fear of rejection. Kotler et al. specifically refer to:

- finding out whether or not a lump is cancerous
- saying no to a second glass of wine
- having a cup of morning tea without a cigarette
- using sunscreen and returning from Hawaii looking pale.

The cost associated with physical discomfort includes activities such as having a mammogram, suffering nicotine withdrawal or taking exercise.

Hastings (2007) draws on Rangun et al. (1996) to propose systematically assessing the level of cost in relation to the production of tangible or intangible benefits (see Table 8.2). He suggests that change is relatively easy for low cost/tangible benefits and communication would be the key element of a social marketing strategy. In contrast, the high cost/intangible benefits quadrant is the most difficult and may need to rely on moral persuasion and social influence rather than marketing. When both the cost is high and benefits are tangible and personal, 'push marketing' approaches may be needed providing support and augmented products to reduce the cost to the individual. For the remaining quadrant, low cost/intangible benefits, convenience should be emphasized along with the benefits to the individual and society.

Table 8.2   Cost–benefit assessment

	Tangible personal benefits	**Intangible societal benefits**
Low cost	Using the stairs rather than lifts to increase personal fitness	Separating household rubbish for separate collection and recycling
High cost	Giving up smoking	Stopping taking holidays which involve air flights to reduce carbon emissions

Based on Hastings, 2007: 75

Place in commercial marketing would generally refer to distribution channels for goods, for example retail outlets. In social marketing, place refers to where tangible products or services are provided or where the behaviour occurs. However, it also includes where people might receive information.

Promotion is rather wide-ranging. It includes campaign publicity and, more importantly, the complexities of message design and dissemination, together with monitoring and modification. As Solomon (1989: 94) notes:

> Promotion is far more than simply and superficially placing advertisements. It is actively reaching out to the right people with the right message at the right time in order to obtain the right effects. And this is not easy to achieve, especially with the large number of competing messages and media.

Clearly, it depends on detailed understanding of other elements of the marketing mix, the audience and communication channels.

Positioning is sometimes added as a fifth 'P'. It is substantially concerned with the psychological location of products. It involves framing products or social issues so that target groups will perceive certain characteristics, and believe and remember them rather than alternative, less desirable frames.

While the marketing mix provides a useful starting point, the National Social Marketing Centre (2007) contends that it may not be sufficient to fully address complex behaviours.

Understanding the competition

Anti-health competition is not difficult to find – as the running battle between public health and the tobacco industry over many years has demonstrated. As well as direct anti-health messages, there may be other 'competing offers' – either external such as competition for time and attention or internal such as addiction, habit or pleasure (National Social Marketing Centre, 2007: 36).

Planning and implementation

One of the undoubted strengths of marketing in general and social marketing in particular is its commitment to systematic planning. There is no fundamental difference between the approach to health promotion planning set out in this book and the various planning strategies that appear in social marketing practice (see, for instance, 'The Montana Model of Systematic Coordination' (Linkenbach and D'Atri, 1998) or the Total Process Planning Model (National Social Marketing Centre, 2006)).

The initial stage involves a thorough assessment of needs. The National Social Marketing Centre (2007) refers to this as scoping. It involves behavioural analysis, developing insight into the customer's perspective and audience segmentation as well as bringing together stakeholders and developing partnerships. It culminates in agreeing which ideas to take forward for further development. Although scoping is critical to success, the National Social Marketing Centre notes that in practice there has been a tendency to sidestep efforts to fully understand what would 'move and motivate' the audience (2007: 129).

Programme development should be based on *formative research* which involves the 'consumer'. Formative research allows ideas to be pre-tested prior to implementation and enables consumers' views to be incorporated into the development of products and services and the design of messages.

Lefebvre and Flora (1988) note the importance of process tracking during the process of implementation and Solomon (1989) the need for information and rapid feedback systems. Such monitoring systems allow checks to be made on programme delivery and the progress of campaigns. They provide important evaluation data and also the opportunity to adjust the programme. In our later discussions of evaluation, we use the more conventional terms of 'process' and 'formative evaluation'.

Clearly, evaluation is an integral part of the planning process – including summative as well as formative and process elements. The key question is: what level of success can be expected? The emphasis in social marketing is on achieving behavioural goals including preventing the emergence of problem behaviours, sustaining existing desired behaviours, and changing existing problem behaviours (National Social Marketing Centre, 2005). However, the hierarchy of communication effects would indicate a number of intermediate outcomes beginning with awareness of the programme through to the final stage of the hierarchy, which would be adoption of the behaviour. Perhaps one of the most useful lessons to be learned from commercial marketing is its recognition that behavioural goals are difficult to achieve, even with the expenditure of large sums of money. Expectations must be realistic if they are to be achievable.

Realistic expectations derive from research, previous experience and a sound theoretical understanding of what is involved in achieving results of a particular kind with the specified target group. A case study of a successful social marketing initiative is provided in the box.

Case study: the West of Scotland Cancer Awareness Project (WoSCAP) – oral cancer

Behavioural goals

To encourage individuals among the target group with signs and symptoms of mouth cancer to consult the health services earlier.

Partnership

Health Boards and health care professionals

Target group

- men and women over the age of 45
- particularly high risk groups such as men over 50, heavy smokers and living in deprived areas.

Developmental research revealed

- low awareness of oral cancer and its symptoms
- low awareness was equated with perceptions of low prevalence
- there was familiarity with the notion of early detection and treatment being associated with better outcomes but …
- at the same time, personal fears may prevent individuals from seeking advice about possible symptoms
- while rationally they would advise others to seek help, their own emotional response might make them personally more hesitant.

Theoretical framework

Stages of change, social cognitive theory, exchange theory

The campaign

Mass media advertising based on strategic research and qualitative pre-testing

- objectives

  - to raise awareness of mouth cancer and the importance of early detection
  - to inform people about the signs to look out for and what action to take should they find something

(Continued)

(Continued)

- personal testimony from real people was found to be effective in getting the message across
- the end line 'If in doubt, get it checked out' was used.

Public relations

Local interventions

- photographic exhibition
- awareness days.

Communication with health professionals via websites, newsletter

Training of over 2000 health professionals

Review of referral pathways and service redesign

Dentists agreeing to see patients not registered with them

Effectiveness

- awareness of the campaign was high (83 per cent prompted awareness)
- people were more aware of mouth cancer and more prepared to talk about it
- of the patients who had seen the campaign, 68 per cent reported that it had encouraged them to seek advice more quickly
- one third of mouth cancers and half the premalignant conditions diagnosed were among people who had come forward as a result of the campaign.

Derived from West of Scotland Cancer
Awareness Project, undated; Hastings and
McDermott, 2006; NSMS Case Study Database, 2008

The relationship between health promotion and social marketing

Notwithstanding their separate origins, there are clear commonalities between social marketing and health promotion. Nonetheless, there are technical lessons to be learned from social marketing's close adherence to systematic planning, especially detailed analysis of the determinants of the behaviour in question, understanding the audience and its motivations, developing messages which tap into these motivations and pretesting all materials.

The early development of social marketing for health focused on achieving specific behavioural goals. The emphasis on individual behaviour made it vulnerable to criticisms of victim-blaming in the same way as the preventive model of health promotion. Social marketing has responded by acknowledging the importance of considering and addressing the social determinants of health behaviour. It attempts to understand individuals within their wider social context and gain insight into the reality of people's lives (see National Social Marketing Centre, 2007). This strand has become more evident as social marketing has developed over time, along with its contribution to tackling inequality. Further, its role in policy development has been recognized. For example, the National Social Marketing Centre distinguishes between *operational social marketing* which 'is applied as a process and worked through systematically to achieve specific behavioural goals' and *strategic social marketing* where the approach is used 'to inform and enhance strategic discussions, and guide policy development and intervention option identification' (2006: 24).

This clearly echoes health promotion's concern to address the wider determinants of health. The territory of social marketing appears to be expanding and becoming remarkably similar to health promotion itself. Moreover, the promise that it offers for achieving designated behavioural outcomes is attractive to public health managers and those responsible for achieving defined health targets (see, for example, Department of Health, 2008a). This raises a number of key questions. Is social marketing an alternative to health promotion? What, if any, are the differences?

While there are undoubted similarities, there are also distinct differences in emphases and values. The primary focus for social marketing is on achieving behavioural goals, whereas for health promotion – and certainly the model espoused by this book – it is on empowering individuals and communities to achieve control over their health. Health promotion would, therefore, have a wider remit in working towards individual and community empowerment, in seeking to create supportive environments for health and tackling power imbalances. For some critics, this has been at the expense of supporting individual behaviour change. However, comprehensive health promotion should include enabling individual behaviour change – not as an end in itself, but as instrumental to achieving the wider goal of empowerment.

Notwithstanding social marketing's claims to be consumer-led, there appears to be an element of top-down paternalism both in defining the agenda and in addressing all the requisite variables to achieve desired behavioural outcomes. Health promotion, in contrast, is more concerned with facilitating choice rather than securing adherence to prescribed behaviours. This is reflected in ways of working which include engaging individuals and communities, participation, building individual and community capacity and addressing the structural determinants of health and health-related behaviour.

Social marketing recognizes the importance of tackling structural factors and advocacy is included within its repertoire of activity. However, advocacy in this context tends to be undertaken on behalf of client groups rather than involving individuals and communities and enabling them to take action, which would be more typical of an empowerment approach.

The development of social marketing has confounded early concerns that marketing approaches are inappropriate for health and inconsistent with health promotion. Social marketing methods can clearly be successful in achieving designated behavioural outcomes. The wisdom of extending its remit beyond this is debatable. We contend that it is not an alternative to health promotion. However, to see health promotion and social marketing as competitors is unhelpful. Social marketing methods can have an important place within health promotion, provided, of course, that they facilitate voluntary adoption of behaviours. Equally, locating social marketing within health promotion capitalizes on the synergy between the two, enhancing the capacity to achieve both behavioural and empowerment goals. A recent analysis of the relationship between health promotion and social marketing (Griffiths et al., 2008: 3) concluded that:

By coming together, specialised health promotion and social marketing for health can ensure that health improvement strategies and practice are as effective as they possibly can be.

ADVOCACY FOR HEALTHY PUBLIC POLICY – THE ROLE OF MASS MEDIA

Traditionally, mass media have been associated with attempts to inform, influence and persuade. One of the more vitriolic condemnations of the persuasive use of mass communication has been provided by Rakow (1989: 169–70) in her discussion of critical theory and information campaigns. She reiterates a point that we made earlier in our discussions of ideology when she comments that:

> Bureaucratic organizations are ... selective about the information they provide, which exposes the myth that simply providing information is a commendable activity. Organizations control which information will be made available to whom because their goal is not really to inform but rather to control ... That one can presume to have even the *right* to persuade someone else, let alone the *responsibility* to do so is never questioned ... [this] cultural preoccupation with persuasion reflects a conquest mentality that justifies the 'violence' [invasiveness] of strategies to change others, reflecting a larger cultural – masculine – propensity to dominate and conquer.

Rakow (1989: 169–70) also forcefully challenges the downstream tendency to utilize media in the service of individual behaviour change, rather than addressing the root causes and determinants of unhealthy outcomes:

> What information is a potential client of a social service agency going to be given? How to beat the system that put her in the situation in the first place? Why are behaviours such as drug use or teenage pregnancy portrayed as the country's most important problems and not militarism, violence against women, or homelessness? Why is the medical profession targeting individuals with health messages such as restriction of cholesterol intake rather than targeting government and industry who are responsible for the actions and policies that put carcinogens in our food, pollute our planet, determine whose health problems get research attention, and the like?

The alternative strategies advocated by Rakow involve community development and participation. Wallack and colleagues (1993) concur but also consider that mass media may make a substantial contribution, in tandem with community work, in advocating for healthy public policy. However, before examining this role more closely, we will consider how mass media might address the fundamental health issue of inequalities.

The health divide – contributions of mass media

In 1997, a working group was established by the English Health Education Authority to consider the most efficient use of mass media for tackling inequality in health (Hastings et al., 1998). Two conflicting approaches to addressing this fundamental issue for health promotion were identified.

The first of these centres on the use of audience segmentation and careful targeting of health messages to reach disadvantaged groups. The techniques involved are exemplified by the tobacco industry's practice of directly marketing brands to specific target groups on the basis of characteristics such as their socio-economic status and personal traits, particularly by direct mail. Strategies used include 'relationship marketing' – that is, the attempt to build a relationship with customers. As Hastings et al. (1998: 49) explain:

> Loyal customers ... buy more ... products, are easier to satisfy, are less price-sensitive and make positive recommendations to their friends and family. ... acquiring new customers through research, promotion and other marketing is up to five or six times more expensive than retaining existing ones. Similarly, research indicates that the average company loses 10 per cent of its customers each year ... by contrast unhappy customers are a considerable liability — they stop buying the company's products — usually without warning — often support the competition and complain to their friends and family.

'Emotional branding' is also considered to play a major part in selling commercial or social products. As Hastings et al. (1998) note, 'customers buy products to satisfy not only objective, functional needs, but also symbolic needs'. For example, a new smoker does not actually need nicotine, or cigarettes, but may be acquiring luxury from attractively packaged cigarettes, association with people who use the same brand or merely demonstrating independence.

Social marketers should, therefore, ensure that product 'tonality' matches the needs of their target audience and particularly lower socio-economic status and disadvantaged groups (Hastings et al., 1998: 52):

> There is also evidence that branding may be a particularly effective way to reach people in deprived communities. Research into how working-class populations use cultural symbols in advertising found that these groups are often poorly informed about the objective merits of different products and therefore tend to rely more heavily than other groups on 'implicit meanings' — context, price, image — to judge products (Durgee, 1986). ... de Chernatony (1993) and Cacioppo and Petty (1989) found that people in deprived communities are less likely to evaluate products on a rational objective basis, but look for clues as to the product's value in terms of its price or its image. They argued that the symbolic appeal of brands is particularly effective in targeting those individuals who do not have the time, skills or motivation to evaluate the objective attributes and benefits of a particular campaign.

The alternative strategy to address the 'health divide' is to use media advocacy to challenge the social and political system that results in the disadvantage in the first place!

Defining media advocacy – social justice and market justice

The Health Communication Unit (2000: 1) defines media advocacy as:

> the strategic use of media (usually the news media) to shape public opinion, mobilize community activists, and influence decision makers to create a change in policy.

Freudenberg (2005) also refers to its role in changing corporate practices which impact negatively on health.

Wallack et al. (1993), in their classic text, challenge individualistic, victim-blaming approaches and assert that advocacy:

> is necessary to steer public attention away from disease as a personal problem to health as a social issue ... [It] is a strategy for blending science and politics with a social justice value orientation to make the system work better, particularly for those with the least resources.

Wallack et al. (1993: 7) make a succinct and coherent distinction between market justice and social justice in a number of observations that chime with our discussion of voluntarism in Chapter 2.

> Market justice suggests that benefits such as healthcare, adequate housing, nutrition, and sustainable employment are rewards for individual effort (on a level playing field), rather than goods and services that society has an obligation to provide. Market justice depends on enlightened self-interest as a guarantor of the distribution of necessary goods and services to those in need.

Wallack illustrates this philosophy, which is so deeply embedded in the USA (and, indeed, many European societies), by citing Galbraith's (1973: 5–6) classic and maverick approach to economics and his critique of large American corporations:

> The corporate economic is not responsible — or is only minimally responsible — for what it does ... If the goods that it produces or the services it renders are frivolous or lethal or do damage to air, water, landscape or the tranquility of life, the firm is not to blame. This reflects public choice. If people are abused, it is because they choose self-abuse.

Social justice, on the other hand, 'is concerned with whether conditions in society are fair and whether resources are distributed equitably. Too often they are not' (Galbraith, 1973).

A healthy society is a democratic society founded on social justice (Krieger, 1990: 414, cited by Wallack et al., 1993: 15):

> Democracy is about having a stake because you are a real participant. It is about knowing whom to hold accountable, and it is about having the power to hold them accountable. Democracy is not about letting priorities be set by a bureaucratic or technocratic élite, or by the 'blind forces' of the market (which always turn a blind eye toward human suffering); it is about constructing a social agenda, based on human need, through informed and active popular participation at every level.

Subscribing to the 'religious mystique' of individualism and market forces is uncontroversial, so social marketing is entirely acceptable within the dominant ideology. The use of media advocacy is not!

Advocacy – the struggle

If there is no struggle, there is no progress. Those who profess to favour freedom, and yet deprecate agitation, are men who want crops without ploughing up the ground. They want rain without thunder and lightning. They want the ocean without the awful roar of its many waters. This struggle may be a moral one; or it may be a physical one; or it may be both moral and physical; but it must be a struggle. Power concedes nothing without a demand.

Frederick Douglass, 1857, cited by Wallack et al., 1993: 39

Distinctions between traditional media use and media for advocacy

Media advocacy shifts the focus from individual responsibility to social responsibility and the goal away from individual behaviour to social and environmental change (The Health Communication Unit, 2000). The main differences between traditional media practices in health promotion and the practice of media advocacy are summarized as follows (which draws on Wallack et al., 1993: 60–75).

Traditional mass media direct messages from a central source to a mass audience. They involve one-way communication and, typically, limit audience involvement to pretesting and segmentation. Media advocacy, on the other hand, has close links with communities and 'seeks to provide community groups with skills to communicate their own story in their own words'. Accordingly, media advocacy has been considered to involve 'narrow-casting' rather than broadcasting and is targeted at relatively small audiences and individual decision makers. Community members are viewed as potential advocates and change agents. The focus of traditional mass communication is on *individual* attitude and behaviour change, whereas media advocacy seeks to develop 'healthy public policy'. Its role can therefore include, in ascending order of radicalism:

- gaining unpaid advertising by providing newsworthy information
- agenda setting about health issues as a precursor to later action
- consciousness raising to stimulate actions having a focus on disease and inequalities in health
- critical consciousness raising about social, economic and environmental issues which influence health and equity.

Although advocacy addresses short-term, pressing issues, the goal is to set this within the broader context of general policy change designed to address social and environmental determinants of health. A particular feature of media advocacy is its concern with agenda setting and critical consciousness raising. Media advocates are health activists who confront social rather than individual 'pathogens'. They therefore seek to make full use of news channels by reacting to news and creating it. They present themselves as 'partners in the news-making and gathering processes'. The use of news may be supplemented by appropriate use of paid media placements. However, public service announcements (PSAs) are viewed with suspicion as they rarely have access to prime-time programming and controversial issues are likely to be censored. In short, media advocacy aims to fill the 'power gap' rather than the 'information gap'.

Agenda setting

Our earlier comments about the 'aerosol model' and mass media strengths and limitations have received support over the years from many distinguished theoreticians and practitioners. Cohen (1963: 13), for example, commented on the power of the press as follows:

> [the press] may not be successful much of the time in telling people what to think, but it is stunningly successful much of the time in telling people what to think *about*. [*An observation also attributed to Ed Murrow, the distinguished American journalist and radio reporter*]

Cohen continues with an apt observation that both supports the uses and gratification theory and indicates the role of media producers in shaping opinion:

> the world looks different to different people, depending not only on their personal interests but also on the map that is drawn for them by the writers, editors, and publishers of the papers they read.

A major function of media advocates is thus to 'draw particular maps' that highlight key social issues following the now well-recognized strategy of 'agenda setting'. Wallack et al. (1993: 61) offer a nice image (from Lippmann, 1965) of the process of agenda setting as 'directing the searchlight':

> Mass media are like the beam of a searchlight that moves restlessly about, bringing one episode and then another out of darkness into vision.

The short-term goals are therefore to generate increased media coverage of the issues and to 'frame the coverage in ways that support policy solutions' (Niederdeppe et al., 2007: 47).

The empowerment model of health promotion, discussed in Chapter 1, emphasized the importance of agenda setting. It placed particular emphasis on the process of 'critical consciousness raising' (CCR) as a more potent device than simple agenda setting – one that often seeks to bring about quite radical political change. CCR will be revisited in our discussion of community development in Chapter 9.

Narrow casting

Reference was made above to media advocacy's 'narrow-casting' approach. This is an important characteristic of advocacy's employment of media. It asserts that, although, ultimately, the general population is the ultimate beneficiary, the primary goal will typically be decision makers, legislators, community leaders and community groups. As Wallack et al. (1993: 78) observe:

> Media advocacy isn't about a mass audience. It's not about reaching everybody. It's about targeting the two or three per hundred who'll get involved and make a difference. It's about starting a chain reaction.

They also illustrate the narrow-casting function of media advocacy in relation to attempts to challenge the impact of the giant McDonald's chain on the nation's diet. They (1993: 118–19) describe a radio spot produced by Schwartz that:

> addressed the CEO of McDonald's by name and told him he could be a hero to children all over the world if he just changed the way his company fried its food. ... when people hear their names or the names of their organizations mentioned in a spot, they not only pay attention but imagine everyone else hearing the spot is paying attention as well. Schwartz wanted to change the behaviour of only one man; his radio message had an intended audience of one.

Media advocacy and civil disobedience – the case of BUGA UP

BUGA UP was an Australian movement that followed a particularly vigorous and radical pathway, adopting tactics that were, on occasions, of dubious legality and included civil disobedience.

The acronym stands for Billboard Utilizing Graffitists Against Unhealthy Promotions and activists set out to alter advertising messages on billboards and other displays with spray cans to replace them with more appropriate healthy messages. Examples of the finished products included changing the messages on a very large billboard located on top of a building at one of Sydney's crossroads. The original was an advertisement for Marlborough cigarettes. After the 'spray can surgery', it read 'It's a Bore'. A rather more risqué facelift was given to a poster advertising Winfield cigarettes, which incorporated the emblematic term 'Anyhow' (see the discussion on page 366 of myth creation). After the improvements, it read, 'anyhow ... have a Wank IT'S HEALTHIER'.

The activists were accused of defacing private property. They claimed that they were 're-facing' it.

Chesterfield-Evans and O'Connor (1986: 241) indicate the effects of this 'civil disobedience':

> The group has attracted hundreds of people of all ages. Among about fifty arrests there have been five doctors and a university professor. The charges have generally been along the lines of 'malicious damage'. But the definition of 'malicious' involves 'indifference to human life and suffering' and this has been used by the graffitists to deny malicious intent and maintain that the advertisement was malicious prior to its message being altered. Hence the graffiti 'improved' the ad.

An example of the re-facing of posters can be seen in Figure 8.3.

The quotation from Chesterfield-Evans and O'Connor indicates two of the main strengths of BUGA UP's approach. The activists were eminently respectable people

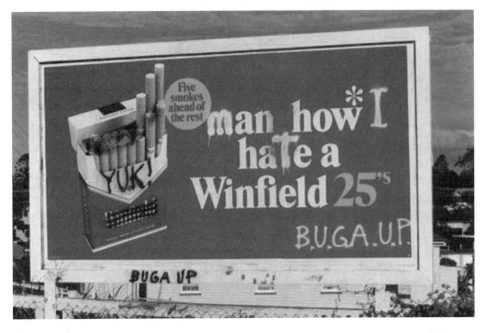

Figure 8.3   An example of the work of BUGA UP's media advocay work (see www.bugaup.rg/gallery.htm)

and their facing up to the giant tobacco corporations was readily 'framed' in terms of the myth of David and Goliath. Chapman's description of the origins of BUGA UP reveals that the reasons for its members' dissatisfaction was that existing health education approaches to smoking were having little effect and they felt that they should 'refocus upstream'.

It is important to note at this point that media advocacy is one particular strategy within the general armamentarium of public health advocacy (see Chapter 6). However, as with all effective mass media use, it is important to supplement media with interpersonal methods. Chapman and Lupton (1994), in their 'A–Z of public health advocacy', describe a full range of detailed tactics that can be employed (see box).

Ten tactics from an A–Z of public health advocacy

Be there! The first rule of advocacy
Crank letters (or how to put your opposition's worst foot forward)
Demonstrations
Gatecrashing
Jargon and ghetto language
Media cannibalism (how media feed off themselves)

(Continued)

(Continued)

Networks and coalitions
'Piggy backing'
Shareholders
Talkback (access) radio

Chapman and Lupton, 1994

An early example from the UK, which was effective in attracting (unpaid) media attention, was a demonstration to raise consciousness about tobacco advertising. The demonstration was associated with the tobacco-sponsored John Player Portrait Award and exhibition at the National Portrait Gallery in London. A UK advocacy organization, AGHAST, decided to enter a specially commissioned portrait entitled 'The Early Death of Jack Filbert'. It showed an emaciated man in his early thirties propped up in a hospital bed, complete with oxygen cylinder. He held a cigarette in his hand. The picture was shortlisted but, unsurprisingly, did not make it to the final round.

Accordingly, AGHAST held its own alternative exhibition entitled 'The Lung Slayer Portrait Award' outside the National Portrait Gallery. Good press coverage was achieved and *The Guardian* newspaper printed a photograph of the Jack Filbert portrait, but not the actual tobacco award winner.

Chapman and Wakefield (2001) summarize some of the techniques used by the Australian anti-tobacco movement to attract media attention. These include:

- test cases involving ordinary individuals suing employers, airlines and nightclubs for not providing smoke-free areas
- making passive smoking an occupational health issue by equating it to asbestos exposure
- publication of expert retorts and the views of international experts
- use of sound bites such as 'a non-smoking section in a restaurant is about as much use as a non-urinating section in a swimming pool'
- commissioning of opinion polls
- challenging misleading press statements on environmental tobacco smoke made by the tobacco industry and reports produced by their scientists which downplayed the risk.

Some of the 'highlights' of the advocacy campaign against tobacco advertising included:

- the six-year civil disobedience billboard graffiti campaign
- finding and supporting sports and cultural celebrities to speak out against the use of their sport for tobacco sponsorship
- picketing the tobacco-sponsored Australian Open Tennis Championship
- levying of a 5 per cent state tobacco tax used to replace sponsorship with public health messages.

Maintaining media interest over a sustained period is undoubtedly challenging. Reflecting on 30 years' experience of tobacco control advocacy in Australia, Chapman and

Wakefield (2001: 276) conclude that 'properly conducted advocacy rests on analytic precision drawn from both theoretical perspectives and empirical trial-and-error experience'. Further, effective public health advocates have the capacity to frame issues in ways which attract public and political support. They note, for example, tapping into myths such as David and Goliath – the small person taking on the might of the tobacco industry and The Pied Piper – the tobacco industry leading children to take up a dangerous habit.

MASS MEDIA AND HEALTH PROMOTION

The mass media are still frequently seen as a panacea and can give the illusion that action is being taken – even if it may not always be effective action! However, properly planned mass media interventions can have a place in health promotion, ideally as part of comprehensive programmes which also include interpersonal influences. The use of mass media for advocacy is entirely consistent with an empowerment model of health promotion. In addition to achieving the primary goal of social and policy change, media advocacy can also help to mobilize communities and contribute to community development – an issue that will be discussed in the next chapter.

KEY POINTS

o Mass media can successfully raise awareness, transmit relatively simple information and influence attitudes. However, they are less successful in developing complicated understandings, teaching the skills needed to support health-related behaviour, or promoting the adoption of beliefs and attitudes which are inconsistent with existing value systems and motivations.

o Mass media are more effective when combined with methods that use personal interaction and as part of comprehensive, community-wide programmes.

o In addition to being a channel for specific campaigns, the media offer other (no cost) opportunities for health promotion such as inclusion of health issues in entertainment programmes like soap operas or in news coverage.

o Over and above the deliberate use of mass media to persuade, the media also have a considerable background influence on social norms.

o Drawing on the principles of social marketing, mass media work should follow tried and tested marketing principles, in particular:

   – systematic planning
   – understanding the target group and its needs, motivations and priorities
   – analysing the cost–benefit implications for the individual as a basis for constructing messages and putting strategies in place to deal with barriers
   – audience segmentation

(Continued)

(Continued)

- designing and pretesting messages which appeal to the audience and are simple, clear and appropriately branded
- using an appropriate source who is credible and attractive
- ensuring that the programme is delivered through appropriate channels and is of sufficient intensity in relation to number of individuals reached, number of times individuals are exposed to the message, and duration of the programme
- using multiple media is more likely to be effective. Repetition is useful – provided it does not become boring!

○ Media advocacy can shape public opinion and bring about policy change through its direct influence on decision makers and/or by creating a groundswell of public opinion.

9

WORKING WITH COMMUNITIES

Go to the people
Live with them
Learn from them
Love them
Start with what they know
Build with what they have
But with the best leaders
When the work is done
The task accomplished
The people will say
'We have done this ourselves'

Lao Tsu, 700BC

OVERVIEW

This chapter considers ways of working with communities. It will:

- consider the meaning of community
- identify different types of community health work
- focus particularly on community development and empowerment as approaches consistent with the values of health promotion
- discuss aspects of good practice in working with communities
- consider some of the challenges in aligning the rhetoric of community development and empowerment with practice.

RODUCTION

hout this text, we have emphasized the centrality of community participation
promotion and have referred to WHO's repeated endorsement of the

primacy of equity and the importance of active participating communities. We have also argued in favour of an empowerment model of health promotion. This chapter focuses on ways of working with communities and developing their capacity to participate, and particularly on community development as a means of achieving community empowerment.

WORKING WITH COMMUNITIES: DEFINITIONS AND CONCEPTS

The concept of community

The notion of community is frequently linked to place. For example, the Calouste Gulbenkian Foundation (1984) defined it as:

> A grouping of people who share a common purpose, interest or need, and who can express their relationship through communication face to face, as well as by other means, without difficulty. In other words, in the majority of cases we see a community as being related to some geographic locality where the propinquity of the inhabitants has relevance for those interests or needs that they share.

The English health policy document *Our Healthier Nation* defined a healthy community as one that 'contains or enables access to all things which allow people to live a full life'.

A community is a 'setting':

- where diversity and local character are celebrated
- where everyone is valued equally, regardless of race, age and gender
- where people are responsible citizens and support each other
- with ready access to the necessities of everyday life, including good work prospects, adequate shops and high-quality public services, such as schools, and medical and social care
- where people like to be and where they can and do join in
- which is safe and environmentally sound
- which provides healthy housing
- with good transport links
- which has good opportunities for play and recreation. (Department of Health, 2002: 1)

While the sentiments are undoubtedly worthy and the implications for creating supportive environments for health and social capital are of interest, it is misleading to conflate 'community' with 'neighbourhood', as has happened here. In the early days of community development, understanding of community tended to be associated with neighbourhood and traditionally much community development work operated within relatively small and self-contained geographical locations of similar size to a neighbourhood.

Boutilier et al. (2000) note the absence of clear definitions of community in both health promotion policy initiatives and in more general bureaucratic usage, together with the tendency to infer the existence of community in the occupation of a geographic space.

The term itself is often tagged on as a descriptor (for example, 'community health initiatives') or vague references are made to the 'community' as a solution, for example in such phrases as 'we just need to work more with the community' (2000: 252). They contend that such imprecise and abstract notions of community can give them an idealized quality which fails to address the 'realities of citizen participation' (2000: 252). The assumption is that communities are homogenous and inclusive, whereas in fact there may be disparate groups, vested interests and conflict and some groups will be more able to participate than others.

De Leeuw (2000: 289) argues that 'it is not just living (in the sense of dwelling) arrangements (in terms of spatially defined localities) that determine "communities", but, rather, ways in which people relate to each other' and proposes 'communication arrangements' as a core definition. New types of interaction are emerging to challenge traditional ideas of community. The development of modern communication technology has in many ways removed the geographical constraints that formerly limited communication and opened up a range of 'virtual communities'. De Leeuw is critical of the distinction between real and virtual communities, contending that virtual communities are real to those who feel they belong. Note, for example, publicity for the 'Taking Liberties' exhibition at the National Library in London which posed the question: 'Why do more young people vote during the X Factor [the TV programme to choose a pop star by viewer votes] than the general election?'.

Over and above issues of location and communication, social bonds and a sense of connectedness are central to the concept of community. A community is characterized by the existence of a network of vertical and horizontal relationships and a shared sense of identity, predicament and, in some instances, purpose. The Standing Conference for Community Development (2001: 4) defines community as:

> the web of personal relationships, groups, networks, traditions and patterns of behaviour that exist amongst those who share physical neighbourhoods, socio-economic conditions or common understandings and interests.

Having a shared sense of identity is important to notions of community, for example groups based on culture, faith, gender, sexuality, disability and service use. McMillan and Chavis (1986: 9) identify the following elements of a sense of community:

- Membership – a feeling of belonging
- Influence – 'making a difference to the group and of the group mattering to its members'
- Integration and fulfilment of needs – 'a feeling that members' needs will be met by the resources received through their membership in the group'
- Shared emotional connection – 'the commitment and belief that members have shared and will share history, common places, time together and similar experiences'.

Henderson et al. (2004: 70) note that people 'define for themselves which communities they feel part of and this cannot be imposed on them'. Further, individuals may align themselves with a number of different communities and when assessing health needs, it may be helpful to think in terms of communities rather than a single community, for example:

- specific small localities
- communities of interest (gender, disability, age, faith)
- service users
- general public.

Rissel and Bracht (1999: 61) identify four broad areas that should be included in an analysis of community:

Space or boundaries — or their absence

Social institutions — such as health, education, religious, business, labour, recreation and local government

Social interaction — the presence of coalitions, influence networks and social support including divisions and discriminatory practices

Social control mechanisms — community institutions such as schools, religious institutions and the police along with values, norms and customs.

Community health work

The initial challenge in discussing ways of working with communities is terminology. There is considerable semantic confusion stemming from the variety of different terms (see box), subtle differences, the absence of universal definitions, the tendency to use terms interchangeably, differences in terminology in different parts of the world and changes in terminology over time. NICE's review (2008a: 12) noted that 'no two definitions of the same approach are the same' and that different terms have been used to describe very similar approaches.

Community work and health: terms in common use

- citizenship
- community action
- community activity
- community capacity building
- community development
- community empowerment
- community engagement
- community involvement
- community mobilization
- community organization
- community participation
- social action.

Community level health promotion interventions are of many and various types. A major point of distinction is between *working in communities* and *working with communities*. The former refers to a location or target for health promotion activity to address an externally defined agenda – and frequently behavioural targets. It is therefore often referred to as 'community-based' and associated with 'top-down' interventions. In contrast, the latter signals a commitment to involving communities in developing their own agenda and working collectively to improve the health of the community. Our focus here is on the latter. An early classic example is provided by the Tenderloin project (see box).

Case study: the Tenderloin project

Origin

Initially set up in 1979 as a university project using student volunteers to tackle social isolation, poor health and powerlessness among the elderly residents of Single Room Only (SRO) hotels in the Tenderloin area of San Fransisco.

Goals

'To improve the physical, mental, and emotional health of elderly residents by increasing social support and providing relevant health education

and

To facilitate, through dialogue and participation, a process through which residents are encouraged to identify common problems or needs and to individually and collectively seek solutions to these problems.' (Minkler, 1985: 304)

Theoretical basis

- Social support theory – developing social support networks to improve health and increase sense of control.
- Freirean philosophy – development of critical consciousness among participants using problem–posing techniques to facilitate discussion and culture circles (see Chapter 7).
- Alinsky's approach to community organization – mobilizing action to tackle issues identified by the community members and empowering disadvantaged and low income communities.

Phases

1 Gaining entry and legitimacy
2 Initial community development within single hotels
3 Coalition building between different hotels and social action
4 Organizational incorporation facilitating continued growth

Volunteers initially provided free blood pressure checks to establish contact and trust.
   After a year, an informal group of twelve residents and two outside facilitators had been set up. Residents began to share concerns and the group atmosphere met social needs. Seven additional groups were set up and common features were:

(Continued)

(Continued)

- decreased reliance on the external facilitator over time and the emergence of indigenous leaders – although groups did not become fully autonomous
- recognition of the need to work together with groups in other hotels.

Actions/achievements

Crime and victimization were identified by residents as a key problem and recommendations for dealing with it in a non victim-blaming way were developed and presented to city officials. The outcomes were:

- increased police patrols in the neighbourhood
- police visits to SRO hotels to make contact with residents
- a Safehouse Project which recruited local businesses and other organizations as places of refuge for people in times of danger and medical emergencies
- reduction in crime by 18 per cent within the first year of the Safehouse Project.

Over time, the project changed in structure from a grass-roots organization to a non-profit organization with safeguards to ensure continued community control. Subsequent activity included:

- seeking funding
- a leadership training programme
- a comprehensive nutrition programme which focused on removing the barriers to accessing food rather than nutrition education:
  - minimarkets in SRO hotels to increase access to fresh food and to provide the opportunity for residents to run a small business
  - bulk food buying club
  - weekly community breakfast
  - buddy shopping for frail residents
  - advocacy to provide food storage and cooking facilities in the hotels.

Throughout, an important element of the project was social contact and the development of social support networks.

see Minkler (1985) for a full account

In a general sense, this latter type of approach has been referred to as community development. The term community organization has also been used, particularly in the North American context, and was defined in the Younghusband Report (1959) as:

primarily aimed at helping people within a local community to identify social needs, to consider the most effective ways of meeting these and to set about doing so, in so far as their available resources permit. (cited by Smith, 2006)

Community ownership and empowerment are key elements. The central role of the community rather than external agents is emphasized in Bracht et al.'s (1999: 86) definition.

Community organisation is a planned process to activate a community to use its own social structures and any available resources to accomplish community goals that are decided on primarily by community representatives and that are generally consistent with local values. Purposive social change interventions are organized primarily by individuals, groups, or organisations from within the community to attain and sustain community improvements and/or new opportunities.

Table 9.1 characterizes the differences between community-based and community development approaches.

Table 9.1   Key differences between community-based and community development approaches

Issue	Community-based	Community development
Community organizing model	Social planning	Locality development; social action
Root metaphor	Individual responsibility	Empowerment
Approach/orientation	Weakness/deficit Solve problem	Strength/competence Capacity building
Definition of problem	By agencies, government or outside organization	By target community
Primary vehicles for health promotion and change	Education, improved services, lifestyle change, food availability, media	Building community and control, increasing community resources and capacity, economic and political change
Role of professionals	Key, central to decision making	Resource
Role of participation by target community members and institutions	Providing better services, increasing consumption and support	To increase target community control and ownership, improve social structure
Role of human service agencies and formal helpers	Central mechanism for service delivery	One of many systems to respond to needs of a community's members
Primary decision makers	Agency representatives, business leaders, governmental representatives, 'appointed' community leaders	Indigenous elected leaders
View of community	Broad site of the problem, technically and externally defined, consumers	Specific, targeted source of solution, internally defined, subjective, a place to live
Target community control of resource	Low	High
Community member ownership	Low	High

Source: Boutilier et al., 2000, based on Felix et al.,1989

The focus on the collective rather than the individual is emphasized in the Global Consortium on Community Health Promotion's view that community health promotion refers to 'health promotion action initiated with community members by community members and for community members' (Ritchie, 2007: 96). Further, a core principle is that:

> Community participation is essential and must drive every stage of health promotion actions — setting priorities, making decisions, planning strategies and conducting evaluation. (Nishtar et al., 2006: 7)

Before considering contemporary terminology and definitions, we will briefly explore the range of activity that might be included in community health work.

Some time ago, Rothman (1979) developed a typology of different types of community intervention which provides a useful framework. The types of intervention are:

- **locality development** – self-help, community capacity and integration (process goals)
- **social planning** – problem solving with regard to community problems (task goals)
- **social action** – shifting of power relationships, achievement of social change (task/process goals).

Twelvetrees (1982) provides another related classification system which identifies three overlapping approaches to community work:

- **community development** – proper
- **political action** – similar to Alinsky's social action approach
- **social planning** – collaboration between voluntary bodies and the state to change and improve services.

Social planning is generally led by organizations external to the community and involves the community, to a greater or lesser extent, primarily in order to increase effectiveness in solving the community's problems and improve service provision. Social action, on the other hand, attempts to shift the distribution of power and resources and influence policy and practice in the public or private sector. It is a movement embodying protest and often associated with the work of Alinsky (1969, 1972). Kirklin and Franzen (1974: 5) offer a succinct description:

> Large numbers of people are organized to bring into being a new power aggregate (or community organization) to force the existing political/economic power structure to change public and private policies. The battle is classically seen to be between the 'power haves' and the 'power have nots'.

The terms 'locality development', 'community development' and 'community organization' have, in the past, been used to describe ways of working that are concerned with developing the capacity of the community to identify its own priorities and work towards them. These approaches tend to be based on collaboration with statutory organizations and authorities. As Kindervatter notes:

> ... social action strategies aim to enable people to jointly challenge and change existing community power relationships. In terms of the relationship between community members and outside authorities, locality development assumes collaboration and co-operation, whereas social action assumes either competition or conflict. (Kindervatter, 1979, cited by Tones and Tilford, 2001: 399)

However, for some, community development is more political in intent and has a more overarching meaning encompassing developing the capacity – and indeed the motivation – to take social action.

Kickbush and O'Byrne (1995) distinguish between different levels of participation in community-based efforts to improve health:

- **marginal** – where community participation is limited and has little effect on the outcome
- **substantive** – where there is considerable community participation in identifying priorities and activities to address them within a context where there may still be high levels of external control
- **structural** – where there is an ideological commitment to community participation and it is a fundamental requirement of programmes.

Laverack (2007) identifies three roles for practitioners which reflect these different levels: directive, telling communities what to do; facilitative, supporting communities to identify and achieve their own goals; working with communities, to achieve social and political change.

In practice, 'pure' forms of the various approaches referred to rarely exist (see, for example, the analysis by the Community Development Project Information and Intelligence Unit, 1974). Furthermore, as projects mature and evolve, there may be a shift in approach. For example, the Tenderloin project (see box on pages 402–3) began as a social action project in Rothman's terminology. However, following its incorporation as a non-profit organization, it also took on a social planning role.

Regardless of the label used to describe different ways of working, a number of key conceptual strands emerge. These are the extent to which approaches:

1   are controlled by external agencies or from within the community
2   meet community or externally defined goals
3   enable communities to participate
3   build capacity and empower communities
5   challenge power relationships
6   seek social and political change.

The balance between these elements will vary from project to project.

Figure 9.1 provides an overview of different types of community health work.

Contemporary definitions

Latterly, the terms community participation and engagement have come into more frequent use and have some commonalities with community development.

Community participation refers to:

a process by which people are enabled to become actively and genuinely involved in defining the issues of concern to them, in making decisions about factors that affect their lives, in formulating and implementing policies, in planning, developing and delivering services and in taking action to achieve change. (WHO, 2002a: 10)

Community engagement has been similarly defined as:

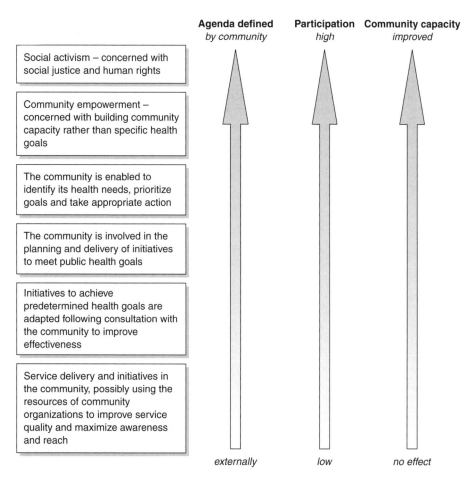

Figure 9.1 Typology of community health work

the process of getting communities involved in decisions that affect them. This includes the planning, development and management of services, as well as activities which aim to improve health or reduce health inequalities. (Popay, 2006, cited by NICE, 2008a: 5)

The term **community development** predates the use of community participation and community engagement. It was defined by the Calouste Gulbenkian Foundation (1984) as:

a strategy for the attainment of social policy goals. It is concerned with the worth and dignity of people and the promotion of equal opportunity ... [it] is most needed in communities where social skills and resources are at their weakest. [It] involves working with those most affected by poverty, unemployment, disability, inadequate housing and education, and with those who for reasons of class, income, race or sex are less likely than others to be, or to feel, involved and significant in local community life.

This definition draws attention to the focus on disadvantaged and excluded communities and the need to increase their capacity to participate. Over and above developing skills and motivation among the community, tackling power imbalances is clearly a key issue as emphasized in the following definition.

> Community development is about building active and sustainable communities based on social justice and mutual respect. It is about changing power structures to remove the barriers that prevent people from participating in the issues that affect their lives. (Standing Conference for Community Development, 2001: 5)

Community development is accordingly based on a number of core values and commitments – see box.

Community development – values and commitments

Values

Social justice
Participation
Equality
Learning
Cooperation

Commitments

Challenging discrimination and oppressive practices within organizations, institutions and communities.
Developing practice and policy that protects the environment.
Encouraging networking and connections between communities and organizations.
Ensuring access and choice for all groups and individuals within society.
Influencing policy and programmes from the perspective of communities.
Prioritizing the issues of concern to people experiencing poverty and social exclusion.
Promoting social change that is long term and sustainable.
Reversing inequality and the imbalance of power relationships in society.
Supporting community-led collective action.

Standing Conference for Community Development, 2001: 5

The role of community development in enabling community action is recognized in Henderson et al.'s (2004: 6) definition:

> Community development: the process of change in neighbourhoods and communities. It aims to increase the extent and effectiveness of community action, community activity and agencies' relationships with communities.

Strengthening community action is one of the five action areas identified by the Ottawa Charter (see box) which also identifies community development as the means of increasing the capacity to take action. Community action is interpreted here as the range of actions needed to achieve change which will improve the health of the community. This contrasts with the narrower interpretation as political activism, aligned with the notion of social activism mentioned above.

Ottawa Charter: Strengthen Community Actions

Health promotion works through concrete and effective community action in setting priorities, making decisions, planning strategies and implementing them to achieve better health. At the heart of this process is the empowerment of communities – their ownership and control of their own endeavours and destinies. Community development draws on existing human and material resources in the community to enhance self-help and social support, and to develop flexible systems for strengthening public participation in and direction of health matters. This requires full and continuous access to information, learning opportunities for health, as well as funding support.

WHO, 1986

Community development is not new (for a review of its history, sees Tones and Tilford, 2001; Smith, 2006). Bivins (1979) described it as an old and reliable grass-roots approach to health education and gave examples of its use in the 1940s, although its principles and applications were in use at a much earlier date. For instance, Hilton (1988: 3–4), using the synonym 'community organization', sees its origins in the Antigonish movement in the 1920s. The movement's principles, set out below, are entirely consistent with community development and the emphasis on the importance of adult education is of particular interest:

- each person is endowed by God with intellectual, volitional (act of will) and physical faculties that must be developed to obtain full and abundant life for all
- major social institutions of society must be transformed to guarantee equal opportunity and full development of all people
- adult education and group action are the most effective means whereby the common people themselves will be able to transform social institutions and this will be done by defining and controlling the nature and direction for social change
- the process begins when common people use adult education and group action to solve their immediate social and economic problems.

Kindervatter (1979: 71) also referred to the origin of community development in the 1920s:

Community organization first appeared in US social work textbooks in the 1920s and 1930s; however, not until the War on Poverty in the sixties did the concept and its application receive much attention. [Its] purpose is to enable communities to improve and change their socio-economic milieu and/or their position in that milieu. [It] developed largely as a response to the conditions of poor people in Western urban settings, but is now practised in a variety of forms in urban and rural locales, in Third World as well as technologically advanced contexts.

Henderson et al. (2004) note that community development has been taken up and championed by other professions – initially, education, particularly youth and community work and community-based adult education, followed by social work in the late 1960s and 70s. Latterly, it has received considerable attention in the context of economic development and regeneration, and it has also been used in public health, housing and community arts. The development of community health work has been substantially informed by community development and also the self-help movement and human rights movements (Jones and Sidell, 1997).

In the UK, there has recently been increasing commitment among the statutory sector to working with communities, driven by the New Labour government's emphasis on participation. Gilchrist (2000) notes that despite this commitment, the government has seemed reluctant to use the term community development. She speculates that this may be, in part, a response to community development's emphasis on achieving goals defined by the community rather than contributing to service delivery and the formulation of solutions to externally defined problems. She further comments that 'community development promotes a participatory form of democracy which sits uneasily alongside the UK's tradition of representation and paternalism' (Gilchrist, 2000: 3).

NICE (2008a: 3) sees community development and engagement as 'complementary, but different terms' preferring the use of community engagement as the umbrella term. The CDX (undated) notes that community development, community capacity building and community involvement all include attention to enabling communities to participate by developing skills and confidence. However, community involvement, participation and engagement tend to be used to refer to efforts to encourage communities to work with other agencies. In contrast, community development is concerned with addressing the issues the community defines for itself – and indeed enabling it to do so.

Conceptualizations of community development generally encompass the notion of empowerment. Laverack (2007: 22), however, in identifying community empowerment as the ultimate goal of community-based interaction, provides a separate definition which places emphasis on social action:

> A process by which communities gain control over their lives, including the determinants of health. The key difference is the sense of struggle and liberation that is bound in this process of gaining power.

Ideology

There are clear similarities between community development and an empowerment model of health promotion. For many, the empowering potential of community development makes it the strategy of choice for health promotion. The very existence of a genuine community is frequently seen as a desirable goal in its own right – that is, a social system where there is a shared sense of purpose, a coherent network of social relationships and the capacity to work together to achieve collective goals. Where a community possesses an additional fund of competences such that it can offer social support to its members, it can also be said to be healthy. The currently popular description of this 'fund of competences' is, of course, social capital.

As we observed in Chapter 2, there is considerable evidence that social support contributes not only to health and wellbeing, but also to disease prevention. It could reasonably be argued, therefore, that the mere fact of creating or building communities having social capital where none existed before is quintessentially health-promoting. However, the ultimate ideological goal of health promotion and community development is the achievement of equity and the reduction of inequalities in health. Particular attention therefore needs to be paid to ensuring that marginalized and disadvantaged groups are able to participate and that their needs are met. Furthermore, commitment to empowerment demands that individuals and communities are able to establish control over factors which influence their health.

Braunack-Mayer and Louise (2008) contend that community empowerment is aligned with bottom-up approaches and favoured as an alternative to top-down paternalistic approaches whether or not they are coercive. It is characterized as the community having a central role in decision making. However, marginalized and disadvantaged communities may lack the power to exercise autonomous choice – or, indeed, influence policy. They argue that this may 'create a licence for paternalistic intervention' (2008: 6) or for an alternative form of paternalism which is concerned with developing community capacity. They therefore reject simplistic divisions between paternalistic top-down approaches and autonomous bottom-up ones. They see the inclusion of some top-down elements as the 'inevitable response' (2008: 7) to the ethical dilemmas presented by community empowerment.

Laverack and Labonte point out the contradiction that those involved in health promotion exercise 'expert power over the community through "top-down" programmes while at the same time using an emancipatory "bottom-up" discourse' (2000: 261). They argue for the inclusion of community empowerment as a parallel track in all health promotion programme planning, even top-down behaviourally orientated programmes (see Figure 4.8).

Ends and means

There may be a variety of different motivations underpinning the use of community-based strategies to improve health. At one extreme, it may involve little more than cosmetically concealed top-down, authoritarian attempts at persuasion to achieve externally defined goals. It may also serve to shift responsibility from the state to the community. For example, the community can become the scapegoat for problems which are the product of wider social, economic and environmental factors – victim-blaming at the collective level! Alternatively, the community can be seen as a resource to respond to inadequacies in state provision. Boutilier et al. (2000) comment critically on the use of community rhetoric as a response to fiscal crises in the North American context and a means of legitimizing the transfer of responsibility to the community.

Clearly, such cynical misappropriation is entirely inconsistent with the definition of community development set out above and its attendant values. Other, more consistent goals, range in intent from the conservative to the more radical, for example:

- improving service delivery to meet the community's needs
- developing self-reliance and the capacity for self-help in the community
- enabling people to achieve their personal health goals
- activism to tackle the structural determinants of health and create healthier environments
- activism to defend the rights of disadvantaged groups and challenge oppression and oppressive practices.

Naidoo and Wills (1994) comment on the dual accountability of community development workers – to their employers and to the communities they serve (see box for example). Gilchrist (2000: 2) notes the inherent tension in community development 'between the goals of the state and the aspirations of the "target" community, with no guarantee that they would necessarily be aligned'. Even at the community level, there may be tensions between achieving the collective goals of the community as opposed to meeting the needs of specific groups or vocal individuals.

Case study: community development projects 1969–1977

The Community Development Project was set up as a Home Office Initiative in 1969 to identify ways of meeting the needs of local people in areas of high social need.

Many, though not all, CDPs developed radical critiques of the economic and political policies underlying poverty and deprivation. Some came into conflict with the local authorities because of their involvement in tenants and other local community groups which opposed council policies on housing and other issues. There was also conflict with the Home Office who closed down the central unit in 1976 and became increasingly concerned at what was going on. Some projects closed early after government and local authority pressure. There were also internal conflicts within some CDP teams.

Working Class Movement Library (undated); see also Smith, 2006

NICE (2008a) acknowledges that approaches which are limited to informing or consulting the community have relatively little impact on health. In contrast, approaches in which communities are partners or have delegated or total control have more positive effects on health and other aspects of people's lives, such as sense of community and social capital along with empowerment and wellbeing.

Claims about the contribution of community participation to health promotion include:

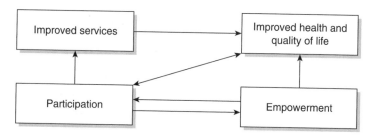

Figure 9.2 Pathways to community empowerment

- increasing democracy
- combating exclusion
- empowering people
- mobilizing resources and energy
- developing holistic and integrated approaches
- achieving better decisions and more effective services
- ensuring the ownership and sustainability of programmes. (WHO, 2002a: 12)

There are often complex and reciprocal relationships between participation and its anticipated effects. See, for example, Figure 9.2 which indicates that the process of participation can be empowering, but equally empowerment can enhance participation. Furthermore, participation can impact directly on health and quality of life or indirectly through its empowering effect and improving services.

From a pragmatic perspective, those involved in planning health promotion interventions should be explicit about what their ultimate goal is and the change pathway leading towards it – i.e. what the intended outcome is and what the strategy for achieving it is. Is developing active participating communities a goal in its own right or a strategy for increasing the likelihood of adopting healthy behaviours? Is participation a way of improving service provision or a means of empowering individuals and communities?

Moreover, it is important to be clear about the approach being used and its underpinning values (NICE, 2008a). Commitment to the principles of community development requires critical attention to process as well as outcomes to ensure that it is empowering. The Global Consortium on Community Health Promotion states that

> it is the participatory, empowering and equity focused *process* that forms the fundamental bedrock of community health promotion. (Nishtar et al., 2006: 7)

Furthermore, processes should ensure that members of the community are able to participate on an equal footing with professionals.

Henderson et al. (2004) distinguish between consultation which seeks the opinion of local people, participation which involves mobilizing people to become involved, and empowerment which strengthens individuals and communities. Communities may

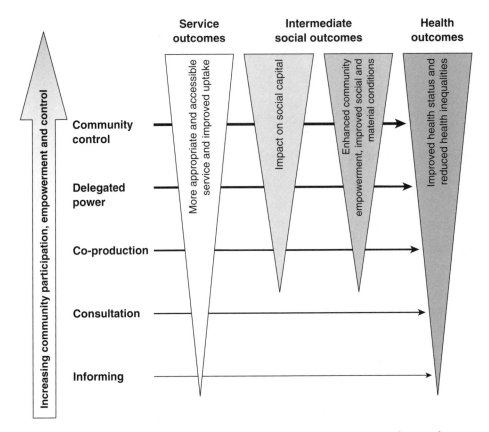

Figure 9.3   Pathways from community participation, empowerment and control to health improvement (NICE, 2008a: 8, based on Popay, 2006)

become involved in a number of different ways which will vary in relation to the amount of power and control that they have. These various levels of participation are usually depicted as ladders ascending from being told nothing, up to being informed, consulted, advising, planning jointly, having some delegated responsibility and, finally, the highest stage of having control (for example, Arnstein, 1969; and Brager and Specht, 1973 – see Figures 5.6 and 5.7). We noted in Chapter 1 that greater levels of participation are linked to higher levels of empowerment (see Figure 1.6). These levels are also incorporated into the framework in Figure 9.3 showing the pathways from participation to empowerment and health.

The use of ladders as a form of representation implies a hierarchy and the superiority of higher levels over lower. While this may be the case in relation to their empowering potential, there may equally be situations when it is appropriate to use information-giving approaches (NICE, 2008a).

There is some debate about whether empowerment is an end in itself or the means of improving other health outcomes. Braunack-Mayer and Louise (2008) challenge the view of 'empowerment as an end' on two grounds. First, improved health outcomes are often invoked as justification for empowerment approaches. Second, health promotion's concern to address 'social, political and economic powerlessness' (2008: 7) stems from the fact that they have a bearing on health.

We have argued in Chapters 1 and 3 that empowerment is central to definitions of health and is a primary goal of health promotion. We do not see any contradiction with the fact that having power and control can at the same time be a means of enabling individuals or communities to achieve other health outcomes.

GOOD PRACTICE IN COMMUNITY HEALTH PROMOTION

While communities may come together spontaneously to tackle a health issue (see, for example, the Entabeni project on page 420), it is more common for an external agent to be involved in initiating community involvement and activity. Efforts to involve communities in health promotion may fail for a number of different reasons – not least poor past experience of involvement. It is important that those involved in community health promotion are aware of current standards of good practice and incorporate these into their initial planning and as a frame of reference for ongoing reflection and evaluation of the process. Not only is this a fundamental ethical requirement, it is also likely to lead to more successful practice.

Henderson et al. (2004) draw on a review by The Health Education Authority and Labyrinth Consulting and Training (1998) to identify good practice for community development and health work – see Table 9.2.

National standards for community engagement to ensure quality and improve the experience of all involved have also been developed in Scotland in collaboration with communities. The standards, each of which has a number of supplementary indicators, are listed in the box (Communities Scotland, 2005: 6) and are based on the following principles:

- Fairness, equality and inclusion must underpin all aspects of community engagement, and should be reflected in both community engagement policies and the way that everyone involved participates.
- Community engagement should have clear and agreed purposes, and methods that achieve these purposes.
- Improving the quality of community engagement requires commitment to learning from experience.
- Skill must be exercised in order to build communities, to ensure practice of equalities principles, to share ownership of the agenda and to enable all viewpoints to be reflected.
- As all parties to community engagement possess knowledge based on study, experience, observation and reflection, effective engagement processes will share and use that knowledge.
- All participants should be given the opportunity to build on their knowledge and skills.
- Accurate, timely information is crucial for effective engagement.

(Communities Scotland, 2005: 5)

Table 9.2 Good practice for community development and health work

	Good practice requires
Clear and realistic role and remit	• Projects to work within a wide definition of health and to establish health as an important community issue • Clarity and consensus about participatory principles and values and their implications • Community participation at all stages of a project • Changes in the culture and ways of working with the statutory sector • A realistic remit for community projects and initiatives based on the time and resources available and the needs and history of the community/users • Respect for minority and different needs and the need for mainstream as well as specific project work
Adequate and appropriate resources to meet the project remit	• Secure, adequate and long-term funding • Accessible and appropriate premises • Experienced, long-term staff with community development skills • Reliable, committed and properly supported volunteers and activists
Adequate and appropriate management and evaluation to support the project	• Effective and supportive project management (through a management committee or line management model) by people with appropriate time, skills and experience • Clearly defined structural arrangements between projects and key agencies to avoid relying too heavily on individuals and to feed in community needs and concerns • Community involvement in project management and decision making • Appropriate monitoring and evaluation to inform project planning and development
Recognition of the importance of the wider environment within which projects operate	• Building on the past history and experience of communities and local agencies and developing new projects within that context • Harnessing the support of local politicians and linking projects to new national policies that endorse community participation • Effective inter-agency and sector links and partnership at local and district or city-wide levels
Building in long-term sustainability	• Linking community health projects into agendas for change that are emerging in the health and social policy fields • Projects achieving real change and gains, and promoting these to communities, funders and agencies • Building community capacity in terms of skills, information access points, networks and groups • Making sure that local agencies and professionals have the skills, knowledge and commitment to support local community participation work, to build community needs and views into their planning, policy and prioritizing and to respond appropriately to community identified needs for change • Seeing sustainability as an integral part of project work, not a final stage.

Source: Henderson et al., 2004

National standards for community engagement

1 **Involvement**: we will identify and involve the people and organisations who have an interest in the focus of the engagement.
2 **Support**: we will identify and overcome any barriers to involvement.
3 **Planning**: we will gather evidence of the needs and available resources and use this evidence to agree the purpose, scope and timescale of the engagement and the actions to be taken.
4 **Methods**: we will agree and use methods of engagement that are fit for purpose.
5 **Working Together**: we will agree and use clear procedures that enable the participants to work with one another effectively and efficiently.
6 **Sharing Information**: we will ensure that necessary information is communicated between the participants.
7 **Working With Others**: we will work effectively with others with an interest in the engagement.
8 **Improvement**: we will develop actively the skills, knowledge and confidence of all the participants.
9 **Feedback**: we will feed back the results of the engagement to the wider community and agencies affected.
10 **Monitoring and Evaluation**: we will monitor and evaluate whether the engagement achieves its purposes and meets the national standards for community engagement.

Communities Scotland, 2005: 6; for detailed indicators, see: www.communitiesscotland.gov.uk/stellent/groups/public/documents/webpages/otcs_008411.pdf

The principles developed by the Centers for Disease Control (CDC) (1997) distinguish different stages in the process of engagement.

Before starting ...

1 Be clear about the purposes or goals of the engagement effort, and the populations and/or communities you want to engage.
2 Become knowledgeable about the community in terms of its economic conditions, political structures, norms and values, demographic trends, history and experience with engagement efforts. Learn about the community's perceptions of those initiating the engagement activities.

For engagement to occur, it is necessary to ...

3 Go into the community, establish relationships, build trust, work with the formal and informal leadership, and seek commitment from community organizations and leaders to create processes for mobilizing the community.
4 Remember and accept that community self-determination is the responsibility and right of all people who comprise a community. No external entity should assume it can bestow on a community the power to act in its own self-interest.

For engagement to succeed ...

5   Partnering with the community is necessary to create change and improve health.
6   All aspects of community engagement must recognize and respect community diversity. Awareness of the various cultures of a community and other factors of diversity must be paramount in designing and implementing community engagement approaches.
7   Community engagement can only be sustained by identifying and mobilizing community assets, and by developing capacities and resources for community health decisions and action.
8   An engaging organization or individual change agent must be prepared to release control of actions or interventions to the community, and be flexible enough to meet the changing needs of the community.
9   Community collaboration requires long-term commitment by the engaging organization and its partners.

Mobilizing communities

One of the major challenges in community health promotion is mobilizing the community and ensuring that all groups are represented. A report by the Joseph Rowntree Foundation (Blake et al., 2008) noted, for example, that community engagement policies do not take sufficient account of the diversity of communities, population turnover and the needs of migrants. Groups least likely to have their views heard were asylum seekers, refugees and economic migrants – and among them particularly women and young people. The study identified a number of barriers to 'getting heard':

- practical barriers such as lack of information and understanding of relevant decision-making processes, lack of transport to meetings and lack of childcare;
- personal barriers such as lack of confidence and/or feelings of discomfort in formal meetings and/or difficulties in the use of English;
- socio-economic barriers including the lack of rights for asylum seekers and the reality of refugees needing to have several jobs to try to support themselves and families back home;
- motivational barriers such as scepticism as to whether involvement is likely to make any difference, cynicism as a result of previous negative experiences, or simply doubts as to whether the desired outcomes could be achieved via local structures of governance at all rather than via some other route (such as through the local MP);
- barriers relating to legitimacy, recognition and acceptance – recognition that is sometimes gained from established organisations or council officers and in other instances by the fact of moving from informal organisation towards formal constitution.

(Blake et al., 2008: 31-2)

Individuals and community groups which have good understanding of local governance structures and political processes are more likely to be successful at having their views heard. Blake et al. (2008) note that key individuals groups and organizations can provide a link between communities and the structures of local governance. They are held to provide bridging social capital.

Burton et al. noted that the types of people involved in area-based initiatives vary according to the nature of the initiative. Strategic level involvement tends to place greater reliance on 'proxy representatives' (2004: 32), such as community leaders or community development workers. In contrast, grass-roots initiatives involve local residents to a greater extent. Burton et al.'s review of area-based initiatives found that involvement could be better planned in relation to approach, structures, roles, processes, methods and resources. In particular, the role of the community needs to be 'clearly articulated at the outset' (2004: 30) and the diversity of the community recognized. Flexibility is also needed to allow 'strategic goals to be changed in the light of community involvement' (2004: 30). Too strong a central commitment to particular policies could lead to alternative community suggestions being dismissed as intransigent.

Some of the barriers to community involvement included structures such as partnership boards run along formal lines characterized by formal agendas, limited opportunity for discussion, rapid decision making and the use of jargon. Clearly, attention needs to be given to ensuring that processes, rather than being intimidating, encourage involvement (see box). Lack of commitment to community involvement among some public sector partners was also an issue and the importance of respecting the 'different but equally valuable contributions of different partners' (Burton et al., 2004: 31) was emphasized. The review noted that effective involvement requires capacity building among all members – not just community.

Case study: enabling parents to participate

Sure Start Local Programmes were a ground-breaking initiative to improve children's start in life in some of the most deprived areas of England. Parental involvement was a central feature of these programmes. One such programme in Leeds had a number of parent members on its partnership board. Meetings were run on quite formal lines although efforts were made to avoid the use of jargon. To facilitate parent participation, a pre-meeting was held with them at a convenient time to discuss agenda items, read through relevant papers, clarify issues as required and provide time to think things through.

Green et al., 2004

The Health Communication Unit (THCU) (2003: 1) defines community mobilization as:

a means of generating interest in, and commitment to, health related matters in a community, and encouraging involvement in developing and implementing health promotion activities to address local health concerns.

Although health communication is generally associated with attempts to educate or persuade, THCU emphasizes its potential contribution to community mobilization by:

- increasing awareness of shared health concerns
- developing the capacity of community groups to take action.

We will return to the issue of awareness raising at a later point in this chapter. However, it is clear that individuals, groups and organizations who are both aware of and concerned about health problems, and who see that they can contribute in some way to resolving them, are more likely to become involved.

Involving communities in coalitions and partnerships with statutory agencies is generally premised on the view that problems in relation to involvement are likely to be due to reluctance on the part of the community. Nair and Campbell, importantly, remind us that the converse can be the case. The Entabeni project (see box), for example, experienced difficulty in mobilizing external partners and found that:

> Most often it is the external partners — particularly those in the public and private sectors — that lack the capacity or skills or organisational systems that would enable them to support the community responses. Our experience is directly in contrast to that presented in the general literature about community development, which often depicts willing and able partners battling to mobilise reluctant communities. (Nair and Campbell, 2008: 51)

Case study: the Entabeni project

The Entabeni project was conceived by local people in a remote rural community in South Africa. Local health volunteers provided assistance to the large numbers of people with AIDS in this deprived community. A three-year project was set up with an NGO to strengthen the community's response.
It aims:

> to empower local volunteers to lead HIV-prevention and AIDS-care,

and

> to make public services more responsive to local needs. (Nair and Campbell, 2008: 45)

The role of the external change agent was to 'facilitate grassroots community responses to AIDS' (2008: 50). They also provided bridging social capital.

The project was successful in providing training for health volunteers in home-based care, peer education, project management and procedures for obtaining grants and services.

One year into the project, attempts to mobilize public and private organizations as partners was proving to be more challenging.

see Nair and Campbell, 2008, for more details

Progress was assessed using Campbell's (2003) criteria for effective partners:

- commitment to HIV/AIDS management and partnership
- conceptualization of HIV/AIDS as a social/developmental issue
- mechanisms for partner accountability to target communities
- incentives to be involved in partnership
- agency capacity.

Particular difficulties included the absence of formal systems to ensure accountability to service users, along with limited capacity due to shortages of funding and trained personnel. Over and above addressing these issues, Nair and Campbell identify the need for positive morale and confidence among prospective partners and the institutionalization of partner roles.

COMMUNITY HEALTH PROJECTS: EXAMPLES

There are clearly numerous different types of community projects. By way of example, we will briefly consider two drawn from opposite ends of the spectrum of participation.

Community-wide interventions

There are a number of meticulously designed and evaluated community-wide interventions which would conform to Rothman's social planning approach. They include the classic demonstration projects such as the Stanford Five City Project, North Karelia Project, Pawtucket Heart Health Programme and Minnesota Heart Health Programme.

It is no coincidence that the major focus of these various interventions is on the prevention of heart disease. This reflects the medical importance of the disease and its general cost to (Western) societies. The agenda is thus predetermined. It would, however, be churlish not to acknowledge that programme designers have recognized the importance of community involvement – both for reasons of ethics and, perhaps more importantly, to maximize the programme's effectiveness. In fact, Minkler (1990), in a very useful review of community organization and radical community movements, acknowledges the way in which the Minnesota Heart Health Programme (targeting a population of some 250,000 residents) was committed to developing 'community partnerships'.

Attempts to involve community members typically include community representation in broad-based coalitions of the great and good and their involvement in 'citizen boards' and various taskforces (Bracht and Gleason, 1990). Bracht and Kingsbury (1990) exemplify the composition of these citizen boards as comprising local government officials, local media personnel, schools, commercial and business organizations, unions, health professionals, minority and voluntary groups, hospitals, churches and community groups. However, the extent to which such initiatives are really representative of the community is somewhat questionable and it is highly unlikely that disadvantaged groups will be substantially empowered.

On the other hand, Minkler (1990: 279) regards the Minnesota Heart Health Programme's achievements as praiseworthy:

Community participation and involvement has been critically integrated into each step of the process by means of a series of small group structures (board membership, functional taskforces, and committees) used as vehicles through which residents have played major roles in generating action areas to be addressed, specific activities to be undertaken, and appropriate groups to be targeted. Moreover, participation on taskforces and committees has not only enabled community residents to share their knowledge of community needs and resources in the design of concrete strategies, but also promoted the continued diffusion of awareness of and interest in heart disease prevention in the community.

Interestingly, Mittelmark, one of the most significant figures in the Minnesota Heart Health Programme, produced a rather bleak assessment of the effectiveness of the 'flagship' heart disease prevention programmes: 'in the final analysis, the main objectives of these studies were not achieved. Risk factors did not on the whole differ between intervention and control communities, and all communities tended to show improvement' (1999b: 11).

A discussion of the effectiveness of the programme is not appropriate here, but it is not unreasonable to speculate that the limited success of these well-designed interventions has something to do with failure to address fundamental structural issues and the root social and political determinants of the problem.

Social action

At the other end of the spectrum are social action projects. A well-known example is the Chipko Movement (Dickens, 1996; Porter, 1998) which originated in the Uttaranchal region of India in 1973 as a grass-roots attempt to challenge government policy awarding logging rights to commercial companies. Activists concerned about deforestation and consequent environmental degradation, with increased risk of flooding and landslides, intervened to prevent trees from being felled by forming a human barrier – hugging the trees. The movement was about more than just saving trees and was concerned with reclaiming forest rights and maintaining traditional ways of life. Sustainability and the judicious use of forests as a resource were also key issues. A particular feature of the movement was the involvement of large numbers of women and it has been widely held to be an example of eco-feminism. Dickens, however, argues from a critical realist perspective that interpretations should be more complex including 'class, property relations and other structures of power' (1996: 68).

On a much smaller scale and at an earlier stage of project development, Laverack (2007) provides an example of efforts by elderly residents to tackle poor housing standards in a deprived inner-city area in England characterized by high levels of unemployment and anti-social behaviour. Poor living conditions were recognized to be linked with poor health and the sense of 'hopelessness, isolation and self blame' (2007: 107) among people living in such conditions. Representatives met with a local health promotion practitioner to consider the way forward. The initial step was to improve community participation, develop a plan of action and seek funding to allow the elderly residents to regain some sense of control and begin to take action.

CHALLENGES AND DILEMMAS

We have argued that health initiatives which actively engage communities in partnership are consistent with the principles of health promotion and particularly the empowerment model which we have advocated. However, in practice, a number of challenges arise.

A key issue is the role of community health workers. Henderson et al. distinguish between two broad categories of role – first, those that are associated with an objective, neutral or democratic approach and would include 'interpreter, communicator, enabler, guide, facilitator, encourager, catalyst, broker, animator (nurturing leadership from within the group), or mediator' and secondly, more directive roles including 'stimulator, expeditor, organiser, negotiator, bargainer, advocate, expert or activist' (2004: 84).

The rhetoric of community development would support the use of non-directive approaches whenever possible. Yet there are situations when more directive approaches may be called for, either to meet the needs of the target group, to suit the stage of the project, or to achieve externally or professionally defined outcomes. For example, the most marginalized and powerless groups may not have their voice heard unless health workers adopt an advocacy or activist role or focus on capacity building. The important issue is that directive approaches should not further disempower these groups by creating dependency, but rather that they should actively contribute to empowering them.

Boutilier et al. (2000) point out that community development workers may initially occupy a position of power vis-à-vis those with whom they are working by virtue of greater income, professional status and their ability to influence political agendas. However, exercising this power becomes 'transformative' if the process enables community members to acquire power as a consequence. As the authors note – this transfer of power classically results in community workers working themselves out of a job. Their role will change through the course of an initiative from being directive at the outset to becoming progressively non-directive as the community assumes control.

Clearly, it is incumbent on community health workers to ensure that all members of the community and diverse interest groups are represented. Their ability to do so will depend on their understanding of the community and insight into the factors that would encourage the participation of different groups – issues that should inform initial planning. Some groups will be more able to participate than others. Ongoing critical reflection to assess the extent to which initiatives are successful in engaging different groups is essential and strategies should be put in place to reach out to under-represented groups. Nonetheless, the views of more powerful groups may come to dominate. NICE (2008a: 23) notes the need to:

> Recognise that some groups and individuals (from the public, community and voluntary sectors) may have their own agendas and could monopolise groups (so inhibiting community engagement).

Situations may also arise when the priorities and needs expressed by the community may differ from those of professionals. Bolam (2005: 447) notes that while lay people have a complex understanding of health, there is a tendency, especially in lower social groups, to focus on 'agency and strength of character' rather than structurally orientated explanations of health inequalities. Furthermore, there is concern among these groups about the 'potential stigma associated with being seen as a victim'. Clearly, then, there may be a conflict of interest between professionals seeking to engage in social action to tackle the upstream structural determinants and some community groups which may prefer more downstream solutions. Commitment to evidence-based practice may also prove to be problematic if the evidence conflicts with the community's views.

There is no easy answer to resolving these issues. Bolam suggests that media advocacy may be needed at the outset to raise awareness of the social determinants of health among such community groups. Yet again, this implies the need for initial paternalistic interventions and assumes that professionals have greater overall strategic insight. We will consider the issue of professionals attempting to subtly influence the agenda to conform with their own views – so-called facipulation – at a later point in this chapter. Commitment to the principles of community development would demand that all positions are respected, fully discussed, additional information sought and a collective decision reached by democratic processes.

There is a view that collective decisions and action can militate against individual freedom of choice and action. We argued in Chapter 1 that an unbridled free for all is inconsistent with the values of health promotion. While individuals have the right to self-fulfilment, this should not be at the expense of the rights of others and the wellbeing of the community more generally. The overarching principle is that fundamental human rights must be respected, whether or not they are recognized by specific groups. Clearly, prejudice and discriminatory practice in all its forms should be challenged.

Gilding the ghetto? Some limitations of community development

Although criticisms have been directed at community-based health work that operates in a top-down fashion with predetermined agendas, it cannot be assumed that community development is a panacea for addressing social-structural health problems. Indeed, although an advocate of community development, Constantino-David (1982) provides a very thoughtful critique listing the following limitations and potential threats.

- Community members are at risk of becoming dependent on the community workers and when the workers withdraw and/or funding is withdrawn, the project collapses.
- A new elite might be created from indigenous workers/opinion leaders recruited by change agents.
- Community workers may face a dilemma: the community's felt needs may be relatively insignificant in the long term and more fundamental goals, such as empowerment or political change, may be deferred or ignored.
- Following on from this last point, community workers must be on their guard to avoid imposing their own political agenda on the community. They therefore face a 'facilitation v. manipulation' dilemma. Their role is to facilitate community decision making in the interest of empowerment. They may, however, yield to the temptation to manipulate or subtly steer the community in the direction of their own choosing. Constantino-David refers to this process as 'facipulation'.

A more important question mark hanging over community development is whether or not it can really have any significant influence on major structural problems such as inequality. The activities of communities and their successes have been described by such metaphors as 'tidying the deckchairs on the Titanic'. Loney (1981), for example, makes this point when referring to the report of the Community Development Project (1977) (referred to in the case study on page 412) which was aptly titled *Gilding the Ghetto*.

Rahman (1995: 32) discusses the problems associated with the failure of successive approaches to Third World development initiatives and comments specifically on what he describes as a 'new worldwide culture of development action termed "popular participation in development" or simply "participatory development"'. He has severe reservations about small-scale participatory efforts that 'seem to be serving the purpose mainly of providing a "safety net" and do not promise fundamental movement toward people's liberation' and do not reflect 'the values of social activism, building towards a more genuinely participatory approach to transformation'.

Serrano-Garcia discusses the effect of a community development programme in Esfuerzo, a poor rural community in Puerto Rico, and asks the question, 'Did our intervention facilitate the empowerment of the residents of Esfuerzo? What are the limits of empowerment efforts within our colonial context?' She (1984: 197) concludes that:

> the community members had gained new skills, feelings of competency, and insights that should enable them to achieve greater control over some aspects of their community life. [They would probably have] ... a different, more affirmative, perspective on their role in their community.

Her writing, however, reflects concern that they might have 'fostered the illusion' that their society allows for empowerment. She then questions the possibility of creating real social change using community development techniques. Her (1984: 197–8) review of the nature of the society, its power structure and barriers to change is illuminating and iterates the recurring observations we have made throughout this book:

> I am convinced that our society does not allow [empowerment]. Ours is a society which, along with the economic and political facts previously presented, is characterized by an ideology of conservatism and pro-American values. These emphasize (a) an electoral definition of democracy, (b) the prevalence of a conservative vision of law and order, (c) uncritical acceptance of United States dominance over Puerto Rico, (d) rigid value stances that acknowledge only clear-cut definitions of right and wrong, (e) individualism, (f) veneration of the right to private property, (g) the belief in the governmental duty to protect this right, (h) protection of the free market, and (i) intolerance toward dissidence ... demonstrated through the constant and active persecution of pro-independence group members.

In the more developed parts of the world, considerable support has been expressed for the potential contribution of participation to tackling inequality in health. The Mayor of London's paper on health inequalities (Smith, 2007), for example, identifies the particular relevance of participation to health inequalities for four reasons:

1   It enables people to take greater control of their health, both individually and collectively.
2   Taking part in decision making can help the most excluded groups to feel that they have more control, decrease their sense of loneliness and isolation and enhance self-esteem.
3   Policy makers can draw on local expertise to achieve better decisions.
4   Using the expertise of community and voluntary groups to deliver some public services can be more successful in reaching vulnerable and excluded groups.

Bentley includes in the ten major lessons learned to date about tackling health inequalities the need to 'capitalise on community engagement' and specifically to:

> Support local authority partners in the development of neighbourhood and community infrastructures to engage residents, particularly those 'seldom seen, seldom heard' in services. Use to ensure that services are responsive to needs, but also to help motivate and support appropriate health-seeking behaviour. Establish effective links with frontline services, utilising the potential of VCF [voluntary, community and faith] sector agencies as valuable catalysts for dialogue, mutual understanding and empowerment. (2008: 5)

While in no way undermining the undoubted value of participation and engagement, the general tenor of all of these documents is located within the mainstream and lacks the radical edge required to address the primary determinants of health inequalities. Ledwith (2007) argues that those involved in community development 'are allowing ourselves to be redefined as a tool of government policy at the expense of our transformative purpose'. As Dixon (1989: 84) observed some time ago, unless it can be redefined to become more politically aware and radical, community development is unlikely to bring about necessary fundamental change in society to address 'class, race or gender struggles to transform the existing economic and power structures' – such sentiments might equally be applied to health promotion more generally. Bridgen (2007: 257) notes that any attempt to genuinely empower communities, as opposed to capacity building or developing social capital, must involve 'some attempt to increase the influence of the community over the external policy developments that affect it'. Attention must therefore be paid to '(i) the relationship between community empowerment programmes and their external political environment, and (ii) the types of processes that would be required if the former was significantly to alter the latter' (2007: 263).

It is our intention below to consider how community health programmes can contribute to wider development and social action goals.

DEVISING COMMUNITY PROGRAMMES FOR DEVELOPMENT AND SOCIAL ACTION

We noted above the importance of shared awareness of health issues for mobilizing communities, and, indeed, potential partners. Bracht et al. (1999: 85) describe stimulation or activation as the process by which a community:

- becomes aware of a condition or problem that exists within a community
- identifies that condition as a priority of community action
- institutes steps to change the condition
- establishes structures to implement and maintain program solutions.

Batten (1967) focuses in on a process of awareness raising and changing group members' perceptions of their situation that parallels aspects of Freirean critical consciousness raising (see Table 9.3).

A Freirean perspective

As we noted in our general discussion of critical education in Chapter 7, Freirean approaches provide quite detailed suggestions for practice. These are consistent with community development (CD) and the analysis offered by Batten. However, as we emphasized earlier in the discussion centring on the phenomenon of 'ghetto gilding', there are substantial limitations to the potential of CD to effect radical change.

Kindervatter (1979) reinforces these doubts and uncertainties in her discussion of the effectiveness of two projects in Indonesia and Thailand. She asks, is it really possible to empower, 'in political settings not committed or even antagonistic to a more equitable sharing of power and resources?' She also raises the important

Table 9.3   Stages of awareness leading to group action

Actions of community worker	Reactions of group members
I Stimulates people to think why they are dissatisfied and with what	Vaguely dissatisfied but passive
II Stimulates people to think about what specific changes would result in these needs being met	Now aware of certain needs
III Stimulates people to consider what they might do to bring such changes about by taking action themselves	Now aware of wanting changes of some specific kinds
IV If necessary, stimulates people to consider how best they can organize themselves	Decide for, or against, trying to meet to do what they now want to do for themselves
V Stimulates people to consider and decide in detail just what to do, who will do it, and when and how they will do it	Plan what to do and how they will do it
VI Stimulates people to think through any unforeseen difficulties or problems that they may encounter in the course of what they do	Act according to their planning
VII Satisfied with the results of what they have achieved	

After Batten (1967)

question of the 'balance of power between conflicting parties' and the need for confrontation by less powerful parties. She (1979: 240) makes an important cultural point, too – namely that cultural norms in the two projects she studied were inimical to confrontation:

> Confrontation has been employed by some groups in Asian contexts, such as squatters in the Philippines, but only in reaction to grossly oppressive conditions. In most cases, people would probably seek other means to solve a problem, and if that failed, possibly leave the problem unsolved.

She observes that although some gains were achieved in the Thai and Indonesian projects, 'these gains were not those which significantly altered existing power structures or relationships'. In those countries:

> people know that posing real challenges to the political or economic system can have serious consequences [and] people themselves must balance the possible risks and sacrifices with achieving a particular gain, and decide what course of action to follow.

An expanded model of community development is needed to take account of these several difficulties. It also needs to emphasize the importance of identifying ways to actively support community members' commitment to action. Figure 9.4 seeks to identify key elements of this expanded model.

In short, community workers act as catalysts and occupy a kind of combined counselling and catalyst role. They employ such typical counselling skills as active listening and providing reflective feedback and act in accordance with the 'holy trinity' of counselling – demonstrating respect, empathy and genuineness. Their credibility and perceived status is clearly important. As we noted in our earlier discussion of communication of innovations theory, the quality of homophily is important in establishing a trusting relationship.

The major feature of this expanded model of community development centres on the kinds of support provided to the dialogic process of consciousness raising and praxis. Before the action plans resulting from praxis can be translated into successful actions, community members will need a range of appropriate life skills and action competences if they are to work effectively in groups, act as lobbyists and deploy a range of other confrontational techniques.

Media advocacy – following the precepts described in Chapter 8 and associated with Wallack's formulation – enables community activists to raise consciousness in the community as a whole. They might, for instance, use media messages based on creative epidemiology or, as described by Wang and Burris (1994), create their own images of community life and predicaments using photography. As Wallack and others have demonstrated, media advocacy is typically associated with the development of coalitions of like-minded people, both within and outside the community. Although the main focus of action might be on a relatively small scale, such as the development of food cooperatives or credit unions, by collaborating with broader-based coalitions, local communities may contribute to a more substantial movement for addressing issues such as health inequalities. As Taylor (1995: 109–10) remarks:

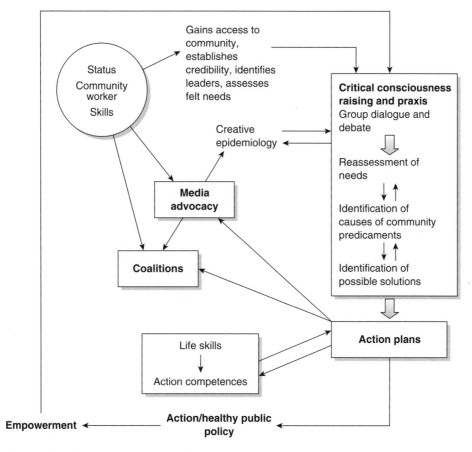

Figure 9.4 An expanded model of community development to include advocacy, praxis and healthy public policy

it is likely that in a more fragmented 'postmodern' environment, networks and alliances will be the foundation on which empowerment is built. Community work needs to develop a practice which can work with allies across the institutional map to find the possibilities for change in an increasingly turbulent environment.

The expert's task

Experts should be on tap not on top!

Kindervatter, 1979

The educational dimension

One of the main themes of this book is our assertion that education (broadly defined) is at the epicentre of health promotion. Its contribution to community development and its variants is probably self-evident. However, Kindervatter's philosophy and practice is of particular interest as she more or less equates community development/organization with what she calls 'non-formal education'. She (1979: 87–8) defines community development as:

- attempting to build local capability by nurturing grass-roots organizations and creating coalitions of organizations
- utilizing natural groups or structures
- starting from people's interests and moving at their pace
- emphasizing the identification and development of 'native' leaders – that is, opinion leaders
- promoting peer support and mutual help
- having an open-ended agenda and aiming to activate people to work together
- building cooperative community problem-solving capacity and a power base from which existing power relationships can be confronted
- emphasizing discussion methods, democratic procedures and action
- having an organizer who serves as a 'process guide' and resource person
- enabling the transfer of initiative and responsibility from community worker to the people to achieve local autonomy.

The *raison d'être* of non-formal education (NFE) is identical to WHO's definition of empowerment as people gaining control over their lives (and their health) or, in Kindervatter's words, gaining 'understanding of and control over social, economic, and/or political forces'. Its methodology includes small group 'teaching' with a community worker as a facilitator rather than instructor, the transfer of responsibility from teacher to participants and an emphasis on participant leadership, as well as the integration of reflection and action (praxis).

We have already discussed the radical philosophy of Freire's empowering educational approach and its imperative for sociopolitical change in pursuit of equity. Kindervatter (1979: 149) incorporates Freire's principles and practice, together with those of Charnofsky (1971), Curle (1972) and Wren (1977), and summarizes them under the rubric 'education for justice' (see box):

- development of critical consciousness
- small group discussion (culture circles)
- utilization of a problem stimulus for circle members to decode
- utilization of tools, such as games, to help people reflect on their realities
- a focus on 'system blame' rather than 'person blame' as a cause of problems
- the aim to achieve conflict resolution with a win–win outcome
- emphasis on non-hierarchical methods and relationships, dialogue and shared leadership
- utilization of facilitators who are committed to liberation, have faith in people, are humble and who act primarily as problem and question posers.

Education for justice

Justice calls for the establishment of a society on both a global and national scale where each person has an equal right to the most extensive basic liberties compatible with a like liberty for all, where social and economic inequalities are so arranged that they are to the greatest benefit of the least advantaged, and where they are linked with position and appointments which are open to all through fair equality of opportunity.

Wren, 1977: 55

Ledwith (2007) emphasizes the need for community development to be both critical and vigilant to retain its radical edge and concern for social justice rather than 'slipping into some feel-good, ameliorative, sticking plaster on the wounds of injustice'. She argues that:

> the full collective potential of community development is threatened by a resistance to praxis, a theory–practice divide which results in 'actionless thought' on one hand, and 'thoughtless action' on the other (Johnston cited in Shaw, 2004: 26). If we fail to generate theory in action, and move towards a unity of praxis where theory and practice are synthesised, we give way to anti-intellectual times which emphasize 'doing' at the expense of 'thinking'; we react to the symptoms rather than root causes of injustice – and leave the structures of discrimination intact – dividing people through poverty, creating massively different life chances by blaming the victims of an unjust system.

KEY POINTS

○ Understanding the nature of community and the characteristics of specific communities is fundamental to community health work.

○ Community health work can be broadly divided into working in communities to achieve externally defined targets or working with communities to enable them to identify their own targets and the best means of achieving them.

○ Notwithstanding problems with terminology, we have identified a number of features which characterize community health work. Key among these is the extent to which communities actively participate in decision-making and whether the focus is on achieving social action to address the structural determinants of health.

(Continued)

(Continued)

o Efforts to engage communities should pay particular attention to ensuring that disadvantaged and socially excluded groups are able to participate and have their voice heard.

o Initiatives which involve communities can serve a range of purposes from improving service provision and achieving behaviour change through to tackling the structural determinants of health and radical social change.

o Practitioners working with communities should have a clear view of their goals and should reflect critically on the process, particularly in relation to power relationships.

o Education has a central role in community development/empowerment which includes increasing the capacity to participate and consciousness raising leading to praxis.

o Community development is an important means for achieving empowerment, equity and tackling social injustice. It requires a critical approach rooted in the core values of mutual respect and cooperation.

10

SETTINGS FOR HEALTH

Change is not made without inconvenience, even from worse to better.

Samuel Johnson (1780–84)

OVERVIEW

This chapter focuses on the settings approach. It will:

- identify key elements of the settings approach drawing on examples from a range of different settings
- consider factors supportive of the successful implementation of the settings approach
- focus on the health promoting school to exemplify the settings approach in more depth
- make further observations about different settings for health.

INTRODUCTION

We have already considered macro-level strategies for influencing health, notably policy and mass media. At the meso level, we have also considered community-based approaches. While the community might well be regarded as a setting for health, in Chapter 9, we focused on issues relating to community development and empowerment. We now turn attention to the settings approach itself.

The emergence of the settings approach has generally been attributed to the Ottawa Charter's (WHO, 1986) assertion that 'health is created and lived by people within the settings of their everyday life; where they learn, work, play and love'. It involves a shift from individual behavioural approaches towards considering the contribution of major settings to health. Not only do settings impact directly on health and wellbeing, but individual choices about health and health behaviour are taken in the settings encountered in day-to-day life – the home, community, workplace and school (WHO, 1999b). As Kickbush (1996: 5) notes, the settings approach shifts 'the focus from the deficit model of disease to the health potentials inherent in the social and institutional settings of everyday life'.

Commitment to the settings approach was also strongly endorsed by the Jakarta Declaration (WHO, 1997):

> comprehensive approaches to health development are the most effective ... particular settings offer practical opportunities for the implementation of comprehensive strategies. These include megacities, islands, cities, municipalities, local communities, markets, schools, the workplace, and health care facilities.

THE SETTINGS FOR HEALTH APPROACH

It is self-evident that access to individuals or groups is a fundamental requirement for health education. The opportunity afforded by different settings for gaining entry has therefore been of considerable interest. The notion of a health career, to which we referred in Chapter 2, is one means of identifying points of contact and a list of key questions for assessing their potential is provided in the box.

Key questions for working in settings

Regarding access

- What kind of target group is accessible via this setting?
- How many people will be reached?
- How easy will it be to reach them?

Regarding the philosophy and purpose

- Has the institution with which the strategy is associated a particular philosophy or goal?

Regarding commitment

- How committed are the institution and its members to the preventive philosophy underpinning the aims (of health education)?

Regarding credibility

- How credible are the institution and the people in it who will act as health educators? How will the public respond to them?

Regarding competence

- Irrespective of commitment, do the potential health educators have the necessary knowledge and communication/education/training skills to promote efficient learning?

After Whitehead and Tones, 1990: 19–20

However, there is an important distinction to be made between seeing a setting merely as a location that offers opportunities for delivering health education – that is, 'health education in a setting'– and the 'settings for health approach', which involves a more comprehensive and coordinated response.

A key feature of the settings approach is that it involves ensuring that the ethos of the setting and all the activities are mutually supportive and combine synergistically to improve the health and wellbeing of those who live, or work, or receive care there. It involves integrating health promotion into all aspects of the setting and including within its remit all those who come into contact with that setting.

To illustrate the difference, Table 10.1 provides a comparison of health education provided in a school and the health promoting school.

Table 10.1 Moving from traditional school health education to the health promoting school

Traditional health education	The health promoting school
Considers health education only in limited classroom terms	Takes a wider view, including all aspects of the life of the school and its relationship with the community – for example, developing the school as a caring community
Emphasizes personal hygiene and physical health to the exclusion of the wider aspects of health	Based on a model of health that includes the interaction of physical, mental, social and environmental aspects
Concentrates on health instruction and acquisition of facts	Focuses on active pupil participation with a wide range of methods, developing pupils' skills
Lacks a coherent, coordinated approach that takes account of other influences on pupils	Recognizes the wide range of influences on pupils' health and attempts to take account of pupils' pre-existing values, beliefs and attitudes
Tends to respond to a series of perceived problems or crises on a one-off basis	Recognizes that many underlying skills and processes are common to all health issues and that these should be pre-planned as part of the curriculum
Takes limited account of psycho-social factors in relation to health behaviour	Views the development of positive self-image and individuals taking increasing control of their lives as central to the promotion of good health
Recognizes the importance of the school and its environment only to a limited extent	Recognizes the importance of the physical environment of the school in terms of aesthetics and also direct physiological effects on pupils and staff
Does not consider actively the health and wellbeing of staff in the school	Views health promotion in the school as relevant to staff wellbeing and recognizes the exemplar role of staff
Does not involve parents actively in the development of a health education programme	Considers parental support and cooperation as central to the health promoting school
Views the role of school health services purely in terms of health screening and disease prevention	Takes a wider view of the school health services, which includes screening and disease prevention, but also attempts actively to integrate services within the health education curriculum and helps pupils to become more aware as consumers of health services

Source: Young and Williams, 1989: 32

The importance of settings was recognized by Target 13 of the European Health for All Policy Framework, *Health 21* (WHO, 1999b: 100):

> By the year 2015, people in the region should have greater opportunities to live in healthy physical and social environments at home, at school, at the workplace and in the local community.

It notes that taking a settings approach:

- focuses attention on where health is promoted and sustained (where people live, work, learn, play and receive health care);
- sets easily recognized boundaries of action;
- makes it easy to identify potential partners;
- provides the opportunity to observe and measure the impact of interventions for health gain;
- offers excellent potential both for pilot testing and as a 'vehicle' for sustainable change in society. (WHO, 1999b: 97)

The document recognizes that a number of different groups will influence the nature of settings, including those not traditionally involved in 'health' who may or may not be aware of their potential contribution in this regard. They include, for example, engineers, urban planners and the retail sector. In some instances, natural grouping and partnerships may already exist. However, attention may need to be given to identifying all key players to ensure adequate representation and to building new partnerships.

The earliest WHO healthy settings initiative was the 'Healthy Cities' project, set up in 1987 and involving some 11 European cities. The settings approach has subsequently expanded rapidly. There are Healthy Cities Networks in all six WHO regions and in the European region there are now over 1200 healthy cities and towns. The principles of the approach have been applied to other settings – some of them linked internationally via WHO networks (see the box).

Examples of settings for health

Healthy cities
Healthy villages
Healthy islands
Health promoting hospitals
Health promoting schools
Health in prisons
Healthy marketplaces
Workplace health promotion

Dooris (2006) notes that settings occupy different levels which may be nested within each other or have cross links with other settings. For example, health promoting schools may exist within healthy cities and be linked to healthy communities. He refers to Galea et al.'s (2000) distinction between elemental and contextual settings and the need to maximize the 'synergy' between different settings.

Denman et al. (2002) draw attention to subtle semantic differences in terminology – health promoting schools and hospitals in contrast to healthy cities and prisons. Latterly, there has been some alignment of terminology, with a trend towards using the term 'healthy' schools and hospitals.

Within the UK, the strategic importance of healthy schools, healthy workplaces and healthy neighbourhoods/communities has been recognized as a means of improving health and tackling inequalities (Department of Health, 1999). These settings were identified as providing access to substantial proportions of the population – schools focusing on children, workplaces on adults and neighbourhoods on older people (Department of Health, 1998a) – with subsequent recognition that a focus on the community could be relevant to young families, older people, people on low incomes, with disabilities and ethnic minority communities (Department of Health, 2002).

A key consideration, however, is who is left out. Clearly, these settings have limited potential for reaching the unemployed, those who do not or cannot attend school (and, even within schools, those who feel alienated are less likely to be influenced), the homeless – that is, the most disadvantaged groups in society and those who have the greatest health needs. Green et al. (2000: 25) contend that:

> health promotion has chosen to privilege some settings (e.g. workplaces, schools, communities) as being more 'legitimate' sites of practice than others (e.g. bingo halls, nightclubs, street corners, public washrooms and other 'sites of resistance').

If the settings approach is to avoid the risk of increasing the health gap in society, it will need to address the needs of marginalized groups and include (as yet) unconventional and challenging settings. Linnan and Owens Ferguson (2007) provide an example of the use of beauty salons as a setting for addressing the well-known health disparities among African American women. Important features include accessibility and frequency of use which achieve both reach and reinforcement. The relationship between staff and clients, characterized by loyalty, trust, support and comfort, is also conducive to discussing personal and health-related issues. Further, a number of key macro-level factors influence the capacity of a setting to influence health. Drawing on a political economy of health theoretical perspective, the authors note that:

> the important role that beauty salons hold from a historical, economic, political, and social context helped us consider the underlying power that this setting may hold for promoting health among African American women. (2007: 524)

A further example is an initiative in north-west England to develop the potential of sports stadia as health promoting settings using a whole systems approach. Healthy Stadia are described as:

> ... those which promote the health of visitors, fans, players, employees and the surrounding community ... places where people can go to have a positive healthy experience playing or watching sport. (Healthy Settings Development Unit, 2007)

A setting has been defined (Nutbeam, 1998b) as:

> where people actively use and shape the environment and thus create, or solve problems relating to, health. Settings can normally be identified as having physical boundaries, a range of people with defined roles, and an organizational structure.

Green et al. (2000: 23) draw on critical theory to provide a broader conceptualization. They caution against taking a simple, instrumental view of settings as neutral, self-contained environments containing 'target audiences' and argue that settings are more than 'physically bounded space–times in which people come together to perform specific tasks (usually oriented to goals other than health)'. Instead, consideration needs to be given to the variability between settings, pre-existing social relationships in the setting and the permeability of its boundaries. Furthermore, settings themselves are culturally constructed and mediated via individual interaction and activity – 'Settings are both the medium and the product of human social interaction' (Green et al., 2000: 23). The view of settings can, therefore, be expanded to also include the following:

> arenas of sustained interaction, with pre-existing structures, policies, characteristics, institutional values, and both formal and informal social sanctions on behaviours. (2000: 23)

This view resonates with a postmodern conceptualization of organizations that acknowledges the complex interplay of factors that shape them (see the box for Charles Handy's description of the culture of organizations). In contrast, a modernist view would see organizations as structured and predictable. This clearly has implications for attempts to introduce change. Postmodern interpretations of organizations cast doubt on the capacity of top-down directives to achieve the commitment required to make them become more health promoting and demand a more complex multilevel response.

The culture of organizations

In organizations there are deep-set beliefs about the way work should be organized, the way authority should be exercised, people rewarded, people controlled. What are the degrees of formalization required? How much planning and how far ahead? What combination of obedience and initiative is looked for in subordinates? Do work hours matter, or dress, or personal eccentricities? ... Do committees control, or individuals? Are there rules and procedures or only results? These are all part of the culture of an organization.

Handy, 1993: 181

Ziglio et al. (1995: 2) identify the main features of settings as follows:

- known boundaries of action
- defined populations

- a common 'culture' affecting all who learn, work or receive care
- a defined set of stressors and resources to reduce or overcome them
- an opportunity to observe and measure the impact of health promotion actions.

Baric (1993) suggests that, to achieve the status of a health promoting setting, the following conditions should be met:

- the creation of a healthy working and living environment
- the integration of health promotion into the daily activities of the setting
- the creation of conditions for reaching out into the community.

The settings approach is consistent with an ecological view of health. Green et al. (2000: 16) contend that it sees health as dependent on the interaction between 'individuals and subsystems of the ecosystem'. The settings approach therefore offers the potential for shaping these elements to maximize health gain. It shifts the goals away from specific behaviour change towards creating the conditions that are supportive of health and wellbeing more generally, with a corresponding shift in focus of activity from risk factors and population groups towards organizational change. Furthermore, it is anticipated that the organizational change will be sustainable so that 'the wheel does not have to be reinvented with each new generation of workers, teachers, nurses' (WHO, 1998a). The emphasis on process is illustrated in the description of a healthy city provided in the box.

Baric (1993) contends that the settings approach requires an extension of the conceptual framework of health promotion to include:

- organizations as systems
- the interactions, behaviour and roles of people in organizations
- accountability – including social responsibility.

What is a healthy city?

A healthy city is defined by a process, not an outcome.

- A healthy city is not one which has achieved a particular health status.
- It is conscious of health and striving to improve it. Thus, any city can be a 'healthy' city, regardless of its current health status.
- What is required is a commitment to health and a process and structure to achieve it.
- A healthy city is one that is continually creating and improving the physical and social environments and expanding the community resources that enable people to mutually support each other in performing all the functions of life and in developing to their maximum potential.

WHO Regional Office for Europe, 2005

(Continued)

(Continued)

What is the 'healthy cities' approach?

Successful implementation of this approach requires innovative actions addressing all aspects of health and living conditions, and extensive networking between cities across Europe and beyond. This entails:

- explicit political commitment;
- leadership;
- institutional change;
- intersectoral partherships.

These are characterized as the four elements for action.

A. Explicit political commitment at the highest level to the principles and strategies of the 'Healthy Cities' project.
B. Establishment of new organizational structures to manage change.
C. Commitment to developing a shared vision for the city, with a health plan and work on specific themes.
D. Investment in formal and informal networking and cooperation.

WHO Regional Office for Europe, 2006

Denman et al. (2002) locate the settings approach within Beattie's (1991) model (referred to in Chapter 5) by characterizing it as having a collective focus and negotiated style of working. Similarly, drawing on Caplan and Holland (1990), they see it as concerned with radical change rather than social regulation and based on the view that knowledge is subjective rather than objective – that is, it is consistent with a radical humanist position.

Dooris (2006: 2) identifies three key elements of the approach:

- an ecological model of health
- a systems perspective
- whole system organization development and change focus.

Kickbush (1995: 6) notes that views about healthy organizations equate with modern management theory and that the characteristics of such organizations include:

- goal focus
- communication adequacy
- optimal power equalization
- resource utilization/distribution
- cohesiveness
- morale
- innovativeness
- autonomy
- adaptation.

Consideration of the respective contributions of behaviour and environment to health – or alternatively agency and structure – has been a major concern of health promotion, as we have noted on a number of occasions. Green et al. (2000) draw attention to the reciprocal determinism between environment and behaviour that is integral to ecological perspectives of health promotion and the settings approach. In short, behaviour is influenced by environment and the behaviour of individuals and groups shapes the environment. The settings approach does not, therefore, subscribe to a simple input–output view of intervention and effect, but, rather, presupposes a complex web of interaction between multiple layers of inputs. Poland et al. (2000b: 346) identify the key characteristics of settings for health projects as 'integrated, comprehensive, multifaceted, participatory, empowering, partnership, responsive, and tailored'. Whitelaw et al. (2001: 341) suggest that activity in the settings approach is concerned with:

- development of personal competences
- policies
- reshaping environments
- building partnerships
- bringing about sustainable change by means of participation
- developing empowerment
- ownership of change throughout the setting.

Wenzel (1997) contends that, despite the rhetoric, the settings approach has amounted to little more than a rebadging of traditional health education and that settings are simply a vehicle for individualistic health promotion. There are certainly some signs of this in England. Despite support for the settings approach expressed in *Saving Lives: Our Healthier Nation* (Department of Health, 1999), subsequent documents such as *Choosing Health* (Department of Health, 2004) and *Health Challenge England* (Department of Health, 2006c) have tended to view settings as a means of achieving behavioural targets such as exercise uptake and smoking cessation rather than fully subscribing to the principles of the approach. Dooris (2006: 2) also notes that despite a high level of support, the settings approach has 'not gained as much influence as it might have – in terms of either guiding wider international policy or driving national-level public health strategy'. Referring to Kickbush (1996, 2003), he suggests that this may be attributable to the need to understand the settings approach in terms of a political and social process, and the essentially non-medical logic which underpins it may make the approach less accessible to health professionals than, for example, members of the community or political decision makers.

Mittelmark (1997), however, takes a different view and argues that the post Ottawa era has been characterized by awareness among practitioners of the complex interaction between settings and behaviour. Furthermore, Green et al. (2000) suggest that any failure to achieve full health promoting setting 'status' may derive not so much from the inherent sophistication of the concept and the lack of comprehension on the part of practitioners, but from practical limitations within the setting. These include the 'competing interests, agendas and interpretations of key "gatekeepers"' (2000: 24). Whitelaw et al. (2001) attribute the relatively modest achievements to health promotion being only one element within the context of wider organizational development and identify a number of practical difficulties:

- competing forces
- translating the philosophy of the approach into practical activity within the setting
- the credibility and status of health promoters as agents of change
- lack of sufficient support.

Whitelaw et al. (2001) note the variation in what is being attempted under the settings banner and the difficulty faced by practitioners in moving beyond a focus on projects and towards achieving broader change across the setting and sustaining activity over a significant period. They raise the issue of whether or not there should be a consensus on what constitutes a settings approach – a one size fits all – given the differences in:

- the scale of what is attempted
- the nature of the setting – from nation states to prisons
- the range of outcomes and emphases.

While a consensus contributes to achieving a common vision, Whitelaw et al. (2001: 341) note that allowance should be made for practical reality failing to live up to the theoretical ideal. Poland et al. (2000a: 346) also suggest that 'a one size fits all approach (the use of identical protocols in similar settings)' may be inappropriate and that local autonomy may be required in relation to adaptation to suit specific needs and circumstances.

Whitelaw et al. (2001: 342–4) identify five broad types of settings activity by considering the ways in which problems are framed and solutions identified – in particular, the respective weight attached to the contributions of agency and structure.

- **The passive model** The problem and solution are dependent on the behaviour and actions of individuals. Traditional health education activity takes place within the setting – the setting itself merely has a subservient role.
- **The active model** The primary problem and part of the solution lie with the behaviour of individuals and part of the solution with the setting. The contribution of the setting is therefore needed to facilitate change in behaviour and the achievement of goals.
- **The vehicle model** The problem lies with the setting and the solution with learning from individually based projects. The primary goal shifts from the individual to changing features of the setting. Working on specific topic-focused projects is the 'vehicle' for achieving this – for example, beginning with an issue such as sun protection as a basis for considering the wider health promoting potential of the organization.
- **The organic model** The problem is seen to lie with the system and the solution with the processes and practices that make up the whole. It focuses on the development of individuals and groups throughout the organization, premised on the assumption that overarching systems are the product of individual actions. The overall aim is to improve the ethos or culture of the setting and strengthen collective participation.
- **The comprehensive model** This aims to change the structure and culture of the setting with the assumption that individuals are relatively powerless to do anything about it. It takes more of a deterministic view that systems change is dependent on 'powerful levers', so the emphasis is on policies and strategies for achieving change.

The latter two are clearly more consistent with the 'ideal' interpretation of the settings approach. However, Whitelaw et al. suggest that the distinctions between these five types of activity should be viewed loosely and that they may overlap in a complementary way or operate sequentially to facilitate progression within an organization.

Variations in practice may, therefore, arise from the extent to which organizations aspire, and are able, to achieve the 'ideal'. The particular characteristics of organizations will also undoubtedly influence the way in which the settings approach is operationalized. Denman et al. (2002) observe that differences in the size and complexity of settings will influence the mode of operation of the settings approach. For example, they refer to healthy cities as macro settings that rely heavily on intersectoral collaboration to achieve their goals. Schools, in contrast, are held to be more self-contained and self-sufficient. While collaboration has undoubted benefits (and is a core principle of the approach), schools will be less dependent on this aspect.

Variation also occurs within settings. There is a broad division into types of schemes – prescriptive and needs-led. The former involve working towards predefined criteria, whereas needs-led approaches are more flexible and responsive to local priorities (see, for example, Rivers et al.'s (1999) audit of local healthy schools schemes). The WHO position has been to acknowledge – indeed welcome – diversity in implementation of the settings approach, both between and within settings, provided it is consistent with core principles. In line with notions of subsidiarity, this affords considerable local autonomy and the opportunity to respond to local needs while maintaining the integrity of the approach and commitment to its underpinning values.

Carrots and sticks

A range of factors will impinge on an organization's decision to become a health promoting setting – at the most basic level, these could be the latitude for making change and the resources available. A critical issue is the momentum created by external pressure (or incentives!) and internal motivation. In some instances, formally structured international or national programmes or networks may be in place which may help to create that momentum.

International networks can fulfil an important advocacy role. For example, the European Network of Health Promoting Schools (ENHPS), now re-established as the Schools for Health in Europe (SHE) network, has encouraged a number of countries to adopt the initiative.

Barnekow Rasmussen (2005) notes that the ENHPS launched in 1991 enlarged from an initial small group of seven countries to include 43 by 2005. It encouraged commitment from and cooperation between relevant government departments – in this instance, education and health. Such high level support and cooperation are key factors in developing national initiatives. International networks can also establish core principles and quality standards and be a means of encouraging innovation and disseminating good practice.

Drawing on the experience of involving countries in the ENHPS, Barnekow Rasmussen identifies a number of stages between initial pilot and ultimate incorporation into mainstream policy, which could equally apply to other settings. These are:

- positive identification by decision makers
- disseminating information
- building credibility

- demonstrating relevance
- demonstrating feasibility
- incorporation into government policy. (2005: 171)

The development of 'healthy' settings in the private sector is, perhaps, less amenable to regulation and national or local control than it is in the public sector and, therefore, tends to rely on convincing organizations about the potential benefits. For example, with regard to workplace health promotion, it is possible to regulate health and safety issues. However, the move towards consideration of positive health and addressing the factors that would improve health demanded by the settings for health approach relies more on gaining the commitment of individual employers.

The origins of workplace health promotion lie in the reorientation of traditional occupational health and safety legislation and practice supported by the European Framework Directive on safety and health (Council Directive 89/391/EC) together with recognition of the workplace as an important setting for health (European Network of Workplace Health Promotion (ENWHP), 2007). The Luxembourg Declaration 1997 provided the first definition of workplace health promotion:

> the combined efforts of employers, employees and society to improve the health and well-being of people at work. This can be achieved by a combination of improving the work organisation and the working environment, promoting active participation and by encouraging personal development.

This definition provided a foundation for subsequent declarations (see, for example, ENWHP, 2007).

More recently, workplace health promotion has been described as:

> a modern corporate strategy, which aims to prevent ill-health at the workplace, to enhance health potential and to improve well-being at work. It is based on voluntary action and consensus building among all stakeholders. By including elements such as work organisation, organisational and human resource management, WHP goes beyond the legal requirements and takes on a broader dimension than traditional occupational safety and health. The new understanding encompasses both physical and mental well-being, the quality of life and learning. (ENWHP, undated a: 8)

It involves:

- having an organisational commitment to improving the health of the workforce
- providing employees with appropriate information and establishing comprehensive communication strategies
- involving employees in decision making processes
- developing a working culture that is based on partnership
- organising work tasks and processes so that they contribute to, rather than damage, health
- implementing policies and practices which enhance employee health by making the healthy choices the easy choices
- recognising that organisations have an impact on people and that this is not always conducive to their health and well-being. (ENWHP, undated b)

Clearly, different settings will vary both in their commitment and capacity to prioritize health goals. Again, this might be expected to be a more realistic proposition within the public than the private sector, notwithstanding Kickbush's (1998: 2) assertion that 'almost all organizations have not only a vested interest, but also a social responsibility, in maintaining and improving their members' health'.

Some of the structural barriers to health promotion in the workplace have been identified by the Faculty of Public Health Medicine (1995: 4) as the:

- problem of access to the very large number of small workplaces
- decentralization and fragmentation of larger organizations
- absence of statutory provision for occupational health in the United Kingdom (unlike other countries such as France, Germany and Holland) – such provision ensures that basic requirements of occupational health and safety are met
- organizational cultures that can discourage the implementation and support of health promotion policies
- financial difficulties – in times of recession, health promotion programmes may be among the first company activities to be cash limited
- continuous organizational change, as lack of formal plans and short-term focus prevent the development of longer-term health promotion initiatives
- failure to assign managerial responsibility and accountability for workplace health promotion to a named individual or department – lack of continuity is common
- lack of facilities, including appropriate accommodation, which may impede the implementation of programmes – this is related to the wider issue of funding
- inadequate basic safety and absent or poor occupational health, which may induce cynicism.

Workplace health promotion is unlikely to be a priority for most employers and managers. Convincing arguments will, therefore, be needed to justify investing resources of both time and money in developing the health promoting potential of organizations. Such arguments are frequently couched in economic terms emphasizing the monetary return on investment (see box). While purists might be critical of the narrow focus on servicing the needs of productivity, from the perspective of persuasive communication, framing the argument in this way means that it is likely to appeal to the primary motivation of those working in industry and the private sector.

The economic benefits of workplace health promotion

- A reduction in absenteeism of between 12% and 36% among participants in WHP programmes. Every US Dollar invested in WHP brought a Return on Investment (ROI) of between $2.5 and $4.8 due to reduced absenteeism costs. The ROI for medical costs amounts to 5.9.
- In Finland, it has been demonstrated that every 1 euro invested in programs for maintaining work ability brings a return of €4 to €6 in productivity.
- Cost–benefit ratios established in US studies range from $3 to $8 for every dollar invested in health promotion programs within five years.
- Some companies also make the evaluations of their intervention programs available to the public: The health care costs for participants in intervention programs

(Continued)

(Continued)

at DaimlerChrysler were between $5 and $16 lower per month compared to non-participants. Glaxo Wellcome's health promotion programme saved $1 million in 1 year and cut absence due to medical reasons by 20,000 working days between 1996 and 2003. In a comprehensive workplace health programme, a Canadian company, MDS Nordion, reduced absenteeism from 5.5 to 4 days annually and cut turnover to half the industry average.

- Another study shows that employees who consider their workplaces to be 'healthy' do not only have a lower rate of absenteeism, but statistically show a significantly higher level of job satisfaction and work-morale and are less likely to change their job.

Selected from ENWHP, undated c

An alternative conceptualization of benefits might include improved working relationships, the opportunity to improve the health and wellbeing of the workforce and enhance the corporate image – echoing the tradition of nineteenth-century British industrial philanthropists such as Salt, Cadbury and Rowntree! The report by De Greef and Van den Broek for the ENWHP (2004) emphasizes the need for business to combine 'technical and economic innovation with social innovation' and outlines a broader set of arguments to support workplace health promotion which it is claimed:

- leads to an improved working situation
- improves health-related outcomes
- generates an enhanced image
- improves human resources management
- boosts productivity
- increases health awareness and motivation
- leads to healthy workers
- generates more job satisfaction. (2004: 54)

The report identifies the following main drivers for the business case for workplace health promotion:

- Corporate values that recognize the social and economic relevance of a participatory workplace culture;
- Social and demographic trends with significant impacts on the labour market as external drivers;
- The impacts of workplace health investments along the employee-customer-profit-chain also highlighting the role of workplace health investments for improved business processes. (2004: 55)

De Greef and Van den Broek argue that the case for workplace health promotion needs to be aligned with companies' goals and strategies. This is equally true for settings more generally. Within the educational context, there is clear recognition of the reciprocal relationship between health and education. Children who are healthy are more able to take advantage of education and education contributes to health. As the Department of Health (1999: 4.16) points out:

> Education is vital to health. People with low levels of educational achievement are more likely to have poor health as adults. So by improving education for all we will tackle one of the main causes of inequality in health. Education can build self-esteem and can equip children and young people with the skills to adopt a healthier lifestyle. Education can also contribute to general improvement in health by enhancing people's ability to secure opportunities for work.

For most settings, health and health promotion do not form part of their core business. It might be anticipated that an organization's motivation to become a health promoting setting would be influenced by the level of compatibility with:

- its primary goals
- its core values
- its *modus operandi*.

Hospitals, for example, might appear to be obvious contenders in that the core business of hospitals could loosely be defined as being concerned with health. However, the move to becoming a health promoting hospital (see the box) would require traditional organizations to undergo a major reorientation – from curing disease to promoting health, from patient compliance to empowerment, from a narrow concern with patients to including relatives, staff and the wider community, and from being inward-looking to being outward-looking. Such developments have again been supported by international networks – initially European, but a global network has more recently been established. The definition of a health promoting hospital used in the WHO glossary emphasizes the need to include health promotion in the corporate identity:

> A health promoting hospital does not only provide high quality comprehensive medical and nursing services, but also develops a corporate identity that embraces the aims of health promotion, develops a health promoting organizational structure and culture, including active, participatory roles for patients and all members of staff, develops itself into a health promoting physical environment and actively cooperates with its community. (Nutbeam, 1998b: 11)

Health promoting hospitals (HPHs)

Fundamental principles: The Vienna Recommendations

Within the framework of the health for all strategy, the Ottawa Charter for Health Promotion, the Ljubljana Charter for Reforming Health Care and the Budapest Declaration on Health Promoting Hospitals, a health promoting hospital should:

1 promote human dignity, equity and solidarity, and professional ethics, acknowledging differences in the needs, values and cultures of different population groups

(Continued)

(Continued)

2 be orientated towards quality improvement, the wellbeing of patients, relatives and staff, protection of the environment and a realization of the potential to become learning organizations

3 focus on health with a holistic approach and not only on curative services

4 be centred on people providing health services in the best way possible to patients and their relatives, to facilitate the healing process and contribute to the empowerment of patients

5 use resources efficiently and cost-effectively, and allocate resources on the basis of contribution to health improvement

6 form as close links as possible with other levels of the healthcare system and the community.

WHO Euro, 1997

Standards for health promotion

Management policy
Patient assessment
Patient information and intervention
Promoting a healthy workplace
Continuity and cooperation

Groene, 2006

In contrast, while at first sight schools are primarily concerned with educational rather than health goals, commitment to education as a means of developing the whole person has much in common with a positive, holistic view of health. Furthermore, the emergence of the 'whole school approach' to education in the 1980s was entirely consistent with the settings approach and prepared the ground for the emergence of the health promoting school concept. The 'whole school approach' recognized that a child's learning at school is the product not just of what is taught through the planned formal curriculum, but also their total experience at school, which would include the environment, relationships and practices in the school (the hidden curriculum), the activities organized by the school (the informal curriculum) and contact with the school health service (the parallel curriculum).

We have made some general observations about the key features of the settings approach. We will now consider the health promoting school in more detail as an example. Although there are substantial contextual differences between settings, as we have noted, there are still some parallels to be drawn. We will then conclude by making some brief points of comparison with other settings.

THE HEALTH PROMOTING SCHOOL

Bearing in mind our earlier point about the problems of reaching out of school youth and disaffected young people, schools are widely accepted as having considerable potential for influencing the health of young people and future adults. This is not altogether surprising given that the length of time spent in school in industrialized countries has been estimated to be around 15,000 hours (Rutter et al., 1979). Schools are increasingly recognized as a major setting for health promotion – see, for example, the commitment to schools as a strategic setting by the Health21 policy framework for the European Region set out in the box and the recognition of the importance of school health by the WHO mega countries network. The European Strategy for Child and Adolescent Health and Development also recognizes the influence of schools on health and their importance as a health promoting setting (WHO, 2008a).

Health promoting schools: a strategy for achieving Health21 targets

Schools are an important setting in which health can be created and sustained. Young people's perception of health can be greatly enhanced by the content of the formal teaching curriculum. Action to protect and promote health can be brought to life in the school's physical environment. On a wider level, the school influences the perceptions, attitudes, actions and behaviour not only of pupils but also of teachers, parents, health care workers and local communities. All aspects of organizational life contribute to physical, social and emotional health; moreover, the young learn best about responsibility and empowerment through direct participation in decision-making. The European 'health-promoting school' approach combines these elements, and this concept should be introduced in all schools in the 51 Member States in the Region.

WHO, 1999b: 28

Not only do schools reach a substantial proportion of young people at a formative stage in their development, they also provide opportunities for influencing the health of staff and the wider community. The health promoting school aims to achieve:

healthy lifestyles for the total school population by developing supportive environments conducive to the promotion of health. It offers opportunities for, and requires commitments to, the provision of a safe and health-enhancing social and physical environment. (WHO Euro-EC-CE, 1993)

Furthermore, it is seen to contribute to school improvement by improving 'the whole quality of the school setting. Success here will better equip schools to enhance learning outcomes' (Stewart Burgher et al., 1999: 5).

The 'English National Healthy School Standard' (Department for Education and Employment, 1999) emphasized the dual benefits of the health promoting school – contributing to health gain and raising levels of pupil achievement. This is consistent with the twin national drivers which supported its introduction: 'Saving Lives: Our Healthier Nation' (Department of Health, 1999) and 'Excellence in Schools' (Department for Education and Employment, 1997).

Origins and concepts

Although the roots of the health promoting school can be traced back much further (for a detailed account, see St Leger, 1999; Tones and Tilford, 2001; Denman et al., 2002; Young, 2005), the concept is generally attributed to a consensus conference sponsored by WHO in 1989, which led to the publication of *The Healthy School* (Young and Williams, 1989). This identified three main elements of the health promoting school:

- health education taught through the formal curriculum
- the school ethos and environment
- the relationships between the home, school, the surrounding community and services.

It also established, as a key principle, that the focus should be on addressing the needs of pupils and called for their active involvement. Health education within this context should, therefore, meet the needs of pupils as they mature – revisiting issues at an appropriate level by means of a so-called 'spiral curricular approach' – and use active learning methods. Tones (1996) suggests that a health promoting curriculum should include the following three areas:

- health knowledge to develop awareness and understanding of key issues
- life skills to develop skills and competences
- social education to raise consciousness about the social determinants of health.

Addressing this breadth cannot be achieved by separate classes on health-related topics, but requires integration and consistency across the whole curriculum.

The ethos and environment of the school should complement what is taught and be health-enhancing in their own right. Furthermore, efforts within the school should be strengthened and supported by strong links with parents and the wider community.

Parsons et al. added management and planning to the basic tripartite model, along with desired impact. They also placed the whole within the local, national and international context – referring to it as an eco-holistic model (see Figure 10.1). Management aspects are included in the operational definition offered by Stewart Burgher et al. (1999: 4–5):

> A health promoting school uses its management structures, its internal and external relationships, its teaching and learning styles and its methods of establishing synergy with its social environment to create the means for pupils, teachers and all those involved in everyday school life to take control over and improve their physical and emotional health.

The growth of the health promoting school movement has been supported by local, national and international networks, which provide opportunities for technical support and information exchange and a forum for collaboration (Rowling, 1996). Young (2005) comments on the separate but convergent developments in school health promotion in the USA and Europe and the similarities between the European model – referred to as the health promoting school – and comprehensive school health programs in the USA. However, he notes the greater emphasis on pupil participation in the early European model and, as it has developed, its particular focus on equity

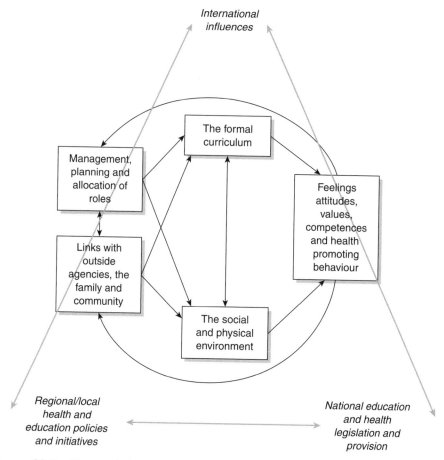

Figure 10.1   The eco-holistic model of the health promoting school (after Parsons et al., 1997)

and democracy. Commitment to democracy, equity and empowerment are among the core principles established by the First Conference of the European Network of Health Promoting Schools (see the box for the full list).

Principles of the health promoting school developed by the First Conference of the ENHPS

Democracy
Equity
Empowerment and action competence

(Continued)

(Continued)

School environment – physical and social
Curriculum
Teacher training
Measuring success
Collaboration
Communities
Sustainability

European Network of Health Promoting Schools, 1997

St Leger (1999) notes the similarity of structural frameworks for health promoting schools adopted by the different WHO regions. Following a review of research, evaluation and practice, he proposes the following principles. The health promoting school:

- promotes the health and wellbeing of students
- upholds social justice and equity concepts
- involves student participation and empowerment
- provides a safe and supportive environment
- links health and education issues and systems
- addresses the health and wellbeing issues of staff
- collaborates with the local community
- integrates into the school's ongoing activities
- sets realistic goals
- engages parents and families in health promotion. (St Leger, 2005: 145)

He also lists the essential elements of health promoting schools, which are: having school policies in place which promote health and wellbeing, attention to the school's physical and social environment, the development of health skills and action competences, and links with the community and health services.

Implementation of health promoting schools should be consistent with the core values. However, the activities carried out in schools under the health promoting school banner vary enormously. Stewart Burgher et al. (1999) identify five broad categories of activity in ENHPS schools:

- improvements to the physical environment
- education on health topics
- building democracy in schools
- development of policies
- teacher training both topic-based and skills-based – for example, in communication, the use of active learning methods, management, cooperation with parents and so on.

Activities in health promoting schools usually span most, if not all, the categories. The box provides examples of the activities undertaken to promote mental health in Hull and the East Riding in the UK.

Examples of activities to promote mental health

- Developing and introducing anti-bullying strategies
- Setting up a school council to give pupils a voice
- Introducing 'circle time' – encouraging pupils to speak, listen and empathize with each other
- Setting up a breakfast club to help pupils concentrate in lessons, socialize and so on
- Improving the staffroom facilities
- Creating a playground area for quiet activities
- Organizing a stress management course for staff
- Introducing a new school uniform to reduce peer pressure to wear designer labels
- Introducing new playtime games and equipment to reduce opportunities for bullying at lunchtime
- Developing and setting up a 'buddy system' to integrate pupils at breaks and lunchtimes, and to assist new children to feel part of the school
- Promoting the 'Baby Think It Over' project to highlight the challenges of parenthood to teenagers
- Introducing a 'skills swap' between pupils and older members of the community to enhance relationships and develop trust.

Cockerill, undated

Developing partnerships is fundamental to the health promoting school way of working – within schools, involving pupils and all staff, and outside schools, working with parents, the community and other agencies.

The emphasis on democratic approaches to education has been spearheaded in Denmark, where the aim of health education is to develop the capacity of pupils to act independently and collectively to promote their own and other's health (Jensen, 1991). This ability to influence one's own life and society is referred to as 'action competence' and its key components have been listed as:

- insight and knowledge
- commitment
- vision
- experience
- social skills. (Jensen, 2000)

Reference to our earlier discussion of empowerment in Chapter 3 will indicate that the notion of action competence links in to the various constructs of empowerment. As we noted in Chapter 7, within the UK, this constellation of competences has been conceived as 'health skills' by Anderson et al. (1994) or, more broadly, as 'life skills' (see Figure 10.2). Bruun Jensen and Simovska (2005) emphasize the importance of genuine student participation on the grounds of ownership, democracy, ethical considerations and meaningfully defining subjective notions of health and wellbeing. A summary of the IVAC approach used by the Danish Network of health promoting schools and an example of its application is provided in the box.

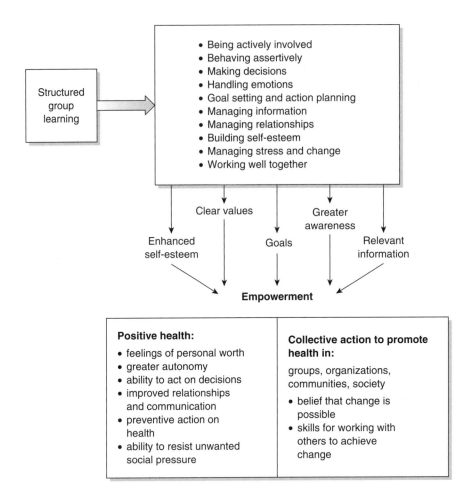

Figure 10.2   Health skills (after Anderson et al., 1994)

Case study: participation in practice – the IVAC approach

Phases

1 Investigation
2 Visions and alternatives
3 Action
4 Change

Example

A team in a health promoting school in Macedonia attempted to improve the psycho-social environment of the school. The team was made up of 35 students

(Continued)

(Continued)

aged 12–15 years, five teachers, the school health promotion coordinator and two consultants.

Investigation: Students considered the holistic concept of health and applied it to the existing school environment, identifying aspects that they did or did not like and reflecting on their relationship with health. Students also conducted a survey of the whole school to explore priorities about the environment and health.

Vision: Students developed a vision of their ideal school using a teacher facilitated process.

Action and change: One of the actions selected was to shorten lessons from 45 to 40 minutes to create more time in the middle of the day for sports activities, socializing and relaxation. Students developed arguments based on the benefits for the health of the whole school and the overall atmosphere to convince staff to introduce the change. Ministerial approval was needed for the change and the students had to learn about policy and decision-making processes, i.e. return to the investigation phase. For some students, who expected change to just happen, this was dispiriting and teachers needed skill to support them through this challenge – achieved by reflecting on the gains and difficulties of earlier phases.

Bruun Jensen and Simovska, 2005

Implementation of the health promoting school concept

The degree to which the state controls education and the level of national and local support for the concept of the health promoting school will clearly be influential in relation to implementation. Similarly, cultural and professional norms about the purpose of education, the role of schools and the way in which they function will shape views about the acceptability of the approach. Lawton (1986), for example, identified key factors that influence views about what should be included in the school curriculum. These derive from a number of perspectives – ideological and philosophical perspectives on the aim of education, sociological perspectives on the nature of society and childhood, and psychological perspectives on development and learning. Although practical and organizational constraints will also have a bearing, the various influences will combine to shape views about what ought to be taught and the methods that should be used. An adaptation of Lawton's model is provided in Figure 10.3 and could equally apply more broadly to views about the health promoting school and receptivity to the concept.

Settings approaches such as the health promoting school can be adopted nationally to establish a supportive context for the adoption of the approach at the individual school level. Young (2005) identifies three main phases in the roll out of such programmes. An initial *experimental phase* (which for some might be called a pilot phase) which involves early innovators, usually from the health sector, attempts to introduce the idea to an often resistant education sector which tends to see health in bio-medical terms. Growing appreciation that the health

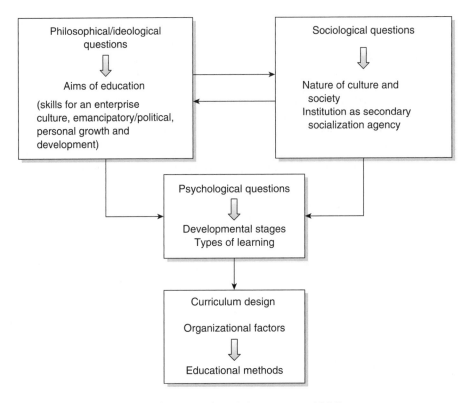

Figure 10.3   Influences on the curriculum (after Lawton, 1986)

promoting school can contribute to both health and education agendas and be of benefit to schools leads to the *strategic development phase*. This involves capacity building through training and staff development and the building of partnerships at all levels. The final *establishment phase* is reached when health promoting schools are recognized by national policy and the concept becomes institutionalized at the school level, i.e. 'it becomes integral to the school's core values and normal ways of working' (2005: 115).

The Egmond Agenda (International Planning Committee, 2002) identified key requirements for building successful initiatives. These are organized around three main components:

1   Conditions

   • analysis to understand the national situation
   • partnership
   • advocacy
   • theoretical base.

2   Programming
  - policy development and long-term objective setting
  - long-term planning
  - teacher education and professional development.
3   Evaluation.

The shift in organizational culture integral to the settings approach requires commitment across the board. Whether or not there is pressure on schools from Ministries or Departments of Education to become health promoting schools, those involved at the individual school level need to fully embrace and adopt the concept. To avoid the tokenism associated with top-down approaches, it follows that staff and pupils should be involved in decisions. Furthermore, staff development may be required to familiarize staff with the principles of the settings approach and the use of participatory approaches. St Leger's (1998) study of teachers in Australia, for example, found that they tended to focus on curricular provision rather than the broader influences of the school on health. Indeed, the basic premise of the health skills project in the UK (Anderson, undated) was that staff training was a prerequisite for the introduction of a whole school approach to developing health skills. A major theme running throughout this text has been the central importance of education, which includes staff training and development. The Egmond Agenda emphasizes that the successful implementation of the health promoting school concept depends on developing the capacity of staff:

> The programme introduces concepts and methodologies that may be unfamiliar to teachers and officials in health and education ministries. Successful health promoting school initiatives have developed extensive education programmes for teachers and health workers. Building the capacity of personnel and providing opportunities for professional development has been shown to be an effective strategy in health promoting school policy. (International Planning Committee, 2002)

There is an extensive body of literature on the curriculum and the factors that shape it (for a brief review of the application to health education, see Ryder and Campbell, 1988; Harrison and Edwards, 1994; Tones et al., 1995; Tones and Green, 2000). However, our purpose here is to focus more specifically on the factors associated with organizational change. Tones et al. (1995) draw on Rogers and Shoemaker (1979) to suggest that the adoption of an innovation by schools will depend on:

  - the nature of the school as a social system
  - the characteristics of individual teachers within the school
  - the extent to which the school feels it owns the innovation
  - the attributes of the innovation
  - the characteristics of the change agents.

The features of an innovation that make it more likely to be adopted are summarized in the box (for a more comprehensive review of diffusion of innovations theory, see Chapter 3).

Features of an innovation that influence the likelihood of adoption

- Simple, flexible and adaptable, rather than complicated, rigid and teacher-proofed
- The opportunity to try it out in a limited way and observe results before making a full-scale commitment
- Compatibility with the existing organization of the school, its timetable and pedagogical practices
- An improvement on the current situation
- Lacking significant costs – material and human.

After Tones et al., 1995

The development of an appropriate strategy for the management of change will depend on a careful reading of the key features of the organization. Anderson (undated) draws on the six-box model developed by Weisbord (1978) to identify these as the:

- purpose of the organization
- structure
- leadership
- rewards
- relationships
- helpful mechanisms.

The role of change agents – either internal or external to the organization – will be important in gaining the support of a critical mass of staff. Tones et al. (1995) note that the change agent or 'product champion' is more likely to be effective if they are perceived to have expertise and be similar in most respects to other members of staff – that is, homophilous.

They also need to identify those whose support it would be most expedient to obtain. Anderson (undated) refers to the matrix developed by Elliott-Kemp (see Figure 10.4) for mapping the people in an organization to identify the key people to persuade or work with. The vertical axis represents power or influence, which can be associated with position, expertise, charisma or the power to punish or reward. The horizontal axis represents the degree of concern or interest. A strategy for building support and influence can be developed from an analysis of the positions of staff on the matrix, bearing in mind the need to obtain senior level support. Where those with considerable position and power have little or no interest, generating a groundswell of commitment among the less powerful may provide sufficient leverage.

Anderson also notes Elliott-Kemp's (1982) warning that people cannot support what they don't understand. It is essential, therefore, that people are drawn into what she terms the 'circle of understanding'. Clarity of purpose and the ability to communicate this to others will therefore be instrumental to success.

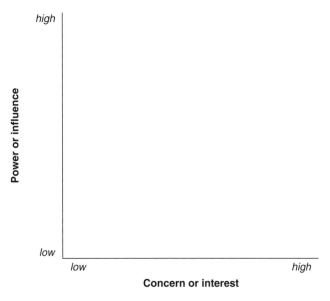

Figure 10.4   The Elliott-Kemp matrix (after Anderson, undated)

Effective implementation – lessons from practice

A number of studies have been undertaken of the implementation of the health promoting school concept. Parsons et al.'s (1997) study involving six European countries found schools that were successful in disseminating ideas and gaining staff commitment valued staff development and training. The involvement of parents was also helpful in generating enthusiasm throughout the school community. Furthermore, celebration of success was important to raise awareness of achievements and sustain motivation.

The evaluation of the ENHPS pilot project in England (Jamison et al., 1998) made a series of recommendations concerning the initiation, implementation and establishment of change. An essential prerequisite for initiation of change was an audit of the current situation, focusing on both strengths and weaknesses. The contribution of key committed individuals was central to success, particularly having a designated coordinator with the capability and standing among other staff to be able to take the initiative forward. Strong management support provided authority and impetus. Setting clear aims and objectives and adopting a systematic approach to planning also contributed to success. However, the need to be realistic was recognized in relation to what is feasible, timescales, and the local and national educational contexts and directives. The flexibility of the settings approach and the ability to adapt it to maximize compatibility with the school's existing priorities was beneficial. The need to consult and keep all stakeholders informed was recognized, along with the importance of good communication mechanisms. The provision of additional funding helped to get activities up and running, but the authors also drew attention to the hidden costs associated with staff putting in a considerable amount of their own time.

In relation to implementation of change, Jamison et al. found that key factors were good communication and management. Allowing time for communication, both within schools and with external agencies, was crucial. Other factors included involving all stakeholders in implementation – pupils, non-teaching staff, parents and outside agencies, as well as teaching staff. Tangible achievements and special events helped to maintain a high profile and provide motivation. This, coupled with time, helped to convince the small core of sceptics within schools who had concerns about the innovation. Flexibility was also important, to respond to new opportunities or competing pressures. Establishing change over the longer term was more likely if linked to the school's development plan. Sustaining ongoing activity was also dependent on having a designated coordinator and ongoing training and support for staff, particularly when there were staff changes. Finally, monitoring and evaluation systems were seen to be important, to check on progress and celebrate achievement.

The audit of healthy schools schemes conducted by Rivers et al. (1999) identified broadly similar factors that facilitated the implementation of healthy schools activities and barriers to success. These are listed in the box. The authors also observed that, frequently, young people are not involved in a systematic way.

Factors affecting the implementation of healthy schools initiatives by schools

Facilitating factors:

staff commitment
support from senior school management
a concern for pupils' health
pupils' awareness of the scheme and its work
outside financial support.

Barriers to success:

lack of time and resources
poor school facilities
curriculum pressures
other pressures of work – preparation for OFSTED (Office for Standards in Education) inspection
ineffective system for internal communication.

Rivers et al., 1999

Denman et al. (2002) identified the important contributory role of school policies, although St Leger's (1999) study of primary schools found that this aspect of the health promoting school received comparatively little attention. Referring to the evaluation of the 'Nottinghamshire Towards Health Project', they noted that key factors influencing success included the school's organizational structure, the level of commitment of staff and awareness of the benefits of being involved. They also identified the characteristics of schools which experienced particular difficulty such as:

- starting from a low level of development
- changing their original objectives
- giving the responsibility for coordination to relatively junior members of staff
- few reserves to deal with unanticipated pressures
- a tradition of responding reactively to pressure and crisis management
- unrealistic initial objectives.

Impact on health

Although evidence of the health impacts of the health-promoting schools approach is not yet strong, Lister-Sharp et al.'s (1999) systematic review found the approach to be promising. This view is endorsed by Jamison et al. (1998), Denman et al. (2002) and Parsons et al. (1997). McBride and Midford (1996) demonstrated that relatively modest interventions can achieve change in the management practices of schools to create a structure that enables schools to promote health in a comprehensive manner. Blenkinsop et al. (2004) also found that involvement in the National Healthy School Standard in England improved health-related work in schools, and pupils valued the improved ethos and social relationships in the school. Nonetheless, demonstrating improved health outcomes remains challenging. Stewart-Brown's review and synthesis of evidence (2006) commented on the lack of evidence relating to initiatives which incorporated all elements of the health promoting schools approach, pointing out the need to evaluate process as well as outcomes. School-based programmes which promoted mental health and encouraged healthy eating and physical activity were found to be most effective. The characteristics of programmes that were effective in influencing health-related behaviour were that they 'were more likely to be complex, multifactorial and involve activity in more than one domain (curriculum, school environment and community)' (2006: 17). Furthermore, intensive, long-duration interventions were more effective. Interventions in schools which incorporated key features of the health promoting schools model were, therefore, more likely to be successful.

Implementation of the concept of the health promoting school clearly has potential for contributing to the health of the whole school community. Kolbe et al. (2005) argue, from a US perspective, that school employee health is an important component of school health programmes and that it can lead to improved staff recruitment, morale, retention and productivity along with reduced risk behaviours, risk factors, illnesses, work-related injuries, absentee days, worker compensation and disability claims, and health care and health insurance costs. Furthermore, while seen as distinct from efforts to improve pupil health, the potential for improved staff health to contribute to pupil health is also recognized. The positive impact of focusing on staff mental health in enabling them to plan whole school programmes and teach young people about mental health is emphasized by Mason and Rowling (2005). The MindMatters national mental health initiative for schools in Australia is based on the health promoting school framework. Staff training was found to not only be beneficial to the individuals involved, but also led to more successful implementation of the programme. The Staff Matters resource was developed to support staff training and is based on five domains – *the interpersonal, the professional* and *the organizational* which interface with *the thriving self* and operate within the context of *the school in the community* (see http://www.mindmatters.edu.au/about/about_landing.html).

The two-way benefits of involving families and communities is emphasized by health promoting schools in Scotland (Learning and Teaching Scotland, 2007). The involvement of families helps to ensure that children get consistent messages at home and school and are supported in efforts to be 'healthy'. Parents can contribute their skills and experience, know more about their children's experience and can be supported in promoting their health. Further, involving the community in partnership with the school helps the community to:

> understand that partnership, with the support and active involvement of local people, services and employers, is valued by the school and is vital to the health and well-being of pupils, staff and parents and all members of the community.

A graphic example comes from Macedonia where, following a period of armed conflict, the health promoting school concept and the principles of democratic participation were used to create a safe and stimulating environment in schools, which allowed young people to 'respond to the challenge of transforming a dangerous environment and threats into experiences shaping their own well-being and the well-being of the community' (Unkowska, 2005: 143). The overall goals were to:

- raise, in conditions of continuous community crisis, the community awareness of the children's needs and rights for the purposes of restoring a feeling of safety and belonging;
- reduce the post traumatic consequences of war in the pupils and teachers, for the purposes of their active involvement in the school and community life;
- build sustainable networks of assistance and support (in the schools and more widely) despite the adverse living conditions. (2005: 142)

OTHER SETTINGS FOR HEALTH

Many of the factors contributing to the successful implementation of health promoting schools are transferable to other settings. For example, awareness and understanding of the concept, and recognizing the advantages for the setting itself and for health are crucial in all settings. Implementation is clearly facilitated if there is top-down support and the allocation of sufficient resources along with the development of appropriate partnerships. At the same time, it is important to encourage grass-roots ownership.

The settings approach requires clear goals and objectives. The process of changing organizational cultures can take time – this needs to be recognized in assessing what is feasible and putting long-term plans in place for further development. Clearly,

Table 10.2   Settings – points of comparison

	Examples	
	High	**Low**
Scale	*Healthy cities* *Healthy islands*	*Healthy prisons*
Supportive national/ international networks	*Healthy cities* *Health promoting schools*	*Beauty salons*
Opportunity for regulation	*Health promoting schools*	*Healthy stadia*
Alignment with core purpose	*Health promoting hospitals*	*Manufacturing industry*
Reach	*Health promoting schools*	*Beauty salons*
Access to disadvantaged groups	*Healthy prisons*	*Health promoting universities*
Funding	*Variable, but generally not generous*	

evaluation to assess achievements is essential. It is helpful to identify some 'early wins' as well as longer-term achievements in order to sustain motivation.

In some instances, partners may share a common view about their goals for a setting. However, given the range of interpretations of health and the diverse professional groups which may be brought together under the settings banner, it is likely that they may have different aspirations. In the early stages, considerable attention will need to be given to partnership building, as discussed in Chapter 4, in order to develop a consensus. Aronson et al. (2007), for example, identified conflicting views at the planning stage of a healthy cities initiative. On the one hand, some partners focused on social factors and living conditions as major determinants, whereas others focused on the role of health care and lifestyle decisions. Towards the end of the project, there was a greater consensus around a broader view of health and evidence that working together on the project had developed common thinking.

Each setting will have its own particular challenges. We do not propose to consider the full range of settings in detail, but rather to draw some brief points of comparison. Some of the key features of different settings are provided in Table 10.2.

Settings will vary in the extent to which they have an inward or outward looking focus and whether the major responsibility for the 'healthy setting' is shared between all stakeholders or held predominantly by one. Healthy cities, for example, are dependent on partnerships between organizations and their respective contribution to a collective enterprise. In contrast, in settings such as the healthy prison, major responsibility for activity within the setting ultimately rests with the prison authorities – notwithstanding the development of partnerships to assist with the process.

Given the emphasis on security, prisons may also appear to be a quintessentially inward looking organization. However, an interesting example of an initiative which crossed the boundaries is provided by the 'Jigsaw Project' which developed a prison visitors' centre into a healthy living centre (see box).

Case study: a 'healthy' prison visitors' centre

Provision included:

For visitors

- Bureaucratic support with the formal processes associated with visiting and responding to visitors' queries.
- Functional support in providing a welcoming environment for visitors, who often travelled considerable distances, to wait and have something to eat and prepare for the visit.
- Stress reduction achieved by the above plus access to peer support, advice from staff and counselling services.
- Other support including access to Citizens' Advice and provision of information on welfare benefits, facilitating (along with prison staff) family days to enable children to visit.

For prisoners

- Courses on drug and alcohol awareness and domestic violence.
- Improved quality of family visits due to support provided for visitors.

For prison staff

- Drop-in centre for prison staff to provide some respite from the prison environment.
- Access to counselling services and information services.

Links with local community

- Offering the use of premises to community groups such as a local youth group and a walking group.

Woodall et al., 2006

The improved quality of visits was one of the positive outcomes of the initiative identified (Woodall et al., 2009). It was anticipated that this would help to maintain family ties and thereby contribute to recognized pathways to resettlement, leading to a reduction in re-offending. Prison officers also experienced less pressure themselves, both on account of the improved atmosphere following visiting time and also because the visitors' centre handled many of the queries which they formerly would have had to deal with themselves.

While detailed implementation will vary, it remains possible to apply the principles of the settings approach across a variety of different settings. This adaptability is perhaps testament to the value of the approach.

THE SETTINGS APPROACH – FUTURE POTENTIAL

Organizations and social systems have an enormous impact on health. The settings approach aims to harness that potential to promote health and wellbeing. The advantages offered by the settings approach are that it:

- offers opportunities for working at least some way upstream to develop conditions supportive of health
- embeds consideration for health within organizational structures
- has an holistic orientation rather than a focus on problems, risks or specific groups.

However, there are also numerous challenges:

- less obvious settings should be considered as well as large-scale mainstream ones to avoid further marginalization of some disadvantaged groups
- the settings approach demands organizational change and commitment – it is not merely a vehicle for more traditional approaches
- it requires a delicate balance between top-down managerial support and the creation of an overall sense of direction on the one hand and, on the other, participation and a sense of ownership at grass-roots level
- it demands new ways of working.

The shift in emphasis from behaviour or policy change to organizational change will necessarily draw on a different combination of professional skills and insights (see the box).

Requirements for achieving organizational change

- Understanding the influence of organizations on the health and illness of their clients and members
- Understanding the special logic and dynamics of organizations in different sectors
- Skills in analysing social structures and processes in organizations
- Ability to shape their own role within the organizations
- Social skills for teamwork and team leadership
- Skills for intervening in organizations

After Scala, 1996

Poland et al. (2000b: 347) provide a useful summary of key factors contributing to the success of the settings approach that depend on a 'reflexive reading of the particular setting and one's role in it'. These include:

- the institutional organizational culture
- the expectations, attitudes and beliefs of key players – workers, management, patients and physicians, students and teachers, parents and children, community groups and state officials
- the nature of the practice environment – such as incentives and disincentives for undertaking health promotion, such as reward structures, pace of work, competing demands, scepticism, regarding the value or relevance or effectiveness of health promotion, training of key staff
- historical developments in the setting – trends in the organization of work, composition of the family or organization of healthcare

- internal politics, leadership (formal and informal), past successes and failures
- who controls access to the setting, who has influence within the setting
- broader social, economic and political context – non-setting factors.

Dooris (2006) identifies the main challenges in taking the settings approach forward and seeking to increase its influence. First, clarifying the theoretical base of the settings approach and secondly developing the evidence base. He also points out the need to keep an eye on the bigger picture, i.e. the social, economic and environmental influences on health.

The emergence of the settings approach acknowledged the interplay of factors that influence health. It moved forward from seeing settings merely as a means of providing access to a target population towards harnessing the potential offered at all levels within a setting – policy, environment (in its widest sense, including social relationships and interaction), along with opportunities for education. Furthermore, the settings approach sees the boundaries of settings as permeable, with opportunities to interact in a mutually beneficial way with the wider community and other settings.

The ultimate indicator of the success of the settings approach will be when giving consideration to health is so firmly embedded into the structure and ways of working of organizations that the qualifying term 'healthy' is no longer needed.

KEY POINTS

○ The settings approach shifts the focus of interventions from the individual to creating the conditions supportive of health and health behaviour.

○ The settings approach involves considering how all aspects of the setting influence the health of all those who come into contact with it.

○ It is important to identify which population groups are reached by specific settings and which are not.

○ Innovative approaches may be needed to ensure that disadvantaged and excluded groups are reached so that the settings approach can contribute to a reduction in health inequalities.

○ The implementation of the settings approach is enhanced by the existence of local, national and international networks.

○ Internal motivation is a key factor in implementing settings for health approaches.

○ Compatibility with the core purpose of the setting, or appreciation of the potential advantages to the setting, increases motivation and favours the development of healthy settings.

○ The settings approach involves organizational change and requires new ways of working and associated professional competences.

(Continued)

(Continued)

o   Changing organizational culture and ways of working takes time.

o   Recognition and celebration of early successes can help to generate and sustain motivation.

o   As with all health promotion initiatives, the settings approach should be based on clear, realistic objectives and sufficient resources, including staffing, should be allocated to achieving them.

o   The evidence base for the settings approach needs to be improved by generating evidence relating to the totality of the setting. It therefore requires attention to process as well as outcomes.

11

EVALUATION

When God made Heaven and God made Earth
He [sic.] formed the seas and gave them birth;
His heart was full of jubilation;
But he made one error – no EVALUATION!
'Oh!' He said, 'That's good!' and He meant it too,
But now we know that that won't do.
Even something that we know is best,
We've got to PROVE by a PRE-POST test.

Apocryphal wisdom from a NASA Newsletter

Evaluation is a vast, lumbering, overgrown adolescent. It has the typical problems associated with this age group too. It does not know quite where it is going and it is prone to bouts of despair. But it is the future after all ...

Pawson and Tilley, 1997: 1

OVERVIEW

This chapter addresses evaluation and the development of an evidence base for health promotion. It also looks at the translation of evidence into practice. It will:

- consider the influence of values on evaluation
- discuss the implications of different research paradigms for health promotion evaluation and the limitations of the RCT
- emphasize the need to look at process and context as well as outcomes
- consider the various types of indicator required
- propose the judicial principle as a means of establishing validity
- identify the types of evidence relevant to evidence-based practice
- consider the contribution of systematic reviews to the evidence base
- consider how evidence informs practice.

INTRODUCTION

Fundamental to all evaluation research is the question of validity – the need to 'prove' that any claims made about the effectiveness and efficiency of interventions are robust and justifiable. It is essential, therefore, to identify appropriate methodology for evaluating health promotion interventions. Traditionally, the randomized controlled trial (RCT) has been viewed as the 'gold standard' for assessing effectiveness. However, there has been considerable debate about its relevance for health promotion. This debate has been characterized by an intense clash of ideologies – earning the description of 'paradigm wars'. In this chapter, we are critical of the use of RCTs for health promotion evaluation and propose a new gold standard based on the 'judicial principle'. We also consider the type of information needed to build an evidence base which can inform future practice and policy.

WHY EVALUATE?

At its simplest, the purpose of evaluation is to assess the extent to which interventions have achieved their goals. In a climate where there is increasing pressure to ensure that public funds are being used to good effect, evaluation is frequently a means of demonstrating accountability (Raphael, 2000). However, it can have a much broader role. Lewis (2001) recognizes the current emphasis on evaluation for accountability and calls for a 'campaign for more evaluation for learning – of both process and impact' (2001: 392).

As we have argued earlier, evaluation is a key element of good health promotion practice and an essential component of the health promotion planning cycle. It allows those implementing interventions to keep a check on progress and introduce any necessary modifications. Importantly, given health promotion's commitment to equity, it can assess whether the benefits reach the most disadvantaged and contribute to a reduction in health inequalities (Barr et al., 1996).

WHO identifies the important role of evaluation in capacity building and increasing the ability of 'individuals, communities, organisations and governments to address important health issues' (WHO, 1998a: 3). Clearly, the development of evaluation evidence is essential for building the evidence base for health promotion. Over and above establishing what works, it is important that such evidence provides insight into how interventions work and under what conditions and in what contexts they succeed or fail.

From an ethical standpoint, evaluation can help to ensure that interventions do no harm either directly, or, in the case of ineffective interventions, indirectly 'by squandering limited resources' or alienating community groups and making them 'more resistant to other attempts to bring about change' (Green and South, 2006: 5).

The purposes of evaluation can therefore be summarized as:

- 'evaluation for accountability
- evaluation for programme management and development
- evaluation for learning
- evaluation as an ethical obligation'. (Green and South, 2006: 5)

VALUES AND EVALUATION

Evaluation is by no means a neutral, technical activity – it is saturated with values, ideological debate and, sometimes, vitriolic argument concerning what should be regarded as evidence of success and the means of assessing it.

WHO (1995) noted that health promotion is an investment and evaluation is concerned to address the costs and benefits of this investment. More specifically, evaluators might measure programme outcomes and processes in order to assess one or more of the following results of this investment:

- contribution to knowledge base/theory of health promotion
- insights that will result in more effective health promotion practice
- relative costs and benefits in financial terms
- levels of stakeholder satisfaction
- evidence to influence policymakers in respect of:
  - development of health policy
  - continued employment of researchers and health promotion departments
- impact on individual and public health.

However, different stakeholders may well differ in their aspirations for health promotion programmes. There is often substantial variation in the views of stakeholders about what would constitute success and, indeed, about the purpose of the evaluation enterprise itself. Figure 11.1 provides an overview of the dynamics of the stakeholder community.

In theory at least, the various stakeholders may all influence evaluation, although the amount of influence different groups bring to bear will vary. Funders are clearly key stakeholders. As the adage reminds us, 'he who pays the piper calls the tune'. Funder power can operate at both ends of the evaluation enterprise. Allocation of funding can be used to control the evaluation research agenda. Funders can also act as gatekeepers

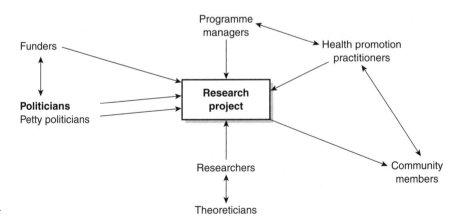

Figure 11.1   The stakeholder community

in relation to the dissemination of research findings – to the extent of withholding unpalatable findings. Some of the less reputable approaches to evaluation are summarized in the box.

> **Pseudo evaluations**
>
> **Eyewash** – focus on surface appearances
> **Whitewash** – covering up programme failure
> **Submarine** – political use of evaluation to undermine a programme
> **Posture** – ritual use of evaluation without any intention to use the findings, for example where evaluation is necessary to secure funding
> **Postponement** – as a means of avoiding or at least postponing action
>
> Newburn, 2001: 9 (drawing on Suchman, 1967, cited by Robson, 1993)

It is, perhaps, not unreasonable that funders should wish to exercise some degree of control. Pawson and Tilley (1997) quote a Department of Health's Code of Practice (see the box) to illustrate this phenomenon.

> **Is the customer always right? The Rothschild Principle**
>
> The main principle governing any Government funding of R&D is the Rothschild principle, laid down in Cmd 4814 and reiterated in the White Paper 'Realising Our Potential: A Strategy for Science, Engineering and Technology': ' ... the customer says what he wants, the contractor does it, if he can, and the customer pays'.
>
> Code of practice, Department of Health, 1993, cited in Pawson and Tilley, 1997: 14

The authors also refer to Stufflebeam's concern at the 'standards' produced by the US Joint Committee on Standards for Educational Evaluation:

[these have] four features ... utility, feasibility, propriety and accuracy [in that order] ... and evaluation should not be done at all if there is no prospect for its being useful to some audience. Second, it should not be done if it is not feasible to conduct it in political terms, or practicality terms, or cost-effectiveness terms. Third, they do not think it should be done if we cannot demonstrate that it will be conducted fairly and ethically. [If it has utility, feasibility and propriety] ... they said we could turn to the difficult matters of the technical accuracy of the evaluation. (Stufflebeam, 1980: 90, cited in Pawson and Tilley, 1997: 13)

The authors object to this kow-towing to customer demands, which, in their view, is characteristic of what they call 'pragmatic evaluation'. This mode of evaluation is criticized as 'methodologically rootless'. Epistemologically speaking, knowledge is considered to be valid only to the extent that it is pragmatically acceptable, so, ontologically, the social world centres on 'power-play'. Political astuteness and technical proficiency rule (Pawson and Tilley, 1997: 14).

The political dimension

The question of power is central to the dynamics of the stakeholder community. Evaluation is inherently political – it is rooted in some stakeholders' concerns to achieve change (and, of course, to justify preferred policies and actions!). In many instances, the political agenda is written large. For example, a critical theory stance in health promotion is manifestly concerned to bring about social change involving, ultimately, a challenge to many aspects of capitalist economies. However, most programmes – even those having a radical agenda – tend to operate within systems rather than directly challenge them. For instance, community development might typically concentrate on creating food cooperatives rather than developing a popular movement designed to confront the power of the web of agencies and government departments involved in food production or, indeed, the retail profit motive. Pawson and Tilley have coined the term 'petty political' to refer to the operations involved in the former, limited pressure for change. We have retained the term in Figure 11.1 and expanded its meaning somewhat to refer to the various minor processes and all actors involved in jostling for power at different levels of influence.

Health promotion values – the seal of approval

While there may be conflicting values, both explicit and implicit, in the stakeholder community, it is worth emphasizing the research-related values that must be upheld if an evaluation is to follow ideological commitments to an empowerment model of health promotion. For example, research carried out on rather than with individuals and the community would be antithetical to the participation imperative inherent in empowerment.

Rootman et al. (2001) argue that although health promotion evaluation has many commonalities with evaluation in general, it should pay due regard to those principles which are particularly relevant to its own domain. Over and above attention to issues such as social justice, equity and empowerment, these include:

- participation to:
  - identify the views of stakeholders
  - increase appreciation of the purpose of the evaluation and acceptance of the findings
  - encourage commitment to act on the findings
- consideration of evaluation from the outset and incorporation into all stages of programme/intervention development and implementation
- communication of evaluation findings to all participants and stakeholders
- harnessing the potential of evaluation to empower individuals and communities.

Green and South (2006) set out ten key principles for evaluating public health interventions (see box).

Key principles for evaluating public health interventions

1 Purpose: evaluation should have a clear purpose.
2 Practicality: evaluation should have practical relevance.
3 Process: evaluation should include attention to process as well as outcomes.
4 Peripheral (contextual) factors: evaluation should consider the effect of contextual factors.
5 Probing: evaluation should go further than attempting to offer simple input–output explanations to provide more complex understanding and contribute to the development of theory.
6 Plural: evaluation should use multiple methods to collect information.
7 Participation: evaluation should involve all stakeholders.
8 Plausibility: findings should reflect the experience of stakeholder groups, i.e. they should make sense.
9 Power: evaluation should recognize the power structures within which it operates, but not be restricted by them. It should include the lay perspective and contribute to empowerment.
10 Politics: evaluation is essentially political, informing decisions at different levels – project, organization, local policy, national policy.

Green and South, 2006: 33

EVALUATION AND PROGRAMME DESIGN

As a key element of systematic programme planning, evaluation should be considered from the outset and integrated at all stages. The model adopted here centres on the key elements described in Figure 11.2.

Three varieties of evaluation are included in Figure 11.2 – summative, formative and process. 'Summative' refers to an end-on assessment of the extent to which the programme has achieved its purpose. It is primarily concerned with the achievement of outcomes. The term 'impact' is generally used to refer to immediate changes which lead to longer term 'outcomes'. However, there is inconsistency in the literature with some authors referring to outcomes leading to impacts. For simplicity, our preference is to use the single term 'outcome' and, if necessary, distinguish short-, medium- and long-term outcomes.

'Process' evaluation consists of recording information collected throughout the programme and will be used for 'illumination'. 'Formative' evaluation also involves using information acquired throughout the programme. However, this information is used during the programme to make changes designed to maximize outcomes.

The construction of objectives formulates specific goals based on intended outcomes and information about the 'client group' or community. The actual selection of research methodology and methods will depend on the nature of the evaluation task and, of course, the ethical/ideological appropriateness of that methodology. At this juncture, we will consider the ideological issues associated with the choice of research methodology. In essence, this will involve discussing approaches that have competing value positions and which have been the subject of considerable debate.

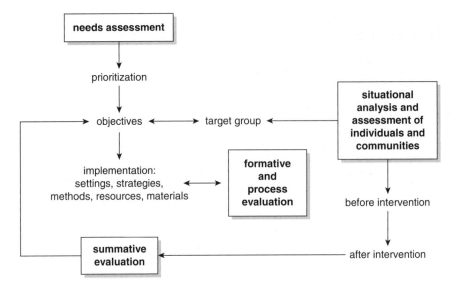

Figure 11.2   Programme planning – the place of research

> ### Paradigm – a definition
>
> A paradigm is a worldview built on implicit assumptions, accepted definitions, comfortable habits, values defended as truths, and beliefs projected as reality. As such, paradigms are deeply embedded in the socialization of adherents and practitioners: paradigms tell them what is important, legitimate, and reasonable. Paradigms are also normative, telling the practitioner what to do without the necessity of long existential or epistemological consideration. But it is this aspect of paradigms that constitutes both their strength and their weakness – their strength in that it makes action possible, their weakness in that the very reason for action is hidden in the unquestioned assumptions of the paradigm.
>
> Patton, 1997: 267

PARADIGM WARS – POSITIVISM AND ITS ALTERNATIVES

Conflicts between different paradigms (see box for definition) not only apply to the nature and philosophy of health promotion, but are reflected in the stance taken about what should or should not constitute appropriate and ethical evaluation. The major debate centres on the battle between positivism and a collection of approaches associated with qualitative methodology.

'Epistemology' is at the very centre of disagreements about which research approach and its concomitant methods are acceptable. Epistemology is concerned with beliefs about knowledge and what constitutes evidence. It is associated with the concept of 'ontology'. Denzin and Lincoln (1994: 99) succinctly describe the relationship between paradigms and the above-mentioned concepts, along with their specific application in methodologies.

> A paradigm encompasses three elements: epistemology, ontology and methodology. Epistemology asks, how do we know the world? What is the relationship between the enquirer and the known? Ontology raises basic questions about the nature of reality. Methodology focuses on how we gain knowledge about the world.

Accordingly, some approaches to evaluation would be considered inherently flawed and incapable of revealing the 'truth'. Furthermore, advocates of some approaches might argue that there are different forms of truth, while others might deny that truth exists.

The positivist paradigm

By way of simplifying a complex field of philosophical analysis and criticism related to conceptualizations of research and practice, three different paradigms will be discussed briefly below. These are positivism, interpretivism and a 'third way' that espouses critical realism and a utilization-focused perspective. The major debate has been between advocates of interpretivism and what has been until recently the dominant paradigm of positivism – notwithstanding the fact that interpretivism itself embraces a number of research traditions. The 'third way' might be subject to challenge, largely because of its alleged compromise position. For health promotion, however, the positivism v. interpretivism debate is of special importance as a positivist approach has characterized the medical model and underwritten the alleged 'gold standard' for evaluating programmes – the randomized controlled trial (RCT).

Positivism defined

Positivist philosophy can be traced to Auguste Comte (1798–1857), who compared and contrasted three constructions of reality – theological, metaphysical and positive. Positivism was equated with science, which was seen as the sole way forward to gaining a true understanding of the world. Comte's ideas were adopted by the logical positivists, whose philosophy rested on the assumption that we could gain an accurate representation of the world through our senses (and various devices that would increase the power of our senses); this 'scientific knowledge' would form the basis for progressive and cumulative advances in knowledge that would be free from partial interpretations and superstitious interpretations of reality.

Positivist science was viewed as having a value-free, 'neutral' status. It was objective rather than subjective. Moreover, the positivist approach was more than mere empiricism – a procedure, 'involving the production of accurate data – meticulous, precise, generalisable – in which the data themselves constitute the end for the research. It is summed up by the catchphrase "the facts speak for themselves"' (Bulmer, 1982). While accurate data collection and generalizability is also characteristic of positivist research, unlike empiricism, it is theory-driven. The ultimate goal is the construction of general laws.

Experiment is central to positivist methodology, although Popper has challenged its capacity to achieve verification. His centrally important concept of falsifiability is now inevitably considered to be at the heart of 'scientific method'. In other words, a theory holds until disproved, so the logical method of science is falsification and continual checking of claims to knowledge. In short, the key features of Popper's perspective are as follows:

- it is critical of 'induction'
- it is impossible to verify a universal theory with any degree of certainty, but it is possible to disprove a theory and therefore only one convincing 'disproof' will result in the rejection of theory regardless of how much supporting evidence already exists
- therefore, theory (a set of hypotheses) only survives until disproved
- accordingly, the method employed by 'science' must be falsification
- therefore, the 'gold standard' results of a properly constructed randomized controlled trial would also only hold until disproved.

Knowledge is therefore always provisional. As the procedure involves deduction rather than induction and is based on the confirmation or falsification of hypotheses, the scientific model adopted has been described as 'hypothetico-deductive' (Popper, 1945, 1959).

Perhaps unsurprisingly, social and behavioural scientists seeking an objective truth looked to the natural sciences and positivism as the way forward. As we have noted, such an approach is central to the medical model. However, its relevance for health promotion has been subject to intense criticism associated with the mounting challenge to medical hegemony.

Interpretivism – an alternative to positivism

While positivism is relatively easy to define, it is much more difficult to pick one's way through the plethora of methodologies and methods that constitute the opposition! Perhaps the most frequently used overarching terms are 'interpretivism' and 'constructivism'.

'Interpretivism' – a concept virtually identical to 'constructivism' (Guba and Lincoln, 1989) – centres on people's ways of interpreting/making sense of reality. It is essentially inductive – theory tends to be generated from data rather than data being used to test theory.

As Holloway (1997: 93) notes, interpretivism:

can be linked to Weber's *Verstehen* (German for 'empathetic' understanding) approach ... 'understanding' in the social sciences is inherently different from 'explanation' in the natural sciences. [Weber] differentiates between nomothetic, rule-governed methods of the latter and idiographic methods focusing on individual cases and not linked to the general laws of nature but to the actions of human beings ... Most qualitative research has its origin in the interpretive perspective.

One of the main traditions within the interpretivist approach has been termed 'hermeneutics' (from the Greek god Hermes, the messenger, who interpreted messages from Zeus to human beings). Holloway (1997: 87) again notes that:

Researchers ... gather data from language, texts and actions. They have to return to the data frequently, and ask the participants what the data mean to them.

Guba and Lincoln (1989) emphasize the importance of a 'dialectic' approach which involves questioning assumptions. As Schwandt (1994: 128) explains:

> They believe that the best means of achieving researcher and client constructions of reality is the 'hermeneutic-dialectic' process, so called because it is interpretive and fosters comparing and contrasting divergent constructions in an effort to achieve a synthesis of same. They strongly emphasize that the goal of constructivist enquiry is to achieve a consensus (or, failing that, an agenda for negotiation) on issues and concerns that define the nature of the enquiry.

Apart from the constructions of the research reality embodied in this latter constructivist approach, it will be apparent that 'subjects' of the research are not 'objects' but, rather, participants. This commitment is also apparent in what Guba and Lincoln (1989) called 'fourth generation evaluation', which entails stakeholder involvement, exploration of different perspectives and issues, negotiation to achieve consensus, development of reports communicating the nature of consensus and proposed actions to participants, and an iterative process of reviewing and revisiting the evaluation to address perceptions, concerns and issues that have not been resolved.

This emphasis on the experience and perspectives of individuals is central to phenomenological enquiry – another major strand within the interpretivist tradition associated with the work of Husserl and later Heidegger. It draws on Hegel's philosophy and particularly the centrality of conscious experience. A key feature of phenomenological research is that it attempts to be free from assumptions, preconceptions and preformed hypotheses.

By way of a resumé of the key features of the paradigms opposed to positivism, we might usefully summarize the 'manifesto' of new paradigm research, according to Reason and Rowan (1981) as shown in the box.

A manifesto of new paradigm research

- Research is never neutral – either it accepts or rejects the status quo.
- Research may be beneficial, but it may also be harmful.
- A close relationship between researcher and researched is essential. Both are equal in the research process. They are partners in defining the scope and nature of the research.
- Researcher and researched should have equal ownership of the products of the research.
- Research should be particularly concerned with knowledge having a practical, action-orientated outcome.
- Research should encourage people to take action – new paradigm research supports the politics of self-determination.
- New paradigm research rejects a traditional 'objective' approach and associated quantitative methods. It seeks a new kind of synthesis of subjectivity and objectivity.
- New paradigm researchers are committed to a holistic view of people and the environments and contexts in which they live their lives.

After Reason and Rowan, 1981

Pawson and Tilley (1997: 19) provide a useful graphic summary of constructivist research and its rationale (see Figure 11.3).

Participatory research

As we noted earlier, the participative convictions of interpretivism chime with health promotion's ideological commitment to involving client and community. Whyte (1997) provides an interesting historical slant on the development of 'participatory research' and 'action research'. He notes the possible confusion between the terms 'action research', 'participatory research' and 'participatory action research' and proceeds to remind us that it is possible to have action research without participation and participatory research without action. Moreover, participation and action can 'emerge' from social research and Whyte recalls how, in his classic research on Street Corner Society (Whyte, 1943), two participants, Doc and Sam Franco, 'became in a very real sense participant observers'. Moreover, 'We all hoped that publication of the book would eventually be helpful to the district and to others like it … (although there were no specific action or policy recommendations). Certain individuals begin as informants, then become key informants and ended up as co-participant observers, helping the professional field worker to interpret what they are learning from interviewing and observation'. Whyte (1991: 20) defined 'participatory action research' (PAR) as follows:

> In participatory action research (PAR), some of the people in the organization or community under study participate actively with the professional researcher throughout the research process from the initial design to the final presentation of results and discussion of action implications.

He subsequently felt that it was necessary to expand this definition to take account of emancipatory values (which he considered had always been implicit in the first definition). The addendum (Whyte, 1997: 111–12) states:

> The social purpose underlying PAR is to empower low-status people in the organization or community to make decisions and take actions which were previously foreclosed to them.

Macauley et al. (1999: 774), discussing research imperatives in the health context, reiterate the nature and importance of participation:

> Participatory research attempts to negotiate a balance between developing valid generalizable knowledge and benefiting the community that is being researched and to improve research protocols by incorporating the knowledge and expertise of community members … these goals can best be met by the community and researcher collaborating in the research as equals … Participatory research began as a movement for social justice in international development settings. It was developed to help improve social and economic conditions, to effect change, and to reduce the distrust of the people being studied. [Participatory research] … provides a framework to respond to health issues within a social and historical context.

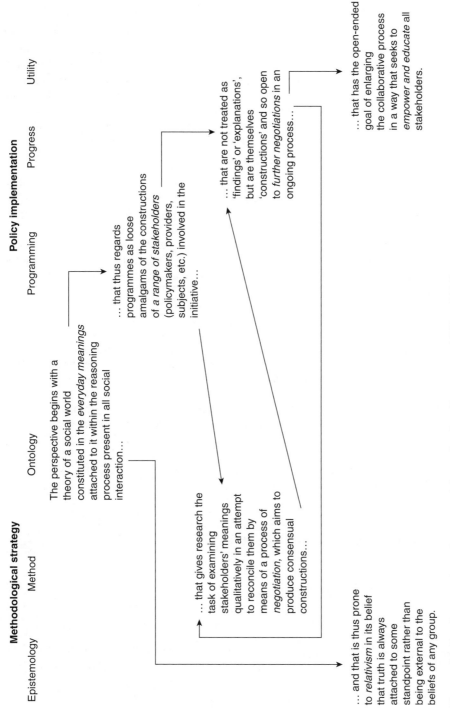

Figure 11.3   An overview of constructivist evaluation (Pawson and Tilley, 1997)

Realistic v. utilization-focused evaluation

Pawson and Tilley (1997) have launched a vigorous, and influential, challenge to both traditional, positivist research paradigms and, at the same time, to the constructivists' equally constraining insistence that, in the words of Guba and Lincoln (1989: 17), 'no accommodation is possible between positivist and constructivist belief systems as they are now formulated'. To do this, they felt, was to throw out the evaluation baby with the positivist bathwater! On the other hand, they questioned what they describe as a purely 'pragmatic approach', which they felt was exemplified in Patton's (1982: 49) alleged lack of interest in the epistemological basis of research and his overemphasis on an all-purpose methodological 'toolbox'. They disapprovingly cite the following statement:

> If a funding mandate calls for a summative outcomes evaluation, then the evaluator had better be prepared to produce such an animal, complete with a final report that includes that terminology right there on the front page, in big letters in the title.

This is perhaps rather unfair. Patton (1997) in a recent text on 'utilization-focused evaluation', acknowledges the value of both positivist and interpretivist paradigms. He considers that discussions about paradigm wars, 'are now primarily about philosophy rather than methods'. He (1997: 296) adds:

> I disagree, then, that philosophical assumptions necessarily require allegiance by evaluators to one paradigm or the other. Pragmatism can overcome seemingly logical contradictions ... the flexible and open evaluator can view the same data from the perspective of each paradigm and can help adherents of either paradigm interpret data in more than one way.

However, Milburn et al. (1995) comment that, in practice, the combination of different methods is often determined solely by pragmatic considerations and more attention needs to be paid to the way findings are combined and the methodological implications.

From our particular perspective on the inherently political nature of health promotion, we should note Patton's belief that evaluation is not value-free and 'politics is omnipresent in evaluation' (see the box).

When is evaluation not political?

Evaluation is not political under the following conditions:

- no one cares about the programme
- no one knows about the programme
- no money is at stake
- no power or authority is at stake
- and no one in the programme, making decisions about the programme, or otherwise involved in, knowledgeable about, or attached to the programme, is sexually active.

Patton, 1997: 352

Patton also adds that, as utilization-focused evaluation is pragmatic (and 'useful'), it can be applied to a variety of situations having different ideological commitments. Accordingly, he (1997: 103) states that: 'Using evaluation to mobilize for social action, empower participants, and support social justice are options on the menu of evaluation process uses'.

An interesting indicator of Patton's 'pragmatic paradigm' is provided by his apparent affection for Rudyard Kipling's (*Just So Stories*, 1902) well-known aphorism:

I keep six honest serving men,
(They taught me all I knew);
Their names are What and Why and When
and How and Where and Who.

He translates this as:

Who is the evaluation for?
What do we need to find out?
Why do we want to find that out?
When will the findings be needed?
Where should we gather information?
How will the results be used?

Further consideration of the philosophy and ideology of pragmatism requires much more space than is at our disposal here. However, we have not seen the end of the debate!

Realistic evaluation

Pawson and Tilley's approach to 'realistic evaluation' has been particularly influential in evaluating 'social programmes' and, thus, is especially relevant to the complex interventions and collaborations characteristic of health promotion. The approach can be termed 'post positive' and recognizes the existence of realities that can be investigated in robust fashion and used to implement social policy. At the same time, the narrow positivist approach epitomized by randomized controlled trials are determinedly discarded. The authors approvingly quote Guba and Lincoln's observation that true experimental design 'effectively strips away the context and yields results that are valid only in other contextless situations' (1989: 60, cited by Pawson and Tilley, 1997: 22). Realistic evaluation rejects this 'successionist' logic and argues for a 'generative logic'. The essence of realistic evaluation is to be found in a simple formula:

Outcome = mechanisms + context

Part of the rationale for Pawson and Tilley's rejection of the simplistic causal underpinning of the RCT is based on the recognition of a 'stratified reality' and inherently complex 'mechanisms'. Observations of 'regularities' in both physical and social science can be understood and influenced only by understanding these mechanisms. We will later, in discussing health promotion programmes, make reference to the 'black box' that must be illuminated if understanding is to be gained and efficient programmes achieved. Moreover, the individual choices resulting from the interplay of 'mechanisms' take place within 'contexts' – in other words, within various settings and their associated sets of norms and social rules. Accordingly:

> Evaluators need to acknowledge that programmes are implemented in a changing and permeable social world, and that programme effectiveness may thus be subverted or enhanced through the unanticipated intrusion of new contexts and new causal powers. Evaluators (also) need to focus on how the causal mechanisms which generate social and behavioural problems are removed or countered through the alternative causal mechanisms introduced in a social programme ... (Pawson and Tilley, 1997: 216–8)

Before leaving our brief description of realistic evaluation, it is worth noting that qualitative/ interpretivist methodology is central to its philosophy and practice. One particularly interesting aspect is the authors' argument that a central part of the collaboration of researcher and participants involves a 'teaching-learning' process: stakeholders are 'taught' by the researchers so that they gain understandings of programmes and their attributes in order to participate fully in (empowered) decision making. Also, of course, the researchers need to be taught by the stakeholders to gain maximum insight into the social and psychological realities and constructions of reality.

Before proceeding to consider the factors associated with selecting indicators of programme success, we should perhaps end this section on paradigm wars by asking where we stand. Which paradigms and ideologies and methodologies would seem to be most appropriate to health promotion? Should the emphasis be on agency or structure? Should we aim to seek an objective truth or recognize that there are different interpretations of reality?

Springett draws on the work of Habermas and Heidegger to identify important considerations for health promotion:

> ... the relationship between organism and the environment, on context, on the whole being greater than the sum of the parts; on connexions and synergy; on emergent systems, complexity and non-linear causality. (2001: 142)

The 'realist' perspective recognizes the existence of structures and institutional factors which are 'independent of the individual's reasoning and desires' (Pawson and Tilley, 1997: 23). At the same time, it acknowledges the importance of including a constructivist or interpretivist perspective in relation to exploring individual experience. Similarly, interpretive approaches are central to critical theory, but it also accepts the existence of structures and processes which shape individual experience (Connelly, 2001) and which could be explored by other forms of enquiry.

We would wish to avoid postmodern pessimism and consider that it is, in fact, possible to develop general understandings of the world. On the other hand, we recognize that multiple interpretations occur as a result of psychological and social constructions of reality. Our stance is thus consistent with the realist and critical theory positions. Life and health are complex and we must gain in-depth understandings drawing on multiple methodologies if we are to exert influence over the development of health promotion. We are firmly committed to participative, emancipatory research designed to empower and address social injustice and health inequalities. We are thus perhaps concerned not so much with an ideology of research but, rather, with research for an ideology of health promotion.

EFFECTIVENESS, EFFICIENCY AND EFFICACY

In the last analysis, evaluation is concerned with whether or not an intervention has been successful notwithstanding alternative conceptualizations and debate about what constitutes success. Two standards are typically used in assessing the extent of success – or failure. These are 'effectiveness' and 'efficiency'. The former term simply refers to the extent to which a programme has achieved its goals, while 'efficiency' is a measure of relative effectiveness – that is, how successful a programme has been in comparison to competing strategies or methods. For instance, if a course of drugs could lower population cholesterol levels more quickly, completely and safely than dietary change, it would be more efficient (although possibly less cost-effective) to prescribe that drug.

The efficacy paradox

The concept of efficacy has also been used, albeit less commonly, as a measure of effectiveness. It describes effectiveness and efficiency when interventions operate under ideal conditions: 'Effectiveness has all the attributes of efficacy except one: it reflects performance under ordinary conditions ... ' (Brook and Lohr, 1985: 711).

The concept of efficacy relates to the notion of programme fidelity, which means the extent to which an intervention is delivered in accordance with recommended best practice. It has particular significance for evaluating health promotion programmes in relation to what we describe here as the 'efficacy paradox'. For instance, if an intervention has been shown to be effective when it has been constructed according to an ideal specification and implemented with complete fidelity, the chances are that ordinary practitioners working under average conditions will not be able to achieve the same degree of success. Indeed, the programme might fail. Conversely, when such a programme has not met its objectives and, consequently, has been considered ineffective, that evaluation judgement is flawed as the programme was doomed to fail due to inadequate implementation. We will consider the implications of such flawed judgement when discussing the question of validity later in the chapter. For now, we should merely note that programme design must clearly identify what might be achieved within existing limitations and set the objectives accordingly. If these limited results are judged to be not worthwhile, the proposed programme should be scrapped. In the last analysis, the decision is grounded in health economics – do the programme gains justify the expenses incurred?

On cost-effectiveness

One of the most important criteria for appraising the efficiency of health promotion programmes involves calculating the relative financial costs of competing interventions. Godfrey (2001) notes the tendency for using 'partial' economic assessments – for example, merely describing the cost of an intervention. Clearly, this situation would be seen as far from satisfactory by health economists and Godfrey lists four different types of 'full' economic evaluation.

- Cost-minimization – the costs of two or more interventions assumed to achieve identical outcomes are calculated. The intervention that minimizes costs is judged to be the intervention of choice.
- Cost-effectiveness analysis – in addition to measuring the cost of programmes, benefits are assessed in quantifiable terms, such as the numbers of individuals exercising regularly or uptake of immunization against childhood diseases. It would, of course, be meaningless to make judgements about relative value for money unless indicators of health common to all programmes are employed (for instance, life years gained).
- Cost utility analysis – this mode of analysis seeks to measure the utility or values attached to particular health gains. QALYs (quality adjusted life years) are typically used to assess utility.
- Cost–benefit analysis (CBA) – this not only states the costs in monetary terms, but also seeks to place a price tag on the benefits accruing from the programme. A calculation of the cost per given benefit is then possible, typically expressed as a cost–benefit ratio.

Following these observations, it is both clear and logical – and indeed ethical – that if two or more programmes prove to be equally effective and acceptable, then the intervention that costs least should be selected. This is in line with Godfrey's (2001) view that the primary purpose of economic evaluation is to maximize what can be achieved by a given budget. The box provides examples of the calculated benefits against costs of selected health promotion measures.

Health promotion – instances of economic effectiveness

- A cost–benefit analysis of using bike/pedestrian trails in Lincoln, Nebraska calculated the annual cost of using trails (including construction, maintenance and equipment) as $209.28 per capita. The direct medical benefit per annum was costed at $564.41 per capita with an overall cost–benefit ratio of 2.94. (Wang et al., 2005)
- The benefits from legislation requiring cycling-helmet use in Israel (over a five-year period) are considerable and exceed costs by a ratio of 3:1 (total benefits were estimated at $40,544,770). (Ginsberg and Silverberg, 1994)
- NHS expenditure on statins, drugs which reduce cholesterol levels, is around £500 million per year. The cost-effectiveness is estimated to be between £4,000 and £8,000 per QALY. This contrasts with £212 and £873 per QALY for smoking cessation. (Wanless, 2002)

Although this type of analysis may, at first sight, be very seductive for those keen to demonstrate effectiveness and cost-effectiveness, there are both technical and ideological concerns. While costing 'input' is relatively unproblematic, the appropriateness of costing 'output' – that is, assessing and assigning a value to life and quality of life – poses major ethical problems, as discussed in Chapter 2. Raphael (2001b) noted in reference to Lindström's (1994) quality of life model, that it questioned the relevance of cost–benefit analysis to more holistic interpretations of health and interventions operating at interpersonal, community, social and environmental levels that are more typical of health promotion.

Green and South (2006) argue that if cost effectiveness is the sole criterion, then interventions targeted at easy-to-change groups would be favoured over those which focused on groups more resistant to change or coping with adverse social circumstances. This would ultimately result in widening health inequalities. Attention therefore needs to be given to 'goals such as equity, regeneration, social inclusion and social justice' (2006: 41).

DISENTANGLING COMPLEXITY – SELECTING INDICATORS OF SUCCESS

The purpose of indicators is 'to capture key aspects of a programme and its effects' (Green and South, 2006: 45). They provide insight into whether programme objectives have been achieved or whether progress is being made towards them. However, the selection of indicators is essentially political and influenced by values and ideologies. Springett (1998) comments on the tendency to use indicators of ill health rather than health, driven by traditional medical norms and managerial concerns.

We noted in Chapter 4 the centrality of objectives to programme planning. The identification of appropriate indicators will be more straightforward if programme objectives are well defined and comprehensive. Rigorously formulated objectives provide a secure basis for identifying indicators of success – particularly if they set out standards and conditions. SMART objectives should lead to SMART indicators (specific, measurable, appropriate, relevant and time related). The acronym SPICED has also been used and incorporates some of the key principles referred to above:

Subjective
Participatory
Interpretable
Cross-checked
Empowering
Disaggregated. (BOND, 2005)

Figure 11.4 provides an overview of a hypothetical, large-scale health promotion programme.

First, it is assumed that the programme has been designed according to the principles of systematic planning discussed earlier in this book. It is launched at a particular time (T1) and will achieve its final goals (if ever) at another point in time (T4). Temporal progress is indicated by a proximal–distal spectrum – that is, activities occurring at T1 are proximal to the start of the programme, whereas final outcomes at T4 and all other events in between will be more or less distal.

Two kinds of final outcomes are shown in Figure 11.4. They include, on the one hand, the traditional goals of a preventive model – namely, primary, secondary and tertiary prevention – and, on the other, the outcomes of a strategy seeking to address

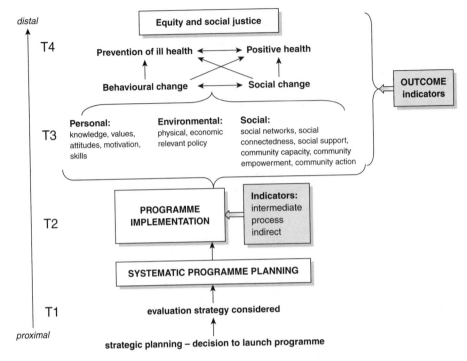

Figure 11.4   An overview of a health promotion programme

'positive health'. The emphasis on the former in many evaluations reflects their respective ease of measurement. However, from a health promotion perspective, it is important to address the challenge and include the positive dimension. The label 'positive health' is used to refer to any outcomes related to 'quality of life' or, even more broadly, 'the good life'. These are not, of course, completely discrete as the quality of life is typically damaged by disease and enhanced by its prevention. Moreover, as has also been clearly demonstrated, the achievement of wellbeing and, more demonstrably, the reduction of inequalities, may have a major impact on preventive outcomes.

There is frequently a substantial time gap between particular health promotion inputs and what might be seen to be final outcomes. For example, it may take many years for the benefits of a school-based healthy eating and exercise programme to become apparent in reduced mortality from coronary heart disease – the gap between T1 and T4 in such a case could well be 30 or 40 years. The use of morbidity and mortality data as indicators to assess the effectiveness of the teaching programme would thus be entirely unrealistic! Green and Tones (1999) are critical of the use of such epidemiological data for evaluating health promotion programmes. They argue that the identification of poor diet and lack of exercise as risk factors for heart disease and epidemiological information about disease prevalence provides the justification for introducing the programme rather than being a means for evaluating it (Green and Tones, 1999). The goal of the health promotion programme would be to alter the known risk factors.

A further objection is based on the fact that many successful health education/ promotion interventions may be necessary, but not sufficient to influence final outcomes. Typically, a complicated web of inputs over time would be needed. For instance, effective life skills training, together with an efficient sex education programme in schools, might only have an impact on sexual risk taking if policy measures have been implemented to ensure ready access to condoms and, say, a user-friendly drop-in centre for young people.

Intermediate, indirect and process indicators

Measuring health outcomes can be difficult, as recognized by the evaluation of the National Healthy School Standard (NHSS):

> It is to be hoped that effective health education will lead ultimately to improved health and the reduction of illness, but this is a very long-term prospect. Within the scope of the evaluation, it is unlikely that NHSS activities would have a direct effect on these outcomes. Therefore we need to focus on health related behaviour, the intermediate step between health promotion activities and impact on health. (Blenkinsop et al., 2004: 52)

Green and South (2006) emphasize that it is important to have realistic aspirations for what might reasonably be achieved within the time frame of a programme when defining outcome indicators. For example, these might include a change in health-related behaviour, or the introduction of a no smoking policy or achievement of environmental change, or development of social capital within a community. To reiterate our earlier point – if strong evidence already exists about the link between such factors and disease reduction or positive health goals, there is no need to revisit this. If there is no such robust relationship with mortality and morbidity – or positive health – then there is no ethical justification for the introduction of the programme in the first place!

Intermediate indicators identify antecedents of the outcomes. They relate to the various stages in the causal pathway between the intervention and the outcomes. Intermediate indicators contribute, in various degrees, to the outcome. Green and South (2006) point out that the classification of indicators as intermediate or outcome is to some extent a matter of definition. Furthermore, this could well vary from programme to programme. For example, self-empowerment and social capital may be deemed to be outcomes worth pursuing in their own right, so evidence of achievement in this regard, provided by measures of confidence and control, could rightly be called outcome indicators. On the other hand, it seems increasingly clear that empowerment is a major determinant of adopting behaviour consistent with preventive outcomes. In this latter case, evidence of empowerment would provide intermediate indicators of success.

Process indicators would be used to record the fidelity and quality of the programme and identify any need for improvement and refinement. Understanding which elements of the process contributed to success – or equally failure – is also important in relation to the wider dissemination and uptake of programmes.

Implementing a programme may involve a number of subsidiary activities such as the development of leaflets or the training of staff. Indicators relating to these are referred to as indirect indicators – for example, pre-testing leaflets to assess their suitability or assessing the capacity of teachers to provide drug education following training. Although necessary to the success of the intervention, these indirect indicators do not form part of the direct causal pathway linking intervention and outcome. Again, the distinction can be blurred. Barnes et al. (2004) recognize the difficulty of separating process, outcomes and systems indicators. For example, the development of good partnerships may be an essential element of the process and also a positive outcome.

Opening the black box

One of health promotion's major requirements is illumination. In other words, we need to know not just whether or not a programme has been effective, but to identify key elements of the process and how these link to outcomes. In line with realist evaluation, we need to understand how an intervention works and why it works, or fails to work within a particular context. The more complicated the programme, the greater the need for illuminative insights.

Again, the significance of illumination in evaluation is not a discovery of health promotion. Workers in the field of educational research who questioned the value of experimental design also argued the case for gaining insights through illumination. Parlett and Hamilton (1972), for example, proposed an 'illuminative, social-anthropological paradigm' that took account of the wider contexts in which educational programmes function. They used an analogy with the theatre to point out that, without such insights, evaluators risk being 'rather like a critic who reviews a production on the basis of the script and applause-meter readings, having missed the performance'!

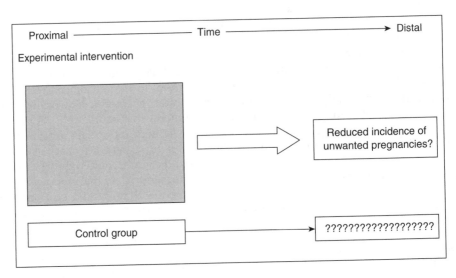

Figure 11.5   The black box problem

Figure 11.5 illustrates what might be called the 'black box problem'. It simulates an experimental evaluation of a school-based programme designed to reduce the incidence of unwanted pregnancies by comparing its long-term results with one of a number of control schools lacking such an intervention. An evaluator would need detailed information about the intervention and its dynamics. Figure 11.6 reveals the kinds of complexity that might be revealed if the black box were opened.

In short, we would expect to observe a complex web of synergistic elements. It also demonstrates that a number of additional, cumulative inputs would be needed over quite a lengthy period of time if success were to be achieved. Moreover, as a school setting might be only one component of a comprehensive community-wide programme, Figure 11.6, in fact, substantially underestimates the level of complexity there could actually be.

Theory of Change and the selection of indicators

Reference to relevant theory and models which shed light on the anticipated change process will help with the identification of appropriate indicators. For example, the use of the Health Action Model (HAM) will shed light on the various factors which inform behavioural intention and those that will affect whether that intention is put into action.

As we have noted above, indirect, intermediate and outcome indicators should be selected to provide evidence at various stages along the complex and often convoluted pathway leading from proximal interventions to ultimate outcomes. Yet, in many instances, the assumptive logic linking an intervention with anticipated effects is either missing or poorly articulated, leading to problems with evaluation as well as compromising the success of an intervention. This is particularly so in the case of complex community initiatives. Weiss put forward the argument that:

> ... a key reason complex programs are so difficult to evaluate is that the assumptions that inspire them are poorly articulated ... stakeholders of complex community initiatives typically are unclear about how the change process will unfold and therefore place little attention to the early and mid-term changes that need to happen in order for a longer term goal to be reached. The lack of clarity about the 'mini-steps' that must be taken to reach a long term outcome not only makes the task of evaluating a complex initiative challenging, but reduces the likelihood that all of the important factors related to the long term goal will be addressed. (ActKnowledge, undated a)

The Theory of Change Approach was developed by the Aspen Institute Roundtable on Community Change to respond to the challenge of evaluating comprehensive community initiatives (CCIs), also referred to as complex community initiatives (see Connell et al., 1995; Fulbright-Anderson et al., 1998). These involve interventions with multiple components leading to multi-level outcomes. The Theory of Change Approach provides a means of unpicking the steps along the pathways of change – or indeed the complex networks. It involves 'surfacing' the latent theory which outlines stakeholders' expectations about the various steps along the pathway linking activities to the achievement of goals. This is done through a guided process which draws on existing knowledge and theory and also the insight of practitioners and other stakeholders. Evaluators and stakeholders work together to 'co-construct' the theory of change for an initiative. The

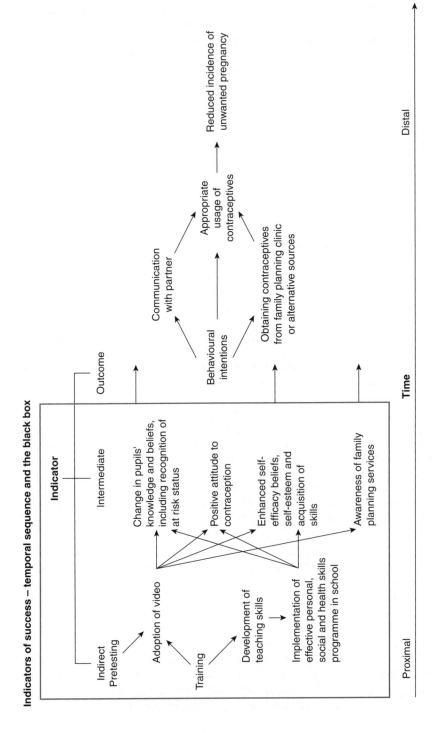

Figure 11.6   The black box, opened

stages are summarized in the box. They start with the identification of long-term goals as, in practice, it has proved easier to reach agreement about these and then work back to intermediate outcomes and activities. The development of indicators for each stage makes the theory testable.

> **The Theory of Change approach: stages in the process**
>
> 1 Identification of long-term goals and the assumptions behind them.
> 2 Backwards mapping to connect to the preconditions or requirements needed to achieve the goal.
> 3 Identification of the actions undertaken to achieve the desired change.
> 4 Developing indicators to measure outcomes to assess the performance of the initiative.
> 5 Writing a narrative explaining the logic of the initiative.
>
> ActKnowledge, undated b

The characteristics of a good theory are held to be that it is:

- plausible
- doable
- testable. (Connell and Kubisch, 1998)

The use of logical frameworks for programme planning is consistent with the Theory of Change. As we noted in Chapter 4, logical frameworks help to ensure that all necessary elements of a programme are in place and also make explicit the assumptions about the way programmes will work. As with the Theory of Change, they help to ensure that programmes are successful as well as identifying key indicators to assess progress. An example of a Theory of Change linking the rationale for the activity (in this case, participatory action research) with anticipated short-, medium- and longer-term outcomes which provide the basis for the development of indicators, comes from the Children's Fund evaluation – see Figure 11.7.

Theory of Change has been a popular approach for evaluating complex social policy programmes. In England, for example, it has been used in national evaluations of Health Action Zones (see Judge, 2000; Judge and Bauld, 2001) and the Children's Fund (see Barnes et al., 2004). Mason and Barnes (2007) distinguish between those programmes which have involved evaluators from the initial stages of programme planning, more typical of the USA where the approach was developed, and those which have not involved evaluators until programmes are under way, more typical of the UK experience. In the latter situation, it is not uncommon for the theory to be constructed retrospectively and, indeed, to be influenced by the need to justify actions.

RELIABILITY, VALIDITY AND THE RCT

Having considered the various types of indicator to include in evaluation, it is important to ensure that resulting evidence is valid. In other words, if the combined results of the

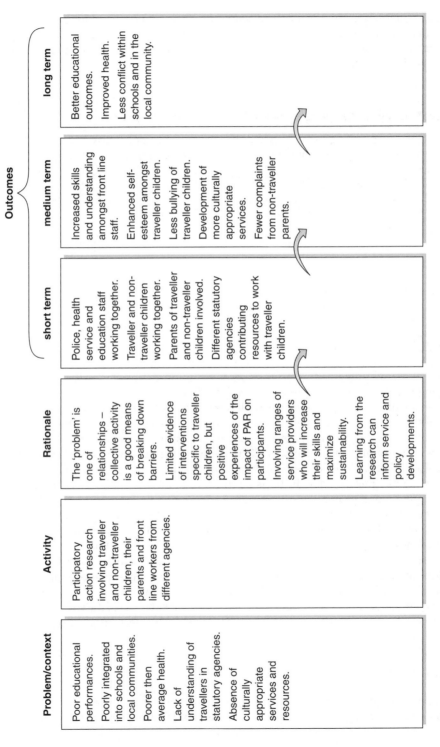

Figure 11.7   A Theory of Change for work with traveller childern (derived from Barnes et al., 2004)

indirect, intermediate and outcome indicators demonstrate a certain level of effectiveness, we must be satisfied that the evidence is robust and any claims of success can be justified.

The two standard criteria for assessing the quality of research measures are reliability and validity. Reliability is concerned with consistency and replicability – that is, the extent to which research techniques will produce consistent results, regardless of how, when and where the research is carried out. For example, a completely reliable questionnaire should yield identical scores, whoever administers the questionnaire. Moreover, if individuals are retested, they should provide the same response (provided, of course, that they have not actually changed during the time that elapses between test and retest). Similarly, if individuals or groups are interviewed or observed, then different interviewers or observers should draw the same conclusions.

Validity is, quite simply, the extent to which investigators and their instruments actually measure what they intend to measure – and nothing else. It describes the truth and authenticity of research findings. An unreliable evaluation cannot be valid. Equally, an evaluation might demonstrate highly reliable results, but lack validity – it might merely have measured the wrong things, but done so very consistently.

In the context of evaluation of research, two varieties of validity are distinguished – internal and external. 'Internal validity' refers to the degree of certainty that the results of an evaluation are due to the intervention under investigation and not to other factors. Granger (1998) makes the useful distinction between outcomes and effects. An outcome is defined as 'a measure of the variables that follow all or some of the intervention'. In contrast, an effect is 'the outcome minus an estimate of what would have occurred without the intervention'. This concern to attribute any change to the intervention in comparison with what would have happened had the intervention not taken place – the so-called counterfactual situation – is central to debates about evaluation methodology.

'External validity' describes the generalizability of the results – that is, the extent to which a given intervention can be expected to produce similar results in other populations and, therefore, be of use to other practitioners and planners.

As we will see, the classic RCT is strong on internal validity, but weak on external validity. On the other hand, interpretivist approaches are, perhaps arguably, more likely to generate results that can be used by other practitioners. However, special efforts must be made to ensure rigour.

The RCT – strengths and limitations

The RCT conforms to the principles of true experimental design. Within the domain of medicine, the popularity of the RCT – and the current movement for evidence-based medicine – have been ascribed to the influential work of Cochrane (1972, cited by McPherson, 1994: 6), who argued that evaluation of effectiveness should be the first priority of the NHS in the UK and decided 'to concentrate on one simple idea – the value of randomized controlled trials in improving the NHS – and to keep the book short and simple'.

Cochrane's rationale was certainly convincing, as was his demonstration that many routinely performed medical interventions were not based on evidence of effectiveness. The argument for evidence-based practice – and the use of experimental method – was by no means confined to medicine. Indeed, as Shacklock Evans (1962) points out, the use of experimental designs of the kind Cochrane espoused can be attributed primarily to Fisher (1949) and the field of agricultural biology and subsequently applied to education by Lindquist (1940). The emphasis of the experimental approach on avoiding threats to internal validity can be seen in Fisher's (1949: 19) observation:

> Whatever degree of care and experimental skill is expended in equalizing the conditions, other than the one under test, which are liable to affect the result, this equalization must always be to a greater or less extent incomplete and in many important practical cases will be grossly defective.

Let us begin by noting some of the obvious limitations of claims that programmes have been effective where the validity of the results can be severely challenged!

Inadequacies in judging programme effectiveness

Situation 1 in Figure 11.8 is so limited in its utility that it cannot really be called a research design, as there is no indication of the status of the group before the intervention (X). The result of the assessment (observation 'O') might therefore be due to a positive effect of the intervention. Alternatively, the intervention might have had no effect at all. Indeed, it might have made things worse!

Situation 2 – a simple pre–post test design – provides more information. However, although it would be possible to record any changes occurring between the pre-test and post-test, it would not be possible to demonstrate with any degree of certainty that the changes were due to the intervention.

Situation 3, on the other hand, uses a control group that does not receive the intervention and, so, assuming that there is a statistically significant difference between pre- and post-test and no such difference in the control group, it is reasonable to conclude that the intervention had had an impact. Unfortunately, there can be no certainty that the experimental and control groups were identical in all key respects before the intervention. Accordingly, the apparently superior performance of the experimental group might, by chance, have been due to differences between the groups rather than the effectiveness of the intervention.

Situation 4, however, is a TRUE experimental design. This is symbolized here by the use of the traditional 'OXO' terminology initiated and elaborated by Campbell and Stanley (1963) and Cook and Campbell (1979). The essential difference is that 'subjects' are randomly assigned to experimental and control situations, thus partialling out differences of any kind. Randomization is the key to the superior status of the RCT and the justification for its gold standard accolade.

Furthermore, the rigour of RCT versions of true experimental design have been enhanced by the use of additional measures, such as the 'double blind trial', in which neither researchers nor subjects know who is receiving the active, experimental ingredient. This helps to minimize researcher bias and avoid placebo effects.

Type 1 and 2 errors and true experimental design

The major strength of true experimental designs is their capacity to avoid 'Type 1 error'. In other words, to avoid claiming that a given intervention has been effective when apparent differences between experimental and control groups might have resulted from

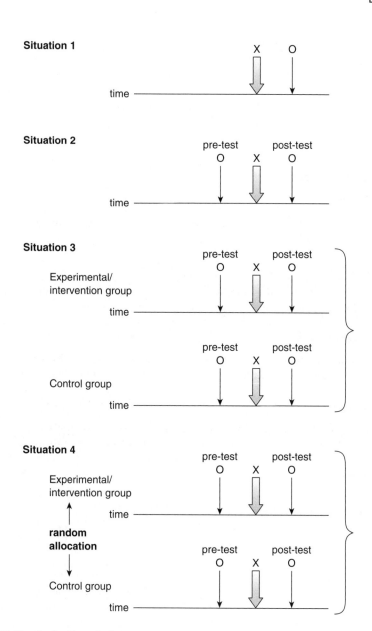

Figure 11.8 Evaluation designs

extraneous factors. The success of the research design lies in its capacity to eliminate alternative causes so that the effects attributable to the intervention can be identified.

This particular virtue may be achieved at the expense of incurring a 'Type 2 error' – that is drawing an erroneous conclusion that an intervention was ineffective when it may, in fact, actually have had an effect. For instance, a programme may actually have had an impact on the target group, but the instruments might have been insufficiently sensitive to discriminate between the effect on experimental and control groups. Similarly, failure to detect change may also occur when there are mixed populations and the positive effect of an intervention in one section of the population is diluted by a zero effect in the rest of the population or even a negative 'reactance' effect. An overview of different types of error is provided in the box.

Five types of error

Type 1 error

An erroneous conclusion that an intervention has achieved significant change when, in fact, it has failed to do so.

Type 2 error

An erroneous conclusion that an intervention has failed to have a significant impact when, in fact, it has actually done so.

Type 3 error

Asserting that an intervention has failed to achieve successful results when it was so poorly designed that it could not possibly have had a desired effect.

Type 4 error

Conducting an evaluation of a programme that no one cares about and is irrelevant to decision makers. Evaluation for the sake of evaluation is central to this error.

Type 5 error

An intervention is shown to produce a genuine statistically significant effect, but the change is so slight as to have no practical significance.

After Basch and Gold, 1986: 300–1

Green and Lewis (1986: 264–7), while cautioning evaluators against the 'fallacy of assuming inexorable forward movement', list the following situations that may also distort understanding of the effectiveness of interventions and contribute to Type 1 and 2 errors.

- Delay of impact (or sleeper effect) – an intervention actually has an impact, but this does not emerge until later – perhaps quite a long time after the evaluation when circumstances are favourable.
- Decay of impact (or backsliding effect) – the intervention produces an effect, but this decays more or less rapidly. Without continuing measurement, the programme might have been judged a success when it had, for all practical purposes, been a failure.

- Borrowing from the future – the intervention triggers changes in behaviour that would have happened anyway, the programme merely hastening the inevitable.
- Secular trends – a positive secular trend may result in overestimating programme effects, while a negative secular trend may result in discounting an influence that had delayed the decline.
- Contrast effects – premature termination of a programme may create a backlash resulting in a slowing or reversal of behavioural outcomes that would have occurred had the programme continued.

Although accepted as standard practice for testing drugs, the limitations of the RCT have been recognized even within a biomedical context. Charlton (1991: 355) argued that the RCT was:

> vital but of restricted applicability to medicine .... it should only be employed in conditions of clinical unpredictability. When an obviously effective treatment emerges there is no need for a controlled trial to establish its usefulness.

On the other hand, he noted that:

> Gain in objectivity is achieved by simplification and at the cost of completeness ... the patient is depersonalized, the doctor is deskilled. (1991: 356)

Are RCTs ever relevant for evaluating health promotion?

We are inclined to respond to this question by saying, 'Well, not never, but hardly ever!' More particularly, we might say that the RCT or, more properly, the true experimental design is only likely to be useful to the extent that the health promotion intervention approximates to the clinical trial. In other words, that, first, the intervention is simple and, second, we do not know the answer already nor have better ways of finding it. This is rare within the overall complexity of the health promotion enterprise. Furthermore, following our earlier discussion of realistic and utilization-focused evaluation, if the trial strips away consideration of contextual factors, the findings will have little relevance to other situations.

We have considered above some of the epistemological concerns about the use of RCTs for health promotion evaluation. There are also technical and practical issues.

Establishing an adequate control group presents a number of difficulties. Interventions are generally complex, frequently multi-sectoral and usually targeted at groups of various size rather than individuals. The allocation of individuals to intervention and control groups, as required by true experimental designs, is therefore simply not practicable. Random assignment of whole groups such as communities or schools is more feasible. However, inherent differences between groups may compromise their use as controls. Such studies are generally held to have a 'comparison group' or 'reference group' rather than a proper control. Studies in which random allocation to control and intervention group is not possible are usually referred to as quasi-experimental. Some of the large-scale community intervention trials such as the Community Intervention Trial for Smoking Cessation (COMMIT) matched communities with regard to key characteristics before randomly allocating them to intervention and comparison groups (COMMIT Research Group, 1991) in order to minimize this problem.

Furthermore, when the impetus for an intervention comes from the community itself, it is virtually impossible to provide an adequate control (Mackenbach, 1997). Similarly, McPherson (1994: 12) notes that the pursuit of objectivity fails to acknowledge the potential influence of volition and decision making. He concludes that 'choice itself can dramatically affect important measures of outcome'. Choice and control are both recognized as central to the health promotion endeavour. Removing these elements by random allocation would, therefore, systematically introduce bias by reducing effectiveness.

Contamination of the reference or control group can also be a problem, especially in large-scale interventions. For example, Nutbeam et al. (1993) reported that reference areas used by the 'Heartbeat Wales' heart disease prevention programme rapidly became independently involved in establishing their own heart health initiatives, thus compromising their value as controls.

Although not unique to RCTs, the emphasis in evaluation design is on assessing outcomes rather than the quality of the intervention itself. A 'Type 3 error' occurs when an intervention could not possibly succeed because of its inherent inadequacy. The Type 3 error relates to the concept of efficacy that was defined earlier in this chapter. Key considerations in relation to the quality of the programme include:

- it has been systematically planned
- it addresses all key determinants derived from theoretical analysis and research into the needs of the target group
- fidelity of implementation
- adequate resources – financial and staffing
- sufficient intensity
- sufficient reach
- supportive materials have been pre-tested with the target group
- staff are properly trained and have the competences needed to implement the programme.

The 'Type 5 error' is a well-known phenomenon, but not normally labelled in this way. It is not unknown for research to yield very respectable p-values by simply using very large numbers of subjects! Practical significance is undoubtedly of more relevance to those working in the field than such artificially constructed statistical significance.

Furthermore, we should emphasize that health promotion does not conform with a simple input–output model. There may be a range of outcomes – anticipated and unanticipated – which are the product of complex pathways of change. The capacity of RCTs to unpick that complexity is open to question – however sophisticated the design and statistical tests. Lang's acerbic comment about using 'statistics as a drunken man uses lampposts – for support rather than illumination' (cited by Cohen and Cohen, 1960) encapsulates over-reliance on statistics. Equally, the complex social interventions needed to tackle contemporary public health problems are not amenable to RCT design. Green and South (2006) conclude that experimental and quasi-experimental methods have limited utility for informing public health policy and practice.

Our concerns about the relevance of the RCT for health promotion evaluation are summarized in the box and we concur with the conclusions of the WHO European Working Group on Health Promotion Evaluation (WHO, 1998a: 3):

Conclusion 4: The use of randomized control [*sic*] trials to evaluate health promotion initiatives is, in most cases, inappropriate, misleading and unnecessarily expensive.

For a better understanding of the impact of health promotion initiatives, evaluators need to use a wide range of qualitative and quantitative methods that extend beyond the narrow parameters of randomized controlled trials.

Limitations of RCTs for health promotion evaluation

- Inability to cope with the complexity of health promotion programmes
- Do not pay sufficient attention to process and the quality of interventions
- Practical difficulties in relation to randomization
- Contamination of control or reference groups
- Statistical significance may be achieved at the expense of practical significance
- Do not provide illumination of the pathways linking intervention and outcomes and the ways in which these are influenced by the various components of complex interventions
- Do not include formative evaluation, which is essential to improving the success of programmes
- Are ideologically incompatible with health promotion in relation to:

  - commitment to 'active' individual and community participation in the research process
  - contributing to its empowering and 'emancipatory' role
  - the use of research as a tool for achieving political and social change

---

A NEW GOLD STANDARD – THE JUDICIAL PRINCIPLE

We have asserted the need for adopting a particular kind of post-positivist paradigm for health promotion research. The rejection of a positivist approach, together with its gold standard RCT design, does not mean that we should abandon the pursuit of reliability and validity. Quite the reverse. A critical realist model, as we have seen, has no difficulty in addressing Type 2 and 3 errors, but it is imperative that it replace the techniques intrinsic to true experimental design with robust alternatives that will maximize internal validity – that is, provide strong evidence that will substantiate claims that programmes or parts of programmes have produced change.

Reliability, replicability, dependability and validity

As qualitative methodology is central to the interpretivist aspects of critical, realistic evaluation, it makes sense to give some thought to the methods recommended by qualitative researchers to achieve reliability and validity. Lincoln and Denzin (1994: 579), for example, comment that:

a text is valid if it is sufficiently grounded, triangulated, based on naturalistic indicators, carefully fitted to a theory [and its concepts], comprehensive in scope, credible in terms of member checks, logical, and truthful in terms of its reflection of the phenomenon in question. The text's author then announces the validity claims to the reader. Such claims now become the text's warrant to its own authoritative representation of the experience and social world under inspection.

Reliability and validity are often assessed simultaneously and qualitative researchers tend to use such terms as 'replicability', 'dependability', 'confirmability', 'trustworthiness', 'transferability' and 'authenticity' to assess the consistency of interventions and the extent to which their results actually measure the constructs that they are claiming to measure.

According to Denzin (1994: 508):

> The foundation for interpretation rests on triangulated empirical materials that are trustworthy. Trustworthiness consists of four components: credibility, transferability, dependability, and confirmability (these are the constructionist equivalents of internal and external validity, reliability and objectivity).

Various specific techniques have also been devised to provide a basis for demonstrating credibility and providing transparent results that allow judgements to be made about reliability and validity. Some examples will be discussed below.

Member checks

In general, the rationale for this technique is testing results of research against the perceptions of audience members. Guba and Lincoln (1981: 316) suggest that the evaluator should, for example:

- draw a sample from informants
- check data derived (from interviews, for example) with the interviewees
- ask them to point out any errors of fact.

Apart from checking reliability and validity, the researcher's categorization of interviewees' responses can be reassessed and incomplete categories can be fleshed out.

Member checks provide what elsewhere might be described as 'respondent validation'.

Thick description

Denzin (1994: 505) compares 'thin description' to 'thick description'. The former:

> simply reports facts, independent of intentions or circumstances. A thick description, in contrast, gives the context of an experience, states the intentions and meanings that organized the experience, and reveals the experiences as a process. Out of this process arise ... claims for truth, [and its] verisimilitude.

In short, thick, rich detail makes it possible to gain illuminative insights and allow others to check a researcher's claims.

Audit trails

This interpretivist research technique is designed to provide a detailed account of how researchers/evaluators have reached their decisions about the categories that they have constructed from raw data and the conclusions they have reached and, perhaps, about the theories they have derived from these. As Morse puts it, 'interested parties can reconstruct the process by which the investigators reached their conclusion'.

She (1994: 230) cites the following list of six types of documentation for an audit trail (developed by Halpern, 1983):

> raw data, data reduction and analysis products, data reconstruction and synthesis products, process notes, materials relating to intentions and dispositions, and instrument development information.

Transferability

This is the alternative version of external validity. Again, thick descriptions can provide sufficiently detailed information for people to make judgements about the relevance of findings to different but related situations and to know how to proceed.

'Purposive/purposeful sampling' is considered to yield the most useful data. Situations and/or individuals are deliberately selected in the expectation that they will prove to be a rich source of relevant data. Deliberate selection implies choosing from alternatives. Choices should be made on the basis of both previous research and, of course, sound theoretical understandings.

Authenticity

Lincoln and Guba (1985) offer authenticity as an alternative concept to validity. Research is not only authentic when the strategies it uses will ensure true reporting of participants' feelings and ideas, it should also demonstrate that it is consistent with these ethical and ideological principles. The components of authenticity would typically include:

- notions such as fairness and equity
- ontological authenticity – that is, participants gain some insight into their human condition
- understandings that help with insight and relating to other people
- catalytic authenticity/validity – the research method itself should achieve its substantive ideological goals so that, for example, in participative health promotion research, it should contribute to empowerment.

The judicial principle – assessing the validity of evidence

The business of evaluating health promotion, with all its complexities, requires a new approach – a new gold standard. Decisions must, of course, still be made on the basis of evidence, but the criteria for making the vigilant decisions that would be used by real people in real life when addressing problems and making policy must be reassessed.

Accordingly, we propose here the use of a 'judicial principle'. As the words suggest, we draw a parallel with the judicial system and argue that decisions should be made on the basis of a pot pourri of evidence derived from different sources. Two degrees of judicial certainty should be employed. Where the level of certainty for action must be of a higher order, the criterion used in criminal law should be used – that is, it must be beyond reasonable doubt. Where the consequences of decision making are less serious and the demand for evidence is, therefore, less stringent, the criterion employed in civil law might be used – that is, take into account the balance of probabilities.

These two levels of probability could loosely be compared with their quantitative equivalents – p-values of $p < 0.01$ (or less if the evidence is especially compelling) and $p < 0.05$ for balance of probability estimates.

Evidence and causality

Although Pawson and Tilley questioned the utility of assumptions based on a successionist logic – that is, the notion that whatever follows an event is presumed to have been caused by it – cause and effect evidence is important in applying the judicial principle. As we noted in Chapter 2, several criteria are generally accepted as providing evidence of causality in the medical arena. In addition to identifying strong, specific, consistent associations that are temporally correct, health promotion research would, ideally, seek evidence that better results were achieved when interventions were relevant, comprehensive and of sufficient intensity – and theoretically plausible.

The question of triangulation

In the last analysis, the question of causality and internal validity rests on the nature and quality of the evidence that has been assembled by the evaluation research. It is our view that the judicial principle should make substantial use of triangulation of evidence to maximize researchers' and decision makers' conviction that cause has been demonstrated to at least the level of a balance of probabilities.

Triangulation is of central significance for qualitative research methodology. Essentially, triangulation is a technique derived from surveying or navigation. It involves two or more sightings of a particular target to then accurately establish its geographical position. In the same way, using different 'research sightings' should contribute to valid interpretations of reality or realities. The idea is both attractive and has the virtue of common sense. However, some researchers and theoreticians have struck a cautionary note. For instance, Blaikie (1991: 131) makes the following point:

> The failure to recognize the implications of using incompatible ontologies and epistemologies has led either to muddy confusions about bias and validity … or false pretensions about what combining quantitative and qualitative methods means … It should also be clear that triangulation means many things to many people and none of the uses in sociology bears any resemblance to its use in surveying.

To provide an extreme illustration, consider a situation in which one group of researchers believes that it is not possible to know the world, but only a variety of different interpretations of it, whereas another group believes that the world is real and knowable. If these contradictory beliefs are well founded, then it has to be admitted that using evidence based on one perspective could not be used to support evidence based on the other! However, as Blaikie implies, researchers adopting a post-positive realist position can legitimately accumulate evidence from many different sources and, in principle, these sources of data can all offer valid insights into whatever issue or problem is under investigation. As is hopefully clear by now, we concur with the realist position. Accordingly, we believe that a considered use of triangulation is justified. A number of varieties have traditionally been identified (Denzin, 1970):

- data triangulation
- investigator triangulation
- theory triangulation
- methodological triangulation.

In short, our confidence in the validity of observations and findings is proportional to the extent that information from different sources is congruent and compatible. For instance, from different data sources (such as GP records of drug use over a period of time, interview data from patients and data from observations of patients in social settings), reports of different investigators (such as interview reports from other investigators), consistency between analyses of findings derived from different (and appropriately selected) theories (such as consistency between communication of innovations theory and the health belief model), and achieving similar results from different methods (such as questionnaire data, semi-structured interviews and sources of 'unobtrusive measures').

As Stake (1995) points out, the acceptance of triangulation has not been limited to qualitative researchers or realist evaluators. He cites Campbell and Fiske (1959: 81, in Stake, 1995: 114): 'The achievements of useful hypothetically realistic constructs in a science requires multiple methods focused on the diagnosis of the same construct from independent points of observation through a kind of triangulation.'

Producing conclusive evidence about what works in relation to tackling complex and enduring social problems such as health inequality is undoubtedly challenging. Judge and Bauld (2006) argue that there are often unrealistic expectations about evaluation and the speed with which findings can be generated. This is particularly so when initiatives are driven by political agendas rather than the need to plan interventions rigorously with sufficient attention to evaluation from the outset to be able to generate robust evidence. The emphasis on outcomes and the pressure to know rapidly if complex initiatives work can also obscure important learning. As Judge and Bauld (2006: 343) comment:

> The challenge when evaluation opportunities arise in this way is to negotiate the best possible research approach that acknowledges inter alia that incontrovertible measures of impact are not the only useful products that can be generated. The value of throwing light on complex processes in reflective and scholarly ways should not be underestimated even if it falls short of what is ideally required.

Finally, in this chapter, we need to consider how evidence might be translated into policy and practice.

EVIDENCE-BASED HEALTH PROMOTION

The movement towards evidence-based practice has been heavily influenced by evidence-based medicine, the origins of which Sackett et al. (1996) trace back to mid-nineteenth-century Paris. Its basic tenets are summarized in the box.

> ### The basic tenets of evidence-based medicine
>
> - Clinical decisions should be based on the best available scientific evidence.
> - The clinical problem determines the evidence to be sought.
> - Identifying the best evidence involves epidemiological and biostatistical ways of thinking.
> - Conclusions based on the available evidence are useful only if put into action for individual patients or for population healthcare decisions.
> - Performance should be constantly evaluated.
>
> Davidoff et al., 1995, in Jacobson et al., 1997: 449

As we noted in Chapter 5, there is increasing recognition of the importance of evidence-based practice within the wider public health arena and considerable current interest in evidence-based health promotion. Nutbeam (1999) points to the significant inclusion of the words 'evidence-based' in the call for member states to 'adopt an evidence-based approach to health promotion policy and practice' in the Resolution on Health Promotion passed at the 51st World Health Assembly (WHO, 1998c). He takes this to imply the need to justify health promotion activity with greater reference to research evidence on effectiveness in achieving 'predetermined outcomes'.

Raphael (2000) suggests that the increasing emphasis on evidence-based practice derives, in part, from 'economic rationalism' and the need to justify expenditure and ensure that funds are deployed to maximum effect. However, there is also a strong ethical imperative to adopt the principles of evidence-based practice to ensure that health promotion does no harm – either directly or indirectly by wasting limited funds on ineffective or inappropriate interventions or by raising unrealistic expectations about what might be achieved. We might also add that incorporating evidence into decisions about practice is a key aspect of 'reflective practice' and fundamental to the provision of quality health promotion. The basic premise of this text is that the systematic planning of health promotion requires a series of decisions to be made at each stage and that these should be informed by a thorough appraisal of available evidence.

Perkins et al. (1999: 4) note that, 'like motherhood and apple pie', evidence-based health promotion has come to be seen as a good thing. However, they identify a number of tensions in implementing it. First, the tension between reflection and action and the issue of how much evidence is required before action can be taken and what level of uncertainty can be tolerated.

Second, the tension between evidence and practice and the theory–practice gap that arises from failure to translate research findings into practice. This, they suggest, can have a number of origins, which include shortcomings on the part of practitioners in accessing, interpreting and acting on relevant evidence or on the part of researchers in addressing relevant issues and disseminating their findings in ways that meet practitioners' needs. An alternative explanation is the lack of acknowledgement of the 'uniqueness of practice contexts and the processes of social, organizational and educational change' (Perkins et al., 1999: 7).

Third, the tension between different types of knowledge – not only between different research paradigms, which we have discussed above, but also between empirical evidence and professional judgement.

Fourth, the tension between values and evidence and the complex interplay between the two, particularly in relation to the selection and interpretation of evidence.

Finally, the tension between inspiration and evidence and the relative emphasis on tried and tested methods in contrast to innovative and creative solutions to problems.

A particular area of contention concerns attempts to apply the principles of evidence-based medicine to health promotion. This derives from a conceptualization of evidence-based medicine as being associated with the use of the RCT as the gold standard of evaluation and taking a narrow biomedical view of outcomes – an interpretation that has been challenged even by the proponents of evidence-based medicine. The key issues that we will consider at this point are what evidence of effectiveness is relevant to health promotion practice and how that evidence can be accessed – in particular via systematic reviews.

What is evidence?

Evidence-based health promotion has been defined (Wiggers and Sanson-Fisher, 1998: 141) as: 'the systematic integration of research evidence into the planning and implementation of health promotion activities.'

We have questioned the utility of experimental methods for assessing the effectiveness of health promotion. MacIntyre and Pettigrew (2000) suggest that resistance to applying the principles of evidence-based medicine – and by this they are essentially referring to systematic reviews and experimental designs – to social or public health settings derives from a number of misconceptions:

- systematic reviews and experimental designs have a biomedical provenance
- the real world is too complex for evidence-based medicine principles
- social and public health interventions do not have the capacity to do harm
- it is sufficient to know that an intervention does good in a general sense without the necessity of analysing how much, for which subgroups and at what cost
- plausibility is an adequate basis for policy making
- experimental methods define outcomes narrowly and use too short a time frame.

A particular concern is the capacity to do harm. The authors cite a study by Carlin and Nolan (1998) that demonstrated that a bicycle safety education programme doubled the risk of injury in boys. Furthermore, they note that plausibility is not necessarily sufficient justification. For example, putting babies to sleep in the prone position would seem to make sense in that it resembles the recovery position, but has been shown to be associated with increased risk of sudden infant death syndrome. They argue that systematic evaluation offers the opportunity to identify the wider effects of interventions, both positive and negative. While agreeing with these concerns and upholding the need for rigour in evaluation research, our contention is that this is best achieved by means of triangulation and the judicial principle. Furthermore, evaluation needs to remain open to unanticipated outcomes.

Sackett et al. (1996: 72) support the use of randomized trials and systematic reviews to assess the effectiveness of therapy: 'It is when asking questions about therapy that we should try to avoid the non-experimental approaches, since these routinely lead to false-positive conclusions about efficacy.' However, they contend that evidence-based medicine is not restricted to randomized trials and meta analyses, but 'involves tracking down the best external evidence with which to answer our clinical questions'.

There is a growing consensus that the best evidence in relation to health promotion interventions includes both quantitative and qualitative research and addresses process and context as well as outcomes. This adoption of a more catholic and methodologically plural approach to evidence runs counter to attempts to create hierarchies of evidence topped by the RCT (see the box on page 242–3, Chapter 5). It also acknowledges that the answer to the simple question 'Does it work?' is not enough and that evidence is needed in relation to process as well as outcomes. A whole series of supplementary questions require answers, such as the following.

- How does it work?
- Were there any unanticipated outcomes?
- What components are essential for success?
- What components are redundant?
- Why does it work in this context (or, equally importantly, not work)?
- Can it be replicated?
- Is this an appropriate and acceptable way of tackling the problem?

A Health Development Agency's (HDA, undated) consultation exercise on the development of an evidence base found support for the inclusion of a broader range of research than that provided by RCTs, notwithstanding some concern among a minority about any overemphasis on 'grey' evidence. The decision to adopt an inclusive approach to sources of information acknowledged the complex interplay of factors that influence health, the need to understand what works in particular contexts, and why, and the inability of narrowly focused experimental methods to capture the breadth of information required. Sources of evidence were identified (HDA, undated) as:

- evidence maps
- expert working groups reports
- literature reviews
- meta analyses
- research summaries
- reviews
- syntheses
- systematic reviews of effectiveness.

Raphael (2000) suggests that even when there is a strong accumulated evidence base, decision making should still draw on local evidence. On the one hand – and particularly at the needs assessment stage – this helps to secure local ownership. On the other hand, it ensures and checks out local relevance.

Wiggers and Sanson-Fisher's definition referred to above presupposes that evidence derives from research. However, Sackett et al.'s (1996: 71) discussion of evidence-based medicine, while calling for the 'conscientious, explicit and judicious use of current best evidence in making decisions about the care of individual patients', also recognizes the importance of integrating evidence with clinical expertise (1996: 72):

> Without clinical expertise, practice risks becoming tyrannized by evidence for even excellent external evidence may be inapplicable or inappropriate for an individual patient. Without current best evidence, practice risks becoming rapidly out of date to the detriment of patients.

They see the application of professional expertise as a means of avoiding evidence-based medicine becoming merely 'cookbook' medicine. Equally, professional judgement that incorporates familiarity with the context and constraints is important in relation to assessing what health promotion interventions are likely to be successful in particular situations and with specific groups.

Sackett et al. also note the importance of integrating guidelines on practice with individual patient preferences and choice. The issue of choice is perhaps particularly relevant to health promotion, given its emphasis on participation and empowerment rather than control and compliance. Making informed choices will necessarily require access to non-prejudicial information and the accurate interpretation of risk. Jacobson et al. (1997) draw attention to the problem of incomplete and partial reporting, citing as an example the media coverage of early research findings on the association between third-generation oral contraceptive pills and venous thrombosis. The selective reporting of risk by the press ignored any protective effects in relation to cardiovascular risk and the increased risks associated with pregnancies arising as a result of discontinuing oral contraception, which tends to occur following such scare stories.

Evidence theory and values

Green (2000: 125) has argued that empirical evidence alone is 'insufficient to direct practice and that recourse to the explanatory and predictive capability of theory is essential to the design of both programmes and evaluations'. When there is no empirical evidence available, then recourse to theory will be the only option. However, even when there is ample empirical evidence, the application of theoretical principles remains important for a number of reasons. Identification of appropriate indicators of outcome and process is reliant on theory. Reference to theory, as we have noted, can also ensure that all the necessary elements of a programme are in place and, therefore, reduce the risk of intervention failure and Type 3 errors in evaluation. Consideration of the extent to which they are based on theory therefore becomes an essential criterion in assessing the quality of interventions and evaluation designs. Not only should evaluation be informed by theory, but the findings of evaluations should contribute to the further development and refinement of theory in a constantly evolving cycle. Without the extraction of general theoretical principles, empirical evidence of effectiveness risks offering little more than a menu of, often context-specific, proven interventions.

General principles will be of more relevance to practitioners in that they allow adaptation to suit specific situations.

Clearly, the interpretation of evidence may be value-laden – note, for example, the different interpretations of ways for achieving better health in the box. Raphael (2000: 335) argues that, given the commitment of health promotion to enabling and empowerment, evidence relevant to health promotion should encompass consideration of whether or not these goals have been achieved, contending that 'ethical health promotion practice requires explicit recognition of the interactions among ideologies, values, principles and rules of evidence'.

Alternative interpretations of the route to better health

Ten tips for better health (Donaldson, 1999)

1 Don't smoke. If you can, stop. If you can't, cut down.
2 Follow a balanced diet with plenty of fruit and vegetables.
3 Keep physically active.
4 Manage stress by, for example, talking things through and making time to relax.
5 If you drink alcohol, do so in moderation.
6 Cover up in the sun and protect children from sunburn.
7 Practise safer sex.
8 Take up cancer-screening opportunities.
9 Be safe on the roads: follow the Highway Code.
10 Learn the First Aid ABC – airways, breathing, circulation.

An alternative ten tips for better health (Gordon, 1999)

1 Don't be poor. If you can, stop. If you can't, try not to be poor for long.
2 Don't have poor parents.
3 Own a car.
4 Don't work in a stressful, low-paid, manual job.
5 Don't live in damp, low-quality housing.
6 Be able to afford to go on a foreign holiday and sunbathe.
7 Practise not losing your job and don't become unemployed.
8 Take up all the benefits you are entitled to, if you are unemployed, retired or sick or disabled.
9 Don't live next to a busy major road or near a polluting factory.
10 Learn how to fill in the complicated housing benefit/asylum application forms before you become homeless and destitute.

Raphael, 2000: 362

A further example of the way in which values may lead to different opinions about evidence is provided by Jacobson et al. (1997) in the context of evidence-based medicine. They refer to the widely quoted study by Russell et al. (1979), which demonstrated that brief advice to stop smoking from a GP during routine consultations with a warning of follow-up, achieved a 5 per cent rate of quitting. This could be interpreted by some as highly effective and worth the small amount of additional time, whereas for others 5 per cent may be seen as too small an effect to justify action. Furthermore, we could speculate that some would see offering such unsolicited advice as intrusive and interfering with individual freedom or, alternatively, as motivating people to give up a demonstrably health-threatening habit. It is interesting to note the Cochrane Collaboration's (2002) disclaimer about Cochrane reviews that acknowledges interpretations of the evidence may vary:

> The results of a Cochrane Review can be interpreted differently, depending on people's perspectives and circumstances. Please consider the conclusions presented carefully. They are the opinions of review authors, and are not necessarily shared by the Cochrane Collaboration.

The Research and Evaluation Division of HEBS (1996: 359) suggests that there are different demands when assessing the outcomes of health promotion interventions in comparison to medical interventions as 'outcomes might be difficult to specify tightly or measure consistently, and indeed differ according to the agendas of particular stakeholders'.

By way of example, let us consider Wight et al.'s (2002) rigorous cluster randomized trial of a theoretically based sex education programme for adolescents (SHARE). The findings were reported by the press as evidence of the ineffectiveness of sex education – for example, *The Independent* had the headline 'Classes in safe sex are ineffective, says study' (Duckworth, 2002). The objective of the study was to compare the effectiveness of the SHARE programme with current practice in reducing unsafe sexual intercourse. The main outcome measures used were self-reported exposure to sexually transmitted disease, use of condoms and contraceptives in most recent sexual intercourse and unwanted pregnancies. The conclusions drawn by the authors were that **'compared with conventional sex education** [our emphasis] this specially designed intervention did not reduce sexual risk taking in adolescents' (2002: 1430). It is worth noting in passing that a process evaluation of the delivery of sex education and the broader features of each school enabled the authors to discount differences in quality of delivery as a factor in the lack of effectiveness. However, they also found that pupils in the intervention arm of the trial were more knowledgeable than those in the control arm of the trial. Furthermore, the SHARE programme was rated more positively by pupils than comparison programmes, did not encourage earlier sexual activity and had some beneficial effects on the quality of young people's sexual relationships – outcomes that may variously be judged as more relevant by teachers and young people than behavioural outcomes.

Nutbeam (2000a) notes that different stakeholders have different perspectives on what constitutes success and may have different views about the evidence needed:

- policymakers and budget managers may be concerned about the likely short-term achievement of returns on the level of investment in relation to health gain
- health promotion practitioners need to assess the feasibility of achieving defined objectives within particular contexts

- the population that is to benefit from health promotion intervention may be concerned about whether or not the programmes address recognized priorities and felt needs and are participatory
- academic researchers may be concerned with epistemological considerations and methodological rigour in making judgements about success.

Evidence of effectiveness

A key requirement for getting evidence into practice involves access to evidence. It is worth noting at this point that there may be a mismatch between the needs and interests of those generating research evidence and the end-users of that evidence. Furthermore, comparatively little attention has been given to the dissemination of research findings.

The development of electronic databases and search tools has done much to improve access to published research papers. However, Jacobson et al. (1997) draw attention to a number of limitations. They note, for example, that databases such as Medline have only 50–80 per cent recall of relevant literature. Furthermore, accessing grey literature, such as unpublished reports, theses and conference proceedings, can be difficult. Given the wide-ranging and multidisciplinary nature of health promotion, the numerous journals that publish papers on relevant issues and the variety of different databases that cover these, locating all published papers on a particular topic can be particularly problematic.

Clearly, journal editors and peer reviewers of articles occupy key gatekeeper positions. Not only do they control quality standards for published material and establish what would be regarded as minimal reporting criteria, but they also arbitrate on matters of current interest. Lister-Sharp et al.'s (1999: v) review of health promoting schools made the following recommendations for these groups:

> Ensure, in publications of studies of school health promotion interventions, that the following are reported: the theoretical basis or assumptions underpinning the interventions; the content of the interventions; and the process of delivery.

Oakley et al. (1995) call for journals to refuse to accept methodologically flawed papers. Jacobson et al. (1997) suggest that negative findings are less likely to be published. Studies that yield negative findings are also less likely to be submitted for publication: 'current emphasis on success stories may deter the dissemination of cautionary tales regarding tales of things that have gone wrong' (Research and Evaluation Division of HEBS, 1996: 360).

Conversely, multiple reporting of some studies can distort the picture. The pressure on academics to publish papers has fuelled the practice of publishing a number of separate papers on different stages of a single project. This so-called 'salami slicing' inflates the visibility of individual projects, but, at the same time, can fail to provide a complete view of the whole.

Even presupposing that information is readily available, coping with the plethora of published material can be problematic for practitioners. Some years ago – well before the information explosion fuelled by developments in information technology – Davidoff et al. (1995) estimated that doctors would need to read 17 articles a day, every day of the year to keep up to date. It is clear that the demands of practice make it impossible for practitioners to keep on top of the ever-growing literature on effectiveness. It is not surprising, therefore, that increasing emphasis is being placed on reviews of evidence that attempt to synthesize the literature.

Tones and Tilford (2001) distinguish between commentary reviews and systematic reviews. The former bring together the findings of available studies and, hence, are subject to the vagaries of access to and selection of information and, in some instances, interpretation. There is clearly a risk that, consciously or unconsciously, such commentaries will be based on studies selected to suit a particular agenda or argument. Clearly, objectivity would demand that an attempt is made to seek out and, if appropriate, discount contradictory findings. Over reliance by commentators on a few key studies can inflate their importance in influencing decisions about practice.

Cummins and MacIntyre (2002) use the term 'factoids' to refer to assumptions or speculations that are reported and repeated until they are considered to be true. They examine the current policy emphasis in the UK on tackling food deserts – areas of deprivation where it is difficult for families on low income to gain access to affordable healthy food – to illustrate that, when the social climate is right, facts can become assumed and decisions made on comparatively little evidence. Without questioning the quality of the studies themselves – or, indeed, the existence of food deserts – the authors are concerned that the evidence is heavily influenced by three key studies. They (2002: 438) conclude that:

> The over interpretation of a few small-scale studies undertaken up to ten years ago could end up being used to make policy decisions supported by major central government groups and agencies, because the findings are understood to fit in with the current way of thinking ...

This paper illustrates how factoids can easily and uncritically become part of the apparatus of government health policy when they fit in with broader policy objectives. The key problem is that the burden of proof, or demand for evidence, may vary according to a policy's perceived fit with the prevailing collective world view about issues of popular topical interest. One of the main messages of the evidence-based movement needs to be emphasized: when making any health policy (or other) decisions, we need to move away from an unquestioning acceptance of conventional wisdom and 'expert' advice and cast a more critical and objective eye over the facts.

Jacobson et al. (1997) suggest that the same papers may be used to support different conclusions or not used at all. To illustrate the point, they note that the same three papers on screening and intensive management in patients over 75 have been used as evidence to demonstrate both benefit and no benefit and that they did not feature at all in other reviews. They (1997: 449) also contend that 'the quality of review articles is inversely related to the expertise of the reviewer in the clinical topic, and practitioners are justified in maintaining some scepticism about their conclusions'. This inverse relationship might at first sight appear surprising. However, a high level of clinical expertise may militate against pure objectivity in reviewing the evidence.

Systematic reviews

Systematic reviews attempt to address the shortcomings of commentary reviews by bringing together all the published and unpublished material on a particular issue and drawing objective conclusions. Both the selection of studies and extraction of data should conform to explicit criteria so that the process is rigorous, transparent and essentially replicable.

The development of the methodology for conducting systematic reviews has been pioneered by the Cochrane Collaboration, which focuses particularly on healthcare interventions. There is also a Cochrane health promotion and public health field. In an attempt to apply similar evidence-based principles to the development of social policy, the Campbell Collaboration has been established more recently. Within the UK, the NHS Centre for Reviews and Dissemination and the Evidence for Policy and Practice Information and Coordinating Centre (EPPI-Centre) have also been involved in the development of systematic reviews.

The process of conducting a systematic review involves a number of stages. An overview of the stages identified by the NHS Centre for Reviews and Dissemination is provided in the box.

Stages in the systematic review process

Stage 1: Planning the review

Phase 0 Establishing the need for a review
Phase 1 Preparation of a proposal for a review
Phase 2 Development of a review protocol

Stage 2: Conducting a review

Phase 3 Identification of research
Phase 4 Selection of studies
Phase 5 Study quality assessment
Phase 6 Data extraction and monitoring progress
Phase 7 Data synthesis

Stage 3: Reporting and dissemination

Phase 8 The report and recommendations
Phase 9 Getting evidence into practice

NHS Centre for Reviews and Dissemination, 2001

Ensuring that the selection of articles is free from bias and replicable is fundamental to the systematic reviewing process. It is therefore important that written criteria for inclusion and exclusion are established at the outset. Guidance on undertaking systematic reviews developed by the Centre for Reviews and Dissemination (2009) suggests that criteria for inclusion should be developed from consideration of the following key elements (referred to by the acronym PICOS):

- Population
- Interventions
- Comparators
- Outcomes
- Study design

The Campbell Collaboration Guidance lists questions that reviewers should consider in establishing criteria about which studies are relevant to the review (Campbell Collaboration, 2001: 4):

- What characteristics of studies will be used to determine whether or not a particular effort was relevant to the topic of interest?
- What characteristics of studies will lead to exclusion?
- Will relevance decisions be based on a reading of report titles, abstracts, full reports?
- Who will make the relevance decisions?
- How will the reliability of relevance decisions be assessed?

The studies ultimately selected should meet all the inclusion and none of the exclusion criteria. Although decisions should be based on explicit criteria, there will inevitably be a certain amount of subjectivity. Reliability is enhanced if papers are independently assessed by more than one reviewer. A further stage in the selection may involve identifying those papers that would be included in a narrative review only and those that might be included in a meta analysis.

Oakley et al.'s (1995) review of sexual health interventions for young people initially identified 270 papers reporting sexual health interventions. Of these, 73 reported evaluations of sexual health interventions examining their effectiveness in changing knowledge, attitudes or behaviour, of which 65 were identified as separate outcome evaluations – 45 (69 per cent) of these lacked random control groups, 44 (68 per cent) failed to present pre-intervention data and 38 (59 per cent) post-intervention data and 26 (40 per cent) omitted to discuss the relevance of loss of data caused by drop-outs. Only 12 (18 per cent) of the 65 outcome evaluations were judged to be methodologically sound.

Similarly, Lister-Sharp et al.'s (1999) review of primary studies of the health promoting school found 1067 titles and abstracts that were initially selected as evaluations of interventions or providing useful background material. However, only 12 finally met the inclusion criteria. Furthermore, of the 200 reviews of the effectiveness of school health promotion, only 32 met the inclusion criteria.

Thus, commenting on the lack of methodologically sound evaluations for inclusion is a common feature of systematic reviews. Notwithstanding the explicit rational basis for rejecting papers, there are questions about the feasibility of drawing generalizable conclusions from the final batch of papers, which frequently, as we have seen, constitute only a minute proportion of the literature available.

Speller et al. (1997b) contend that inclusion tends to be based on the quality of the research only and overlooks the quality of the health promotion intervention. They note that Oakley's systematic review of the effectiveness of sexual health interventions for young people did not use criteria on the appropriateness of the interventions included in the review. Speller et al. also refer to problems arising from 'pooling' dissimilar interventions and cite a comparison of 'brief interventions' on alcohol misuse with more extensive approaches (NHS Centre for Reviews and Dissemination, 1993). The interpretation of what constituted a 'brief' intervention was very broad, ranging from five minutes' advice to structured sessions provided by a general practitioner over six months.

Tilford (2000) also notes the lack of attention to the process of implementation and the tendency for reviews to be conducted on narrowly focused health education interventions rather than more complex initiatives that have come to be more typical of health promotion. This disparity between the types of reviews produced and the types of activity in which practitioners are involved clearly limits their utility.

There are signs that some of these concerns are beginning to be addressed. The Centre for Reviews and Dissemination (CRD) (2009) points out the need to assess the quality of the intervention. This involves two key aspects. First, whether the intervention has been properly defined including its theoretical underpinnings and the use of exploratory studies or needs assessment. Second, the extent to which the intervention has been delivered as intended.

The *Campbell Collaboration Guidelines* (2001: 4) state:

> A Campbell Review can include evidence from studies of the implementation of an intervention. These studies can identify factors that enable/impede the implementation process and they can describe the subjective experience of the people providing and/or receiving the intervention or the process of implementing a particular intervention. This evidence can derive from studies using a range of methods and include both qualitative and quantitative data.

There is increasing emphasis on the importance of including qualitative studies. The *Guidelines* (Campbell Collaboration, 2001: 6) suggest that qualitative research can:

- contribute to the development of a more robust intervention by helping to define an intervention more precisely
- assist in the choice of outcome measures and assist in the development of valid research questions
- help to understand heterogeneous results from studies of effects.

A number of appraisal tools are available for assessing the quality of qualitative research (see the Centre for Reviews and Dissemination (2009) guidance on undertaking reviews). Nonetheless, the guidance notes the considerable debate – even among qualitative researchers themselves – about the suitability and applicability of assessment criteria.

We have focused here particularly on the selection of papers for inclusion in systematic reviews. However, it is worth noting that subjectivity and human error can influence the data extraction process. This can be minimized by using clear data extraction forms and more than one assessor (Khan and Kleijnen, 2001). Synthesizing findings can also be problematic, particularly when there is lack of consistency and wide divergence in the findings. Information about process and context, if available, can offer some insight into the origins of the variation. The issue of contradictory findings arose in a review of the effectiveness of peer-delivered programmes for young people (EPPI-Centre, 1999), which found five studies comparing the effects of peer-delivered and teacher-delivered interventions. Two of these found peers to be more effective than teachers, two found them to be neither more nor less effective and one concluded that neither peers nor teachers were effective.

Pawson and Tilley (1997) refer to the much-quoted review by Martinson (1974) which provides a summary of all published reports on attempts at rehabilitation of offenders between 1945 and 1967 and yet was only able to reach equivocal conclusions. While acknowledging the importance of accumulating sound evidence, Pawson and Tilley contend that answers are both complicated and may lack uniformity.

Clearly, it is important that the reviews bring together robust evidence, which will inevitably be related to the quality of the study design. There has been concern that, despite increasing recognition of the value of qualitative studies, the criteria for inclusion of studies within systematic reviews of health promotion have tended to replicate those adopted by evidence-based medicine, with overemphasis on RCTs and experimental studies (see the box on p. 242–3 in Chapter 5).

Dixon-Woods et al. (2006: 29) argue that the influential methodology promoted by the Cochrane movement, which they refer to as the 'rationalist' model of systematic review, 'focuses exclusively on questions concerned with effectiveness, and almost exclusively on RCTs as a means of answering the question of whether something "works"'. They comment on their experience of incorporating qualitative research into a systematic review of support for breast feeding:

> Throughout our project we experienced difficulty with matching the tasks and epistemological assumptions associated with qualitative research with the template offered by conventional systematic review methodology — even more 'liberal' forms such as that offered by the NHS CRD guidance. We found that it was inappropriate or impossible to specify a clearly focused review question; to use completely reproducible and transparent search and selection strategies; or to construct an inherently reproducible synthesis. (2006: 39)

Tilford (2000) suggests that the selection of studies has, in fact, been broader than is often supposed, while still acknowledging the dominance of positivist studies and criteria relevant to these.

Dixon-Woods et al. recognize the risk that qualitative research may merely be used for enhancement or illumination and thus take on 'a complementary but subsidiary "unequal handmaiden" role to the quantitative research' (2006: 32). The authors consider the difficulties – both technical and epistemological – of attempting to properly integrate qualitative studies. For example, should the review questions be defined from the outset according to conventional practice or should they develop through an interative process involving reflection on issues emerging from the selected studies – with implications for revisiting the search strategy? They also note problems with accessing qualitative studies arising from the indexing of databases and divergent views about what constitutes qualitative research. In relation to synthesis, they distinguish between two broad approaches:

- **aggregative synthesis** (sometimes referred to as integrative synthesis) which focuses on summarizing data when the concepts, categories and variable used for this are 'largely secure and well specified' (2006: 36)
- **interpretive synthesis** which is concerned with the development of concepts.

An overview of the respective merits of different approaches to synthesizing data is provided by Dixon-Woods et al. (2004). These include narrative summary, thematic analysis, grounded theory, meta-ethnography, content analysis, case survey, qualitative comparative analysis, Bayesian meta analysis and other forms of meta analysis. (See also Centre for Reviews and Dissemination, 2009.)

Although systematic reviews aspire to seek out and provide an objective and transparent synthesis of all evidence, we have noted a number of limitations. We might add that the search for evidence is frequently restricted to one language – usually English – which clearly inhibits the international exchange of information and cross-fertilization of ideas.

The utility of reviews to professional, organizational and policy decisions will necessarily be dependent on the reliability of the review process and its relevance to practice. The Centre for Reviews and Dissemination (2009: 170) notes that because of the complexity of public health interventions, 'traditional criteria for producing systematic reviews only partially fulfil the requirements for public health interventions' and a more iterative process may be needed.

Pawson (2002) is critical of the way systematic reviews look at the evidence on widely dissimilar interventions and their potential contribution to achieving broad health outcomes. For example, a review of initiatives to prevent injury might include interventions ranging from the distribution of free smoke alarms to school road safety education. In line with realistic evaluation, he argues that rather than identifying what works or does not work, the key issue is to understand generative mechanisms. Furthermore, the extent to which change takes place will be heavily influenced by the context. A realist synthesis would therefore be concerned with what works, for whom and in what circumstances. Instead of looking at simple cause–effect relationships, a realist synthesis would be reoriented towards identifying generative themes and their applicability in different situations. For example, it might focus on the use of incentives or 'giveaways' such as smoke alarms to establish for what purposes, which groups and in what contexts this type of approach would work.

Evidence into practice

The Centre for Reviews and Dissemination (2009: 90) notes that: 'Simply making research available does not ensure that those that need to know about it get to know about it or can make sense of the findings.' Attention should therefore be given to planning the dissemination process to facilitate 'the transfer of research into practice'. On the one hand, this is dependent upon the quality and relevance of the evidence and, on the other, the dissemination strategy used. We have already commented in Chapter 5 on the way practitioners use evidence. Clearly, it is essential that evidence meets the needs of practitioners and due attention is given to the dissemination of evidence of effectiveness.

Dixon-Woods et al. (2006: 30) draw attention to a key criticism of the evidence-based movement – that 'it results in reductionist and standardized models that fail to acknowledge individual variability or the influence of context' and contrast 'the orderly series of events, decisions and outcomes implied by "the evidence" and the inherently contingent, intuitive and fuzzy realities of practice and experience'. It is important, therefore, that evidence incorporates practitioner experience and expertise along with understanding of contextual factors.

To determine whether an intervention, even one well founded in evidence, is likely to be successful requires an understanding of local contexts and circumstances, of local professionals' knowledge bases, commitment and engagement, and detailed assessment of the population at whom the intervention is aimed. (Kelly et al., 2004: 5)

Furthermore, as we have already argued, the evidence should incorporate theoretical perspectives which allow the implications for different circumstances to be drawn out.

Green and South (2006) identify a number of concerns about the mismatch between the evidence available and both the current health agenda and the needs of practitioners:

1   the evidence base is dominated by simple interventions which focus on changing individual behaviour rather than the more complex 'upstream determinants' of health and health action
2   interventions focus on a small range of risk behaviours
3   programme failures are rarely reported
4   the emphasis of published reviews tends to be on outcomes rather than process and context.

Oldenburg et al.'s (1999) analysis of the extent to which health promotion research provides an empirical basis for the diffusion and institutionalization of effective interventions involved an audit of articles in 12 selected journals. They found that:

- less than 11 per cent of studies could be classified as diffusion or institutionalization research
- most research was on behaviour associated with cardiovascular disease and cancer
- most published research was on interventions directed at behaviour change in individuals or small groups rather than social, environmental, ecological or policy approaches.

They conclude that these findings support the view that health promotion research is not relevant to the issues that practitioners are dealing with and the methods they use and is difficult to apply to real-life practice situations.

It would seem that, to improve the translation of public health intervention and health promotion research into practice and relevant policy, it will be important to encourage:

intervention research directed at those targeted behaviours that have not been studied adequately to date; appropriately staged research to ensure that efficacy and effectiveness are proven prior to policy and community-wide implementation; and, most importantly, research which directly addresses methods of diffusing effective programmes and implementing social and environmental strategies to promote better health. (Oldenburg et al., 1999: 128)

Swann et al. (2005: 20) propose the following 'rules' for judging the quality of evidence:

- Systematicity – does the review apply a consistent and comprehensive approach?
- Transparency – is the review clear about the processes involved?
- Quality – are the appropriate methods and analysis undertaken?
- Relevance – is the review relevant in terms of focus (i.e. populations, interventions and settings)?

Clearly, it is helpful to facilitate access to evidence of effectiveness. In the UK, The National Institute for Health and Clinical Excellence (NICE) regularly publishes guidance on public health issues – both in full and as a quick reference version along with generic implementation tools and support. It is also important that such information is timely if it is to inform key decisions. For example, the Contributors to the Cochrane and Campbell Collaborations (2000) produced summaries of evidence – reviews of reviews – related to implementing the wider public health agenda and, in particular, achieving the targets of the national health strategy 'Saving Lives: Our Healthier Nation'.

The approach to dissemination adopted by the Centre for Reviews and Dissemination (2009) draws explicitly on the principles of communication and dissemination which we have discussed at length in previous chapters. It involves consideration of six key elements. The **message** itself should be relevant and include 'the nature of the intervention, the strength of the evidence, its transferability, the degree of uncertainty and whether the findings confirm or reject existing predispositions or practices' (2009: 87). Attention should be paid to aspects of the **setting** in which the target audience operates, including the organizational, economic, social and political environments, as well as whether the context is likely to be 'hostile or receptive' to the message. The **characteristics of the target audience** should be considered, including their capacity to influence others, and **appropriate communication channels** identified. Attention should also be paid to the source and source credibility. Lastly, **the dissemination strategy** should be selected. The alternatives for this are:

- push strategies – concerned with providing information
- pull strategies – concerned with generating demand for information
- linkage and exchange – based on partnerships between producers and users of research
- integrated approaches that incorporate aspects of all three.

The CRD guidance favours the integrated approach.

Wilson et al. (2001) suggest that it is naïve to suppose that if information is made available to practitioners, it will automatically be accessed, appraised and integrated into practice. Indeed, it is hardly surprising that the forces of inertia affecting changes in professional practice are not dissimilar to those influencing changes in individual behaviour. This resistance to change has been graphically encapsulated by Tyrrell (1951):

> The human mind is in the grip of an unconscious urge which makes it cling desperately to the world of familiar things and resists all that threatens to tear it away from its moorings.

Some time ago, Gibson (undated) developed a checklist, based on his personal experience, of some 50 ploys used to avoid change in the school curriculum (see the box).

How to avoid curriculum change!

It has been done before.
It has never been done before.
The parents wouldn't like it.

(Continued)

(Continued)

It doesn't fit into any syllabus.
It's too vague and I haven't got time anyway.
We don't have suitable staff.
The Head wouldn't go along with it.
I am personally in favour, but the Unions you know ...
It's not a multidisciplinary thing is it?
Not if it means another committee.
Only if we can have another committee.
I don't have the power to implement it.
You don't have the right to suggest it.
Who are you anyway?
Have you had any experience of this sort of thing?
etc.
etc.

Gibson, undated

Plus ça change!!

Various levels of pressure can be applied to encourage professionals to adopt improved practice – including guidance and codes of practice. However, as we noted in relation to individual behaviour change, voluntary adaptation is likely to secure greatest commitment and avoid a subversive backlash. Kelly et al. (2004: 7) draw on the work of Stacey to suggest that the appropriate time to introduce 'planning and control mechanisms such as guidance, application of standards of practice, and performance management' is when there is both:

1 a high level of certainty about interventions based on the availability and strength of evidence
2 a high level of agreement among practitioners about proposed change.

In our earlier consideration of the factors influencing behaviour change in Chapters 3 and 7, we made the important distinction between increasing awareness and actually changing behaviour. Dissemination of information, however effective, cannot be expected in itself to achieve changes in practice. A review of strategies for getting knowledge into practice and improving the quality of healthcare (NHS Centre for Reviews and Dissemination, 1999) concluded that:

- routine mechanisms are essential for achieving individual and organizational change
- individual beliefs, attitudes and knowledge influence professional behaviour, together with other important factors, such as the organizational, economic and community environments in which practitioners are working
- attempts to achieve change should be based on a 'diagnostic analysis' to identify factors that will affect the proposed change
- multifaceted interventions that tackle different barriers to change are more likely to be successful than single interventions

- adequate resources are needed along with people with appropriate knowledge and skills
- systematic strategies for achieving change should include monitoring and evaluation, along with plans to consolidate change.

Evidence-based health promotion holds out the promise of ensuring that energy and resources are directed to maximum effect by enabling effective interventions to be identified. It can also support practitioners' attempts to resist pressure to adopt ill-conceived, although politically appealing, stratagems or programmes. Middleton et al. (2001), for example, made their concerns known to the Home Office about the introduction into the UK of the 'Scared Straight' programme from the USA. They based their objection on the fact that systematic reviews of the programme had shown adverse outcomes. Furthermore, rather than being the cost-cutting exercise that some feared, evidence-based practice enables a realistic assessment to be made of the scope of the intervention necessary to achieve desired effects. It can, therefore, be used to generate arguments to secure sufficient funding. However, whether or not these potential benefits are realized will ultimately be dependent on the quality of the evidence base and in particular:

- its relevance to practitioners
- identification of appropriate outcomes
- attention to process and context as well as outcomes
- recognition of the need for methodological pluralism
- consistency with the core values of health promotion
- effective dissemination.

KEY POINTS

o Evaluation is an essential component of the health promotion planning cycle – evaluation and dissemination should therefore be considered from the very first stages of planning.

o Health promotion evaluation should conform with the key principles, values and ideology of health promotion – notably participation and empowerment.

o RCTs are rarely, if ever, applicable to health promotion evaluation.

o The judicial principle, based on the notion of triangulation, has been proposed as a means of assessing evidence which can cope with the complexity of health promotion and public health interventions.

o Evaluation should address process as well as outcomes.

o The selection of appropriate evaluation indicators is easier if programme objectives are well defined and the anticipated pathway between intervention and the achievement of outcomes is explicitly stated – the so-called Theory of Change.

o Evaluation should not only demonstrate whether an intervention has been successful, but should also identify how the various intervention components lead to outcomes and how contextual factors influence programme delivery and its success – or failure.

(Continued)

(Continued)

o Efforts should be made to actively disseminate evaluation findings along with attention to the factors associated with the uptake of innovations and new ways of working.

o Practitioners are more likely to make use of evidence if it is relevant to their needs and current priorities.

o Evidence should include practitioners' perspectives and theoretical principles as well as research and evaluation studies.

o Systematic reviews are an important device for summarizing research evidence but need to also pay attention to the quality of interventions and include qualitative as well as quantitative studies.

o The findings of evaluation should inform the further development and refinement of health promotion theory.

CONCLUDING COMMENTS

One of our aims in writing this book was to capture the essence of health promotion and its unique contribution to public health. Its emergence as a specialist discipline in the 1980s was accompanied by intense debate as it sought to clarify its core values and purpose. Health promotion practice is characterized by commitment to equity, empowerment and social justice and ways of working which uphold voluntarism, autonomy, participation, partnerships and social justice.

Our basic premise was that systematic planning is fundamental to the effectiveness and efficiency, and indeed, the ethics of health promotion programmes. Hopefully, we have demonstrated that planning is not just a technical process, but provides a framework for action based on core values and for incorporating theory and empirical evidence. We have emphasized the importance of theory throughout and have demonstrated the wide range of theory which can and should inform planning and practice.

MacDonald and Mussi (1998) observed that the distinctive voice of health promotion involved three elements – the theory of the problem, the principles of the solution and integration of response. Following on from this, we can conceptualize health promotion in the following way:

- the theory of the problem – involves a holistic view of health, including wellbeing, a socio-ecological analysis of the determinants of health and an 'upstream approach' to prevention
- the principles of the solution – including empowerment; participation; a collaborative approach to working with individuals, communities and organizations; a comprehensive approach
- integration of response – requires working at all levels and across all sectors.

Rather than planning being a linear process, we see it as iterative, providing the opportunity to work in partnership with key stakeholders in shaping the development of programmes. Further, it should be part of a cyclical process of evolution and development whereby evaluation findings are fed back into the development of both health promotion practice and related theory.

BIBLIOGRAPHY

Aarons, A. and Hawes, H. (1979) *Child-to-child*. London: Macmillan.

Abbasi, K. (1999) 'The World Bank and world health under fire', *British Medical Journal*, 318: 1003–6.

Abel, T. (2007) 'Cultural capital in health promotion', in D.V. McQueen and I. Kickbush, *Health and Modernity: The Role of Theory in Health Promotion*. New York: Springer.

Abel-Smith, B. (1994) *An Introduction to Health Policy: Planning and Financing*. London: Longman.

Abramson, L.Y., Seligman, M.E.P. and Teasdale, J.D. (1978) 'Learned helplessness in humans: critique and reformulation', *Journal Abnormal Psychology*, 87: 49–74.

Acheson, D. (1998) *Independent Inquiry into Inequalities in Health: Recommendations*. London: Department of Health.

ActKnowledge (undated a) *Theory of Change: Origins*. New York: ActKnowledge. (*Website*: http://www.theoryofchange.org/background/origins.html).

ActKnowledge (undated b) *Theory of Change: Process*. New York: ActKnowledge. (*Website:* http://www.theoryofchange.org/process/overview.html).

Adams, L. and Armstrong, E. (1995) *From Analysis to Synthesis II: The Revenge*, Report of the Penrith Symposium. Sheffield: Sheffield Health.

Agostinelli, G. and Grube, J.W. (2002) 'Alcohol counter-advertising and the media: a review of recent research', *Alcohol Research and Health*, 26 (1): 15–21.

Ahmad, O.B., Boschi-Pinto, C., Lopez, A.D., Murray, C.J.L., Kozano, R. and Inoue, M. (2001) *Age Standardization of Rates: A New WHO Standard*. Geneva: WHO, GPE Discussion Paper Series: No. 31.

AHPO (2007) *The HIA Process*. West Midland Public Health Observatory. (*Website:* http://www.apho.org.uk/resource/view.aspx?RID=44532).

Ajzen, I. (1991) 'The theory of planned behavior', *Organizational Behavior and Human Decision Processes*, 50: 179–211.

Alberoni, F. (1962) 'L'élite irresponsable; theorie et recherche sociologique sur "le divismo"', *Ikon*, 12–40/1: 45–62. (Translated by McQuail.)

Aldoory, L. and Bonzo, S. (2005) 'Using communication theory in injury prevention campaigns', *Injury Prevention*, 11: 260–3.

Alinsky, S. (1969) *Reveille for Radicals*. New York: Vintage Books.

Alinsky, S.D. (1972) *Rules for Radicals*. New York: Random House.

American Cancer Society/International Union Against Cancer (2003) *Strategy Planning for Tobacco Control Advocacy*. (*Website:* http://strategyguides.globalink.org/pdfs/guide1_AdvocacyGuide.pdf).

American Heritage Dictionary of the English Language (2000, 4th edn) New York: Houghton Mifflin.

Amidei, N. (1991) *So You Want to Make a Difference: Advocacy is the Key*. Washington, DC: OMB Watch.

Anderson, J. (1975) 'Public policy making', in F. Delaney, 'Policy and Health Promotion', *Journal of the Institute of Health Education*, 32 (1): 5–9.

Anderson, J. (undated) *The HEA Health Skills Dissemination Project: A Whole School Approach to Life Skills and Health Education*. Leeds: Counselling and Career Development Unit.

Anderson, J., Beels, C. and Powell, D. (1994) *Health Skills for Life*. Walton-on-Thames: Nelson.

Annett, H. and Rifkin, S. (1990) *Improving Urban Health*. Geneva: WHO.

Anonymous (1994) 'Population health looking upstream', *Lancet*, 343: 429–30.

Ansari, W.E. (1998) 'Partnerships in health: how's it going to work?' *Target*, 29 July: 18.

Antonovsky, A. (1979) *Health, Stress and Coping*. San Francisco, CA: Jossey-Bass.

Antonovsky, A. (1984) 'The sense of coherence as a determinant of health', in J.D. Matarazzo, S.M. Weiss, J.A. Herd, N.E. Miller and S.M. Weiss (eds), *Behavioural Health: A Handbook of Health Enhancement and Disease Prevention*. New York: John Wiley: 114–29.

Antonovsky, A. (1987) *Unraveling the Mystery of Health*. San Francisco: Jossey-Bass.

Antonovsky, A. (1996) 'The salutogenic model as a theory to guide health promotion', *Health Promotion International*, 11 (1): 11–18.

Appleton, J. (1992) 'Notes from a food and nutrition PRA in a Guinean fishing village', *RRA Notes (No. 16): Special Issue on Applications for Health*: 77–85.

Argyle, M. and Kendon, A. (1967) 'The experimental analysis of social performance', *Advances in Experimental Social Psychology*, 3: 35–98.

Argyle, M. (1978) *The Psychology of Interpersonal Behaviour* (3rd edn). Harmondsworth: Penguin.

Arnstein, S.R. (1969) 'A ladder of citizen participation', *Journal of the American Planning Association*, 35 (4): 216–24.

Aronson, E. (1976) *The Social Animal*. San Francisco: W.H. Freeman.

Aronson, E. and Mettee, D. (1968) 'Dishonest behavior as a function of low levels of self-esteem', *Journal of Personality and Social Psychology*, 9: 121–7.

Aronson, R.E., Norton, B.L. and Kegler, C.K. (2007) 'Achieving a "broad view of health": findings from the California Healthy Cities and Communities evaluation', *Health Education and Behavior*, 34(3): 441–452.

Aronson, R.E. Norton, B.L. and Kegler, M.C. (2007) 'Achieving a "broad view of health": Findings from the California Healthy Cities and Communities Evaluation', *Health Education and Behavior, 43* (3): 441–52.

ASH (1999) *Bad for Business? Smoking and the Hospitality Trade*. London: ASH.

ASH (2001) *Factsheet No. 2: Smoking Statistics: Illness and Death*. London: ASH.

ASH (2002a) *Basic Facts No. 1: Smoking Statistics*. London: ASH.

ASH (2002b) *Fact Sheet No. 19: Tobacco Advertising and Promotion*. London: ASH.

ASH (2002c) *British American Tobacco – The Other Report to Society*. London: ASH

ASH (undated) *Action on Smoking and Health – Home page*. (*Website*: www.ash.org.uk).

Ashton, J. (2007) 'Grasping defeat: health promotion is a doing word not a proper noun', *Journal of the Royal Society of Health*, 127 (5): 207–10.

Ashton, J. and Seymour, H. (1988) *The New Public Health*. Buckingham: Open University Press.

Association of Public Health Observatories (2002) *Focusing on the Health of England: Background*. Stockton on Tees: APHO. (*Website:* www.pho.org.uk).

Babb, P. (2005) *Measurement of Social Capital in the UK National Statistics*. London: National Statistics. (*Website:* http://www.statistics.gov.uk/socialcapital/downloads/Social_capital_measurement_UK_2005.pdf).

Babb, P., Martin, J. and Haezewindt, P. (2004) *Focus on Social Inequalities*. London: TSO. (*Website:* http://www.statistics.gov.uk/downloads/theme_compendia/fosi2004/SocialInequalities_full.pdf).

Bachrach, P. and Baratz, M.S. (1970) *Power and Poverty: Theory and Practice*. New York: Oxford University Press.

Backett-Milburn, K. and McKie, L. (1999) 'A critical appraisal of the draw and write technique', *Health Education Research*, 14 (3): 387–98.

Backett-Milburn, K. and Wilson, S. (2000) 'Understanding peer education: insights from a process evaluation', *Health Education Research*, 15 (1): 85–96.

Baelz, P.R. (1979) 'Philosophy of health education', in I. Sutherland (ed.), *Health Education: Perspectives and Choices*. London: Allen & Unwin.

Ball, S. (1994) 'Theatre and health education: meeting of minds or marriage of convenience?', *Health Education Journal*, 53: 222–5.

Bandura, A. (1977) 'Self-efficacy toward a unifying theory of behavioural change', *Psychological Review*, 64 (2): 191–225.

Bandura, A. (1982) 'Self-efficacy mechanism in human agency', *American Psychologist*, 37 (2): 122–47.

Bandura, A. (1986) *Social Foundations of Thought and Action: A Social Cognitive Theory*. Englewood Cliffs, NJ: Prentice-Hall.

Bandura, A. (1989) 'Human agency in social cognitive theory', *American Psychologist*, 44 (9): 1175–84.

Bandura, A. (1992) 'Exercise of personal agency through the self-efficacy mechanism', in R. Schwarzer (ed.), *Self-Efficacy: Thought Control of Action*. Washington, DC: Hemisphere Publishing.

Banfield, E.C. (1958) *The Moral Basis of a Backward Society*. New York: Free Press.

Banken, R. (2001) *Strategies for Institutionalizing HIA*. ECHP Health Impact Assessment Discussion Papers, No. 1. Brussels: European Centre for Health Policy.

Baric, L. (1969) 'Recognition of the "at-risk" role', *International Journal of Health Education*, XII(1): 2–12.

Baric, L. (1993) 'Health promotion – the settings approach', *Journal of the Institute of Health Education*, 31 (1): 17–24.

Barker, D.J.P. and Rose, G. (1984) *Epidemiology in Medical Practice* (3rd edn). Edinburgh: Churchill Livingstone.

Barnekow Rasmussen, V. (2005) 'The European Network of Health Promoting Schools – from Iceland to Kyrgyzstan', *Promotion & Education*, XII (3–4): 169–72.

Barnes, M. (ed.), Allan, D., Coad, J., Fielding, A., Hansen, K., Mathers, J., McCabe, A., Morris, K., Parry, J., Plewis, I., Prior, D. and Sullivan, A. (2004) *Assessing the Impact of The Children's Fund: The Role of Indicators*. National Evaluation of the Children's Fund. (*Website*: http://www.ne-cf.org/core_files/CF%20indicators%20paper%20final.doc).

Barnes, R. and Scott-Samuel, A. (2000) *Health Impact Assessment – A Ten Minute Guide*. Liverpool: Liverpool Public Health Observatory.

Barr,A., Hashagen, S. and Purcell, R. (1996) *Measuring Community Development in Northern Ireland: A Handbook for Practitioners*. Belfast: Voluntary Activity Unit, Department of Health and Social Services (Northern Ireland).

Barrett-Lennard, G.T. (1998) *Carl Rogers' Helping System: Journey and Substance*. London: Sage.

Bartholomew, L.K., Parcel, G.S., Kok, G. and Gottlieb, N.H. (2001) *Intervention Mapping: Designing Theory and Evidence-Based Health Promotion Programs*. New York: McGraw Hill.

Bartlett, R.V. (1989) 'Policy through impact assessment: institutionalised analysis as a policy strategy', in R. Banken, *Strategies for Institutionalizing HIA*. Brussels: European Centre for Health Policy.

Basch, C.E. and Gold, R.S. (1986) 'Type V errors in hypothesis testing', *Health Education Research*, 1 (4): 299–305.

Basch, P.F. (1990) *Textbook of International Health*. Oxford: Oxford University Press.

BAT (2008) *Sustainability Reporting*. (*Website*: http://www.bat.com/group/sites/uk__3mnfen.nsf/vwPagesWebLive/DO726NTL?opendocument&SKN=1).

Batten, T.R. (1967) *The Non-Directive Approach in Group and Community Work*. Oxford: Oxford University Press.

Bauld, L. and Judge, K. (2000) 'Strong theory flexible methods: emergent approaches to health promotion evaluation', British Heart Foundation Health Promotion Research Group Workshop, 'Evaluating Health Promotion Interventions: Beyond the Dialogue', Ilkley, 8–9 May.

Baum, F. (2001) 'Healthy Public Policy', in T. Heller, R. Muston, M. Sidell and C. Lloyd (eds), *Working for Health*. London: Sage.

Beaglehole, R., Bonita, R. and Kjellström, T. (1993) *Basic Epidemiology*. Geneva: WHO.

Beattie, A. (1991) 'Knowledge and control in health promotion: a test case for social policy and social theory', in J. Gabe, M. Calnan, and M. Bury (eds), *The Sociology of the Health Service*. London: Routledge.

Beattie, A. (1993) 'The changing boundaries of health', in A. Beattie, M. Gott, L. Jones and M. Sidell (eds), *Health and Wellbeing: a Reader*. London: Macmillan.

Beauchamp, D.E. (1976) 'Public health as social justice', *Inquiry*, 13: 3–14.

Beauchamp, T.L. (1978) 'The regulation of hazards and hazardous behaviors', *Health Education Monographs*, 6 (2): 242–56.

Beauchamp, D.E. and Steinbock, B. (eds) (1999) *New Ethics for the Public's Health*. New York: Oxford University Press.

Becker, M.H. (ed.) (1984) *The Health Belief Model and Personal Health Behavior*. Thorofare, NJ: Charles B. Slack.

Belbin, E., Downs, S. and Perry, P. (1981) 'How do I learn?', in J. Anderson, *The HEA Health Skills Dissemination Project: A Whole School Approach to Life Skills and Health Education*. Leeds: Counselling and Career Development Unit.

Bell, S. (2001) *LogFrames: Improved NRSP Research Project Planning and Monitoring*. Hemel Hempstead: DFID, NRSP.

Bennett, P. and Murphy, S. (1997) *Psychology and Health Promotion*. Buckingham: Open University Press.

Bentley, C. (2008) *Systematically Addressing Health Inequalities*. London: Department of Health. (*Website*: http://www.dh.gov.uk/en/Publicationsandstatistics/Publications/PublicationsPolicy AndGuidance/DH_086570).

Berensson, M.K., Carlsson, P., Granath, M. and Urwitz, V. (2001) 'Quality indicators for health promotion pro-grammes', *Health Promotion International*, 16 (2): 187–95.

Berger, A.A. (1991) *Media Analysis Techniques*. Newbury Park, CA: Sage.

Berkman, L.F. and Syme, S.L. (1979) 'Social networks, host resistance, and mortality: a nine-year follow-up study of Alameda County residents', *American Journal of Epidemiology*, 109: 186–203.

Berkman, L.F., Glass, T., Brissette, I., Teresa E. Seeman, T.E. (2000) 'From social integration to health: Durkheim in the new millennium', *Social Science and Medicine*, 51: 843–57.

Berndt, T.J. and Burgy, L. (1996) 'Social self concept', in B.A. Bracken (ed.), *Handbook of Self Concept: Developmental, Social and Clinical Considerations*. New York: Wiley.

Berne, E. (1964) *Games that People Play*. New York: Grove Press.

Bernhard, J. (2001) *Health Education Research: Special Issue on Health Education and the Internet*, 16 (6).

Bivins, E.C. (1979) 'Community organisation – an old but reliable health education technique', in P.M. Lazes (ed.), *Handbook of Health Education*. New York: Aspen.

Blackwell, S. and Kosky, M. (2000) *The Role of 'Citizens' Juries' in Decisions About Equity in Health Care*. Perth, Australia: Medical Council.

Blaikie, N.W.H. (1991) 'A critique of the use of triangulation in social research', *Quality and Quantity*, 25: 115–36.

Blake, G., Diamond, J., Foot, J., Gidley, B., Mayo, M., Shukra, K., and Yarnit, M. (2008) *Community Engagement and Community Cohesion*. York: Joseph Rowntree Foundation. (*Website*: www.jrf.org.uk).

Blane, D., Brunner, E. and Wilkinson, R. (1996) *Health and Social Organization: Towards a Health Policy for the 21st Century*. London: Routledge.

Blaxter, M. (1990) *Health and Lifestyles*. London: Tavistock/Routledge.

Blaxter, M. and Patterson, S. (1982) *Mothers and Daughters: A Three Generational Study of Health Attitudes and Behaviour*. London: Heinemann.

Blazer, D.G. (1982) 'Social support and mortality in elderly community populations', *American Journal of Epidemiology*, 115: 684–94.

Blenkinsop, S., Eggers, M., Schagen, I., Schagen, S., Scott, E., Warwick, I., Aggleton, P. and Chase, E., with Zuurmond, M. (2004) *Evaluation of the Impact of the National Healthy School Standard. Final Report*. (*Website*: http://www.wiredforhealth.gov.uk/PDF/Full_report_2004.pdf).

Bloxham, S. (1997) 'The contribution of interagency collaboration to the promotion of young people's sexual health', *Health Education Research*, 12 (1): 91–101.

Bolam, B.L. (2005) 'Public participation in tackling health inequalities: implications from recent qualitative research', *European Journal of Public Health*, 15 (5): 447.

BOND (2005) *Monitoring and Evaluation: Guidance Notes No. 43*. (*Website*: http://www.allindiary.org/uploads/D4_BOND_monitor_and_evaluate.pdf).

Boster, F.J. and Mongeau, P.A. (1984) 'Fear arousing persuasive messages', in R. Bostrom (ed.), *Communication Yearbook* (Vol. 8): 330–75. Newbury Park, CA: Sage.

Botvin, G.J. (1984) 'The life skills training model: a broad spectrum approach to the prevention of cigarette smoking', in G. Campbell (ed.), *Health Education and Youth: A Review of Research and Developments*. Lewes, East Sussex: Falmer Press.

Boulos, M.N.K. (2005) 'British internet-derived patient information on diabetes mellitus: is it readable?', *Diabetes Technology & Therapeutics*, 7 (3): 528–35.

Bourdieu, P. (1980) *Questions de Sociologie*. Paris: Les Editions des Minuit.

Boutilier, M., Cleverly, S. and Labonte, R. (2000) 'Community as a setting for health promotion', in B.D. Poland, L.W. Green, and I. Rootman (eds), *Settings for Health Promotion: Linking Theory and Practice*. Thousand Oaks, CA: Sage.

Bowling, A. (1997a) *Measuring Health: A Review of Quality of Life Measurement Scales* (2nd edn). Buckingham: Open University Press.

Bowling, A. (1997b) *Research Methods in Health*. Buckingham: Open University Press.

Bracht, N. (ed.) (1999) *Health Promotion at the Community Level: New Advances*. Thousand Oaks, CA: Sage.

Bracht, N. and Gleason, J. (1990) 'Strategies and structures for citizen partnerships', in N. Bracht (ed.), *Health Promotion at the Community Level*. Thousand Oaks, CA: Sage.

Bracht, N. and Kingsbury, L. (1990) 'Community organization principles in health promotion: a five stage model', in N. Bracht (ed.), *Health Promotion at the Community Level*. Thousand Oaks, CA: Sage.

Bracht, N., Kingsbury, L. and Rissel, C. (1999) 'A five-stage community organization model for health promotion', in N. Bracht (ed.), *Health Promotion at the Community Level: New Advances*. Thousand Oaks, CA: Sage.

Bradshaw, J. (1972) 'The concept of social need', *New Society*, 30 March.

Bradshaw, J. (1994) 'The conceptualization and measurement of need: a social policy perspective', in J. Popay and G. Williams (eds), *Researching the People's Health*. London: Routledge.

Brager, C. and Specht, H. (1973) *Community Organizing*. New York: Columbia University Press.

Brandes, D. and Ginnis, P. (1986) 'A guide to student-centred learning', in J. Ryder and C. Campbell, *Balancing Acts in Personal, Social and Health Education*. London: Routledge.

Braunack-Mayer, A. and Louise, J. (2008) 'The ethics of community empowerment: tensions in health promotion theory and practice', *Promotion & Education*, 15 (3): 5–8.

Breed, W. and Defoe, J.R. (1981) 'The portrayal of the drinking process on prime-time television', *Journal of Communication*, 31: 48–58.

Brehm, J.W. (1966) *A Theory of Psychological Reactance*. New York: Academic Press.

Brehm, S.S. and Brehm, J.W. (1981) *Psychological Reactance: A Theory of Freedom and Control*. New York: Academic Press.

Breslow, L. (1999) 'From disease prevention to health promotion', *JAMA*, 281: 1030–3.

Breslow, L. (2004) 'Perspectives: the third revolution in health', *Annual Review of Public Health*, 25 (April): xiii–xviii.

Breslow, L. (2006) 'Health measurement in the third era of health', *American Journal of Public Health*, 96: 17–19.

Bridgen, P. (2007) 'Evaluating the empowering potential of community-based health schemes: the case of community health policies in the UK since 1997', in J. Douglas, S. Earle, S. Handsley, C.E. Lloyd, and S. Spurr (eds), *A Reader in Promoting Public Health: Challenge and Controversy*. London: Sage.

British Standards Institute (1978) 'BS 4778 British Standard quality vocabulary', in Society of Health Education and Health Promotion Specialists, *Developing Quality in Health Education and Health Promotion*. Society of Health Education and Health Promotion Specialists.

Broadcast Committee of Advertising Practice (2004) *Television Advertising Standards Code.* (*Website*: http://www.cap.org.uk/cap/codes/).

Brook, R.H. and Lohr, K.N. (1985) 'Efficacy, effectiveness, variations, and quality: boundary-crossing research', *Medical Care*, 23 (5): 710–22.

Broughton, B. (2001) *How LogFrame Approaches Could Facilitate the Planning and Management of Humanitarian Operations.* (*Website*: http://www.mande.co.uk/docs/bblogframe.pdf).

Brown, E.R. and Margo, G.E. (1978) 'Health education: can the reformers be reformed?', *International Journal of Health Services*, 8 (1): 3–23.

Brown, C. (1984) 'The art of coalition building: a guide for community leaders', in F.D. Butterfoss, R.M. Goodman and A. Wandersman (1993) 'Community coalitions for prevention and health promotion', *Health Education Research*, 8 (3): 315–30.

Brown, I. (2006) 'Nurses' attitudes towards adult patients who are obese: literature review', *Journal of Advanced Nursing*, 53 (2): 221–32.

Bruner, J.S. (1971) *The Relevance of Education.* New York: Norton and Co.

Brunner, E. (1996) 'The social and biological basis of cardiovascular disease in office workers', in D. Blane, E. Brunner and R. Wilkinson, R (1996) *Health and Social Organization: Towards a Health Policy for the 21st Century.* London: Routledge.

Bruun Jensen, B. and Simovska, V. (2005) 'Involving students in learning and health promotion processes – clarifying why/what/and how', *Promotion & Education*, XII (3–4): 150–6.

Buchan, H., Gray, M., Hill, A. and Coulter, A. (1990) 'Needs assessment made simple', *Health Service Journal*, (100): 240–1.

Buchanan, D.R. (1994) 'Reflections on the relationship between theory and practice', *Health Education Research*, 9 (3): 273–83.

Buchanan, D.R. (2000) *An Ethic for Health Promotion: Rethinking the Sources of Human Well-Being.* New York: Oxford University Press.

Buchanan, D.R. (2006) 'A new ethic for health promotion: reflections on a philosophy of health education for the 21st century', *Health Education and Behaviour*, 33: 290–304.

Bulmer, M. (1982) *The Use of Social Research: Social Investigations in Public Policy Making.* London: Allen & Unwin.

Bunting, M. (2007) 'Capital ideas: Robert Putnam discusses the implications of his latest research into community, identity and trust', *The Guardian*, 18 July.

Bunton, R. (1992) 'Health promotion as social policy', in R. Bunton and G. Macdonald (eds), *Health Promotion: Disciplines and Diversity.* London: Routledge.

Bunton, R. and Burrows, R. (1995) 'Consumption and health in the "epidemiological" clinic of late modern medicine', in R. Bunton, S. Nettleton and R. Burrows (eds), *The Sociology of Health.* London: Routledge.

Bunton, R. and Macdonald, G. (eds) (1992) *Health Promotion: Disciplines and Diversity.* London: Routledge.

Burton, P., Goodlad, R., Croft, J., Abbott, J., Hasting, A., Macdonald, G. and Slater, T. (2004) *What works in community involvement in area-based initiatives? A systematic review of the literature.* Home Office Online Reports 53/04. (*Website*: http://www.homeoffice.gov.uk/rds/pdfs04/rdsolr 5304.pdf).

Butcher, K. and Kievelitz, U. (1997) 'Planning with PRA: HIV and STD in a Nepalese mountain community', *Health Policy and Planning*, 12 (3): 253–61.

Butterfoss, F.D., Goodman, R.M. and Wandersman, A. (1993) 'Community coalitions for prevention and health promotion', *Health Education Research*, 8 (3): 315–30.

Cabanero-Verzosa, C. (1996) *Communication for Behavior Change.* Washington, DC: The World Bank.

Cacioppo, J.T. and Petty, R.E. (1989) 'The elaboration likelihood model: the role of effect and affect laden information processing in persuasion', in P. Cafferata and A. Tybout (eds), *Cognitive and Affective Responses to Advertising.* Lexington, MA: Lexington Books.

Calman, K.C. (1997) 'Equity, poverty and health for all', *British Medical Journal*, 314 (7088): 1187–91.

Calnan, M. (1987) *Health and Illness*. London: Tavistock.

Calouste Gulbenkian Foundation (1984) *A National Centre for Community Development* (report of a working party). London: Gulbenkian Foundation.

Campbell, C. (2003) *Letting Them Die: Why HIV/ AIDS Prevention Programmes Often Fail*. Oxford: James Currey; Bloomington: Indiana University Press; and Cape Town: Juta.

Campbell, C., Wood, R. and Kelly, M. (1999) *Social Capital and Health*. London: Health Development Agency.

Campbell Collaboration (2001) *Campbell Systematic Reviews: Guidelines for the Preparation of Review Protocols*. (*Website*: www.campbellcollaboration.org/artman2/uploads/1/C2_Protocols_guidelines. pdf).

Campbell, D. and Fiske, D. (1959) 'Convergent and discriminant validation by the multitrait-multimethod matrix', *Psychological Bulletin*, 56: 81–105.

Campbell, D. and Stanley, J. (1963) *Experimental and Quasi Experimental Evaluations in Social Research*. Chicago: Rand McNally.

Campbell, O., Cleland, J., Collumbien, M. and Southwick, K. (1999) *Social Science Methods for Research on Reproductive Health*. Geneva: WHO.

Canadian Council on Social Development (2001) 'Defining and redefining poverty: a CCSD perspective', Position Paper, Ottawa, Ontario: CCSD. (*Website*: www.ccsd.ca/pubs/2001/poverty pp.htm).

Cantril, H. (1958) 'The invasion from Mars', in E.E. Maccoby, T.M. Newcomb and E.L. Hartley (eds), *Readings in Social Psychology*. New York: Henry Holt.

Caplan, R. and Holland, J. (1990) 'Rethinking health education theory', *Health Education Journal*, 49: 10–12.

Carlin, J.P.T. and Nolan, T. (1998) 'School-based bicycle safety education and bicycle injuries in children', in S. MacIntyre and M. Petticrew, 'Good intentions and received wisdom are not enough', *Journal of Epidemiology and Community Health*, 54: 802–3.

Carlisle (2002) *'Artful Approach to Joint Working', Health Development Today*. (*Website*: www.hda-online.org.uk).

Carr-Hill, R. and Chalmers-Dixon, P. (2002) *A Review of Methods for Monitoring and Measuring Social Inequality, Deprivation and Health Inequalities*. Oxford: South East Public Health Observatory. (*Website*: www.sepho.org.uk)

Carr-Hill, R. and Chalmers-Dixon, P. (2005) *The Public Health Observatory Handbook of Health Inequalities Measurement*. SEPHO. (*Website*: http://www.sepho.org.uk/Download/Public/9707/1/Carr-Hill-final.pdf).

Catford, J. (1983) 'Positive health indicators – towards a new information base for health promotion', *Community Medicine*, 5: 125–32.

Catford, J. (1993) 'Auditing health promotion: what are the vital signs of quality?', *Health Promotion International*, 8 (2): 67–8.

Cattell, R.B. (1966) *The Scientific Analysis of Personality*. Chicago: Aldine.

Cavanagh, S. and Chadwick, K. (2005) *Health Needs Assessment: A Practical Guide*. London: NICE. (*Website*: http://www.nice.org.uk/aboutnice/whoweare/aboutthehda/hdapublications/health_needs_assessment_a_practical_guide.jsp).

CDX (undated) *What is Community Development?* Sheffield: Community Development Exchange (*Website*: http://www.cdx.org.uk/files/u1/what_is_cd.pdf).

Centers for Disease Control (1997) *Principles of Community Engagement: Part 2*. (*Website*: http://www.cdc.gov/phppo/pce/part2.htm).

Centre for Reviews and Dissemination (2009) *Systematic Reviews: CRD's Guidance for Undertaking Reviews in Healthcare*. York: CRD (*Website*: http://www.york.ac.uk/inst/crd/systematic_reviews_book.htm).

Chapman, S. (1994) 'The A–Z of public health advocacy', in S. Chapman and D. Lupton (eds), *The Fight for Public Health: Principles and Practice of Media Advocacy*. London: BMJ Publishing Group.

Chapman, S. and Egger, G. (1983) 'Myth in cigarette advertising and health promotion', in S. Chapman and D. Lupton (1994), *The Fight for the Public Health: Principles and Practice of Media Advocacy*. London: BMJ Publishing Group.

Chapman, S. and Lupton D. (1994) *The Fight for Public Health: Principles and Practice of Media Advocacy*. London: BMJ Publishing Group.

Chapman, S. and Wakefield, M. (2001) 'Tobacco control advocacy in australia: reflections on 30 years of progress', *Health Education and Behavior*, 28 (3): 274–89.

Charlton, B.G. (1991) 'Medical practice and the double-blind, randomized controlled trial' (editorial), *British Journal of General Practice*, 42 (350): 355–6.

Charnofsky, S. (1971) *Educating the Powerless*. Belmont, CA: Wordsworth Publishers.

Chave, S.P.W. (1958) 'John Snow, the Broad Street pump and after', in J. Ashton, *The Epidemiological Imagination*. Buckingham: Open University Press.

Chesterfield-Evans, A. and O'Connor, B. (1986) 'Billboard utilizing graffitists against unhealthy promotions (BUGA UP) – its philosophy and rationale and their application in health promotion', in D.S. Leathar, G.B. Hastings and J.K. Davies (eds), *Health Education and the Media*. London: Pergamon Press.

Chief Medical Office (2003) *Annual Report of the Chief Medical Officer 2003*. London: Department of Health. (*Website*: http://www.dh.gov.uk/en/Publicationsandstatistics/Publications/AnnualReports/Browsable/DH_4875366).

Child Poverty Action Group (2007) *Media Briefing: Meeting the Government's Child Poverty Target: Progress to Date*. (*Website*: http://www.cpag.org.uk/info/briefings_policy/CPAG_briefingHBAI_2006.pdf).

Cochrane, A.C.L. (1972) *Effectiveness and Efficiency: Random Reflections on the Health Service*. London: Nuffield Provincial Hospitals Trust.

Cochrane Collaboration (2002) *Cochrane Collaboration Disclaimer about Cochrane Reviews*. Oxford: Cochrane Collaboration. (*Website*: www.cochrane.org/cochrane/revabstr/mainindex.htm).

Cockerill, A. (undated) *Promoting Mental Health in Schools*. Hull: HAZNET, Hull and East Riding Community Health NHS Trust. (*Website*: www.haznet.org.uk/hazs/hazmap/hull_mental-hlth-schools.pdf).

Coggans, N. and McKellar, S. (1994) 'Drug use amongst peers: peer pressure or peer preference', *Drugs: Education, Prevention and Policy*, 1: 15–26.

Cohen, A.K. (1955) *Delinquent Boys: The Culture of the Gang*. New York: Free Press.

Cohen, B. (1963) *The Press and Foreign Policy*. Princeton, NJ: Princeton University Press.

Cohen, J.M. and Cohen, M.J. (1960) *The Penguin Dictionary of Quotations*. Harmondsworth: Penguin.

Colebatch, H.K. (1998) *Policy*. Buckingham: Open University Press.

Coleman, J. (1988) 'Social capital in the creation of human capital', *American Journal of Sociology*, 94 (supplement): S25–S120.

Coleman, J. (1990) *Foundations of Social Theory*. New York: Free Press.

COMMIT Research Group (1991) 'Community intervention trial for smoking cessation (COMMIT): summary of design and intervention', *Journal of the National Cancer Institute*, 83(22): 1620–8.

Commission on Social Determinants of Health (2007) *Achieving Health Equity: From Root Causes to Fair Outcomes. Interim Statement*. Geneva: WHO. (*Website*: http://www.who.int/social_determinants/resources/interim_statement/en/index.html).

Commission on Social Determinants of Health (2008) *Closing the Gap in a Generation: Health Equity through Action on the Social Determinants of Health*. Geneva: WHO. (*Website*: http://www.who.int/social_determinants/final_report/en/).

Communities and Local Government and Department of Health (2007) *Delivering Health and Well-being in Partnership: The Crucial Role of the New Local Performance Framework*. Wetherby: Communities and Local Government Publications.

Communities Scotland (2005) *National Standards for Community Engagement*. (*Website*: http://www.communitiesscotland.gov.uk/stellent/groups/public/documents/webpages/otcs_008411.pdf).

Community Cohesion Review Team (2001) *Community Cohesion*. London: Home Office.

Community Development Project Information and Intelligence Unit (1974) *Models of Social Change and Possible Strategies on Three Levels of Operation*. London: Community Development Project.

Community Development Project (1977) *Gilding the Ghetto*. London: Community Development Project.

Community Health Scholars Program (2002) *The Community Health Scholars Program: Stories of Impact*. Ann Arbor, MI.

Connell, J.P. and Kubisch, A.C. (1998) 'Applying a theory of change approach to the evaluation of comprehensive community initiatives: progress, prospects and problems', in K. Fulbright-Anderson, A.C. Kunisch and J.P. Connell (eds), *New Approaches to Evaluating Community Initiatives, Vol.2: Theory, Measurement and Analysis*. Washington, DC: Aspen Institute.

Connell, J.P., Kubisch, A.C., Schorr L.B. and Weiss, C.H. (eds) (1995) *New Approaches to Evaluating Community Initiatives: Volume 1 – Concepts, Methods and Contexts*. Washington, DC: Aspen Institute.

Connelly, J. (2001) 'Critical realism and health promotion: effective practice needs an effective theory' (editorial), *Health Education Research*, 16 (2): 115–9.

Conner, M. and Norman, P. (eds) (2005) *Predicting Health Behaviour: Research and Practice with Social Cognition Models* (2nd edn). Maidenhead: Open University Press.

Conner, M. and Sparks, P. (1996) 'The theory of planned behaviour and health behaviours', in M. Conner and P. Norman (eds), *Predicting Behaviour*. Buckingham: Open University Press.

Constantino-David, K. (1982) 'Issues in community orgnization', *Community Development Journal*, 17: 190–201.

Constantino-David, K. (1992) 'The Philippine experience in scaling-up', in G. Walt, *Health Policy: An Introduction to Process and Power*. London: Zed.

Contributors to the Cochrane Collaboration and the Campbell Collaboration (2000) *Evidence from Systematic Reviews of Research Relevant to Implementing the 'Wider Public Health' Agenda*. University of York: NHS Centre for Reviews and Dissemination. (*Website*: www.york. ac.uk/inst/crd/wph.htm).

Cook, T.D. and Campbell, D.T. (1979) *Quasi-Experimentation*. Chicago: Rand McNally.

Cooper, H., Arber, S., Fee, L. and Ginn, J. (1999) *The Influence of Social Support and Social Capital on Health*. London: Health Development Agency.

Cornwall, A., Musyoki, S. and Pratt, G. (2001) *IDS Working Paper 131: In Search of a New Impetus: Practitioners' Reflections on PRA and Participation in Kenya*. University of Sussex, Brighton: Institute of Development Studies. (*Website*: www.ids.ac.uk/ids/bookshop/details.asp?id=639).

Cornwell, J. (1984) *Hard-earned Lives*. London: Tavistock.

Corwin, R.G. (1978) 'Power', in E. Sagarin (ed.), *Sociology: The Basic Concepts*. New York: Holt, Rinehart & Winston.

Cote, S. and Healy, T. (2001) *The Well Being of Nations: The Role of Human and Social Capital*. Paris: Organisation for Economic Co-operation and Development.

Coulthard, M., Walker, A. and Morgan, A. (2001) *Assessing People's Perceptions of Their Neighbourhood and Community Involvement* (Part 1). London: Health Development Agency.

Coulthard, M., Walker, A. and Morgan, A. (2002) *People's Perceptions of Their Neighbourhood and Community Involvement: Results From the Social Capital Module of the General Household Survey 2000*. London: The Stationery Office. (*Website*: www. statistics.gov.uk/products/p9233.asp).

Crawford, R. (1980) 'Healthism and the medicalization of everyday life', *International Journal of Health Services*, 10 (3): 365–88.

Crick, B. and Lister, I. (1978) 'Political literacy', in B. Crick and A. Porter (eds), *Political Education and Political Literacy*. London: Longman.

Croft, S. and Beresford, P. (1992) 'The politics of participation', *Critical Social Policy*, 26: 20–44.

Crossley, M.L. (2002) 'Introduction to the symposium on "health resistance": The limits of contemporary health promotion', *Health Education Journal*, 61: 101.

CSDH (2008) *Closing the gap in a generation: health equity through action on the social determinants of health. Final Report of the Commission on Social Determinants of Health*. Geneva: World Health Organization.

Culyer, A.J. (1977) 'Need, values and health status measurement', in A.J. Culyer and K.G. Wright (eds), *Economic Aspects of Health Services*. London: Martin Robertson.

Cummins, S. and MacIntyre, S. (2002) '"Food deserts" – evidence and assumption in policy making', *British Medical Journal*, 325: 436–8.

Cunningham, G. (1963) 'Policy and practice', *Public Administration*, 41.

Curle, A. (1972) *Education for Liberation*. New York: John Wiley.

Daghio, M.M., Fattori, G. and Ciardullo, A. (2006) 'Evaluation of easy-to-read information material on healthy life-styles written with the help of citizens' collaboration through networking', *Promotion & Education*, XIII (3): 191–6.

Dahlgren, G. and Whitehead, M. (1991) *Policies and Strategies to Promote Social Equity in Health*. Stockholm: Institute of Futures Studies.

Daniel, P. and Dearden, P.N. (2001) *Integrating a Logical Framework Approach to Planning into the Health Action Zone Initiative*. Hull: HAZNET, Hull and East Riding Community Health NHS Trust.

Daniels, N. (1985) *Just Health Care*. New York: Cambridge University Press.

Davey Smith, G. (1996) 'Income inequality and mortality: why are they related?' *British Medical Journal*, 312: 987–8.

Davidoff, F., Haynes, B., Sackett, D.L. and Smith, R. (1995) 'Evidence-based medicine: a new journal to help doctors identify the information they need', *British Medical Journal*, 310: 1085–6.

Davie, R., Butler, N. and Goldstein, H. (1972) *From Birth to Seven*. London: Longman.

Davies, J.B. (1992) *The Myth of Addiction*. Switzerland: Harwood.

Day, I. (2002) '"Putting yourself in other people's shoes": the use of forum theatre to explore refugee and homeless issues in schools', *Journal of Moral Education*, 31 (1): 21–34.

de Chernatony, L. (1993) 'Categorizing brands: evolutionary process underpinned by two key dimensions', *Journal of Marketing Management*, 9 (2): 173–88.

De Greef, M. and Van den Broek, K. (2004) *Making the Case for Workplace Health Promotion: Analysis of the effects of WHP*. Essen: ENWHP (*Website*: http://www.enwhp.org/fileadmin/downloads/report_business_case.pdf).

De Kadt, E. (1982a) 'Ideology, social policy, health and health services: a field of complex interactions', *Social Science and Medicine*, 16: 741–52.

De Kadt, E. (1982b) 'Community participation for health: the case of Latin America', *World Development*, 10 (7): 573–584.

De Leeuw, E. (1993) 'Health policy, epidemiology and power: the interest web', *Health Promotion International*, 8 (1): 49–52.

De Leeuw, E. (2000) 'Commentary – beyond community action: communication arrangements and policy networks', in B. Poland, L.W. Green and I. Rootman (eds), *Settings for Health Promotion*. Thousand Oaks, CA: Sage.

de Vries, H. (1989) *Smoking Prevention in Dutch Adolescents*. Maastricht: University of Limburg.

Defoe, J.R. and Breed, W.R. (1989) 'Consulting to change media contents: two cases in alcohol education', *International Quarterly of Community Health Education*, 9: 257–72.

Delaney, F. (1994a) 'Making connections: research into intersectoral collaboration', *Health Education Journal*, 53: 474–85.

Delaney, F. (1994b) 'Muddling through the middle ground: theoretical concerns in intersectoral collaboration and health promotion', *Health Promotion International*, 9 (3): 217–25.

Delaney, F. (1994c) 'Policy and health promotion', *Journal of the Institute of Health Education*, 32 (1): 5–9.

Delk, J.L. (1980) 'High-risk sports as indirect self-destructive behavior', in N.L. Farberow (ed.), *The Many Faces of Suicide*. New York: McGraw-Hill.

Denman, S., Moon, A., Parsons, C. and Stears, D. (2002) *The Health Promoting School: Policy Research and Practice.* London: Routledge Falmer.

Denzin, N.K. (1970) *The Research Act in Sociology.* London: Butterworths.

Denzin, N.K. (1994) 'The art and politics of interpretation', in N.K. Denzin and Y.S. Lincoln (eds), *Handbook of Qualitative Research.* Thousand Oaks, CA: Sage.

Denzin, N.K. and Lincoln, Y.S. (eds) (1994) *Handbook of Qualitative Research.* Thousand Oaks, CA: Sage.

Department for Education and Employment (1997) *Excellence in Schools.* London: The Stationery Office.

Department for Education and Employment (1999) *National Healthy School Standard: Guidance.* Nottingham: DfEE Publications.

Department for Work and Pensions (2007a) *Households Below Average Income (HBAI) 2005/6.* (*Website*: http://www.dwp.gov.uk/asd/hbai.asp).

Department for Work and Pensions (2007b) *Opportunity for All: Indicators Update 2007.* (*Website*: http://www.dwp.gov.uk/ofa/reports/2007/OpportunityforAll2007.pdf).

Department of Health (1988) *Public Health in England: The Report of the Committee of Inquiry into the Future Development of the Public Health Function. The Acheson Report.* Cm. 289. London: HMSO.

Department of Health (1991) *The Health of the Nation: A Consultative Document for Health in England.* London: HMSO.

Department of Health (1992) *The Health of the Nation.* London: HMSO.

Department of Health (1993) *The Code of Practice for the Commissioning and Management of Research and Development.* London: HMSO.

Department of Health (1995) *Variations in Health: What Can the Department of Health and NHS Do? Report of the Variations Sub-group of the Chief Medical Officer's Health of the Nation Working Group.* London: HMSO.

Department of Health (1996) *Policy Appraisal and Health.* London: Department of Health.

Department of Health (1997) *The New NHS: Modern Dependable.* London: The Stationery Office.

Department of Health (1998a) *Our Healthier Nation.* London: Department of Health. (*Website*: www.ohn.gov.uk/ohn/ohn.htm).

Department of Health (1998b) *Smoking Kills: A White Paper on Tobacco.* London: The Stationery Office.

Department of Health (1998c) *The Health of the Nation – A Policy Assessed.* London: The Stationery Office.

Department of Health (1999) *Saving Lives: Our Healthier Nation.* London: The Stationery Office.

Department of Health (2000) *Information About the Healthy Workplace Initiative.* London: Department of Health. (*Website*: www. signupweb.net/about.htm).

Department of Health (2001a) *The Report of the Chief Medical Officer's Project to Strengthen the Public Health Function.* London: Department of Health.

Department of Health (2001b) *Shifting the Balance of Power Within the NHS: Securing Delivery.* London: Department of Health.

Department of Health (2002) *Our Healthier Nation: Healthy Neighbourhoods* (from website). London: Department of Health. (*Website*: www.ohn.gov.uk/ohn/ people/neighb.htm).

Department of Health (2003) *Health Equity Audit: A Guide for the NHS.* (*Website*: http://www. dh.gov.uk/en/Publicationsandstatistics/Publications/PublicationsPolicyAndGuidance/DH_4084138).

Department of Health (2004) *Choosing Health: Making Healthy Choices Easier. Cm6374.* London: The Stationery Office. (*Website*: http://www.dh.gov.uk/en/Publicationsandstatistics/Publications/PublicationsPolicyAndGuidance/DH_4094550).

Department of Health (2005) *Delivering Choosing Health: Making Healthier Choices Easier. Cm 6374.* London: Department of Health.

Department of Health (2006a) *A Stronger Local Voice.* London: TSO.

Department of Health (2006b) *Factsheet on Health Inequalities*. London: Department of Health. (*Website*: http://www.dh.gov.uk/en/Publicationsandstatistics/Publications/Publications PolicyAndGuidance/DH_4139513).

Department of Health (2006c) *Health Challenge England – Next Steps for Choosing Health*. (*Website*: http://www.dh.gov.uk/en/Publicationsandstatistics/Publications/PublicationsPolicyAnd Guidance/DH_4139514).

Department of Health (2007a) *Guidance on Joint Strategic Needs Assessment*. London: Department of Health. (*Website*: http://www.dh.gov.uk/en/Publicationsandstatistics/Publications/Publications PolicyAndGuidance/DH_081097).

Department of Health (2007b) *Health Impact Assessment*. London: Department of Health. (*Website*: http://www.dh.gov.uk/en/Publicationsandstatistics/Legislation/Healthassessment/index.htm).

Department of Health (2007c) *Health Profile of England*. London: Department of Health. (*Website*: http://www.dh.gov.uk/en/Publicationsandstatistics/Publications/PublicationsStatistics/DH_09716).

Department of Health (2007d) *Health Survey for England – Introduction*. London: Department of Health. (*Website*: http://www.dh.gov.uk/en/Publicationsandstatistics/PublishedSurvey/ HealthSurveyForEngland).

Department of Health (2007e) *Local Involvement Networks*. London: Department of Health. (*Website*: http://www.dh.gov.uk/en/Policyandguidance/Organisationpolicy/PatientAnd Publicinvolvement/DH_076366).

Department of Health (2007f) *Screening questions for Health Impact Assessment*. London: Department of Health. (*Website*: http://www.dh.gov.uk/en/Publicationsandstatistics/Legislation/Health assessment/DH_4093617).

Department of Health (2007g) *The NHS in England: The Operating Framework for 2008/9*. (*Website*: http://www.dh.gov.uk/en/Publicationsandstatistics/Publications/PublicationsPolicyAnd Guidance/DH_081094).

Department of Health (2008a) *Ambitions for Health*. London: Department of Health. (*Website*: http://www.dh.gov.uk/en/Publichealth/Choosinghealth/DH_086106).

Department of Health (2008b) *NHS Health Trainers*. (*Website*: http://www.dh.gov.uk/en/Public health/Healthinequalities/HealthTrainersusefullinks/index.htm).

Department of Health and Social Security (1976) *Prevention and Health: Everybody's Business*. London: HMSO.

Department of Health and Social Security (1980) *Inequalities in Health: Report of a Research Working Group Chaired by Sir Douglas Black*. London: DHSS.

DETR (2000) *Index of Multiple Deprivation 2000*. London: DETR.

DETR (2001) *Local Strategic Partnerships: Government Guidance*. London: DETR. (*Website*: www. local-regions.dtlr.gov.uk/lsp/guidance).

Deviren, F. and Babb, P. (2005) *Young People and Social Capital*. London: National Statistics. (*Website*: http://www.statistics.gov.uk/articles/nojournal/Social_capital_young_people.pdf).

Dewey, J. (1910) *How We Think*. Boston, MA: Heath.

Dewey, J. (1946) *The Public and Its Problems: An Essay in Political Inquiry*. Chicago: Gateway Books.

Dickens, P. (1996) *Reconstructing Nature: Alienation Emancipation and the Division of Labour*. New York: Routledge.

Dickson, D.A., Hargie, O. and Morrow, N.C. (1989) *Communication Skills Training for Health Professionals: An Instructor's Handbook*. London: Chapman & Hall.

Dignan, M.B. and Carr, P.A. (1992) *Program Planning for Health* (2nd edn). Malvern, PA: Lee & Febiger.

Dijkstra, A. and de Vries, H. (2000) 'Subtypes of pre-contemplating smokers defined by different long-term plans to change their smoking behavior', *Health Education Research*, 15 (4): 423–34.

Dixon, J. (1989) 'The limits and potential of community development for personal and social change', *Community Health Studies*, XII (1): 82–92.

Dixon-Woods, M., Agarwal, S., Young, B., Jones, D. and Sutton, A. (2004) *Integrative Approaches to Qualitative and Quantitative Evidence*. London: Health Development Agency. (*Website*: http://www.nice.org.uk/niceMedia/pdf/Integrative_approaches_evidence.pdf).

Dixon-Woods, M., Bonas, S., Booth, A., Jones, D.R., Miller, T., Sutton, A.J., Shaw, R.L., Smith J.A. and Young, B. (2006) 'How can systematic reviews incorporate qualitative research? A critical perspective', *Qualitative Research*, 6 (1): 27–44.

Doll, R. (1992) 'Health and the environment in the 1990s', *American Journal of Public Health*, 82 (7): 933–41.

Doll, R., Peto, R., Wheatley, K., Gray, R. and Sutherland, I. (1994) 'Mortality in relation to smoking: 40 years' observations on male British doctors', *British Medical Journal*, 309: 901–11.

Donald, A. (2001) 'What is quality of life?' *What is… series*, 1(9): 1–4. (*Website*: http://www.jr2.ox.ac.uk/bandolier/painres/download/whatis/WhatisQOL.pdf).

Donaldson, L. (1999) *Ten Tips for Better Health*. London: The Stationery Office. (*Website*: www.archive.official-documents.co.uk/document/cm43/4386/4386-tp.htm).

Donaldson, L. (2009) *150 Years of the Annual Report of the Chief Medical Officer: On the State of Public Health 2008*. London: HMSO (*Website*: http://www.dh.gov.uk/en/Publications andstatistics/Publications/AnnualReports/DH_096206).

Dooris, M. (2006) 'Health promoting settings: future directions', *Promotion & Education*, 13 (1): 2–4.

Dorfman, L., Wallack, L. and Woodruff, K. (2005) 'More than a message: framing public health advocacy to change corporate practices', *Health Education and Behavior*, 32 (3): 320–36.

Dorling, D., Rigby, J., Wheeler, B., Ballas, D., Thomas, B., Fahmy, E., Gordon, D. and Lupton, R. (2007) *Poverty Wealth and Place in Britain 1968–2005*. Bristol: The Policy Press in association with Joseph Rowntree Foundation.

Douglas, M.J., Conway, L., Gorman, D., Gavin, S. and Hanlon, P. (2001) 'Developing principles for health impact assessment', *Journal of Public Health Medicine*, 23 (2): 148–54.

Dowd, E.T. (2002) 'Psychological reactance in health education and promotion', *Health Education Journal*, 61: 113.

Downie, R.S., Tannahill, C. and Tannahill, A. (1996) *Health Promotion Models and Values* (2nd edn). Oxford: Oxford University Press.

Doyal, L. and Gough, I. (1991) *A Theory of Human Need*. London: Macmillan.

Doyal, L. and Pennell, I. (1979) *The Political Economy of Health*. London: Pluto.

Draper, R. (1988) 'Healthy public policy: a new political challenge', *Health Promotion*, 2 (3): 217–18.

Dubos, R. (1979) *The Mirage of Health*. New York: Harper Colophon.

Duckworth, L. (2002) 'Classes in safe sex are ineffective, says study', *The Independent*, 14 June.

Duncan, J.S. and Duncan, N.G. (1992) 'Ideology and bliss: Roland Barthes and the secret history of landscape', in T.J. Barnes and J.S. Duncan (eds), *Writing Worlds: Discourse, Text and Metaphor in the Representation of Landscape*. London: Routledge.

Durfee, W. and Chase, T. (1999) *Brief Tutorial on Gantt Charts*. Minneapolis, MN: University of Minnesota. (*Website*: www.me.umn.edu/courses/ me4054/assignments/gantt.html).

Durgee, J.F. (1986) 'How consumer sub-cultures code reality: a look at some code types', *Advances in Consumer Research*, 13: 332–7.

Durham, J. and Ali, M. (2008) 'Mine risk education in the Lao PDR: time for a public health approach to risk reduction?', *International Journal of Health Promotion and Education*, 46 (1): 27–32.

Duryea, E.J. (1991) 'Principles of non-verbal communication in efforts to reduce peer and social pressure', *Journal of School Health*, 61: 5–10.

Dworkin, G. (1972) 'Paternalism', *Monist*, 56 (1): 64–84.

Eagleton, T. (1991) *An Introduction to Ideology*. London: Verso.

Edgar, A., Salek, S., Shickle, D. and Cohen, D. (1998) *The Ethical QALY: Ethical Issues in Healthcare Resource Allocations*. Haslemere: Euromed Communications Ltd.

Educe Ltd and GFA Consulting (undated) *Five Vital Lessons: Successful Partnerships with Business*. (*Website*: http://fivevital.educe.co.uk/index_1.htm).

Ehrenreich, B. and English, D. (1979) *For Her Own Good: 150 Years of Experts' Advice to Women*. London: Pluto Press.

Eiser, J.R. and Eiser, C. (1996) *Effectiveness of Video for Health Education: A Review*. London: HEA.

Elliott-Kemp, J. (1982) 'Managing organizational change', in J. Anderson, *HEA Health Skills Project*. Leeds: Counselling and Career Development Unit.

ENWHP (2007) *Luxembourg Declaration*. (*Website*: http://www.enwhp.org/fileadmin/rs-dokumente/dateien/Luxembourg_Declaration.pdf).

ENWHP (undated a) *Healthy Employees in Healthy Organisations: For Sustainable Social and Economic Development in Europe*. (*Website*: http://www.enwhp.org/fileadmin/downloads/free/1248_ENWHP_Image_engl_final.pdf).

ENWHP (undated b) *Workplace Health Promotion* (*Website*: http://www.enwhp.org/index.php?id=9).

ENWHP (undated c) *Why Invest in Better Health in European Companies and Organisations*. (*Website*: http://www.enwhp.org/index.php?id=473).

EPPI-Centre (1999) *A Review of the Effectiveness and Appropriateness of Peer-delivered Health Promotion Interventions for Young People*. London: Institute of Education, University of London. (*Website*: http://eppi.ioe.ac.uk/EPPIWeb/home.aspx?page=/hp/reports/peer_health/peer-delivered_health_promotion_ intro.htm).

Etzioni, A. (1967) 'Mixed scanning: a third approach to decision making', *Public Administration Review*, 27: 385–92.

European Centre for Health Policy (1999) *Gothenburg Consensus Paper: Health Impact Assessment*. Copenhagen: WHO Regional Office for Europe. (*Website*: http://www.euro.who.int/document/pae/gothenburgpaper.pdf).

European Network of Health Promoting Schools (1997) *Conference Resolution*. First Conference of the European Network of Health Promoting Schools, Thessaloniki-Halkidiki, 1–5 May, WHO Regional Office for Europe.

Euroqol (undated) *Euroqol EQ-5D*. (*Website*: http://www.advancedinterventions.org.uk/pdf/RatingScales/EQ-5D.pdf).

Evans, D., Head, M.J. and Speller, V. (1994) *Assuring Quality in Health Promotion: How to Develop Standards of Good Practice*. London: HEA.

Evans, G. and Newnham, J. (1992) 'The dictionary of world politics: a reference guide to concepts, ideas and institutions', in G. Walt, *Health Policy: An Introduction to Process and Power*. London: Zed.

Ewart, C.K. (1992) 'Role of physical self-efficacy in recovery from heart attack', in R. Schwarzer (ed.), *Self-efficacy: Thought Control of Action*. Washington: Hemisphere Publishing.

Eysenck, H.J. (1960) *The Structure of Human Personality*. London: Methuen.

Faculty of Public Health Medicine (1995) 'Health promotion in the workplace', *Guidelines for Health Promotion*, 40.

Faden, R.R. and Faden, A.I. (1978) 'The ethics of health education as public health policy', *Health Education Monographs*, 6 (2): 180–97.

Fairclough, N. (1995) *Ideology*. London: Arnold.

Fairclough, N. (2001) 'CDA as a method in social scientific research', in R. Wodak and M. Meyer (eds), *Methods of Critical Discourse Analysis*. London: Sage.

Felix, M., Chavis, D. Florin, P. (1989) Enabling community development: language, concepts and strategies. Presentation sponsored by Health Promotion Branch, Ontario Ministry of Health, Toronto, May 16–18.

Ferlander, S., and D. Timms, (1999) *Social Cohesion and On-line Community*, Brussels: European Commission.

Farrelly, M.C., Davis, K.C., Haviland, M.L., Messeri, P. and Healton, C.G. (2005) 'Evidence of a Dose-response relationship between 'truth' anti-smoking ads and youth smoking prevalence', *American Journal of Public Health*, 95 (3): 425–31.

Farrelly, M.C., Davis, K.C., Duke, J. and Messeri, P. (2008) 'Sustaining "truth": changes in youth tobacco attitudes and smoking intentions after 3 years of a national antismoking campaign', *Health Education Research*, Epub, 17 January.

Feighery, E. and Rogers, T. (1989) 'Building and maintaining effective coalitions', in F.D. Butterfoss, R.M. Goodman and A. Wandersman, 'Community coalitions for prevention and health promotion', *Health Education Research*, 8 (3): 315–30.

Feighery, E., Rogers, T., Thompson, B. and Bracht, N. (1992) 'Coalition problem solving guide', in N. Bracht, *Health Promotion at the Community Level – New Advances*. Thousand Oaks, CA: Sage.

Festinger, L. (1957) *A Theory of Cognitive Dissonance*. Stanford, CA: Stanford University Press.

Fien, J. (1994) 'Critical theory, critical pedagogy and critical praxis in environmental education', in B.B. Jensen and K. Schnack (eds), *Action and Action Competence as Key Concepts in Critical Pedagogy*. Copenhagen: Royal Danish School of Educational Studies.

Fien, J. (2000) 'Education for sustainable consumption: towards a framework for curriculum and pedagogy', in B.B. Jensen, K. Schnack and V. Simovska (eds), *Critical Environmental and Health Education*. Copenhagen: Research Centre for Environmental and Health Education, Danish University of Education.

Fien, J. and Trainer, T. (1993) 'Education for sustainability', in J. Fien (ed.), *Environmental Education: A Pathway to Sustainability*. Geelong, Australia: Deakin University Press.

Finn, P. (1980) 'Attitudes toward drinking conveyed in studio greeting cards', *American Journal of Public Health*, 70: 826–9.

Finnegan, J.R. and Viswanath, K. (1999) 'Mass media and health promotion: lessons learned, with implications for public health campaigns', in N. Bracht (ed.), *Health Promotion at the Community Level*. Thousand Oaks, CA: Sage.

Fishbein, M. (1976) 'Persuasive communication', in A.E. Bennett (ed.), *Communication Between Doctors and Patients*. London: Oxford University Press for Nuffield Provincial Hospitals Trust.

Fishbein, M. and Ajzen, I. (1975) *Belief, Attitude, Intention and Behavior: An Introduction to Theory and Research*. Reading, MA: Addison-Wesley.

Fisher, R. (1949) *The Design of Experiments* (5th edn). Edinburgh: Oliver & Boyd.

Fletcher, C.M. (1973) *Communication in Medicine*. (The Rock Carling Fellowship, 1972.) London: Nuffield Provincial Hospitals Trust.

Foreman, A. (1996) 'Health needs assessment', in J. Percy-Smith (ed.), *Needs Assessments in Public Policy*. Buckingham: Open University Press.

Forrest, R., and A. Kearns, (2000) 'Social cohesion, social capital and the neighbourhood'. Paper presented to ESRC Cities Programme Neighbourhoods Colloquium, Liverpool, 5–6 June.

FOREST (2008) *How Forest Works*. (*Website*: http://www.forestonline.org/output/How-Forest-Works.aspx).

Frank, R.H. (2000) 'Why living in a rich society makes us feel poor', *New York Times Magazine*, 15 October.

Frankel, S., Davison, C. and Davey Smith, G. (1991) 'Lay epidemiology and the rationality of responses to health education', *British Journal of General Practice*, 41: 428–30.

Frankena, W.K. (1970) 'A model for analyzing a philosophy of education', in J.R. Martin (ed.), *Readings in Philosophy of Education: A Study in Curriculum*. Boston, MA: Allyn & Bacon.

Frankham, J. (1998) 'Peer education: the unauthorised version', *British Educational Research Journal*, 24 (2): 179–93.

Freidson, E. (1961) *Patients' Views of Medical Practice*. New York: Russell Sage.

Freire, P. (1972) *Pedagogy of the Oppressed*. Harmondsworth: Penguin.

French, J. (2000) 'Understanding health promotion through its fault lines', PhD thesis. Leeds: Leeds Metropolitan University.

French, J. and Blair-Stevens, C. (2007) *Big Pocket Guide to Social Marketing* (2nd edn). London: National Consumer Council.

French, J. and Milner, S. (1993) 'Should we accept the status quo?', *Health Education Journal*, 52 (2): 98–101.

French, J.R.P. and Raven, B.H. (1959) 'The bases of social power', in D. Cartwright (ed.), *Studies in Social Power*. Ann Arbor, MI: University of Michigan Press.

Freudenberg, N. (1978) 'Shaping the future of health education: from behavior change to social change', *Health Education Monographs*, 6 (4): 372–7.

Freudenberg, N. (1981) 'Health education for social change: a strategy for public health in the US', *International Journal of Health Education*, XXIV (3): 1–7.

Freudenberg, N. (1984) 'Training health educators for social change', *International Quarterly of Community Health Education*, 5 (1): 37–52.

Freudenberg, N. (2005) 'Public health advocacy to change corporate practices: implications for health education practice and research', *Health Education and Behavior*, 32: 298–319.

Friedli, L. (2009) *Mental Health, Resilience and Inequality*. Copenhagen: WHO Regional Office for Europe. (*Website*: http://www.euro.who.int/document/e92227.pdf).

Friedman, M. and Rosenman, R.H. (1974) *Type A Behavior and Your Heart*. New York: Knopf.

Fukuyama, F. (1999) *Social Capital and Civil Society*. Fairfax, VA: The Institute of Public Policy, George Mason University, IMF Conference of Second Generation Reforms. (*Website*: www.imf.org/pubs/ft/seminar/1999/reforms/fukuyama.htm).

Fulbright-Anderson, K., Kubisch, A.C. and Connell, J.P. (1998) *New Approaches to Evaluating Community Initiatives: Volume 2 – Theory, Measurement, and Analysis*. Washington, DC: Aspen Institute.

Gagne, R.M. (1985) *The Conditions of Learning and Theory of Instruction* (4th edn). New York: Holt Saunders.

Galbraith, J. (1973) *Economics and the Public Purpose*. New York: Mentor.

Galea, G., Powis, B. and Tamplin, S. (2000) 'Healthy islands in the Western Pacific – international settings development', *Health Promotion International*, 15 (2): 169–78.

Gallie, W.B. (1955) 'Essentially contested concepts', *Proceedings of the Aristotelian Society*, 56: 167–98.

Garmezy, N. (1983) 'Stressors of childhood', in N. Garmezy and M. Rutter (eds), *Stress, Coping and Development in Children*. New York: McGraw-Hill.

Gibson, M. (undated) 'How to avoid curriculum change', personal communication.

Gibson, R. (1986) *Critical Theory and Education*. London: Hodder & Stoughton.

Giddens, A. (1989) *Sociology*. Cambridge: Polity Press.

Giddens, A. (1991) *Modernity and Self Identity: Self and Society in the Late Modern Age*. Cambridge: Polity Press.

Gilchrist, A. (2000) 'Community work in the UK – an overview', *Talking Point* (Association of Community Workers) No. 191 (Oct/Nov): 1–4.

Gillam, S. and Murray, S. (1996) *Needs Assessment in General Practice*. London: RCGP.

Gillies, P. (1998) 'Effectiveness of alliances and partnerships for health promotion', *Health Promotion International*, 13 (2): 99–120.

Ginn Daugherty, H. and Kammeyer, K.C.W. (1995) *An Introduction to Population* (2nd edn). New York: Guilford.

Ginsberg, G. and Silverberg, D. (1994) 'A cost–benefit analysis of legislation for bicycle safety helmets in Israel', *American Journal of Public Health*, 84 (4): 653–6.

Godfrey, C. (2001) 'Economic evaluation of health promotion', in I. Rootman, M. Goodstadt, B. Hyndman, D.V. McQueen, L. Potvin, J. Springett and E. Ziglio (eds), *Evaluation in Health Promotion: Principles and Perspectives*. Copenhagen: WHO.

Godin, G., Gagnon, H., Alary, M., Levy, J.J. and Otis, J. (2007) 'The degree of planning: an indicator of the potential success of health education programs', *Promotion & Education*, XIV (3): 138–42.

Goodman, R.M., Steckler, A. and Kegler, M.C. (1997) 'Mobilizing organizations for health enhancement: theories of organizational change', in K. Glanz, F.M. Lewis and B.K. Rimer (eds), *Health Behavior and Health Education: Theory, Research, and Practice* (2nd edn). San Francisco: Jossey-Bass.

Gordon, D. (1999) 'An alternative ten tips for staying healthy', in D. Raphael, 'The question of evidence in health promotion', *Health Promotion International*, 15 (4): 355–67.

Gordon, D., Adelman, L., Ashworth, K., Bradshaw, J., Levitas, R., Middleton, S., Pantazis, C., Patsios, D., Payne, S., Townsend, P. and Williams, J. (2000) *Poverty and Social Exclusion in Britain*. York: Joseph Rowntree Foundation.

Gordon, I. (1958) 'That damned word health', *Lancet*, 2: 638–9.

Gottlieb, N. and McLeroy, K.R. (1992) 'Social health', in M.P. O'Donnell (ed.), *Health Promotion in the Workplace* (2nd edn). New York: Delmar Publishing.

Gottlieb, N.H., Brink, S.G. and Levenson Gingis, P.L. (1993) 'Correlates of coalition effectiveness: the "Smoke Free Class of 2000" program', *Health Education Research*, 8 (3): 375–84.

Gough, I. (1992) 'What are human needs?', in J. Percy-Smith and I. Sanderson (eds), *Understanding Local Needs*. London: Institute for Public Policy Research.

Grace, V.M. (1991) 'The marketing of empowerment and the construction of the health consumer: a critique of health promotion', *International Journal of Health Services*, 21 (2): 329–43.

Graham, H. (1987) 'Women's smoking and family health', *Social Science and Medicine*, 25 (1): 47–56.

Graham, H. and Kelly, M.P. (2004) *Health Inequalities: Concepts, Frameworks and Policy*. London: Health Development Agency.

Granger, C. (1998) 'Establishing causality in evaluations of comprehensive community initiatives', in K. Fulbright-Anderson, A.C. Kubisch and J.P. Connell (eds), *New Approaches to Evaluating Community Initiatives, Vol. 2: Theory, Measurement and Analysis*. Washington, DC: Aspen Institute.

Granner, M.L. and Sharpe, P.A. (2004) 'Evaluating community characteristics and functioning: a summary of measurement tools', *Health Education Research*, 19 (5): 514–32.

Green, J. (1995) 'School sex education policies: a qualitative analysis of the process of policy development', *Journal of the Institute of Health Education*, 32 (4): 106–11.

Green, J. (1997) 'A survey of sex education in primary schools in the Northern & Yorkshire Region', *International Journal of Health Education*, 35 (3): 81–6.

Green, J. (1998) 'School sex education and education policy in England & Wales: the relationship examined', *Health Education Research*, 13 (1): 67–72.

Green, J. (2000) 'The role of theory in evidence-based health promotion practice' (editorial), *Health Education Research*, 15 (2): 125–9.

Green, J. (2008) 'Health education – the case for rehabilitation', *Critical Public Health*, 18 (4): 447–56.

Green, J. and South, J. (2006) *Evaluation*. Maidenhead: Open University Press.

Green, J. and Tones, K. (1999) 'Towards a secure evidence base for health promotion', *Journal of Public Health Medicine*, 21 (2): 133–9.

Green, J. and Tones, K. (2000) 'The health promoting school, general practice and the creative arts: an example of inter-sectoral collaboration', *Health Education*, 100 (3): 124–30.

Green, J., South, J. and Newell, C. (2004) *Sure Start Harehills: Evaluation Report Year One*. Leeds: Centre for Health Promotion Research, Leeds Metropolitan University.

Green, L.W. (1974) 'Toward cost–benefit evaluations of health education: some concepts, methods and examples', *Health Education Monographs*, 2: 34–64.

Green, L.W. (1996) 'Bringing people back to health', *Promotion & Education*, III (1): 23–6.

Green, L.W. and Kreuter, M.W. (1991) *Health Promotion Planning: An Educational and Environmental Approach*. Mountain View, CA: Mayfield.

Green, L.W. and Kreuter, M.W. (1999) *Health Promotion Planning: An Educational and Ecological Approach* (3rd edn). Mountain View, CA: Mayfield.

Green, L.W. and Lewis, F.M. (1986) *Measurement and Evaluation in Health Education and Health Promotion*. Palo Alto, CA: Mayfield.

Green, L.W., Poland, B. and Rootman, I. (2000) 'The settings approach to health promotion', in B. Poland, L.W. Green and I. Rootman (eds), *Settings for Health Promotion: Linking Theory and Practice*. Thousand Oaks, CA: Sage.

Green, L.W., Simons-Morton, D. G. and Potvin, L. (1997) 'Education and life-style determinants of health and disease', in R. Detels, W.W. Holland, J. McEwen and G.S. Omenn (eds), *Oxford Textbook of Public Health*. (Vol. 1, 3rd edn). Oxford: Oxford University Press.

Green, L.W., Glanz, K., Hochbaum, G.M., Kok, G., Kreuter, M.W., Lewis, F.M., Lorig, K., Morisky, D., Rimer, B.K. and Rosenstock, I.M. (1994) 'Can we build models on, or must we replace, the theories and models in health education?', *Health Education Research*, 9 (3): 397–404.

Griffiths, J. and Dark, P. (2005) *Shaping the Future of Public Health: Promoting Health in the NHS*. Department of Health and Welsh Assembly Government. (*Website*: http://www.dh.gov.uk/en/Publicationsandstatistics/Publications/PublicationsPolicyAndGuidance/DH_4116526).

Griffiths, J., Clive Blair-Stevens, C. and Thorpe, A. (2008) *Social Marketing for Health and Specialised Health Promotion: Stronger Together – Weaker Apart. A Paper for Debate*. London: Shaping the Future of Health Promotion, Royal Society of Public Health, National Social Marketing Centre.

Groene, O. (2006) *Implementing health promotion in Hospitals: Manual and Self Assessment Forms*. Copenhagen: WHO Regional Office for Europe. (*Website*: http://www.who-cc.dk/library/Manual%20Standard%20Assessment.pdf)

Guba, E.G. and Lincoln, Y.S. (1981) *Effective Evaluation*. San Francisco: Jossey-Bass.

Guba, E.G. and Lincoln, Y.S. (1989) *Fourth Generation Evaluation*. Newbury Park, CA: Sage.

Gunasekera, H., Chapman, S. and Campbell, S. (2005) 'Sex and drugs in popular movies: an analysis of the top 200 films', *Journal of the Royal Society of Medicine*, 2005 (98): 464–70.

Guttman, N. (2000) *Public Health Communication Interventions: Values and Ethical Dilemmas*. Thousand Oaks, CA: Sage.

Hagard, S. (2000) 'Benchmarking to promote better health', *Promotion & Education*, VII (2): 2–3.

Haglund, B., Weisbrod, R.R. and Bracht, N. (1990) 'Assessing the community: its services, needs, leadership, and readiness', in N. Bracht (ed.), *Health Promotion at the Community Level*. London: Sage.

Haglund, B.J.A., Pettersson, B., Finer, B. and Tillgren, P. (1993) *The Sundsvall Handbook, 'We Can Do It!'*, Third International Conference on Health Promotion, Sundsvall, Sweden, 9–15 June 1991.

Haglund, B.J.A., Jansson, B., Pettersson, B. and Tillgren, P. (1998) 'A quality assurance instrument for practitioners', in J.K. Davies and G. Macdonald (eds), *Quality, Evidence and Effectiveness in Health Promotion*. London: Routledge.

Hale, J.L. and Dillard, J.P. (1995) 'Fear appeals in health promotion campaigns: too much, too little, or just right?', in E. Maibach and R.L. Parrott (eds), *Designing Health Messages*. Thousand Oaks, CA: Sage.

Halpern, E.S. (1983) 'Auditing Naturalistic Inquiries: The Development and Application of a Model', unpublished doctoral dissertation, Indiana University.

Hammond, D., Fong, G.T., Borland, R., Cummings, K.M., McNeill, A. and Driezen, P. (2007) 'Text and graphic warnings on cigarette packages: findings from the ITC Four Country Survey', *American Journal of Preventive Medicine*, 32 (3): 210–17.

Hancock, T. (1982) 'Beyond health care', *The Futurist*, August 4–13.

Hancock, T. (1998) 'Caveat partner: reflections on partnership with the private sector', *Health Promotion International*, 13 (3): 193–5.

Handy, C. (1993) *Understanding Organizations* (4th edn). Harmondsworth: Penguin.

Hansen, A. (1986) 'The portrayal of alcohol on television', *Health Education Journal*, 45 (3): 127–31.

Hansen, A. (2003) *The Portrayal of Alcohol and Alcohol Consumption in Television News and Drama Programmes*. London: Alcohol Concern. (*Website*: http://www.alcoholconcern.org.uk/files/20031219_105216_A%20Hansen%20-%20Alcohol%20and%20Television%20Report%20Oct%2003.pdf).

Harris, A. and Harris, T. (1986) *Staying OK*. London: Pan.

Harrison, J. and Edwards, J. (1994) *Developing Health Education in the Curriculum*. London: David Fulton.

Hart, J.T. (1971) 'The inverse care law', *Lancet*, (i): 405–12.

Harter, S. (1985) 'Manual for the self-perception profile of children', unpublished, University of Denver, cited in T.J. Berndt and L. Burgy (1996), 'Social self concepts', in B.A. Bracken (ed.), *Handbook of Self Concept: Developmental, Social and Clinical Considerations*. New York: Wiley.

Harter, S. (1993) 'Causes and consequences of low self-esteem in children and adolescents', in R.F. Baumeister (ed.), *Self-esteem: The Puzzle of Low Self Regard*. New York: Plenum.

Harvey, L. (1990) *Critical Social Research*. London: Unwin-Hyman.

Hastings, G. (2007) *Social Marketing: Why Should the Devil Have All the Best Tunes?* Oxford: Butterworth-Heinemann.

Hastings, G. and McDermott, L. (2006) 'Putting social marketing into practice', *BMJ*, 332: 1210–12.

Hastings, G.B., Stead, M., Whitehead, M., Lowry, R., MacFadyen, L., McVey, D., Owen, L. and Tones, K. (1998) 'Using the media to tackle the health divide: future directions', *Social Marketing Quarterly*, IV (3): 41–67.

Hattie, J. (1992) *Self Concept*. Hillsdale, NJ: Erlbaum.

Hawes, H. and Scotchmer, C. (1993) *Children for Health*. London: Child-to-Child Trust/UNICEF.

Hawks, D., Scott, K. and McBride, M. (2002) *Prevention of Psychoactive Substance Use: a Selected Review of What Works in the Area of Prevention*. Geneva: WHO. (*Website*: http://www.who.int/mental_health/evidence/en/prevention_intro.pdf).

HC Deb (2001–2) 385, col. 123WH. (*Website*: http://www.publications.parliament.uk/pa/cm200102/cmhansrd/vo020508/halltext/20508h04.htm).

HDA (undated) *Putting Public Health Evidence into Practice: Working Definition of Evidence and Criteria for Inclusion*. London: HDA.

HEA (1989) *Health for Life*. London: HEA.

HEA (1991) *Smoking and Me: A Teacher's Guide* (2nd edn). London: HEA.

HEA (1996) *European Network of Health Promoting Schools*. London: HEA.

HEA (1999a) *Art for Health: A Review of Good Practice in Community-based Arts Projects and Interventions Which Impact on Health and Well-being: Report*. London: HDA.

HEA (1999b) *Art for Health: A Review of Good Practice in Community-based Arts Projects and Interventions which Impact on Health and Well-being*. Summary Bulletin. London: HDA.

Health Education Authority/Labyrinth Consulting and Training (1998) *Community Participation for Health. A Review of Good Practice in Community Participation Health Projects and Initiatives. Summary bulletin*. London: Health Education Authority.

Healthy Settings Development Unit (2007) *Stadia*. (*Website*: http://www.uclan.ac.uk/facs/health/hsdu/settings/stadia.htm).

Heaver, R. (1992) 'Participatory rural appraisal: potential application in family planning, health and nutrition programmes', *RRA Notes Number 16: Special Issue on Applications for Health*: 13–21.

Henderson, P., Summer, S. and Raj, T. (2004) *Developing Healthier Communities*. London: Health Development Agency.

Herman, K.A., Wolfson, M. and Forster, J.L. (1993) 'The evolution, operation and future of Minnesota SAFPLAN: a coalition for family planning', *Health Education Research*, 3 (8): 331–44.

Herzlich, C. (1973) *Health and Illness*. London: Academic Press.

Higbee, K.L. and Jensen, L.C. (1978) *Influence: What It Is and How to Use It*. Provo, UT: Brigham Young University Press.

Hilton, D. (1988) 'Community-based or oriented: the vital difference', *Contact*, 106, December: 1–4.

Hirst, P. (1969) 'The logic of the curriculum', *Journal of Curriculum Studies*, 1 (2): 142–58.

Hochbaum, G.M. (1958) *Public Participation in Medical Screening Programs: A Socio-psychological Study*. Washington, DC: Public Health Service Publication No. 572, US Government Printing Office.

Hoge, R.D. and McScheffrey, R. (1991) 'An investigation of self concept in gifted children', *Exceptional Children*, 57: 238–45.

Hogwood, B.W. and Gunn, L.A. (1984) *Policy Analysis for the Real World*. Oxford: Oxford University Press.

Hogwood, B.W. and Gunn, L.A. (1997) 'Why "perfect implementation" is unattainable', in M. Hill (ed.), *The Policy Process: A Reader*. London: Prentice Hall/ Harvester Wheatsheaf.

Holloway, I. (1997) *Basic Concepts for Qualitative Research*. Oxford: Blackwell.

Holman, H. and Lorig, K. (1992) 'Perceived self-efficacy in self-management of chronic disease', in R. Schwarzer (ed.), *Self-efficacy: Thought Control of Action*. Washington, DC: Hemisphere Publishing.

Holt, C.L., Clark, E.M., Kreuter, M.W. and Scharff, D.P. (2000) 'Does locus of control moderate the effects of tailored health education materials', *Health Education Research*, 15 (4): 393–403.

Home Office Community Cohesion Review Team (2001) *Community Cohesion*. London: Home Office.

Hopson, B. and Scally, M. (1981) *Lifeskills Teaching*. Maidenhead: McGraw-Hill.

Hopson, B. and Scally, M. (1980–2) *Lifeskills Teaching Programmes 1–5*. Leeds: Lifeskills Associates.

Horan, J.J. (1977) 'Chapter 5 – Current topics in decision theory', in *Counselling for Effective Decision Making*. (*Website*: http://horan.asu.edu/cfedm/chapter5.php).

Horrobin, D.F. (1978) *Medical Hubris: A Reply to Ivan Illich*. Edinburgh: Churchill Livingstone.

Hospers, H.J., Kok, G.J. and Strecher, V.J. (1990) 'Attributions for previous failures and subsequent outcomes in a weight reduction program', *Health Education Quarterly*, 17: 409–15.

House, J.S., Robbins, C. and Metzner, H.L. (1982) 'The association of social relationships and activities with mortality: prospective evidence from the Tecumseh Community Health Study', *American Journal of Epidemiology*, 116: 123–40.

Hovland, C.I., Janis, I.L. and Kelley, H.H. (1953) *Communication and Persuasion*. New Haven, CT: Yale University Press.

Hubley, J. (1993) *Communicating Health: An Action Guide to Health Education and Health Promotion*. London: Macmillan.

Huckle, J. (1993) 'Environmental education and sustainability: a view from critical theory', in Fien, J. (ed) *Environmental Education: A Pathway to Sustainability*. Melbourne: Deakin University.

Hudson, B. (1987) 'Collaboration in social welfare: a framework for analysis', *Policy and Politics*, 15, 175–182.

Huff, D. (1979) *How to Lie with Statistics*. Harmondsworth: Pelican.

Hughes, J. (1976) *Sociological Analysis: Methods of Discovery*. London: Nelson.

Huitt, W. (1999) 'Conation as an important factor of mind', *Educational Psychology Interactive*. (*Website*: http://chiron.valdosta.edu/whuitt/col/regsys/conation.html).

Huxley, A. (1958) *Brave New World Revisited*. London: HarperCollins.

Hyyppä, M.T. and Mäki, J. (2001) 'Why do Swedish-speaking Finns have longer active life? An area for social capital research', *Health Promotion International*, 16 (1): 55–63.

Ignatieff, M. (1992) 'The grey emptiness inside John Major', in G. Walt, *Health Policy: An Introduction to Process and Power*. London: Zed.

Illich, I. (1976) *The Limits to Medicine–Medical Nemesis: The Expropriation of Health*. Harmondsworth: Penguin.

Impact Information (2005) 'What's with the newspapers?' *Plain Language at Work Newsletter*, 2 May, (*Website*: http://www.impact-information.com/impactinfo/newsletter/plwork15.htm).

International Planning Committee (2002) *Education and Health in Partnership*. A European conference on linking education with the promotion of health in schools. Conference Report, Egmond aan Zee, Netherlands, 25–27 September 2002. Copenhagen, WHO Regional Office for Europe. (*Website*: http://www. euro.who. int/document/E78991.pdf).

International Union for Health Education (1992) *Advocacy for Health*. Paris: International Union for Health Education.

IUHPE and Canadian Consortium for Health Promotion Research (2007) *Shaping the Future of Health Promotion: Priorities for Action*. Paris: IUHPE.

Jackson, R.H. (1983) ' "Play it safe": a campaign for the prevention of children's accidents', *Community Development Journal*, 18: 172–6.

Jackson, S., Cleverly, S., Poland, B., Robertson, A., Burnam, D., Goodstadt, M. and Salsberg, L. (1997) 'Half full or half empty?: Concepts and research design for a study of indicators of community capacity', in N. Smith, L.B. Littlejohns and D. Thompson, 'Shaking out the cobwebs: insights into community capacity and its relation to health outcomes', *Community Development Journal*, 36 (1): 30–41.

Jacobson, L.D., Edwards, A.G.K., Granier, S.K. and Butler, C.C. (1997) 'Evidence-based medicine and general practice', *British Journal of General Practice*, 47: 449–52.

Jamison, J., Ashby, P., Hamilton, K., Lewis, G., Macdonald, A. and Saunders, L. (1998) *The Health Promoting School: Final Report of the ENHPS Evaluation Project in England*. London: HEA.

Janis, I.L. (1975) 'Effectiveness of social support for stressful decisions', in M. Deutsch and H.S. Hornstein (eds), *Applying Social Psychology: Implications for Research, Practice and Training*. Hillsdale, NJ: Erlbaum.

Janis, I.L. and Feshbach, S. (1953) 'Effects of fear-arousing communications', *Journal of Abnormal and Social Psychology*, 48 (1): 78–92.

Janis, I.L. and Mann, L. (1964) 'Effectiveness of role playing in modifying smoking habits and attitudes', *Journal of Experimental Research in Personality*, 1: 84–90.

Janis, I.L. and Mann, L. (1977) *Decision Making: A Psychological Analysis of Conflict, Choice, and Commitment*. New York: Free Press.

Janssen, I., Craig, W.M., Boyce, W.F. and Pickett, W. (2004) 'Association between overweight and obesity with bullying behaviors in school-aged children', *Paediatrics*, 113: 1187–94.

Jenkins, W.I. (1978) *Policy Analysis: A Political and Organisational Perspective*. London: Martin Robertson.

Jensen, B.B. (1991) *The Action Perspective in School Health Education*. Proceedings from Satellite Congress in Copenhagen, 13–14 June, Research Centre for Environmental and Health Education.

Jensen, B.B. (2000a) 'Health knowledge and health education in the democratic health-promoting school', *Health Education*, 100 (4): 146–53.

Jensen, B.B. (2000b) 'Participation, commitment and knowledge as components of pupils' action competence', in B.B. Jensen, K. Schnack and V. Simosvska (eds), *Critical Environmental and Health Education*. Copenhagen: Research Centre for Environmental and Health Education, The Danish University of Education.

Jensen, B. B. and Schnack, K. (1997) 'The action competence approach in environmental education', *Environmental Education Research*, 3(2): 163–78.

Jitsukawa, M. and Djerassi, C. (1994) 'Birth control in Japan: realities and prognosis', *Science*, 2675: 1048–51.

Jochelson, K. (2005) *Nanny or Steward? The Role of Government in Public Health*. London: Kings Fund. (*Website*: http://www.kingsfund.org.uk/publications/kings_fund_publications/nanny_or.html).

John, P. (1998) *Analysing Public Policy*. London: Continuum.

Johns Hopkins Center for Communication Programs (undated) '*A*' *Frame for Advocacy*. Baltimore, MA: Johns Hopkins Bloomberg School of Public Health, Center for Communication Programs. (*Website*: www.jhuccp.org/pr/advocacy).

Jones, L. and Sidell, M. (1997) *The Challenge of Promoting Health*. London: Macmillan.

Jordan, J., Dowsell, T., Harrison, S., Lilford, R.J. and Mort, M. (1998) 'Whose priorities? Listening to users and the public', *British Medical Journal*, 316: 1668–770.

Joseph Rowntree Foundation (2000) *Findings: Poverty and Social Exclusion in Britain*. York: Joseph Rowntree Foundation. (*Website*: www.jrf.org.uk/knowledge/findings/socialpolicy/930.asp).

Joseph Rowntree Foundation (2008) *A Minimum Income Standard for Britain*. (*Website*: http://www.jrf.org.uk/bookshop/eBooks/2226-income-poverty-standards.pdf).

Judge, K. (2000) 'Testing evaluation to the limits: the case of English Health Action Zones', *Journal of Health Services Research and Policy*, 5 (1), January. (*Website*: www.haznet.org.uk/hazs/evidence/judge.asp).

Judge, K. and Bauld, L. (2001) 'Strong theory, flexible methods: evaluating complex community-based initiatives', *Critical Public Health*, 11 (1): 19–38.

Judge, K. and Bauld, L. (2006) 'Learning from policy failure? Health action zones in England', *European Journal of Public Health*, 16 (4): 341–4.

Jusot, F., Gringon, M. and Dourgnon, P. (2007) *Psychosocial Resources and Social Health Inequalities in France: Exploratory Findings from a General Population Survey*. (*Website*: http://www.irdes.fr/EspaceAnglais/Publications/WorkingPapers/DT6PPsychosocialSocialHealthFrance.pdf).

Kahneman, D. and Tversky, A. (1979) 'Prospect theory: an analysis of decisions under risk', *Econometrica*, 47: 263–91.

Kanfer, F.H. and Karoly, P. (1972) 'Self-control: a behavioristic excursion into the lion's den', *Behavior Therapy*, 3: 398–416.

Kaplan, G.A., Salonen, J.T., Cohen, R.D., Brand, R.J., Syme, L. and Puska, P. (1988) 'Social connections and mortality from all causes and cardiovascular disease: prospective evidence from eastern Finland', *American Journal of Epidemiology*, 128: 370–80.

Kaplan, G.A., Wilson, T.W., Cohen, R.D., Brand, R.J., Syme, L. and Puska, P. (1994) 'Social functioning and overall mortality: prospective evidence from the Kuopio ischemic heart disease risk factor study', *Epidemiology*, 5: 495–500.

Karasek, R.A. and Theorell, T. (1990) *Healthy Work: Stress, Productivity, and the Reconstruction of Working Life*. New York: Basic Books.

Kasperson, R.E., Renn, O., Slovic, P., Brown, H.S. (1988) 'The social amplification of risk: a conceptual framework', *Risk Analysis*, 8: 177–87.

Katz, E. and Lazarsfeld, P. (1955) *Personal Influence: The Part Played by People in the Flow of Mass Communication*. Glencoe, IL: Free Press.

Kawachi, I. (1997) 'Long live community', *The American Prospect*, 8 (35).

Kawachi, I., Colditz, G.A. and Ascherio, A. (1996) 'A prospective study of social networks in relation to total mortality and cardiovascular disease in relation to men in the USA', *Journal of Epidemiology and Community Health*, 50: 245–51.

Keith, L.K. and Bracken, B.A. (1996) 'Self concept instrumentation: a historical and evaluative review', in B.A. Bracken (ed.), *Handbook of Self Concept: Developmental, Social and Clinical Considerations*. New York: Wiley.

Kelleher, D., Gabe, J. and Williams, G. (1994) 'Understanding medical dominance in the modern world', in J. Gabe, D. Kelleher and G. Williams (eds), *Challenging Medicine*. London: Routledge.

Kelly, M. (2006) 'Editorial: new NICE and public health', *Health Education*, 103 (3): 181–4.

Kelly, M.P. and Charlton, B. (1995) 'The modern and the postmodern in health promotion', in R. Bunton, S. Nettleton and R. Burrows (eds), *The Sociology of Health Promotion*. London: Routledge.

Kelly, M., Speller, V. and Meyrick, J. (2004) *Getting Evidence into Practice in Public Health*. London: HDA. (*Website*: http://www.nice.org.uk/niceMedia/pdf/evidence_into_practice.pdf).

Kemm, J.R. (1993) 'Towards an epidemiology of positive health', *Health Promotion International*, 8 (2): 129–34.

Kemm, J. (2001) 'Health impact assessment: a tool for healthy public policy', *Health Promotion International*, 16 (1): 79–85.

Kemm, J. (2007) *More than a Statement of the Crushingly Obvious: A Critical Guide to HIA*. West Midlands Public Health Observatory. (*Website*: http://www.apho.org.uk/resource/item.aspx?RID=44422).

Kerrison, S. and Macfarlane, A. (2000) *Official Health Statistics: An Unofficial Guide*. London: Arnold.

Khan, K.S. and Kleijnen, J. (2001) 'Phase 6: data extraction and monitoring progress', in NHS Centre for Reviews and Dissemination, *Undertaking Systematic Reviews of Research Effectiveness*. York: NHS Centre for Reviews and Dissemination.

Kickbush, I. (1995) *An Overview of the Settings Approach to Health Promotion*. In 'The Settings-based Approach to Health Promotion', An International Working Conference in Collaboration with WHO Regional Office for Europe, 17–20 November 1993. London: NHS Executive/HEA.

Kickbush, I. (1996) 'Tribute to Aaron Antonovsky – what creates health', *Health Promotion International*, 11: 5–6.

Kickbush, I. (1997) 'Think health: what makes the difference?' Address at the Fourth International Conference on Health Promotion, Jakarta 21–25 July, in E. Ziglio, S. Hagard, L. McMahon, S. Harvey and L. Levin, 'Principles methodology and practices of investment for health', *Promotion & Education*, VII (2): 4–12.

Kickbush, I. (1998) 'Health promotion in the 21st century: an era of partnerships to achieve health for all', *Press Release* (WHO/47). Geneva: WHO.

Kickbush, I. (2003) 'The contribution of the World Health Organization to a new public health and health promotion', *American Journal of Public Health*, 93: 383–8.

Kickbush, I. (2007) 'The move towards a new public health', *Promotion & Education*, supp. 2: 9.

Kickbush, I. and O'Byrne, D.O. (1995) 'Community as the focus for health and health changes', *Promotion & Education*, II: 17–20.

Kidd, R. and Kumar, K. (1981) 'A critical analysis of pseudo-Freirean adult education', *Economic and Political Weekly*, 3–10 January: 27–36.

Kieffer, C. (1984) 'Citizen empowerment: a developmental perspective', in J. Rappaport, C. Swift and R. Hess (eds), *Empowerment: Steps Toward Understanding and Action*. New York: Haworth Press.

Kindervatter, S. (1979) *Non-formal Education as an Empowering Process*. Amherst, MA: University of Massachusetts, Center for International Education.

Kingdon, J. (1984) 'Agendas, alternatives and public policies', in G. Walt, *Health Policy: An Introduction to Process and Power*. London: Zed.

Kings Fund (2004) *Public Attitudes to Public Health Policy: Summary*. London: Kings Fund. (*Website*: http://www.kingsfund.org.uk/publications/kings_fund_publications/public_attitudes.html).

Kirklin, M.J. and Franzen, L.E. (1974) *Community Organization Bibliography*. Chicago, IL: Institute on the Church in Urban Industrial Society.

Kirscht, J.P. (1972) 'Perceptions of control and health beliefs', *Canadian Journal of Behavioral Science*, 4: 225–37.

Klapper, J.T. (1960) *The Effects of Mass Communication*. Glencoe, IL: Free Press.

Klapper, J.T. (1995) 'The effects of mass communication', in O. Boyd-Barrett and C. Newbold (eds), *Approaches to Media: A Reader*. London: Arnold.

Knowles, M.S., Holton, F. and Swanson, R.A. (1998) *The Adult Learner: The Definitive Classic in Adult Education and Human Resource Development* (5th edn). Houston, TX: Gulf Publishing.

Kobasa, S.C. (1979) 'Stressful life events, personality and health: an inquiry into hardiness', *Journal of Personality and Social Psychology*, 37: 1–11.

Kok, G., Den Broer, D-J., De Vries, H., Gerards, F., Hospers, H.J. and Mudde, A.N. (1992) 'Self-efficacy and attribution theory in health education', in R. Schwarzer (ed.), *Self-Efficacy: Thought Control of Action*. Washington, DC: Hemisphere Publishing.

Kolb, D.A., Rubin, I.M. and McIntyre, J.M. (1971) *Organisational Psychology: An Experiential Approach*. London: Prentice-Hall.

Kolbe, L.J., Tirozzi, G.N., Marx, E., Bobbitt-Cooke, M., Riedel, S., Jones, J. and Schmoyer, M. (2005) 'Health programmes for school employees: improving quality of life, health and productivity', *Promotion & Education*, XII (3–4): 157–61.

Kotler, P. and Zaltman, G. (1971) 'Social marketing and public health intervention', *Journal of Marketing*, 45 (2): 3–12.

Kotler, P., Roberto, N. and Lee, N. (2002) *Social Marketing: Improving the Quality of Life*. Thousand Oaks, CA: Sage.

Kreuter, M.W. and Skinner, C.S. (2000) 'Tailoring: what's in a name?' (editorial), *Health Education Research*, 15 (1): 1–4.

Kreuter, M.W., Oswald, D.L., Bull, F.C. and Clark, E. (2000) 'Are tailored health education materials always more effective than non-tailored materials?' *Health Education Research,* 15 (3): 305–15.

Krieger, N. (1990) 'On becoming a public health professional: reflections on democracy, leadership, and accountability', *Journal of Public Health Policy,* 11: 412–19.

Krieger, N. (2001) 'A glossary for social epidemiology', *Journal of Epidemiology and Community Health,* 55: 693–700.

Krisberg, K. (2005) 'Anti-smoking campaign lowers youth smoking rates with "truth": funding threatened', *The Nation's Health,* 35 (3). (*Website:* http://www.medscape.com/viewarticle/502009).

Krisher, H.P., Darley, S.A. and Darley, J.M. (1973) 'Fearprovoking recommendations, intentions to take preventive actions, and actual preventive actions', *Journal of Personality and Social Psychology,* 26 (2): 301–18.

Kroeger, A. (1997) *The Use of Epidemiology in Local Health Planning: A Training Manual.* London: Zed.

Kuhn, T.S. (1970) *The Structure of Scientific Revolutions* (2nd edn). Chicago: University of Chicago Press.

Labonte, R. (1993) 'Community development and partnerships', in L. Jones and M. Sidell, *The Challenge of Promoting Health.* London: Macmillan.

Labonte, R. and Laverack, G. (2001a) 'Capacity building for health promotion, Part 1: for whom? And for what purpose?', *Critical Public Health,* 11 (2): 112–27.

Labonte, R. and Laverack, G. (2001b) 'Capacity building in health promotion, Part 2: whose use? and with what measurement?', *Critical Public Health,* 11 (2): 129–38.

Lalonde, M. (1974) *A New Perspective on the Health of Canadians.* Ottawa: Ministry of National Health and Welfare.

Larkey, L.K., Alatorre, C., Buller, D.B., Morrill, C., Klein Buller, M., Taren, D. and Sennott-Miller, L. (1999) 'Communication strategies for dietary change in a worksite peer educator intervention', *Health Education Research,* 14 (6): 777–90.

Lasswell, H.D. (1948) 'The structure and function of communication in society', in L. Bryson (ed.), *Communication of Ideas.* New York: Harper.

Last, J.M. (1963) 'The iceberg: completing the clinical picture in general practice', *Lancet:* 28–31, reprinted in J. Ashton (1994), *The Epidemiological Imagination.* Buckingham: Open University Press.

Last, J.M. (1988) *A Dictionary of Epidemiology* (2nd edn). Oxford: Oxford University Press.

Laverack, G. (2007) *Health Promotion Practice.* Maidenhead: Open University Press/McGraw Hill Education.

Laverack, G. and Labonte, R. (2000) 'A planning framework for community empowerment goals within health promotion', *Health Policy and Planning,* 15 (3): 255–62.

Lawton, D. (1986) *School Curriculum Planning.* London: Hodder & Stoughton.

Lazarsfeld, P.F. and Merton, R.K. (1955) 'Mass communication, popular taste and organized social action', in W. Schramm (ed.), *Mass Communications.* Urbana, IL: University of Illinois Press.

Lazenbatt, A. and McMurray, F. (2004) 'Using participatory rapid appraisal as a tool to assess women's psychosocial health needs in Northern Ireland', *Health Education,* 104 (3): 174–87.

Learning and Teaching Scotland (2007) Health promoting schools: family and community. (*Website:* http://www.ltscotland.org.uk/healthpromotingschools/familyandcommunity/yourrole.asp0).

Ledwith, M. (2007) 'Reclaiming the radical agenda: a critical approach to community development', *Concept,* 17 (2): 8–12.

Lee, K., Lock, K. and Ingram, A. (2006) *The Role of Health Impact Assessment.* London: The Nuffield Trust.

Lefebvre, R.C. and Flora, J.A. (1988) 'Social marketing and public health intervention', *Health Education and Behavior,* 15 (3): 299–315.

Leichter, H.M. (1979) 'A comparative approach to policy analysis: healthcare policy in four nations', in G. Walt, *Health Policy: An Introduction to Process and Power.* London: Zed.

Lenin, I. (1969) *Collected Works* (volume 42). London: Lawrence & Wishart.

Leon, D.A., Walt, G. and Gilson, L. (2001) 'International perspectives on health inequalities and policy', *British Medical Journal*, 322: 591–4.

Lerer, L.B. (1999) 'How to do (or not to do) … health impact assessment', *Health Policy and Planning*, 14 (2): 198–203.

Leventhal, H. (1980) 'The common sense representation of illness danger', in S. Rachman (ed.), *Contribution to Medical Psychology* (Vol. II). London: Pergamon.

Levin, L. and Ziglio, E. (1997) 'Health promotion as an investment strategy: a perspective for the 21st century', in M. Sidell, L. Jones, J. Katz and A. Peberdy (eds), *Debates and Dilemmas in Promoting Health*. London: Macmillan.

Lewin, R.W. (1951) *Field Theory in Social Science*. New York: Harper.

Lewis, F.M. (1987) 'The concept of control: a typology and health-related variables', *Advances in Health Education and Promotion*, 2: 277–309.

Lewis, I.M., Watson, B., White, K.M. and Tay, R. (2007) 'Promoting public health messages: should we move beyond fear-evoking appeals in road safety?', *Qualitative Health Research*, 17 (1): 61–74.

Lewis, J. (2001) 'Reflections on evaluation in practice', *Evaluation*, 7 (3): 387–94.

LGpartnerships – Smarter Partnerships (undated a) *Digging Deeper – Finding Answers reviewing your Partnerships and Making them Work Better*. (*Website*: http://www.lgpartnerships.com/digging.asp).

LGpartnerships – Smarter Partnerships (undated b) *Eight Tests of a Healthy Partnership*. (*Website*: http://www.lgpartnerships.com/howhealthy.asp).

Lichtenstein, S., Slovic, P., Fischoff, B., Layman, M. and Combs, B. (1978) 'Judged frequency of lethal events', *Journal of Experimental Psychology: Human Learning and Memory*, 4 (6): 551–78.

Lincoln, Y.S. and Denzin, N.K. (1994) 'The fifth moment', in N.K. Denzin and Y.S. Lincoln (eds), *Handbook of Qualitative Research*. Thousand Oaks, CA: Sage.

Lincoln, Y.S. and Guba, E.G. (1985) *Naturalistic Inquiry*. Beverly Hills, CA: Sage.

Lindblom, C.E. (1979) 'Still muddling, not yet through', *Public Administration Review*, 39: 517–25.

Lindblom, C.E. (1987) 'How to think about the policy-making process', in F. Delaney, 'Muddling through the middle ground: theoretical concerns in intersectoral collaboration and health promotion', *Health Promotion International*: 9 (3): 217–25.

Lindblom, C.E. and Woodhouse, E.J. (1993) *The Policy-making Process* (3rd edn). Englewood Cliffs, NJ: Prentice Hall.

Lindeman, E. (1926) *The Meaning of Adult Education*. New York: New Republic.

Lindquist, E.F. (1940) *Statistical Analysis in Educational Research*. New York: Houghton Mifflin.

Lindström, B. (1994) *The Essence of Existence: On the Quality of Life of Children in the Nordic Countries*. Gothenburg: Nordic School of Public Health.

Linkenbach, J. and D'Atri, G. (1998) *The Montana Model*. Unpublished training manual for the Montana Social Norms Project.

Linnan, L.A. and Owens Ferguson, Y. (2007) 'Beauty salons: a promising health promotion setting for reaching and promoting health among African American women', *Health Education and Behavior*, 34: 517–30.

Lippmann, W. (1965) *Public Opinion*. New York: Free Press. (Originally published 1922.)

Lipsky, M. (1997) 'Street-level bureaucracy: an introduction', in M. Hill (ed.), *The Policy Process: A Reader* (2nd edn). Hemel Hempstead: Prentice-Hall/Harvester Wheatsheaf.

Liss, P.-E. (1990) *Health Care Need: Meaning and Measurement*. Linkoping: Linkoping Studies in Arts and Science 53.

Lister-Sharp, D., Chapman, S., Stewart-Brown, S. and Sowden, A. (1999) 'Health promoting schools and health promotion in schools: two systematic reviews', *Health Technology Assessment*, 3 (22).

Local Government Data Unit – Wales (2003) *Updating and Revising the Welsh Index of Multiple Deprivation*. (*Website*: http://www.dataunitwales.gov.uk/Documents/Project/Deprivation/WDE02000_031200_WIMD_Study_Report_eng.pdf).

London Health Economics Consortium (1996) *Local Health and the Vocal Community*. London: London Primary Health Care Forum.

Loney, M. (1981) 'The British community development projects: questioning the state', *Community Development Journal*, 16: 55–67.

Lucy, F., Angie, P., Dieter, W. and Jeremy, H. (2004) 'Obesity, bullying and self-esteem in pre-adolescent children', *International Journal of Obesity*, 28 (supp: 1): 193.

Ludbrook, A., Bird, S. and van Teijlingen, E. (2005) *International Review of the Health and Economic Impact of the Regulation of Smoking in Public Places: Summary report. Health Scotland.* (*Website*: http://www.healthscotland.com/uploads/documents/InternationalReviewShortReport.pdf).

Lukes, S. (1974) *Power: A Radical View*. London: Macmillan.

Lupton, D. (1992) 'Discourse analysis: a new methodology for understanding the ideologies of health and illness', *Australian Journal of Public Health*, 16: 145–50.

Lupton, D. and Chapman, S. (1994) 'Two studies of public health news', in S. Chapman and D. Lupton (eds), *The Fight for the Public Health: Principles and Practice of Media Advocacy*. London: BMJ Publishing.

Lynch, J., Davey Smith, G., Kaplan, G.A. and House, J.S. (2000) 'Income inequality and mortality: importance to health of individual income, psycho-social environment, or material conditions', *British Medical Journal*, 320: 1200–4.

Lyng, S. (1990) 'Edgework: a social psychological analysis of voluntary risk taking', *American Journal of Sociology*, 95 (4): 851–86.

Macauley, A.C., Commanda, L.E., Freeman, W.L., Gibson, N., McCabe, L., Robbins, C.M. and Twohig, L. (1999) 'Participatory research maximises community and lay involvement', *British Medical Journal*, 319: 774–8.

MacDonald, G. and Mussi, A. (1998) *Health Promotion Specialists: The Key Profession for Unlocking the Health Agenda Beyond 1998*. Managing Health Promotion: 8th National Conference, Penrith, October.

Macdonald, J.U. and Warren, W.G. (1991) 'Primary health care as an educational process: a model and a Freirean perspective', *International Quarterly of Community Health Education*, 12 (1): 35–50.

MacDonald, M.A. and Green, L.W. (2001) 'Reconciling concept and context: the dilemma of implementation in school-based health promotion', *Health Education and Behavior*, 28 (6): 749–68.

Mackenbach, J. (1997) 'Beyond the RCT? CIT!', *Report of the Expert Meeting Beyond the RCT – Towards Evidence-based Public Health*. Rotterdam: GGD.

MacIntyre, S. and Pettigrew, M. (2000) 'Good intentions and received wisdom are not enough', *Journal of Epidemiology and Community Health*, 54: 802–3.

Maddock, J., Maglione, C., Barnett, J.D., Cabot, C., Jackson, S. and Reger-Nash, B. (2007) 'Statewide implementation of the 1% or less campaign', *Health Education and Behavior*, 34 (6): 953–63.

Mager, R.F. (1975) *Preparing Instructional Objectives*. Belmont, CA: Fearon.

Manderson, L. and Aaby, P. (1992) 'An epidemic in the field? Rapid assessment procedures and health research', *Social Science and Medicine*, 35: 839–50.

Mao Tse-tung (1967) 'Selected works of Mao Tse-tung, (1967)' (Vol. III), *The United Front in Cultured Work*. Peking.

Mappes, T.A. and Zembary, J.S. (1991) *Biomedical Ethics* (3rd edn). New York: McGraw-Hill.

Marmot, M. (2005) 'Social determinants of health inequalities', *Lancet*, 365: 1099–104.

Marmot, M. (2006) 'Harveian Oration: Health in an unequal world', *Lancet*, 368: 2081–94.

Marrow, A.J. (1969) *The Practical Theorist: The Life and Work of Kurt Lewin*. New York: Basic Books.

Marsh, A. and Matheson, J. (1983) *Smoking Attitudes and Behaviour*. London: HMSO.

Marsh, H.W. and Holmes, I. (1990) 'Multidimensional self-concepts: construct validation of responses by children', *American Educational Research Journal*, 27: 89–118.

Martinson, R. (1974) 'What works? Questions and answers about prison reform', in R. Pawson and N. Tilley, *Realistic Evaluation*. London: Sage.

Maslow, A.H. (1954) *Motivation and Personality.* New York: Harper.

Maslow, A.H. (1970) *Motivation and Personality* (2nd edn). New York: Harper & Row.

Mason, J. and Rowling, L. (2005) 'Look after the staff first – a case study of developing staff health and wellbeing', *Promotion & Education*, XII (3–4): 140–1.

Mason, P. and Barnes, M. (2007) 'Constructing theories of change: methods and sources', *Evaluation*, 13 (2): 151–70.

Matarasso, F. (2001) 'The health and social impact of participation in the arts', in T. Heller, R. Muston, M. Siddell and C. Lloyd (eds), *Working for Health.* London: Sage.

Mathers, J., Parry, J. and Wright, J. (2005) 'Participation in health impact assessment: objectives, methods and core values', *Bulletin of the World Health Organization*, 83 (1): 58–64.

Maton, K.I. and Rappaport, J. (1984) 'Empowerment in a religious setting: a multivariate investigation', in J. Rappaport, C. Swift and R. Hess (eds), *Studies in Empowerment: Steps Toward Understanding and Action.* New York: Haworth Press.

May, T. (1993) *Social Research: Issues, Methods and Processes.* Buckingham: Open University Press.

Maycock, B., Howat, P. and Slevin, T. (2001) 'A decision-making model for health promotion advocacy: the case for advocacy of drunk driving control measures', *Promotion & Education*, VIII (2): 59–64.

Mayo, M. and Craig, G. (1995) 'Community participation and empowerment: the human face of structural adjustment or tools for democratic transformation?', in G. Craig and M. Mayo (eds), *Community Empowerment: A Reader in Participation and Development.* London: Zed Books.

McBride, N.T. and Midford, R. (1996) 'Assessing organisational support for school health promotion', *Health Education Research*, 11 (4): 509–18.

McCubbin, M., Labonte, R., and Dallaire, B. (2001) *Advocacy for Healthy Public Policy as a Health Promotion Technology.* Centre for Health Promotion (online archives). (*Website*: http://www.utoronto.ca/chp/symposium.htm).

McDougall, W. (1926) *An Introduction to Social Psychology.* Boston, MA: John W. Luce.

McGuire, G. (1970) 'A vaccine for brainwash', *Psychology Today*, 3: 36–9.

McGuire, G. (1989) 'Theoretical foundations of campaigns', in R.E. Rice and C.K. Atkin (eds), *Public Communication Campaigns* (2nd edn). Newbury Park, CA: Sage.

McKeown, T. (1979) *The Role of Medicine: Dream, Mirage or Nemesis?* Oxford: Blackwell.

McKeown, T. and Lowe, C.R. (1974) *An Introduction to Social Medicine.* London: Blackwell.

McKinlay, J.B. (1975) 'A case for refocusing upstream: the political economy of illness', in A.J. Enelow and J.B. Henderson (eds), *Applying Behavioral Science to Cardiovascular Risk.* Washington, DC: American Heart Association.

McLeroy, K. (1992) 'Editorial: health education research: theory and practice – future directions', *Health Education Research*, 7: 1–8.

McLeroy, K. (1996) 'Community capacity: what is it? How do we measure it? What is the role of the Prevention Centers and CDC?', in L.K. Bartholomew, G.S. Parcel, G. Kok and N.H. Gottlieb, *Intervention Mapping: Designing Theory- and Evidence-based Health Promotion Programs.* Mountain View, CA: Mayfield.

McLeroy, K., Steckler, A.B., Simons-Morton, B., Goodman, R M., Gotlieb, N. and Burdine, J.N. (1993) 'Editorial: social science theory in health education: time for a new model', *Health Education Research*, 8 (3): 305–11.

McMillan, D.W. and Chavis, D.M. (1986) 'Sense of community: a definition and theory', *Journal of Community Psychology*, 16: 6–23.

McPhail, P., Ungoed-Thomas, J.R. and Chapman, H. (1972) 'Moral education in the secondary school', in J. Ryder and C. Campbell, *Balancing Acts in Personal, Social and Health Education.* London: Routledge.

McPherson, K. (1994) 'The best and the enemy of the good: randomised controlled trials, uncertainty, and assessing the role of patient choice in medical decision making', *Journal of Epidemiology and Community Health*, 48: 6–15.

McQuail, D. (ed.) (1972) *Sociology of Mass Communications*. Harmondsworth: Penguin.

McQuail, D. (1994) *Mass Communication Theory: An Introduction* (3rd edn). London: Sage.

Mendelsohn, H. (1968) 'Which shall it be? Mass education or mass persuasion for health?', *American Journal of Public Health*, 58: 131–7.

Michell, L. (1997) 'Loud, sad or bad: young people's perceptions of peer groups and smoking', *Health Education Research*, 12 (1): 1–14.

Michell, L. and West, P. (1996) 'Peer pressure to smoke: the meaning depends on the method', *Health Education Research*, 11 (1): 39–49.

Michener, J. (1971) *Kent State: What Happened and Why*. New York: Random House.

Middleton, J., Reeves, E., Lilford, R., Howie, F. and Hyde, C. (2001) 'Collaboration with the Campbell Collaboration', *British Medical Journal*, 323: 1252.

Miilunpalo, S., Nupponen, R., Laitakari, J., Martila, J. and Paronen, O. (2000) 'Stages of change in two modes of health-enhancing physical activity: methodological aspects and promotional implications', *Health Education Research*, 15 (4): 435–48.

Milburn, K. (1995) 'A critical review of peer education with young people with special reference to sexual health', *Health Education Research*, 10 (4): 407–20.

Milburn, K., Secker, E.F. and Pavis, S. (1995) 'Combining methods in health promotion research: some considerations about appropriate use', *Health Education Journal*, 54: 347–56.

Milgram, S. (1963) 'Behavioral study of obedience', *Journal of Abnormal and Social Psychology*, 67: 371–8.

Milio, N. (1981) *Promoting Health Through Public Policy*. Philadelphia: F.A. Davis.

Milio, N. (1986) 'Promoting health through public policy', in B. Abel-Smith, *Introduction to Health: Policy, Planning and Financing*. Harlow: Longman.

Milio, N. (1988) 'Making healthy public policy: developing the science by learning the art: an ecological framework for policy studies', *Health Promotion*, 2 (3): 263–74.

Mill, J.S. (1961) *On Liberty*, reprinted in *Essential Works of John Stuart Mill*. New York: Bantam Books.

Miller, I. and Norman, W. (1979) 'Learned helplessness in humans: a review and attribution theory model', *Psychological Bulletin*, 86: 93–118.

Mills, C.W. (1959) *The Sociological Imagination*. New York: Oxford University Press.

MIMAS (2001) *Health Survey for England*. Manchester: MIMAS, The University of Manchester (available from the UK Data Archive *website*: www.data-archive.ac.uk).

Mindell, J., Hansell, A., Morrison, D., Douglas, M. and Joffe, M. (2001) 'What do we need for robust, quantitative health impact assessment?', *Journal of Public Health Medicine*, 23 (3): 173–8.

Minkler, M. (1985) 'Building supportive ties and sense of community among the inner-city elderly: the Tenderloin Senior Outreach Project', *Health Education and Behavior*, 12 (4): 303–14.

Minkler, M. (1990) 'Improving health through community organization', in K. Glanz, F.M. Lewis and B.K. Rimer (eds), *Health Behavior and Health Education: Theory, Research and Practice*. San Francisco: Jossey-Bass.

Minkler, M. and Wallerstein, N. (1997) 'Improving health through community organization and community building', in K. Glanz, F.M. Lewis and B.K. Rimer (eds), *Health Behavior and Health Education: Theory, Research, and Practice* (2nd edn). San Francisco: Jossey-Bass.

Minkler, M., Breckwich Vasquez, V., Rains Warner, J., Steusey, H. and Facente, S. (2006) 'Sowing the seeds for sustainable change: a community-based participatory research partnership for health promotion in Indiana, USA and its aftermath', *Health Promotion International*, 21 (4): 293–300.

Mittelmark, M.B. (1997) 'Health promotion settings' (editorial), *Internet Journal of Health Promotion*. (*Website*: http://elecpress.monash.edu.au/IJHP).

Mittelmark, M.B. (1999a) 'Social ties and health promotion: suggestions for population-based research' (editorial), *Health Education Research*, 14 (4): 447–51.

Mittelmark, M.B. (1999b) 'Health promotion at the community-wide level: lessons from diverse perspectives', in N. Bracht (ed.) *Health Promotion at the Community Level: New Advances*. Thousand Oaks, CA: Sage.

Mittelmark, M.B. (2001) 'Promoting social responsibility for health: health impact assessment and healthy public policy at the community level', *Health Promotion International*, 16 (3): 269–74.

Mittelmark, M.B. (2008) 'Editorial. Health promotion: a professional community for social justice', *Promotion & Education*, 15(2): 3–5.

Mogensen, F. (1997) 'Critical thinking: a central element in developing action competence in health and environmental education', *Health Education Research*, 12 (4): 429–36.

Molleman, G.R.M., Ploeg, M.A., Hosman, C.M.H. and Peters, L.H.M. (2006) 'Preffi 2.0 – a quality assessment tool', *Promotion & Education*, XIII (1): 9–14.

Monahan, J.L. (1995) 'Using positive affect when designing health messages', in E. Maibach and R.L. Parrott, *Designing Health Messages*. Thousand Oaks, CA: Sage.

Mongeau, P.A. (in press) 'Fear-arousing persuasive messages: a meta-analysis re-visited', in M. Allen and R. Preiss (eds) (1998) *Persuasion: Advances Through Meta-Analysis*. Thousand Oaks, CA: Sage.

Moon, G. and Gould, M. (2000) *Epidemiology: An Introduction*. Buckingham: Open University Press.

Mooney, G. and Leeder, S.R. (1997) 'Measuring health needs', in R. Detels, W.W. Holland, J. McEwen and G.S. Omenn (eds), *Oxford Textbook of Public Health* (Vol. 3, 3rd edn). Oxford: Oxford University Press.

Morgan, D. (1998) 'Health and environmental impact assessment', in J. Kemm, 'Health impact assessment: a tool for healthy public policy', *Health Promotion International*, 16 (1): 79–85.

Morrow, V. (2001) 'Using qualitative methods to elicit young people's perspectives on their environments: some ideas for community health initiatives', *Health Education Research*, 16 (3): 255–68.

Morse, J.M. (1994) 'Designing funded qualitative research', in N.K. Denzin and Y.S. Lincoln (eds), *Handbook of Qualitative Research*. Thousand Oaks, CA: Sage.

Munro, G. (2006) 'A decade of failure: self-regulation of alcohol advertising in Australia', *The Globe*, 3: 15–18.

Murphy, S. and Bennett, P. (2004) 'Health psychology and public health: theoretical Possibilities', *Journal of Health Psychology*, 9: 13–27.

Murphy, S.T. and Zajonc, R.B. (1993) 'Affect, cognition, and awareness: affective priming with suboptimal and optimal stimulus', *Journal of Personality and Social Psychology*, 64 (5): 723–39.

Murray, S.A. (1999) 'Experiences with "rapid appraisal" in primary care: involving the public in assessing health needs, orienting staff, and education medical students', *British Medical Journal*, 318: 440–4.

Murray, S. and Graham, L.J.C. (1995) 'Practice-based health needs assessment: use of four methods in a small neighbourhood', *British Medical Journal*, 310: 1443–8.

Musgrave, R. (1959) *The Theory of Public Finance*. New York: McGraw-Hill.

Naidoo, J. and Wills, J. (1994) *Health Promotion Foundations for Practice*. London: Baillière Tindall.

Naidoo, J. and Wills, J. (2005) *Public Health and Health Promotion: Developing Practice*. London: Bailliere Tindall.

Nair, Y. and Campbell, C. (2008) 'Building partnerships to support community-led HIV/AIDS management: a case study from rural South Africa', *African Journal of AIDS Research*, 7 (1): 45–53.

Nancholas, S. (1998) 'How to do (or not to do) … a logical framework', *Health Policy and Planning*, 13 (2): 189–93.

National Assembly for Wales (1999) *Developing Health Impact Assessment in Wales*. Cardiff: National Assembly for Wales.

National Assembly for Wales (2002) *Health Impact Assessment*. Cardiff: National Assembly for Wales.

National Cancer Institute (1997) *Theory at a Glance: A Guide for Health Promotion Practice*. Bethesda, MD: National Cancer Institute. (*Website*: http://oc.nci.nih.gov/services/Theory_at_glance/ HOME. html).

National Cancer Institute (1998) *Making Health Communication Programs Work: A Planners Guide*. Bethesda, MD: Information Project Branch Office.

National Cancer Institute (2005) *Theory at a Glance: A Guide for Health Promotion Practice* (2nd edn). Bethesda: NCI. (*Website*: http://www.nci.nih.gov/PDF/481f5d53-63df-41bc-bfaf-5aa48ee1da4d/TAAG3.pdf).

National Cancer Institute (undated) *Making Health Communication Programs Work*. National Cancer Institute. (*Website*: http://www.cancer.gov/pinkbook).

National Civic League (2002) *A New Approach to Improving Community Life*. Denver, CO: National Civic League. (*Website*: www.ncl.org/cs/articles/okubo1.html).

National Curriculum Council (1990) *Curriculum Guidance 5: Health Education*. York: National Curriculum Council.

National Social Marketing Centre (2005) *Social Marketing Pocket Guide*. London: National Social Marketing Centre. (*Website*: http://www.nsms.org.uk/images/CoreFiles/NSMC_SOCIAL_MARKETING_POCKET_GUIDE_Dec2005.pdf).

National Social Marketing Centre (2006) *Its Our Health*. London: National Social Marketing Centre. (*Website*: http://www.nsms.org.uk/images/CoreFiles/itsourhealth.pdf).

National Social Marketing Centre (2007) *Big Pocket Guide to Social Marketing* (2nd edn). London: National Social Marketing Centre. (*Website*: http://www.nsms.org.uk/images/CoreFiles/NSMC_Big_Pocket_Guide_Aug_2007.pdf).

National Statistics (2001) *The National Statistics Socioeconomic Classification*. London: National Statistics. (*Website*: www.statistics.gov.uk/nsbase/methods_quality/ns_sec/default.asp).

National Statistics (2003) *Social Capital: Measuring Networks and Shared Values*. (*Website*: http://www.statistics.gov.uk/CCI/nugget.asp?ID=314&Pos=&ColRank=1&Rank=374).

National Statistics (2007) *National Statistics Socio-economic Classification*. (*Website*: http://www.statistics.gov.uk/methods_quality/ns_sec/).

National Statistics (undated a) *Factsheet 4: Counting Everyone In – The Big Challenge*. London: National Statistics. (*Website*: www.statistics.gov.uk/census2001/ Introfactsheets.asp).

National Statistics (undated b) *Factsheet 9: The Census Questions*. London: National Statistics. (*Website*: www.statistics.gov.uk/census2001/Introfactsheets.asp).

Navarro, V. (1976) 'The underdevelopment of health of working America: causes, consequences and possible solutions', *American Journal of Public Health*, 66: 538–47.

New Policy Institute (undated) *Choices of Low Income Thresholds*. (*Website*:http://www.poverty.org.uk/summary/income%20intro.shtml).

Newburn, T. (2001) 'What do we mean by evaluation?', *Children and Society*,15 (1): 5–13.

Newcastle Healthy City Project (1997) 'Taking a whole systems approach or why elephants matter', *Whole Systems Newsletter*, 2.

Newman, D.L and Brown, R.B. (1996) *Applied Ethics for Program Evaluation*. Thousand Oaks, CA: Sage.

NHS Centre for Reviews and Dissemination (1993) 'Brief interventions and alcohol use', in V. Speller, A. Learmonth and D. Harrison, 'The search for evidence of health promotion', *British Medical Journal*, 315: 361–3.

NHS Centre for Reviews and Dissemination (1996) *Undertaking Systematic Reviews of Research on Effectiveness: CRD Guidelines for Those Carrying Out or Commissioning Reviews*. York: NHS Centre for Reviews and Dissemination.

NHS Centre for Reviews and Dissemination (1999) 'Getting evidence into practice', *Effective Health Care*, 5 (1).

NHS Centre for Reviews and Dissemination (2001) *Undertaking Systematic Reviews of Research Effectiveness*. CRD Report No. 4 (2nd edn). York: NHS Centre for Reviews and Dissemination. (*Website*: www.york.ac.uk/inst/crd/report4.htm).

NICE (2005) *Public Health Guidance Methods Manual version 1*. London: NICE. (*Website*: http://www.nice.org.uk/niceMedia/pdf/Boardmeeting/brdsep05item42.pdf).

NICE (2007) *NICE Public Health Guidance 6: Behaviour Change*. London: National Institute for Health and Clinical Excellence.

NICE (2008a) *Community Engagement to Improve Health. NICE Public Health Guidance 9*. London: NICE.

NICE (2008b) *Smoking Cessation Services*. (*Website*: http://www.nice.org.uk/PH010)

Nichols, T. (1979) 'Social class: official, sociological and Marxist', in R. Levitas and W. Guy (eds), *Interpreting Official Statistics*. London: Routledge.

Nicholson, C. (2007) 'Framing science: advances in theory and technology are fuelling a new era in the science of persuasion', *APS Observer*, 20 (1). (*Website*: http://www.psychologicalscience.org/observer/getArticle.cfm?id=2118).

Niederdeppe, J., Farrelly, M.C. and Wenter, D. (2007) 'Media advocacy, tobacco control policy change and teen smoking in Florida', *Tobacco Control*, 16 (1): 47–52.

Nikku, N. (1997) *Informative Paternalism: Studies in the Ethics of Promoting and Predicting Health*. Linkoping, Sweden: University of Linkoping.

Nishtar, S., Akerman, M., Amuyunzu-Nyamongo, M. Becker, D. Carroll, S. Goepel, E., Hills, M., Lamarre, M.-C., Mukhopadhyay, A., Perry, M. and Ritchie, J. (2006) 'The statement of the Global Consortium on Community Health Promotion', *Promotion & Education*, XIII (1): 7–8.

Nkosi Johnson AIDS Foundation (undated) 'About Nkosi' and 'Nkosi's speech'. Johannesburg, South Africa: Nkosi Johnson AIDS Foundation. (*Website*: http://nkosi.iafrica.com).

Noar, S.M. and Zimmerman, R.S. (2005) 'Health behaviour theory and cumulative knowledge regarding health behaviours: are we moving in the right direction?', *Health Education Research*, 20 (3): 275–90.

Norman, P. and Bennett, P. (1996) 'Health locus of control', in P. Conner and M. Norman (eds), *Predicting Health Behaviour*. Buckingham: Open University Press.

NRU (2003) *Factsheet 3: Health and Neighbourhood Renewal*. London: ODPM.

NRU (2004) *The English Indices of Deprivation 2004: Summary (revised)*. (*Website*: http://www.communities.gov.uk/documents/communities/pdf/131206).

NSMS Case Study Database (2008) *Spreading the Word about Mouth Cancer*. London: National Social Marketing Centre. (*Website*: http://www.nsms.org.uk/public/CSView.aspx?casestudy=68&menu ID=1).

Nuffield Council on Bioethics (2007) *Public Health: Ethical Issues*. (*Website*: nuffieldbioethics.org).

Nuffield Institute for Health (1993) *Directions for Health: New Approaches to Population Health Research and Practice – The Leeds Declaration*. Leeds: Nuffield Institute for Health.

Nutbeam, D. (1996) 'Achieving "best practice" in health promotion: improving the fit between research and practice', *Health Education Research*, 11 (3): 317–26.

Nutbeam, D. (1998a) 'Evaluating health promotion – progress, problems and solutions', *Health Promotion International*, 13 (1): 27–43.

Nutbeam, D. (1998b) *Health Promotion Glossary*. Geneva: WHO.

Nutbeam, D. (1999) 'The challenge to provide "evidence" in health promotion', *Health Promotion International*, 14 (2): 99–101.

Nutbeam, D. (2000a) 'Health promotion effectiveness – the questions to be answered', in International Union for Health Promotion and Education, *The Evidence of Health Promotion Effectiveness: Shaping Public Health in a New Europe*. Paris: IUHPE.

Nutbeam, D. (2000b) 'Health literacy as a public health goal: a challenge for contemporary health education and communication strategies into the 21st century', *Health Promotion International*, 15 (3): 259–67.

Nutbeam, D. and Harris, E. (eds) (2004) *Theory in a Nutshell: a Guide to Health Promotion Theory* (2nd edn). Sydney, Australia: McGraw-Hill Book Company.

Nutbeam, D., Smith, C., Murphy, S. and Catford, J. (1993) 'Maintaining evaluation designs in long-term community-based health promotion programmes', *Journal of Epidemiology and Public Health*, 47: 127–33.

Oakley, A., Fullerton, D., Holland, J., Arnold, S., France-Dawson, M., Kelley, P. and McGrellis, S. (1995) 'Sexual health education interventions for young people: a methodological review', *British Medical Journal*, 310 (6973): 158–62.

O'Brien, M.O. (1995) 'Health and lifestyle: a critical mess?', in R. Bunton, S. Nettleton and R. Burrows (eds), *The Sociology of Health Promotion*. London: Routledge.

Office of the Deputy Prime Minister and Department of Health (2005) *Creating Healthier Communities: a Resource Pack for Local Partnerships*. Wetherby: ODPM Publications.

OHCHR (1966) *International Covenant on Social, Economic and Cultural Rights*. Geneva: OHCHR. (*Website*: http://www.unhchr.ch/html/menu3/b/a_cescr.htm).

Oldenburg, B., Hardcastle, D.M. and Kok, G. (1997) 'Diffusion of innovations', in K. Glanz, F.M. Lewis and B.K. Rimer (eds), *Health Behavior and Health Education: Theory, Research, and Practice* (2nd edn). San Francisco: Jossey-Bass.

Oldenburg, B.F., Sallis, J.F., French, M.L. and Owen, N. (1999) 'Health promotion research and the diffusion and insitutionalization of interventions', *Health Education Research*, 14 (1): 121–30.

O'Neill, O. (2002) *Reith Lectures 2002: A Question of Trust*. London: BBC. (*Website*: www.bbc.co.uk/radio4/reith2002/5.shtml).

Ong, B.E., Humphris, G., Annett, H. and Rifkin, S. (1991) 'Rapid appraisal in an urban setting, an example from the developed world', *Social Science and Medicine*, 32 (8): 909–15.

ONS (2005) *Summary of Main Topics Included in GHS Questionnaires: 1971–2005*. (*Website*: http://www.statistics.gov.uk/downloads/theme_compendia/GHS05/GHS2005_AppxF.pdf).

Orth-Gomér, K. and Johnson, J.V. (1987) 'A six-year follow-up study of a random sample of the Swedish population', *Journal of Chronic Disease*, 40: 949–57.

Packard, V. (1981) *The Hidden Persuaders: A New Edition for the 1980s*. Harmondsworth: Penguin.

Pahl, R. (1995) 'Friendly society', in C. Campbell, R. Wood and M. Kelly, *Social Capital and Health*. London: Health Education Authority.

Palmer, G., MacInnes, T. and Kenway, P. (2007) *Monitoring Poverty and Social Exclusion*. York: Joseph Rowntree Foundation. (*Website*: http://www.poverty.org.uk/reports/mpse%202007.pdf).

Parcel, G.S. and Meyer, M.P. (1978) 'Development of an instrument to measure children's health locus of control', *Health Education Monographs*, 6 (2): 149–59.

Parcel, G.S., Perry, C.L. and Taylor, W.C. (1990) 'Beyond demonstration: diffusion of health promotion innovations', in N. Bracht (ed.), *Health Promotion at the Community Level*. Newbury Park, CA: Sage.

Parlett, M. and Hamilton, D. (1972) *Evaluation as Illumination: A New Approach to the Study of Innovatory Programmes*, Occasional Paper No. 9. Edinburgh: Centre for Research in the Educational Sciences, University of Edinburgh.

Parsons, C., Stears, D., Thomas, C., Thomas, L. and Holland, J. (1997) *The Implementation of ENHPS in Different National Contexts*. Canterbury: Centre for Health Education and Research, Canterbury Christchurch College.

Parsons, T. (1958) 'Definitions of health and illness in the light of American values and social structure', in E. Jaco (ed.), *Patients, Physicians and Illness*. New York: Free Press.

Parsons, T. (1967) *Sociological Theory and Modern Society*. New York: Free Press.

Paterson, D. (1999) *Augusto Boal: A Brief Biography*. Omaha, NE: Pedagogy and Theatre of the Oppressed. (*Website*: www.unomaha.edu/~pto/ augusto.htm).

Patton, M.Q. (1982) *Practical Evaluation*. Beverly Hills, CA: Sage.

Patton, M.Q. (1997) *Utilization Focused Evaluation*. Thousand Oaks, CA: Sage.

Pawson, R. and Tilley, N. (1997) *Realistic Evaluation*. London: Sage.

Pawson, R. (2002) 'Evidence-based policy: the promise of a 'realist synthesis', *Evaluation*, 8(3): 340–58.

Peltzer, K. and Promtussananon, S. (2003) 'Evaluation of Soul City School and mass media lifeskills education among junior secondary school learners in South Africa', *Social Behavior and Personality*, January.

Performance and Innovation Unit (2002) *Social Capital: a Discussion Paper*. (*Website*: http://www.cabinetoffice.gov.uk/upload/assets/www.cabinetoffice.gov.uk/strategy/socialcapital.pdf).

Perkins, E.R., Simnett, I. and Wright, L. (1999) *Evidence-based Health Promotion*. Chichester: John Wiley.

Petersen, A. and Lupton, D. (1996) *The New Public Health: Health and Self in the Age of Risk*. London: Sage.

Petty, R. and Cacioppo, J. (1986) 'The elaboration likelihood model of persuasion', in L. Berkowitz (ed.), *Advances in Experimental Social Psychology, Vol. 19*: 123–205. Orlando, FL: Academic Press.

Pfau, M. (1995) 'Designing messages for behavioral inoculation', in E. Maibach and R.L. Parrott (eds), *Designing Health Messages*. Thousand Oaks, CA: Sage.

Pfau, M. and Van Bockern, S. (1994) 'The persistence of inoculation in conferring resistance to smoking initiation among adolescents: the second year', *Human Communication Research*, 20: 413–30.

Piaget, J. and Inhelder, B. (1969) *The Psychology of the Child*. London: Routledge & Kegan Paul.

Pickin, C. and St Leger, S. (1993) *Assessing Health Needs: Using the Lifecycle Framework*. Buckingham: Open University Press.

Poland, B., Green, L.W. and Rootman, I. (2000a) 'Reflections on settings for health promotion', in B. Poland, L.W. Green and Rootman, I. (eds), *Settings for Health Promotion: Linking Theory and Practice*. Thousand Oaks, CA: Sage.

Poland, B., Green, L.W. and Rootman, I. (2000b) *Settings for Health Promotion: Linking Theory and Practice*. Thousand Oaks, CA: Sage.

Pollard, M.R. and Brennan, J.T. (1978) 'Disease prevention and health promotion initiatives: some legal considerations', *Health Education Monographs*, 6 (2): 211–22.

Pool, H. (1992) *Illness Behaviour and Utilisation of the INF TB Clinic in Surkhet, Nepal*. Unpublished MSc dissertation. Leeds: Leeds Metropolitan University.

Popham, W.J. (1978) 'Must all objectives be behavioural?', in D. Hamilton and M. Parlett (eds), *Beyond the Numbers Game*. London: Macmillan.

Popper, K. (1945) *The Open Society and Its Enemies*. London: Routledge.

Popper, K. (1959) *The Logic of Scientific Discovery*. London: Hutchinson.

Porter, C. (2006) 'Ottawa to Bangkok: changing health promotion discourse', *Health Promotion International*, 22 (1): 72–9.

Porter, P.W. (1998) *A World of Difference: Society, Nature and Development*. New York: Guilford Press.

Potvin, L. and McQueen, D. (2007) 'Modernity, public health and health promotion: a reflexive discourse', in D.V. McQueen and I. Kickbush, *Health and Modernity: The Role of Theory in Health Promotion*. New York: Springer.

Pawson, R. (2002) 'Evidence-based policy: the promise of a 'realist synthesis', *Evaluation*, 8(3): 340–58.

Powles, J. (1988) 'Victoria's food and nutrition policy', *Health Promotion*, 2 (3): 240–2.

Prashar, A., Abrahams, D., Taylor, D. and Scott-Samuel, A. (2004) *Merseytram Line 1: A Health Impact Assessment of the Proposed Scheme*. Liverpool: The International Health Impact Assessment Consortium. (*Website*: http://www.apho.org.uk/resource/item.aspx?RID=53280).

Pressman, J. and Wildavsky, A. (1973) *Implementation: How Great Expectations in Washington are Dashed in Oakland*. Berkeley, CA: University of California Press.

Pridmore, P. (1996) 'Visualising health: exploring perceptions of children using the draw and write method promotion and education', *Promotion & Education*, III (4): 11–15.

Prochaska, J.O. and DiClemente, C.C. (1983) 'Stages and processes of self-change of smoking: toward an integrative model of change', *Journal of Consulting and Clinical Psychology*, 51: 390–5.

Prochaska, J.O. and DiClemente, C.C. (1984) *The Trans-theoretical Approach: Crossing Traditional Boundaries of Therapy*. Homewood, IL: Dow Jones Irwin.

Prochaska, J.O., Redding, C.A. and Evers, K.E. (1997) 'The transtheoretical model and stages of change', in K. Glanz, F.M. Lewis and B.K. Rimer (eds), *Health Behavior and Health Education: Theory, Research, and Practice* (2nd edn). San Francisco: Jossey-Bass.

Pruger, R. and Specht, H. (1972) 'Assessing theoretical models of community organization practice: Alinsky as a case in point', in G. Zaltman, P. Kotler and I. Kaufman (eds), *Creating Social Change*. New York: Holt, Rinehart & Winston.

Public Health Resource Unit and Skills for Health and Public Health Resource Unit (2008) *Public Health Skills and Career Framework Multidisciplinary/Multi-Agency/Multi-Professional*. (*Website*: http://www.phru.nhs.uk/Doc_Links/PHSkills&CareerFramework_Launchdoc_April08.pdf).

Putnam, R.D. (1993) *Making Democracy Work: Civic Traditions in Modern Italy*. Princeton, NJ: Princeton University Press.

Putnam, R.D. (1995) 'Bowling alone: America's declining social capital', *Journal of Democracy*, 6 (1): 65–79.

Putnam, R.D. (1996) 'The strange disappearance of civic America', *The American Prospect*, 7 (24). (*Website*: www.prospect.org/print/V7/24/putnam-r.html).

Quinn, S.C. (1999) 'Teaching community diagnosis: integrating community experience with meeting graduate standards for health educators', *Health Education Research*, 14 (5): 685–96.

Radical Statistics Health Group (1987) *Facing the Figures*. London: Radical Statistics Health Group.

Radius, S.M., Galer-Unti, R.A. and Tappe, M.K. (2008) 'Educating for advocacy: recommendations for professional preparation and development based on a needs and capacity assessment of health education faculty', *Health Promotion Practice OnlineFirst*, 1 April.

Raeburn, J. and MacFarlane, S. (2003) 'Putting the public into public health: towards a more people-centred approach', in R. Beaglehole (ed.), *Global Public Health: a New Era*. Oxford: Oxford University Press.

Raeburn, J.M. and Rootman, I. (1989) 'Towards an expanded health field concept: conceptual and research issues in an era of health promotion', *Health Promotion*, 3 (4): 383–92.

Rahman, M.A. (1995) 'Participatory development: toward liberation or co-optation', in G. Craig and M. Mayo, (eds) *Community Empowerment*. London: Zed Books.

Rahman, M., Kenway, P. and Howarth, C. (2000) *Monitoring Poverty and Social Exclusion 2000*. York: Joseph Rowntree Foundation.

Rainey, R.C. and Harding, A.K. (2005) 'Acceptability of solar disinfection of drinking water treatment in Kathmandu Valley, Nepal', *International Journal of Environmental Health Research*, 15 (5): 361–72.

Rakow, L.F. (1989) 'Information and power: toward a critical theory of information campaigns', in C.T. Salmon (ed.), *Information Campaigns: Balancing Social Values and Social Change*. Newbury Park, CA: Sage.

Rangun, V.K., Karim, S. and Sandberg, S.K. (1996) 'Do better at doing good', *Harvard Business Review*, 74 (3): 42–54.

Rankin, S.H. and Stallings, K.D. (2001) *Patient Education: Principles and Practice*. Philadelphia: Lippincott.

Raphael, D. (2000) 'The question of evidence in health promotion', *Health Promotion International*, 15 (4): 355–67.

Raphael, D. (2001a) *Inequality is Bad for Our Hearts: Why Low Income and Social Exclusion are Major Causes of Heart Disease in Canada*. Toronto: North York Heart Health Network.

Raphael, D. (2001b) 'Evaluation of quality-of-life initiatives in health promotion', in I. Rootman, M. Goodstadt, B. Hyndman, D.V. McQueen, L. Potvin, J. Springett and E. Ziglio (eds), *Evaluation in Health Promotion: Principles and Perspectives*. Copenhagen: WHO.

Raphael, D. (2008) 'Grasping at straws: a recent history of health promotion in Canada', *Critical Public Health*, 18 (4): 483–95.

Rappaport, J. (1987) 'Terms of empowerment/exemplars of prevention: toward a policy for community psychology', *American Journal of Community Psychology*, 15 (2): 121–47.

Rawson, D. (1992) 'The growth of health promotion theory and its rational reconstruction', in R. Bunton and G. Macdonald (eds), *Health Promotion: Disciplines and Diversity*. London: Routledge.

Reardon, K.K. (1981) *Persuasion: Theory and Context*. Beverley Hills, CA: Sage.

Reason, P. and Rowan, J. (eds) (1981) *Human Enquiry: A Sourcebook of New Paradigm Research*. Chichester: Wiley.

Reich, M.R. (2002) *The Politics of Reforming Health Policies*. 5th European Conference on Effectiveness and Quality of Health Promotion, London, 11–13 June.

Research and Evaluation Division of HEBS (1996) 'How effective are effectiveness reviews?' (editorial), *Health Education Journal*, 55: 359–62.

Rhodes, A. (1976) *Propaganda: The Art of Persuasion, World War II*. London: Angus & Robertson.

Rifkin, S. (1992) 'Rapid appraisals for health: an overview', *RRA Notes Number 16: Special Issue on Applications for Health*: 7–12.

Rigler, M. (1996) *Withymoor Village Surgery – a Health Hive*. Dudley: Dudley Priority Health NHS Trust.

Rissel, C. and Bracht, N. (1999) 'Assessing community needs, resources and readiness', in N. Bracht (ed.), *Health Promotion at the Community Level: New Advances* (2nd edn). Thousand Oaks, CA: Sage.

Ritchie, J.E. (2007) 'Criteria and checkpoints for better community health promotion', *Promotion & Education*, XIV (2): 96–7.

Rivers, K., Aggleton, P., Chaise, E., Downie, A., Milvihill, C., Sinkler, P., Tyrer, P. and Warwick, I. (1999) *Learning Lessons: A Report on Two Research Studies Informing the National Healthy School Standard*. London: Department of Health and Department for Education and Employment.

Roberts, A.H. (1969) 'Self control procedures in modification of smoking behaviors: replication', *Psychological Reports*, 24: 675–6.

Roberts, H. (1990) *Women's Health Counts*. London: Routledge.

Roberts, H. (1998) 'Empowering communities: the case of childhood accidents', in S. Kendall (ed.), *Health and Empowerment*. London: Arnold.

Roberts, I. and Power, C. (1996) 'Does the decline in child injury mortality vary by social class? A comparison of class-specific mortality in 1981 and 1991', *British Medical Journal*, 313: 784–6.

Robinson, J. and Elkan, R. (1996) *Health Needs Assessment: Theory and Practice*. London: Churchill Livingstone.

Robinson, S. (2006) 'Victimisation of obese adolescents', *Journal of School Nursing*, 224: 201–6.

Robson C. (1993) *Real World Research*. Oxford: Blackwell.

Rogers, A. and Whyms, D. (1995) 'A broader horizon for health promotion', *Health Matters*, 21: 12–13.

Rogers, C. (1967) 'The interpersonal relationship in the facilitation of learning', in H. Kirschenbaum and V.L. Henderson (eds) (1990 edn), *The Carl Rogers Reader*. London: Constable.

Rogers, C. (1983) 'Freedom to learn for the eighties', in J. Ryder and L. Campbell, *Balancing Acts in Personal, Social and Health Education: A Practical Guide for Teachers*. London: Routledge.

Rogers, E.M. (1995) *The Diffusion of Innovations* (4th edn). New York: The Free Press.

Rogers, E.M. (2003) *Diffusion of Innovation Theory* (5th edn). New York: The Free Press.

Rogers, E.M. and Shoemaker, F.F. (1971) *Communication of Innovations*. New York: The Free Press.

Rogers, E.M. and Shoemaker, F.F. (1979) *Communication of Innovations: A Cross-Cultural Approach*. New York: The Free Press.

Rogers, R.W. (1975) 'A protection motivation theory of fear appeals and attitude change', *Journal of Psychology*, 91: 93–114.

Rogers, T., Howard-Pitney, B., Feighery, E.C., Altman, D.G., Endres, J.M. and Roeseler, A.G. (1993) 'Characteristics and participants' perceptions of tobacco control coalitions in California', *Health Education Research*, 8 (3): 345–57.

Rokeach, M. (1965) 'The nature of attitudes', in D.L. Sills (ed.), *International Encyclopaedia of the Social Sciences*. New York: Macmillan and The Free Press.

Rokeach, M. (1973) *The Nature of Human Values*. New York: The Free Press.

Rollnick, S., Heather, N. and Bell, A. (1992) 'Negotiating behavior change in medical settings: the development of brief motivational interviewing', *Journal of Mental Health*, 1: 25–37.

Rootman, I. (2001) 'Introduction', in I. Rootman, M. Goodstadt, L. Potvin and J. Springett, in 'A framework for health promotion evaluation', in I. Rootman, M. Goodstadt, B. Hyndman, D.V. McQueen, L. Potvin, J. Springett and E. Ziglio (eds), *Evaluation in Health Promotion: Principles and Perspectives*. Copenhagen: WHO.

Rootman, I., Goodstadt, M., Potvin, L. and Springett, J. (2001) 'A framework for health promotion evaluation', in I. Rootman, M. Goodstadt, B. Hyndman, D.V. McQueen, L. Potvin, J. Springett and E. Ziglio (eds), *Evaluation in Health Promotion: Principles and Perspectives*. Copenhagen: WHO.

Rose, G. (1992) *The Strategy of Preventive Medicine*. Oxford: Oxford Medical Publications.

Rosenstock, I.M. (1966) 'Why people use health services', *Millbank Memorial Fund Quarterly*, 44: 94–124.

Rosenstock, I.M. (1974) 'Historical origins of the health belief model', *Health Education Monographs*, 2: 1–8.

Rosenthal, H. (1983) 'Neighbourhood health projects: some new approaches to health and community work in parts of the UK', *Community Development Journal*, 13: 122–31.

Ross, H.S. and Mico, P.R. (1980) *Theory and Practice in Health Education*. Palo Alto, CA: Mayfield.

Ross, M.G. and Lappin, B.W. (1967) *Community Organization: Theory, Principles and Practice*. New York: Harper & Row.

Rothman, A.J. and Salovey, P. (1997) 'Shaping perceptions to motivate healthy behavior: the role of message framing', *Psychological Bulletin*, 121: 3–19.

Rothman, J. (1979) 'Three models of community organization in practice', in F.M. Cox, J.L. Erlich, J. Rothman and J.E. Tropman (eds), *Strategies of Community Organization: A Book of Readings* (3rd edn). Itasca, IL: Peacock.

Rotter, J.B. (1966) 'Generalized expectancies for internal versus external control of reinforcement', *Psychological Monographs*, 80 (1): 1–28.

Rowling, L. (1996) 'The adaptability of the health promoting school concept: a case study from Australia', *Health Education Research*, 11 (4): 519–26.

Royle, J. and Speller, V. (1996) 'Assuring quality in health promotion', paper presented at 'Quality Assessment in Health Promotion and Education', the Third European Conference on Effectiveness, Turin, Italy, September 1996, in V. Speller, L. Rogers and A. Rushmere, 'Quality assessment in health promotion settings', in J.K. Davies and G. Macdonald, *Quality Evidence and Effectiveness in Health Promotion*. London: Routledge.

Russell, M.A.H., Wilson, C., Taylor, C. and Baker, C.D. (1979) 'Effect of general practitioners' advice against smoking', *British Medical Journal*, 2: 231–5.

Rutter, M., Maughan, B., Mortimore, P. and Ouston, J. (1979) *Fifteen Thousand Hours*. London: Open Books.

Ryan, W. (1976) *Blaming the Victim*. New York: Vintage Books.

Rychetnik, L. and Wise, M. (2004) 'Advocating evidence-based health promotion: reflections and a way forward', *Health Promotion International*, 19 (2): 247–57.

Ryder, J. and Campbell, L. (1988) *Balancing Acts in Personal, Social and Health Education: A Practical Guide for Teachers*. London: Routledge.

Saan, H. and de Haes, W. (undated) *HP Framework*. (*Website*: http://www.nigz.nl/index. cfm?act=esite.tonen&pagina=105&a=6&b=105)

Sacker, A., Firth, D., Fitzpatrick, R., Lynch, K. and Bartley, M. (2000) 'Comparing health inequality in men and women: prospective study of mortality 1986–96', *British Medical Journal*, 320: 1303–7.

Sackett, D.L., Rosenberg, W.M.C., Gray, J.A.M., Haynes, R.B. and Richardson, W.S. (1996) 'Evidence-based medicine: what it is and what it isn't', *British Medical Journal*, 312: 71–2.

Saracci, R. (1997) 'The world health organisation needs to reconsider its definition of health', *British Medical Journal*, 314: 1409.

Sarafino, E.P. (1990) *Health Psychology: Biopsychosocial Interactions*. New York: John Wiley.

Sarbin, T.R. and Allen, V.L. (1968) 'Role theory', in G. Lindzey and E. Aronson, *Handbook of Social Psychology* (Vol. 1). Reading: Addison-Wesley.

Sarler, C. (1996) 'Dear Marje!', *The Independent*, 15 November.

SAS (2008) *Return to Offender*. Surfers Against Sewage. (*Website*: http://www.sas.org.uk/campaign/ marine_litter/return_to_offender.php).

Saussure, F. de (1915) *Course in General Linguistics*. London: Peter Owen. (English translation, 1960.)

Scala, K. (1996) *Health Promotion as Intervention in Social Settings*. Late European Summer School: Stratechniques for Health Promotion, 6–11 October, Zeist, The Netherlands, NIGZ.

Scheeran, P. and Abraham, C. (1996) 'The health belief model', in M. Conner and P. Norman (eds), *Predicting Health Behaviour*. Buckingham: Open University Press.

Schnack, K. (2000) 'Action competence as a curriculum perspective', in B.B. Jensen, K. Schnack and V. Simovska, *Critical Environmental and Health Education: Research Issues and Challenges*. Copenhagen: Danish University of Education.

Schramm, W. and Roberts, D.F. (1972) *The Process and Effects of Mass Communication*. Urbana, IL: University of Illinois Press.

Schwandt, T.A. (1994) 'Constructivist, interpretivist approaches to human inquiry', in N.K. Denzin and Y.S. Lincoln (eds), *Handbook of Qualitative Research*. Thousand Oaks, CA: Sage.

Schwartzer, R. and Leppin, A. (1992) 'Possible impact of social ties and support on morbidity and mortality', in M.B. Mittelmark, 'Editorial: Social ties and health promotion: suggestions for population-based research', *Health Education Research*, 14 (4): 447–51.

Sciacca, J. (1987) 'Student peer health education: a powerful yet inexpensive helping strategy', *The Peer Facilitator Quarterly*, 5: 4–6, in K. Milburn, 'A critical review of peer education with young people with special reference to sexual health', *Health Education Research*, 10 (4): 407–20.

Scott, B.E., Schmidt, W.P., Aunger, R., Garbrah-Aidoo, N. and Animashaun, R. (2008) 'Marketing hygiene behaviours: the impact of different communication channels on reported handwashing behaviour of women in Ghana', *Health Education Research*, 23 (3): 392–401.

Scottish Government DG Health and Wellbeing (2007) *Towards a Mentally Flourishing Scotland: The Future of Mental Health Improvement in Scotland 2008–11*. (*Website*: http://www.wellscotland.info/uploads/post-2008.pdf).

Scott-Samuel, A. and O'Keefe, E. (2007) 'Health impact assessment, human rights and global public policy: a critical appraisal', *Bulletin of the World Health Organisation 2007*, 85 (3): 211–17.

Scott-Samuel, A. and Springett, J. (2007) 'Hegemony or health promotion? Prospects for reviving England's last discipline', *Journal of the Royal Society of Health*, 127 (5): 211–14.

Scriven, A. (2007) 'Guest editorial: shaping the future has become the rallying cry for health promoters in the first decade of the 21st century', *The Journal of the Royal Society for the Promotion of Health*, 127 (5): 206.

Scriven, A. and Speller, V. (2007) 'Global issues and challenges beyond Ottawa: the way forward', *Promotion & Education*, XIV (4): 194–8.

Secretary of State for Social Security (1999) *Opportunity for All: Tackling Poverty and Social Exclusion*. London: The Stationery Office.

Seligman, M.E.P. (1975) *Helplessness: On Depression, Development and Death*. San Francisco: W.H. Freeman.

Serrano-Garcia, I. (1984) 'The illusion of empowerment: community development within a colonial context', in J. Rappaport (ed.), *Studies in Empowerment: Steps Toward Understanding and Action*. New York: The Howarth Press.

Settle, D. and Wise, C. (1986) 'Choices: materials and methods for personal and social education', in J. Ryder and C. Campbell, *Balancing Acts in Personal, Social and Health Education*. London: Routledge.

Shacklock Evans, E.G. (1962) 'The design of teaching experiments in education', *Educational Research*, V (1): 37–52.

Shavelson, R.J. and Marsh, H.W. (1986) 'On the structure of self concept', in RT. Schwarzer (ed.), *Anxiety and Cognitions*. Hillsdale, NJ: Erlbaum.

Shaw, M., Dorling, D. and Davey Smith, G. (1999) 'Poverty, social exclusion and minorities', in M. Marmot and G. Wilkinson (eds), *Social Determinants of Health*. Oxford: Oxford University Press.

Shaw, M (2004) *Community Work: Policy, Politics and Practice*. Hull: Universities of Hull and Edinburgh.

Shilton, T., Howat, P., James, R., Burke, L., Hutchins, C. and Woodman, R. (2008) 'Health promotion competencies for Australia 2001–5: trends and their implications', *Promotion & Education*, 15 (2): 21–6.

Signal, L. (1998) 'The politics of health promotion: insights from political theory', *Health Promotion International,* 13(3): 257–63.

Sills, D.L (ed.) (1965) *International Encyclopaedia of the Social Sciences.* New York: Macmillan and The Free Press.

Sindall, C. (1997) 'Intersectoral collaboration: the best of times, the worst of times', *Health Promotion International,* 12 (1): 5–6.

Sindall, C. (2002) 'Does health promotion need a code of ethics?' *Health Promotion International,* 17 (3): 201–3.

Skills for Health and Public Health Resource Unit (2009) *Public Health Skills and Career Framework Multidisciplinary/Multi-Agency/Multi-Professional.* (*Website*: http://www.skillsforhealth.org.uk/workforce-design-development/workforce-design-and-planning/tools-and-methodologies/career-frameworks/~/media/Resource-Library/PDF/Public_Health_Report_Web-April_09.ashx).

Skinner, B.F. (1971) *Beyond Freedom and Dignity.* New York: Knopf.

Slovic, P., Fischoff, B. and Lichtenstein, S. (1982) 'Why study risk perception?', *Risk Analysis,* 2 (2): 89–93.

Smith, B.J., Tang, K.C. and Nutbeam, D. (2006) 'WHO health promotion glossary: new terms', *Health Promotion International,* 21 (4): 340–5.

Smith, M.K. (2006) *Community Work.* (*Website*: http://www.infed.org/community/b-comwrk.htm).

Smith, N.J. (1997) 'Policy networks', in M. Hill (ed.), *The Policy Process: A Reader.* London: Prentice Hall/Harvester Wheatsheaf.

Smith, N., Littlejohns, L.B. and Thompson, D. (2001) 'Shaking out the cobwebs: insights into community capacity and its relation to health outcomes', *Community Development Journal,* 36 (1): 30–41.

Smith, R. (2007) *Reducing Health Inequalities – Issues for London and Priorities for Action.* London: Greater London Authority. (*Website*: http://www.london.gov.uk/mayor/health/docs/finalissuesforlondon2007.pdf).

Smoke Free Movies (undated) *Big Tobacco's Secret History in Hollywood.* (*Website*: http://smokefreemovies.ucsf.edu/problem/bigtobacco.html).

Sobel, M.E. (1981) *Lifestyle and Social Structure: Concepts, Definition, Analyses.* New York: Academic Press.

Social Exclusion Unit (1999) *Teenage Pregnancy.* London: The Stationery Office.

Social Marketing Institute (undated) *About Us.* (*Website*: http://www.social-marketing.org/aboutus.html).

Society of Health Education and Health Promotion Specialists (1997) *Code of Professional Conduct for Health Education and Health Promotion Specialists.* Principles and Practice Standing Committee, Society of Health Education and Health Promotion Specialists.

Solomon, D.S. (1989) 'A social marketing perspective on communication campaigns', in R.E. Rice and C.K. Atkin (eds), *Public Communication Campaigns* (2nd edn). Newbury Park, CA: Sage.

Song, I.S. and Hattie, J.A. (1984) 'Home environment, self concept and academic achievement: a causal modeling approach,' *Journal of Educational Psychology,* 76: 1269–81.

SOPHE (Society for Public Health Education) (1976) *Code of Ethics.* Washington, DC: SOPHE.

SOPHE (2001) *Code of Ethics for the Health Education Profession.* Washington, DC: SOPHE. (*Website*: www. sophe.org/about/ethics.html).

SOPHE (2008) *Toward Domains of Core Competency for Building Global Capacity in Health Promotion: The Galway Consensus Conference Statement.* (*Website*: http://www.sophe.org/upload/Galway%20Consensus%20Conference%20Statement%20-%20Final_84911642_6302008111733.pdf).

Soul City Institute (2008) *Soul Beat Africa.* Soul City Institute Health and Development Communication. (*Website*: http://www.comminit.com/en/africa/about-soul-city.html).

South, J. and Tilford, S. (2000) 'Perceptions of research and evaluation in health promotion', *Health Education Research,* 15 (6): 729–41.

Speller, V. (1998) 'Quality assurance programmes: their development and contribution to improving effectiveness in health promotion', in D. Scott and R. Weston (eds), *Evaluating Health Promotion*. Cheltenham: Stanley Thornes.

Speller, V., Evans, D. and Head, M.J. (1997a) 'Developing quality assurance standards for health promotion practice in the UK', *Health Promotion International*, 12 (3): 215–24.

Speller, V., Learmonth, A. and Harrison, D. (1997b) 'The search for evidence of effective health promotion', *British Medical Journal*, 315: 361–3.

Speller, V., Rogers, L. and Rushmere, A. (1998) 'Quality assessment in health promotion settings', in J.K. Davies and G. Macdonald (eds), *Quality, Evidence and Effectiveness in Health Promotion*. London: Routledge.

Springett, J. (1998) 'Quality measures and evaluation of healthy city policy initiatives', in J.K. Davies and G. Macdonald (eds), *Quality, Evidence and Effectiveness in Health Promotion*. London: Routledge.

Springett, J. (2001) 'Appropriate approaches to the evaluation of health promotion', *Critical Public Health*, 11 (2): 139–51.

St Leger, L. (1998) 'Australian teachers' understanding of the health promoting school concept and the implications for the development of school health', *Health Promotion International*, 13 (3): 223–35.

St Leger, L. (1999) 'The opportunities and effectiveness of the health promoting primary school in improving child health – a review of the claims and evidence', *Health Education Research*, 14 (1): 51–70.

St Leger, L. (2001) 'Building and finding the new leaders in health promotion', *Health Promotion International*, 16 (4): 301–3.

St Leger, L. (2005) 'Protocols and guidelines for health promoting schools', *Promotion & Education*, XII (3–4): 145–7.

Stacey, M. (1994) 'The power of lay knowledge', in J. Popay and J. Williams (eds), *Researching the People's Health*. London: Routledge.

Stainton Rogers, W. (1991) *Explaining Health and Illness: An Exploration of Diversity*. London: Harvester Wheatsheaf.

Stake, R.E. (1995) *The Art of Case Study Research*. Thousand Oaks, CA: Sage.

Standing Conference for Community Development (2001) *Strategic Framework for Community Development*. Sheffield: SCCD. (*Website*: http://www.cdx.org.uk/files/u1/sframepdf.pdf).

Stansfield, S.A. (1999) 'Social support and social cohesion', in M. Marmot and R.G. Wilkinson (eds), *Social Determinants of Health*. Oxford: Oxford University Press.

Stenhouse, L. (1975) 'A critique of the objectives model', in L. Stenhouse, (ed.), *An Introduction to Curriculum Research and Development*. London: Heinemann.

Sternberg, P. (2002) *Nicaraguan Men's Involvement in Sexual and Reproductive Health Promotion*, unpublished PhD thesis. Leeds: Leeds Metropolitan University.

Stewart-Brown, S. (2006) *What is the Evidence on School Health Promotion in Improving Health or Preventing Disease and, Specifically, What is the Effectiveness of the Health Promoting Schools Approach?* Copenhagen: WHO Regional Office for Europe, Health Evidence Network report. (*Website*: http://www.euro.who.int/document/e88185.pdf).

Stewart Burgher, M., Rasmussen, V.B. and Rivett, D. (1999) *The European Network of Health Promoting Schools: The Alliance of Education and Health*. Copenhagen: WHO Regional Office for Europe.

Stufflebeam, D. (1980) 'An interview with Daniel L. Stufflebeam', *Educational Evaluation and Policy Analysis*, 2 (4).

Suchman, E.A. (1967) *Evaluative Research: Principles in Public Service and Action Programs*. New York: Russell Sage.

Summerfield, L.M. (1995) 'National standards for school health education', *ERIC Digest* (ED 387483). ERIC Clearinghouse on Teaching and Teacher Education, Washington, DC. (*Website*: www.ericfacility.net/data-bases/ ERIC-Digests/index).

Supplementary Benefits Commission (1979) *Annual Report for 1978.* London: HMSO.

SureStart (2005) *SureStart Homepage.* (*Website*: http://www.surestart.gov.uk/).

Sutcliffe, T. (1994) 'Don't blame him, he's just a poor sex addict', *The Independent,* June.

Sutherland, E.H. and Cressy, D.R. (1960) *Principles of Criminology.* Philadelphia: Lippincott.

Sutherland, I. (1979) *Health Education: Perspectives and Choices.* London: Allen & Unwin.

Sutherland, I. (1987) *Health Education: Half A Policy: The Rise and Fall of the Health Education Council.* Cambridge: National Extension College.

Sutton, S.R. (1982) 'Fear-arousing communication: a critical examination of theory and research', in J.R. Eiser (ed.), *Social Psychology and Behavioural Medicine.* London: Wiley.

Swann, C., Falce, C., Morgan, A., Kelly, M., Powel, G., Carmona, C., Taylor, L. and Taske, N. (2005) *HDA Evidence Base Process and Quality Standards Manual for Evidence Briefings* (3rd, edn). London: NICE. (*Website*: http://www.nice.org.uk/niceMedia/docs/Process_And_Quality_Standards_Manual_For_Evidence_Briefings-March2005[1].pdf).

Swinburn, B.A. (2008) 'Obesity prevention: the role of policies, laws and regulations', *Australia and New Zealand Health Policy,* 5 (12). (*Website*: http://www.anzhealthpolicy.com/content/5/1/12).

Talbot, R.J. (1991) 'Underprivileged areas and healthcare planning: implications of use of Jarman indicators of urban deprivation', *British Medical Journal,* 302: 383–6.

Tannahill, A. (1992) 'Epidemiology and health promotion: a common understanding', in R. Bunton and G. Macdonald (eds), *Health Promotion Disciplines and Diversity.* London: Routledge.

Taylor, L. and Blair-Stevens, C. (2002) *Introducing Health Impact Assessment (HIA): Informing the Decision-making Process.* London: Health Development Agency.

Taylor, M. (1995) 'Community work and the state: the changing context of UK practice', in G. Craig and M. Mayo (eds), *Community Empowerment: A Reader in Participation and Development.* London: Zed Books.

Teenage Pregnancy Unit (2000) *A Guide to Local Campaigning: Information on Using the Media.* London: Department of Health.

Terence Higgins Trust (2001) *Social Exclusion and HIV: A Report.* London: Terence Higgins Trust.

Terris M. (1983) 'The complex tasks of the second epidemiologic revolution', *Journal of Public Health Policy,* 4(1): 8–24.

Terris, M. (1996) 'Concepts of health promotion: dualities in public health theory', in J. French, *Understanding Health Promotion Through Its Fault Lines.* PhD thesis. Leeds: Leeds Metropolitan University.

Tesh, S., Tuohy, C., Christoffel, T., Hancock, T., Norsigian, J., Nightingale, E. and Robertson, L. (1988) 'The meaning of healthy public policy', *Health Promotion,* 2 (3): 257–62.

The Communication Evaluation Expert Panel (2007) 'Guidance for evaluating mass media communication health initiatives: summary of an expert panel discussion sponsored by the Centers for Disease Control and Prevention', *Evaluation and the Health Professions,* 30 (3): 229–53.

The Health Communication Unit (2000) *Media Advocacy Workbook.* Toronto: Health Communication Unit. (*Website*: http://www.thcu.ca/resource_db/pubs/497736921.pdf).

The Health Communication Unit (2001) *Logic Models Workbook Version 6.1.* (*Website*: http://www.thcu.ca/infoandresources/publications/logicmodel.wkbk.v6.1.full.aug27.pdf).

The Health Communication Unit (2003) *Health Communication and Community Mobilisation: Complementary Strategies for Health Promotion.* The Health Communication Unit, University of Toronto. (*Website*: www.thcu.ca/infoandresources/publications/Health_Comm_and_Comm_Mob.v2.0.content%20Dec%2095_format_June.13.03.doc).

The Informatics Review (undated) *Comprehension and Reading Level.* (*Website*: http://www.informatics-review.com/FAQ/reading.html).

The Poverty Site (undated) *Choice of Low Income Threshold.* (*Website*: http://www.poverty.org.uk/summary/income%20intro.shtml).

The Welsh Health Impact Assessment Support Unit (2004) *Improving Health and Reducing Inequalities: A Practical Guide to Health Impact Appraisal.* (*Website*: http://www.wales.nhs.uk/sites3/Documents/522/improvinghealthenglish.pdf).

Thoresen, C.E. and Mahoney, M.J. (1974) *Behavioral Self-control*. New York: Holt, Rinehart & Winston.

Thuen, F. (1994) 'Injury-related behaviours and sensation seeking: an empirical study of a group of 14-year-old Norwegian schoolchildren', *Health Education Research*, 9 (4): 465–72.

Tilford, S. (2000) 'Evidence-based health promotion', *Health Education Research*, 15 (6): 659–63.

Tilford, S., Green, J. and Tones, K. (2003) *Values, Health Promotion and Public Health*. Leeds: Centre for Health Promotion Research, Leeds Metropolitan University.

Tones, B.K. (1979) 'Past achievement, future success', in I. Sutherland (ed.), *Health Education: Perspectives and Choices*. London: Allen & Unwin.

Tones, B.K. (1981) 'Affective education and health', in J. Cowley, K. David and T. Williams (eds), *Health Education in Schools*. London: Harper & Row.

Tones, B.K. (1987) 'Health promotion, affective education and the personal–social development of young people', in K. David and T. Williams (eds), *Health Education in Schools*. London: Harper & Row.

Tones, K. (1974) 'A systems approach to health education', *Community Health*, 6: 34–9.

Tones, K. (1986) 'Preventing drug misuse: the case for breadth, balance and coherence', *Health Education Journal*, 45 (4): 223–30.

Tones, K. (1993) 'Changing theory and practice: trends in methods, strategies and settings in health education', *Health Education Journal*, 52 (3): 125–39.

Tones, K. (1996) 'The health promoting school: some reflections on evaluation', *Health Education Research*, 11 (4): i–viii.

Tones, K. (2002) 'Health literacy: new wine in old bottles?', *Health Education Research*, 17 (3): 287–90.

Tones, K. and Delaney, F. (1995) *Commissioning Health Promotion: A Consultancy Document*. Cambridge: Cambridge and Huntingdon Health Commission.

Tones, K. and Green, J. (1999) *A Case Study of Withymoor Village Surgery – a Health Hive: Health Promotion and Creative Arts in General Practice*. Leeds: Health Promotion Design.

Tones, K. and Green, J. (2000) 'Health education and the health-promoting school: addressing the drugs issue', in B. Moon, M. Ben-Peretz and S. Brown (eds), *Companion to Routledge International Education*. London: Routledge.

Tones, K. and Tilford, S. (1994) *Health Education: Effectiveness, Efficiency and Equity*. London: Chapman & Hall.

Tones, K. and Tilford, S. (2001) *Health Promotion: Effectiveness, Efficiency and Equity* (3rd edn). London: Nelson Thornes.

Tones, K., Dixey, R. and Green, J. (1995) 'Developing and evaluating the curriculum of the health-promoting schools', in European Network of Health Promoting Schools (eds), *Towards an Evaluation of The European Network of Health-Promoting Schools: The EVA Project*. Copenhagen: European Network of Health Promoting Schools, WHO Regional Office for Europe, European Commission and Council for Europe.

Totten, C. (1992) *Developing Quality in Health Education and Health Promotion*. Society of Health Education and Health Promotion Specialists.

Trower, P., Bryant, B. and Argyle, M. (1978) *Social Skills and Mental Health*. London: Methuen.

Truth (undated) *Truth: About Us*. (*Website*: http://www.thetruth.com/aboutUs.cfm).

Turner, C.M. (1978) *Interpersonal Skills in Further Education*. Blagdon: Further Education Staff College, Coombe Lodge.

Turner, G. and Shepherd, J. (1999) 'A method in search of a theory: peer education and health promotion', *Health Education Research*, 14 (2): 235–47.

Twelvetrees, A. (1982) *Community Work*. London: Macmillan.

Tyrrell, G.N.M. (1951) *Homo Faber*. London: Methuen.

UK Health for All Network (2001) *Briefing Paper 9: Health Impact Assessment*. (*Website*: http://independent.livjm.ac.uk/healthforall/data/Briefing9.doc).

UNDP (2008) *Human Development Report 2007/8*. (*Website*: http://hdrstats.undp.org/countries/country_fact_sheets/cty_fs_GMB.html).

UNDP (undated) *Millenium Development Goals*. (*Website*: http://www.undp.org/mdg/basics.shtml).

UNESCO-EPD (1997) *Educating for a Sustainable Future: A Transdisciplinary Vision for Concerted*

Action. Background document prepared for the UNESCO International Conference on Environment and Society: Education and Public Awareness for Sustainability, Thessaloniki, Greece, 8–12 December.

UNICEF (2007a) *'Will you Listen?' Young Voices from Conflict Zones*. (*Website*: http://www.unicef.org/voy/media/Will_You_Listen_090607.pdf).

UNICEF (2007b) *Child Poverty in Perspective: An Overview of Child Well-being in Rich Countries, Innocenti Report Card 7*. Florence: UNICEF Innocenti Research Centre.

United Nations (1948) *Universal Declaration on Human Rights*. (*Website*: www.un.org/Overview/rights.html).

United Nations Economic Commission for Europe and Statistical Office of the European Communities (undated) *Recommendations for the 2000 Censuses of Population and Housing in the ECE Region*. Statistical Standards and Studies (No. 49). Geneva: United Nations. (*Website*: www/unece.org/stats/documents/census/ 2000).

United Nations Statistics Division (2002) *World Population Housing and Census Programme*. New York: United Nations Statistics Division. (*Website*: http://unstats.un.org/unsd/demographic/census/index.htm).

Unkowska, L.K. (2005) 'Empowering children for risk taking – children's participation as a health promoting strategy in the "Safe Schools in a Community at Risk" project', *Promotion & Education*, XII (304): 142–3.

U.S. Department of Health and Human Services (2000) *Healthy People 2010* (2nd edn). Washington, DC: U.S. Government Printing Office. (*Website*: http://www.healthypeople.gov/Document/tableofcontents.htm).

Unwin, N., Carr, S., Leeson, J. and Pless-Mulloli, T. (1997) *An Introductory Study Guide to Public Health and Epidemiology*. Buckingham: Open University Press.

Vallely, A., Scott, C. and Hallums, J. (1999) 'The health needs of refugees: using rapid appraisal to assess needs and identify priority areas for public health action', *Public Health Medicine*, 1 (3): 103–7.

Verma, T., Adams, J. and White, M. (2007) 'Portrayal of health-related behaviours in popular UK television soap operas', *Journal of Epidemiology and Community Health*, 61: 575–7.

Victorian Smoking and Health Program (1995) *Tobacco in Australia: Facts and Issues – Chapter 15.7 – Product Placement*. Victoria: Victorian Smoking and Health Program (Quit Victoria). (*Website*: http://www.quit.org.au/quit/fandi/prefack.htm).

Vlassoff, C. and Tanner, M. (1992) 'The relevance of rapid assessment to health research and interventions', *Health Policy and Planning*, 7 (1): 1–9.

VSO Netherlands (undated) 'Position paper: VSO Netherlands–the current status.' Utrecht, The Netherlands: VSO Netherlands. (*Website*: www. vso.nl/download/Samenvatting_discussie.doc).

Wallack, L.M. (1980) *Mass Media Campaigns: The Odds Against Finding Behavior Change*. Berkeley, CA: University of California Social Research Group.

Wallack, L. (1998) 'Media advocacy: a strategy for empowering people and communities', in M. Minkler (eds), *Community Organizing and Community Building for Health*. New Brunswick: Rutgers University Press.

Wallack, L., Dorfman, L., Jernigan, D. and Makani, T. (1993) *Media Advocacy and Public Health: Power for Prevention*. Thousand Oaks, CA: Sage.

Wallerstein, N. and Bernstein, E. (1988) 'Empowerment education: Freire's ideas adapted to health education', *Health Education Quarterly*, 15 (4): 379–94.

Wallerstein, N. and Sanchez-Merki, V. (1994) 'Freirian praxis in health education: research results from an adolescent prevention program', *Health Education Research*, 9 (1): 105–18.

Wallston, B.S., Wallston, K.A., Kaplan, G.D. and Maides, S.A. (1976) 'A development and validation of the health locus of control (HLC) scale', *Journal of Consulting and Clinical Psychology*, 44: 580–5.

Wallston, K.A. (1991) 'The importance of placing measures of health locus of control beliefs in a theoretical context', *Health Education Research*, 6 (2): 251–2.

Wallston, K.A. and Wallston, B.S. (1982) 'Who is responsible for your health?: The construct of health locus of control', in G.S. Sanders and J. Suls (eds), *Social Psychology of Health and Illness*. Hillsdale, NJ: Erlbaum.

Wals, A.E.J. and Jickling, B. (2000) 'Process-based environmental education seeking standards without standardizing', in B.B. Jensen, K. Schnack and V. Simovska, *Critical Environmental and Health Education*. Copenhagen: Danish University of Education.

Walt, G. (1994) *Health Policy: An Introduction to Process and Power*. London: Zed.

Wang, C. and Burris, M.A. (1994) 'Empowerment through photo novella: portraits of participation', *Health Education Quarterly*, 21 (2): 171–86.

Wang, G., Macera, C.A., Scudder-Soucie, B., Schmid, T., Pratt, M. and Buchner, D. (2005) 'A cost–benefit analysis of physical activity using bike/pedestrian trails', *Health Promotion Practice*, 6 (2): 174–9.

Wanless, D. (2002) *Securing Our Future Health: Taking a Long-term View*. London: HM Treasury. (*Website*: www. hm-treasury.gov.uk/Consultations_and_Legislation/wanless/consult_wanless_final.cfm).

Wanless, D. (2004) *Securing Good Health for the Whole Population*. (*Website*: http://www.hm-treasury.gov.uk/consultations_and_legislation/wanless/consult_wanless04_final.cfm).

Warner, K.E. (1981) 'Cigarette smoking in the 1970s: the impact of the anti-smoking campaign on consumption', *Science*, 211: 729–31.

Warwick, D.P. and Kelman, H.C. (1973) 'Ethical issues in social intervention', in G. Zaltman (ed.), *Processes and Phenomena of Social Change*. New York: Wiley.

Watson, J., Speller, V., Markwell, S. and Platt, S. (2000) 'The Verona benchmark: applying evidence to improve the quality of partnership', *Promotion & Education*, VII (2): 16–23.

Watson, M.C. (2002) 'Normative needs assessment: is this an appropriate way in which to meet the new public health agenda?', *International Journal of Health Promotion and Education*, 40 (1): 4–8.

Weber, M. (1968) *Economy and Society* (Vol. 1). New York: Bedminster Press.

Weinstein, N.D. (1982) 'Unrealistic optimism about susceptibility to health problems', *Journal of Behavioral Medicine*, 5 (4): 441–60.

Weinstein, N.D. (1984) 'Why it won't happen to me: perceptions of risk factors and susceptibility', *Health Psychology*, 3 (5): 431–57.

Weisbord, M. (1978) 'Organisational diagnosis: a workbook of theory and practice', in J. Anderson, *HEA Health Skills Project*. Leeds: Counselling and Career Development Unit.

Welin, L., Tibblin, G. and Tibblin, B. (1985) 'Prospective study of social influence on mortality: the study of men born in 1913 and 1923', *Lancet*, 1: 915–18.

Wellings, K. and Macdowall, W. (2000) 'Evaluating mass media approaches to health promotion', *Health Education*, 100 (1): 23–32.

Wenzel, E. (1997) 'A comment on settings in health promotion', *Internet Journal of Health Promotion*, http://www.monash.edu.au/health/IJHP/1997/1.

Werner, D. (1980) 'Health care and human dignity', in S.B. Rifkin (ed.), *Health, the Human Factor: Readings in Health, Development and Community Participation*. (CONTACT Special Series No. 3). Geneva: WCC.

Werner, E.E. (1987) 'Resilient children', in E.E. Fitzgerald and M.G. Walraven (eds), *Annual Editions Human Development 87/88*. Guilford, CT: Dushkin.

West of Scotland Cancer Awareness Project (undated) *How Henry Helped Save Lives (and Save the NHS £695k)*. (*Website*: http://www.tunaweb.com/MarketingAwardsScotlandNominees/casestudies/Strat-CRM-HowHenrySaved.pdf).

Whitehead, M. (1987) *The Health Divide*. London: Health Education Council.

Whitehead, M. (1990) *The Concepts and Principles of Equity and Health*. Copenhagen: WHO.

Whitehead, M. (1992) *Policies and Strategies to Promote Equity*. Copenhagen: WHO.

Whitehead, M. and Tones, K. (1990) *Avoiding the Pitfalls: Notes on the Planning and Implementation of Health Education Strategies and the Special Role of the HEA*. London: HEA.

Whitelaw, S., Baxendale, A., Bryce, C., MacHardy, L., Young, I. and Witney, E. (2001) '"Settings"-based health promotion: a review', *Health Promotion International*, 16 (4): 339–53.

WHO (1946) *Constitution*. Geneva: WHO.

WHO (1978) *Declaration of Alma Ata*. International Conference on Primary Health Care, Alma Ata, 6–12 September. Geneva: WHO.

WHO (1984) *Health Promotion: A Discussion Document on the Concepts and Principles*. Copenhagen: WHO.

WHO (1985) *Targets for Health for All*. Copenhagen: WHO Regional Office for Europe.

WHO (1986) *Ottawa Charter for Health Promotion*. First International Conference on Health Promotion, Ottawa, 17–21 November. Copenhagen: WHO Regional Office for Europe.

WHO (1988) *The Adelaide Recommendations*. Geneva: WHO. (*Website*: www.who.int/hpr/archive/docs/ ade-laide.html).

WHO (1991) *Sundsvall Statement on Supportive Environments for Health*. Geneva: WHO.

WHO (1995) *Securing Investment in Health: Report of a Demonstration Project in the Provinces of Bolzano and Trento*. Copenhagen: WHO.

WHO (1997) *The Jakarta Declaration on Leading Health Promotion into the 21st Century*. Geneva: WHO. (*Website*: www/who.int/hpr/archive/docs/jakarta/english.html).

WHO (1998a) *Health Promotion Evaluation: Recommendations to Policymakers: Report of the WHO European Working Group on Health Promotion Evaluation*. Copenhagen: WHO Regional Office for Europe.

WHO (1998b) *Health Promotion in the 21st Century: An Era of Partnerships to Achieve Health for All (WHO/47)*. Geneva: WHO.

WHO (1998c) *Fifty-first World Health Assembly (WHA51.12): Health Promotion*. Copenhagen: WHO.

WHO (1998d) *The WHO Approach to Health Promotion: Settings for Health*. Geneva: WHO.

WHO (1998e) *Health for All in the Twenty-first Century* (A51/5). Geneva: WHO.

WHO (1998f) *Health Promotion Glossary*. Geneva: WHO. (*Website*: http://www.who.int/hpr/NPH/docs/hp_glossary_en.pdf).

WHO (1999a) *World Health Report 1999*. Geneva: WHO.

WHO (1999b) *Health21: The Health for All Policy Framework for the WHO European Region. (European Health for All Series No. 6)*. Copenhagen: WHO Regional Office for Europe. (*Website*: http://www.euro.who.int/document/health21/wa540ga199heeng.pdf).

WHO (2000a) *Mexico Ministerial Statement for the Promotion of Health: From Ideas to Action*. Fifth Global Conference on Health Promotion: Bridging the Equity Gap, Mexico, 5–9 June. Geneva: WHO.

WHO (2000b) *Report of the Technical Programme*. Fifth Global Conference on Health Promotion: Bridging the Equity Gap, Mexico, 5–9 June. Geneva: WHO. (*Website*: www.who.int/hpr/NPH/docs/mxconf_report_en.pdf).

WHO (2000c) *The World Health Report 2000 – Health Systems: Improving Performance*. Geneva: WHO.

WHO (2001) 'Climate and health', Factsheet 266. Geneva: WHO.

WHO (2002a) *Community Participation in Local Health and Sustainable Development: Approaches and Techniques. European Sustainable Health and Development Series 4*. Copenhagen: WHO Regional Office for Europe. (*Website*: www.euro.who.int/document/e78652.pdf).

WHO (2002b) *World Health Report 2002 – Reducing Risks, Promoting Healthy–Life, Chapter 3–Perceiving Risks*. Geneva: WHO. (*Website*: http://www.who.int/whr/2002/en/).

WHO (2003) *World Health Report 2003*. Geneva: WHO.

WHO (2005) *The Bangkok Charter for Health Promotion in a Globalised World*. Geneva: WHO. (*Website*: http://www.who.int/healthpromotion/conferences/6gchp/bangkok_charter/en/index.html).

WHO (2006) *Constitution of the World Health Organisation. Basic Documents 45th edition*. Geneva: WHO. (*Website*: http://www.who.int/governance/eb/who_constitution_en.pdf).

WHO (2007a) *Disability Adjusted Life Year*. Geneva: WHO. (*Website*: http://www.who.int/healthinfo/boddaly/en/).

WHO (2007b) *Global Climate Change: Implications for International Public Health Policy*. (*Website*: http://www.who.int/bulletin/volumes/85/3/06-039503/en/).

WHO (2007c) *International Classification of Diseases*. Geneva: WHO. (*Website*: http://www.who. int/classifications/icd/en/).

WHO (2007d) *The Right to Health*. Geneva: WHO. (*Website*: www.who.int/mediacentre/factsheets/ fs323/en/index.html).

WHO (2008a) *European Strategy for Child and Adolescent Health and Development: From Resolution to Action 2005–2008*. Copenhagen: WHO Euro. (*Website*: http://www.euro.who.int/document/ e91655.pdf).

WHO (2008b) *WHO Framework Convention on Tobacco Control*. Geneva: WHO. (*Website*: http://www. who.int/fctc/en/).

WHO Euro (1997) *The Vienna Recommendations on Health Promoting Hospitals*. Copenhagen: WHO Euro. (*Website*: http://www.euro.who.int/document/IHB/hphviennarecom.pdf).

WHO Euro-EC-CE (1993) *The European Network of Health Promoting Schools*. Copenhagen: WHO European Region.

WHO Health Education Unit (1993) 'Lifestyles and health', in A. Beattie, M. Gott, L. Jones and M. Sidell (eds), *Health and Wellbeing: A Reader*. London: Macmillan.

WHO Health Promoting Hospitals Network (1997) *The Vienna Recommendations on Health Promoting Hospitals*. Copenhagen: WHO European Region. (*Website*: www.univie.ac.at/hph/vierec.html).

WHO Regional Committee for Europe (1998) *Regional Health for All Targets*. Copenhagen: WHO European Region. (*Website*: alpha.mpl.uoa.gr/aspasia/Documents/ Regional%20Health.htm).

WHO Regional Committee for Europe (2002) *Technical Briefing: Health Impact Assessment*. Copenhagen: WHO. (*Website*: www.euro.who.int/document/rc52/ ebd3.pdf).

WHO Regional Office for Europe (2005) *Introduction to Healthy Cities*. (*Website*: http://www.euro. who.int/healthy-cities/introducing/20050202_1).

WHO Regional Office for Europe (2006) *What is the Healthy Cities Approach?* (*Website:* http:// www.euro.who.int/healthy-cities/introducing/20050202_2).

WHO Statistics (2006) *Core Health Indicators*. Geneva: WHO. (*Website*: http://www.who.int/ whosis/database/core/core_select_process.cfm).

WHO, UNEP and WMO (2003) *Climate Change and Human Health – Risks and Responses*. Geneva: WHO.

WHOSIS (2007) *Healthy Life Expectancy (HALE) at Birth (Years)*. Geneva: WHO. (*Website*: http://www.who.int/whosis/indicators/2007HALE0/en/).

Whyte, W.F. (1943) *Street Corner Society*. Chicago: Chicago University Press.

Whyte, W.F. (1991) *Social Theory for Action: How Individuals and Organizations Learn to Change*. Thousand Oaks, CA: Sage.

Whyte, W.F. (1997) *Creative Problem Solving in the Field: Reflections on a Career*. Walnut Creek, CA: Alta Mira Press.

Wiebe, G. (1952) 'Merchandising commodities and citizenship on television', *Public Opinion Quarterly*, 15: 679–91.

Wiggers, J. and Sanson-Fisher, R. (1998) 'Evidence-based health promotion', in R. Scott and R. Weston (eds), *Evaluating Health Promotion*. Cheltenham: Stanley Thornes.

Wight, D., Raab, G.M., Henderson, M., Abraham, C., Buston, K., Hart, G. and Scott, S. (2002) 'Limits of teacher-delivered sex education: interim behavioural outcomes from randomised trial', *British Medical Journal*, 324 (7351): 1430.

Wikler, D.I. (1978) 'Coercive measures in health promotion: can they be justified?', *Health Education Monographs*, 6 (2): 223–41.

Wilkinson, G. (1994) 'Divided we fall', *British Medical Journal*, 308: 1113–14.

Wilkinson, R.G. (1997) 'Socio-economic determinants of health: health inequalities: relative or absolute material standards', *British Medical Journal*, 314 (7080): 591–5.

Wilkinson, R. and Marmot M. (2003) *The Solid Facts*. Copenhagen: World Health Organization.

Wilkinson, R. and Pickett, K. (2009) *The Spirit Level: Why More Equal Societies Almost Always Do Better*. London: Allen Lane.

Williams, A. (2007) 'Skilled worker fails fat test for immigration', *The National Business Review,* 16 November.

Williams, A. and Kind, R. (1992) 'The present state of play about QALYS', in A. Hopkins (ed.), *Measure of the Quality of Life and the Uses to Which Such Measures May be Put.* London: Royal College of Physicians.

Williams, G. and Popay, J. (1994) 'Lay knowledge and the privilege of experience', in J. Gabe, D. Kelleher and G. Williams (eds), *Challenging Medicine.* London: Routledge.

Williams, R. and Wright, J. (1998) 'Epidemiological issues in health needs assessment', *British Medical Journal,* 316 (2 May): 1379–82.

Williams, R.G.A. (1983) 'Concepts of health: an analysis of lay logic', *Sociology,* 17 (2): 185–204.

Williams, T., Wetton, N. and Moon, A. (1989a) *A Picture of Health.* London: HEA.

Williams, T., Wetton, N. and Moon, A. (1989b) *A Way In: Five Key Areas of Health Education.* London: HEA.

Wills, J. and Douglas, J. (2008) 'Health promotion: still going strong?', *Critical Public Health,* 18 (4): 431–4.

Wilson, D. and Colquhoun, A. (1998) 'Influences in the decision to breast-feed: a study of pregnant women and their feeding intentions', *Nutrition & Food Science,* 98 (4): 185–92.

Wilson, P., Richardson, R., Sowden, A.J. and Evans, D. (2001) 'PHASE 9: Getting evidence into practice', in NHS Centre for Reviews and Dissemination, *Undertaking Systematic Reviews of Research Effectiveness* (CRD Report, No. 4, 2nd edition). York: NHS Centre for Reviews and Dissemination.

Winton, W.M. (1987) 'Do introductory textbooks present the Yerkes-Dodson law correctly?', *American Psychologist,* (42): 202–3.

Wise, M. (2001) 'The role of advocacy in promoting health', *Promotion & Education,* VIII (2): 69–74.

Witte, K. and Allen, M. (2000) 'A meta-analysis of fear appeals: implications for effective public health campaigns', *Health Education and Behavior,* 27(5): 591–615.

Woodall, J., Dixey, R., Green, J., Newell, C. (2006). *An Evaluation of the Jigsaw Visitors Centre.* Leeds: Centre for Health Promotion Research.

Woodall, J., Dixey, R., Green, J. and Newell, C. (2009) 'Healthier prisons: the role of a prison visitors' centre', *International Journal of Health Promotion and Education,* 47 (1): 12–18.

Woolcock, M. (2001) 'The place of social capital in understanding social and economic outcomes', *Canadian Journal of Policy Research,* 2 (1): 11–17.

Working Class Movement Library (undated) *Community Development Projects 1969–1977.* Salford: WCML. (*Website:* http://www.wcml.org.uk/group/cdp.htm).

World Bank (1993) *World Health Report 1993.* New York: Oxford University Press.

Wren, B. (1977) *Education for Justice.* London: SCM Press.

Wright, C. and Whittington, D. (1992) *Quality Assurance: An Introduction for Health Care Professionals.* London: Churchill Livingstone.

Yanovitzky, I. and Stryker, J. (2001) 'Mass media, social norms, and health promotion efforts: a longitudinal study of media effects on youth binge drinking', *Communication Research,* 28 (2): 208–239.

Yerkes, R.M. and Dodson, J.D. (1908) 'The relation of strength of stimulus to rapidity of habit formation', *Journal of Comparative Neurology and Psychology,* (18): 459–82.

Young, I. (2005) 'Health promotion in schools – a historical perspective', *Promotion & Education,* XII (3–4): 112–17.

Young, I. and Williams, T. (1989) *The Healthy School.* Edinburgh: Scottish Health Education Group.

Zacharakis-Jutz, J. (1988) 'Post-Freirean adult education: a question of empowerment and power', *Adult Education Quarterly,* 39 (1): 41–7.

Zajonc, R.B. (1980) 'Feeling and thinking: preferences need no inferences', *American Psychologist,* 35: 151–75.

Zeedyk, M.S. and Wallace, L. (2003) 'Tackling children's road safety through edutainment: an evaluation of effectiveness', *Health Education Research*, 18(4): 493–505.

Ziglio, E., Rivett, D. and Rasmussen, V.B. (1995) *The European Network of Health Promoting Schools: Managing Innovation and Change*. Copenhagen: WHO Regional Office for Europe.

Ziglio, E., Hagard, S. and Griffiths, J. (2000a) 'Health promotion development in Europe: achievements and challenges', *Health Promotion International*, 15 (2): 143–54.

Ziglio, E., Hagard, S., McMahon, L., Harvey, S. and Levin, L. (2000b) 'Principles, methodology and practices of investment for health', *Promotion & Education*, VII (2): 4–15.

Ziglio, E., Hagard, S., McMahon, L., Harvey, S. and Levin, L. (2001) *Investment for Health*. Geneva: WHO. (*Website:* www.who.int/hpr/conference/products/ Techreports/Investment.pdf).

Zimmerman, R.S., Palmgreen, P.M., Noar, S.M., Lustria, M.L.A., Lu, H.-Y. and Horosewski, M.L. (2007) 'High-sensation-seeking and impulsive-decision-making young adults effects of a televised two-city safer sex mass media campaign targeting', *Health Education and Behavior*, 34: 810–26.

Zuckerman, M. (1990) 'The psychophysiology of sensation seeking', *Journal of Personality*, 58 (1): 313–45.

INDEX